CHINA AND COVID-19

Domestic & External Dimensions

送走瘟神 - 新冠下中国内外形势

CHINA AND COVID-19

Domestic & External Dimensions

送走瘟神 - 新冠下中国内外形势

Editors

Srikanth Kondapalli

Shaheli Das

PENTAGON PRESS LLP

China and Covid-19: Domestic & External Dimensions

Editors: Srikanth Kondapalli and Shaheli Das

First Published in 2020

ISBN 978-93-90095-09-4

Published by
PENTAGON PRESS LLP
206, Peacock Lane, Shahpur Jat,
New Delhi-110049
Phones: 011-64706243, 26491568
Telefax: 011-26490600
email: rajan@pentagonpress.in
website: www.pentagonpress.in

Printed at Aegean Offset Printers, Greater Noida, U.P.

Dedicated

to

the Valliant Spirit of Covid-19 Victims

and to Doctors and Nurses

in India and Abroad

CONTENTS

List of Tables, Figures and Graphs

TABLES

FIGURES

GRAPHS

Abbreviations

ADB	Asian Development Bank
ADIZ	Air Defence Identification Zone
AI	Artificial Intelligence
AIDDD	AI-Driven-Drug-Design
AIIB	Asian Infrastructure Investment Bank
AIV	Avian Influenza Viruses
AMMS	Academy of Military Medical Sciences
ASEAN	Association of Southeast Asian Nations
AU	African Union
BRI	Belt and Road Initiative
BSL-4	Biosafety Level-4
BW	biological warfare
BWC	Biological Weapons Convention
CC	Central Committee
CCP/CPC	Communist Party of China
CDC	Center for Diseases Prevention and Control
CDDD	Computational-Driven-Drug-Design
CECC	Central Epidemic Command Center
CEEC	Central and Eastern European Countries
CERP	COVID-19 Economic Relief Plan
CEWC	Central Economic Work Conference
CMC	Central Military Commission
CMEC	China-Myanmar Economic Corridor

COSCO	China Ocean Shipping Company Limited
COVID-19	Coronavirus Disease-2019
CPCPD	CPC Propaganda Department
CPEC	China Pakistan Economic Corridor
CPPCC	China People's Political Consultative Conference
CWC	Chemical Weapons Convention
DPP	Democratic Progressive Party
ECLAC	Economic Commission for Latin America and the Caribbean
EEZ	Exclusive Economic Zone
EU	European Union
FDI	Foreign Direct Investment
FOCAC	Forum on China-Africa Cooperation
FONOP	Freedom of Navigation Operations
G20	Group of 20
GDP	Gross Domestic Product
GMOA	Government Medical Officers Association
ICTV	International Committee on Taxonomy of Viruses
ICU	Intensive Care Unit
IHR	International Health Regulations
IMF	International Monetary Fund
LACs	Latin American Countries
LDP	Liberal Democratic Party
MERS	Middle East Respiratory Syndrome
MFA	Ministry of Foreign Affairs
MHLW	Ministry of Health, Labour and Welfare
MOFCOM	China's Ministry of Commerce
MOOTW	Military Operations Other Than War
NBS	National Bureau of Statistics
NDB	New Development Bank [of the BRICS]
NHCC	National Health Command Center
NHI	National Health Insurance
NHIA	National Health Insurance Administration

NIV	National Institute of Virology
NML	National Microbiology Laboratory
NPC	National People's Congress
ODA	Official Development Assistance
PAPF	People's Armed Police Force
PBC	People's Bank of China
PCR	Polymerise Chain Reaction
PD	People's Daily
PEPP	Pandemic Emergency Purchase Programme
PLA	People's Liberation Army
PMI	Purchasing Managers Index
PPE	Personal Protective Equipment
PRC	People's Republic of China
RKATM	rapid kit antigen test machines
RMG	ready-made garment
ROC	Republic of China
RT-PCR	Reverse Transcription Polymerase Chain Reaction
SAARC	South Asian Association for Regional Cooperation
SADS-CoV	Severe Acute Diarrhoea Syndrome Coronavirus
SARS	Severe acute respiratory syndrome
SARS-CoV	Severe Acute Respiratory Syndrome Coronavirus
SEIR	Susceptible Exposed Infectious Recovered Model
SMEs	Small and Medium Enterprises
SOE	State Owned Enterprise
UAVs	Unmanned Aerial Vehicles
UNSC	United Nations Security Council
USA	United States of America
WHA	World Health Assembly
WHO	World Health Organization
WTO	World Trade Organization

List of Contributors

Dr. Abhishek Kumar Darbey is currently Research Associate at the Centre for China Analysis & Strategy (CCAS), New Delhi, India. He received his Ph.D. degree in 2018; B.A. in Chinese language in 2008; M.A. in Chinese language in 2010; and M. Phil in 2013 from the School of Language, Literature & Cultural Studies (SLL&CS) and School of International Studies (SIS), JNU, New Delhi, India, and also, Master of Arts (M.A.) in Political Sciences, IGNOU, New Delhi in 2015. From September 2013 till date, he works at Centre for China Analysis & Strategy (CCAS), New Delhi. His publications include: "Southern Tibet (Zangnan): PRC's Balancing Card against India" World Focus, September 2012, New Delhi; "Can Chinese Dream Resonate African Dream?" World Focus, March 2014, New Delhi; "China's "21st Century Maritime Silk Road" and its implications on India" World Focus, June 2015, New Delhi; His recently published work is a chapter tilted "China and South Africa: Balancing or Bandwagoning?" in book titled, "China and the BRICS: Setting up a Different Kitchen"; "The African Safari" in book titled, "One Belt One Road: China's Global Outreach" and "Indian Perspective on Indo-Pacific Strategy", April 2020, Eurasian Studies Quarterly.
Email: abhishekdarbey@gmail.com

Dr. Ambuj Thakur currently serves as Assistant Professor in the Department of History, Assam Royal Global University, Guwahati. He was a faculty member in the UGC Centre for Studies on Bangladesh & Myanmar, Dibrugarh University, Dibrugarh from 2016-19. Under the mandate of the University Grant's Commission's Area Study Programme, he has undertaken an overland research trip from Imphal (India) to Yangon (Myanmar) on the trails of the Southern Silk Route in early 2019. Earning his doctorate in China Studies from Jawaharlal Nehru University in 2015, he has published his work in many national and international journals, books, newspapers and online portals. A part of the Government of India's 500-member

Youth Delegation to China in 2011, he has also been a Visiting Fellow to the Yunnan Academy of Social Sciences in 2014. His interests lie in exploring the history and politics of the frontier regions of China straddling South and Southeast Asia.
E-mail: ambujtoday@gmail.com

Dr. Amrita Jash is Research Fellow and Managing Editor of *CLAWS Journal* at the Centre for Land Warfare Studies. She co-edited a book titled *COVID-19 & Its Challenges: Is India Future Ready?* with Lt Gen VK Ahluwalia (*Pentagon Press*, 2020). Dr. Jash is a *Pavate Fellow* and has been a Visiting Fellow at the Department of Politics and International Studies, University of Cambridge. She holds a Ph.D in Chinese Studies from Jawaharlal Nehru University. She has been an Adjunct Faculty at the School of Global Affairs-Ambedkar University and a Visiting Faculty at the Department of Chinese-Sikkim Central University; a UGC Graduate Fellow (2012-2017); a *US-INDIA-CHINA Initiative* Fellow *SAIS-Johns Hopkins University* (2013); a researcher under *China's Ministry of Commerce* (2014); a researcher under *Harvard-Yenching-NanchingProgramme* (2015). She has been awarded by the COAS Gen Bipin Rawat for her contribution to Chinese Studies (2019). Dr. Jash's research has appeared in 11 edited books, Peer-Reviewed Journals such as *East Asian Policy*, *Review of Global Politics*, *Strategic Analysis*, *Yonsei Journal*, *China Report*, *Maritime Affairs* and *Strategic Vision*. She has published with *CSIS, RUSI, RSIS, Pacific Forum, ThinkChina, Huffington Post, E-IR, Asia Times, Munk School, Crawford School, ISDP, China-India Brief, SADF* and others. Her expertise include: China's foreign policy, strategic and security issues; Chinese military, India-China relations and China-Japan relations.
Email: ajash108@gmail.com

Dr Jigme Yeshe Lama is currently an Assistant Professor in the Department of Political Science, University of Calcutta. He has a PhD from the Centre for East Asian Studies, School of International Studies, Jawaharlal Nehru University, New Delhi. He has presented papers in several international and national conferences and had edited a volume titled "Changes on the Roof of the World – Reflections on Tibet" published in 2016 by Pentagon Press, New Delhi.
Email: yeshijigme@gmail.com

Dr M.S. Prathibha is an Associate Fellow at the East Asia Centre in Manohar Parrikar Institute for Defence Studies and Analyses. Dr Prathibha is a Member of the Editorial Board of Strategic Analysis (Routledge) and published in various peer-

reviewed journals and international publications. She is a recipient of the Human Resource Development (India) and China Government Scholarship from 2009-2011 at the School of Political Science and International Studies, Beijing Normal University, where she completed her study in Chinese Language and Political Theory.
Email: prathibha.idsa@gmail.com

Mrittika Guha Sarkar is a research scholar at the Centre for East Asian Studies, School of International Studies, Jawaharlal Nehru University (JNU), New Delhi. Her research areas are India-China relations, geopolitics and strategic affairs of East Asia focusing on China, Japan and the Korean Peninsula. She writes for several journals, newspapers and magazines such as *Eurasia Review*, *WION*, *Business Today*, *World Focus*, *Defense and Security Alert (DSA)* and *The Pioneer*. She has been a Project Assistant for the East Asia Centre at the Manohar Parrikar Institute for Defence Studies and Analyses (MP-IDSA), New Delhi. She is also an editorial assistant for the Series Editor of the Routledge Studies on Think Asia.
Email: mrittika11@gmail.com

Munish Sharma was a Consultant at Manohar Parikkar Institute for Defence Studies & Analysis, New Delhi. He analyses technologies such as quantum computing and encryption, blockchain, Artificial Intelligence and 5G from geopolitical perspective and concepts like cyber power, cyber espionage and cyber deterrence in the context of China. He had published several monographs and articles on the subject. He is UK Next Generation Scholar and a Chevening Cyber Security Fellow (2018).
Email: munish.juit@gmail.com

Dr. Priyanka Pandit is Research Fellow at the Indian Council of World Affairs, New Delhi. She holds Ph.D. in Chinese Studies from Jawaharlal Nehru University, New Delhi. Her research focuses on China's political economy, its engagements with multilateral economic institutions and comparative politics. She was formerly a visiting fellow at the Chongyang Institute for Financial Studies in Renmin University, Beijing and Research Institute for Indian Ocean Economies in Yunnan University of Finance and Economics, Kunming where she pursued a year-long course in Mandarin. She co-edited a volume on 'China and BRICS: Setting up a Different Kitchen' and her research has featured in international journals, magazines and newspapers.
E-mail: panditpriyanka5@gmail.com

Dr. Rajasimman Sundaram teaches history, politics, and culture and a member of the BRICS Advanced Studies Institute at Sichuan International Studies University, Chongqing, People's Republic of China. He worked for several think-tanks in India including Manohar Parikkar Institute for Defence Studies & Analysis and Centre for Air Power Studies and Universities at Shanghai and Changchun in China.
Email: simman1981@hotmail.com

Rukmani Gupta is a Consultant with Janes Aerospace and Defence, and a Senior Analyst for Asia-Pacific on the Janes Military Capabilities Desk. Her research is focused on China's pursuit and exercise of power in the international sphere. Prior to joining Janes, Ms Gupta was an Associate Fellow at the Manohar Parrikar Institute for Defence Studies and Analyses, New Delhi where she examined security and foreign policy issues in Asia. Ms Gupta holds an MPhil in Chinese Studies and MA in International Relations from the School of International Studies at Jawaharlal Nehru University, New Delhi. As a recipient of the China-India government scholarship she undertook language training at Liaoning Normal University, Dalian and subsequently at the Beijing Language and Culture University, Beijing.
Email: rukmani.gupta@gmail.com

Sakshi Anand, former full time Assistant Professor at the Centre for Far East Languages, Central University of Jharkhand. She holds the Confucius Scholarship for the study of Chinese language. She did her B.A. and M.A. in Chinese language and M.Phil in Chinese Studies at Jawaharlal Nehru University. Her area of interest includes foreign policy, China-Russia relationship and Belt and Road Initiative.
Email: sakshianand4u@gmail.com

Sana Hashmi is Taiwan Fellow at the Institute of International Relations, National Chengchi University. She is a former Consultant in the Ministry of External Affairs (MEA), Government of India, where she worked on the ASEAN region and the Indo-Pacific with a special reference to China from 2016-19. Her primary research focuses on China's foreign policy, Taiwan's foreign relations, China's territorial disputes, and Asian security.

Before her stint at the MEA, she worked with the Centre for Air Power Studies (CAPS), an autonomous think tank under the Indian Air Force (IAF), from 2011-2016. She has also worked at South Asia Forum for Human Rights (SAFHR), Central Tibetan Administration (CTA), and Institute for Defence Studies and Analyses (IDSA). She holds MPhil and PhD (defence awaited) from Jawaharlal Nehru University, New Delhi. She has published several book chapters, articles in journals, magazines,

web portals and newspaper articles. She is the author of the book, *China's Approach towards Territorial Disputes: Lessons and Prospects* (New Delhi: Knowledge World, 2016).
Email: sanahashmi2@gmail.com

Shaheli Das is a Strategic Sector Cooperation Program Officer at Royal Danish Embassy in New Delhi. She has worked as a researcher at premier think tanks in India such as Centre for Air Power Studies and Observer Researcher Foundation. She is also a Visiting Fellow to Fudan Development Institute in Shanghai. She has also been a recipient of the prestigious Chinese Government Scholarship 2017-18. She has presented papers at various national and international conferences. Further, she has published papers in several reputed journals and magazines such as Strategic Vision for Taiwan Security Journal, The Diplomat, Liberal Studies Journal and BRICS Post, to name a few.
Email: shaheli02@gmail.com

Srikanth Kondapalli is Professor in Chinese Studies at Jawaharlal Nehru University. He was Chairman of the Centre for East Asian Studies, SIS, JNU from 2008-10, 2012-14, 2016-18 and 2018-20. He is educated in Chinese studies in India and China with a Ph.D. in Chinese Studies. He learnt Chinese language at Beijing Language & Culture University and was a post-Doctoral Visiting Fellow at People's University, Beijing from 1996-98. He was a Visiting Professor at National Chengchi University, Taipei in 2004, a Visiting Fellow at China Institute of Contemporary International Relations, Beijing in May 2007, an Honorary Professor at Shandong University, Jinan in 2009, 2011, 2013, 2015, 2016, 2017 and 2019; at Jilin University, Changchun in 2014 and at Yunnan University of Finance and Economics, Kunming in 2016 and 2017, a Non-Resident Senior Fellow at People's University since 2014 and a Fellow at Salzburg Global Seminar in 2010. He wrote two books (*China's Military: The PLA in Transition* in 1999 & *China's Naval Power* in 2001), two monographs, co-edited five volumes (*Asian Security & China* in 2004; *China and its Neighbours* in 2010; *China's Military and India* in 2012, *China and the BRICS: Setting up a Different Kitchen* in 2016) and *One Belt One Road – China's Global Outreach* (New Delhi: Pentagon, 2017) and a number of articles in journals and edited volumes – all on China. He received the *K. Subramanyam Award* in 2010 for *Excellence in Research in Strategic and Security Studies.*
Email: srikondapalli@gmail.com

Dr. Sriparna Pathak is an Assistant Professor and Assistant Academic Dean in the Jindal School of International Affairs of O.P. Jindal Global University, Sonipat, Haryana, India. Prior to this she was a Visiting Faculty at the Centre for Southeast Asian Studies, Gauhati University in Assam, India. She has also been an Assistant Professor at Assam Don Bosco University, prior to which she was a Consultant at the Policy Planning and Research Division at the Ministry of External Affairs, New Delhi. She is also a Fellow at the South Asia Democratic Forum in Brussels, Belgium.

Awarded a Doctorate degree from the Centre for East Asian Studies, Jawaharlal Nehru University (JNU) in 2015, she has also worked with the Observer Research Foundation in Kolkata and New Delhi respectively, UNICEF India and the Centre for Armed Forces Historical Research, New Delhi. She has also been a journalist at the Indian Express, New Delhi and the Avenue Mail, Jharkhand respectively.

She has also been a recipient of the joint fellowship awarded by the Ministry of Human Resources Development, India and the China Scholarship Council, Government of the People's Republic of China. She spent two years in China, actively researching various aspects of China's domestic economy. Besides English, Hindi, Bengali and Assamese, she is also fluent in Mandarin. Her areas of interest are China's domestic economy, trade and economic relations between India and China and China's foreign policy and economic linkages with the world.

Email: sriparnapathak@gmail.com Twitter: @Sriparnapathak

Supriya Sharma is a research scholar at the Centre for East Asian studies, School of International Studies, Jawaharlal Nehru University. Supriya has worked with IDSA and Observer Research Foundation, New Delhi in the past and has published a book chapter and several articles in reputed books and online news portals. Her present research focuses on China's sports diplomacy.

Email: supriyasharma6794@gmail.com

Tenzin Lhadon completed her doctoral dissertation, titled "The Normative Issues in China – EU Relations: A case study of Tibet, 1988–2015", from the Center for East Asian Studies, Jawaharlal Nehru University. She is currently working at the Tibet Policy Institute, Dharamsala, as a Research Fellow, with a focus on China–EU–US relations and the centrality of Tibet as a geopolitical issue between these nations. She has published various commentaries and opinion pieces as well as a chapter titled "The Tibet Factor in China's Foreign Policy" in the edited volume "Reflections on the Roof of the World". She has also been invited as a panelist on various news media channels such as Voice of Tibet, Radio Free Asia and Tibet TV as well as presented papers in various academic conferences.

Email: tenzinlhadon7910@gmail.com

Dr. Tilak Jha is currently working as an Assistant Professor at Times School of Media, Bennett University. He teaches journalism and offers an Open Elective on China to engineering, management and law grads. He last worked as a China Specialist with the BBC where he covered the country's annual parliament session and the Sino-US trade war, among others. Dr. Jha was also a Bai Xian Scholar on the Asian Future Leaders Scholarship between 2014-2016 at China's Zhejiang University, Hangzhou. Dr. Tilak has nearly a dozen book chapters in edited volumes on China by reputed publishers and is a regular contributor to media and policy forums both at the national and the international level. His most recent publication is a chapter on "Welfare Communication and Poverty eradication in India, China", (to be published in September 2020), in Jianguo Gao, Baikady, R., Lakshmana., G., Sheng Li, C. (Eds.), Social Welfare in India and China- A Comparative Perspective (2020), ISBN 978-981-15-5647-0, Palgrave Macmillan, Beijing, China
Email: tilakjha@gmail.com

Introduction

> *"The people of a weak and backward country, however strong and healthy they may be, can only serve to be made examples of, or to witness such futile spectacles; and it doesn't really matter how many of them die of illness."*
>
> **Lu Xun**, "Preface to Call to Arms" *Selected Works of Lu Hsun*
>
> December 3, 1922[1]

Since late 2019, a highly pathogenic novel Coronavirus, now renamed as Coronavirus Disease – 2019 (COVID-19 in short), originated in Wuhan in central China and spread to the rest of the country as well as to most parts of the globe within no time – thus affecting billions of lives, their health and wealth[2]. In its trail are millions of patients across the globe, hundreds of thousands of deaths and turmoil and dislocations all around. By mid-July 2020, according to the World Health Organisation (WHO) estimates, there were more than 13 million infections of COVID-19, over half-a-million deaths in 216 countries. It disrupted on a large scale as well travel, transportation networks, economies and the political systems. Despite advances in scientific knowledge and medicines, as with the other strains of Coronaviruses, COVID-19 did not witness the development of a vaccine yet, thus complicating the hopes of millions of lives across the globe. China and the world literally came to a standstill for several days, weeks and months as nation after nation resorted to complete or partial shutdowns, enforced quarantines and unforeseen restrictions on travel as the contagion spread to the nooks and corners of the world. In the recent living memory, no other disease has had so much of negative impact on the humanity. As China's Premier Li Keqiang told the National People's Congress on May 22, 2020 COVID-19 "is the fastest spreading, most extensive, and most challenging public health emergency" since the People's Republic of China (PRC) was established in 1949[3]. This applies to other countries as well.

Thus, COVID-19 in all likelihood will go down in human history as one of the most decisive events in terms of its global scale, the unprecedented fear that it generated across vast swathes of the world, the kind of economic destruction that it inflicted across the board, barring a few sectors (such as pharmaceuticals, environment etc) and for the comprehensive dislocation it brought about, including in the regional and global orders[4]. An estimated three billion people are in some form or the other of lockdown in the nooks and corners of the world so as to break the chain of contagion.

Viruses and pandemics are not new to the human civilisation. Many variants of the viruses have spread before taking a toll of millions.[5] COVID-19 is one among the many Coronavirus (CoVs) strains that is said to infect human beings mainly the respiratory tract leading to further health complications and even to death. Six strains of the CoVs have been identified by the scientists[6], viz.,

- the globally prevailing 229E, NL63 and OC43 viruses;
- the severe acute respiratory syndrome (SARS) that broke out in Guangdong Province of China in 2002-03 and taking a toll of 775 people with 9 percent fatality rate;
- HKU1 that erupted in Hong Kong in 2005, and
- the Middle East respiratory syndrome (MERS), with acute renal failure, was reported first in Saudi Arabia and affected the entire West Asian region since 2012, taking a toll of 584 deaths in 26 countries[7].

SARS and MERS are said to spread to animals like bats, camels, civet cats or others and then to humans. A recombination of these viruses results in the emergence of novel CoVs, such as the current COVID-19.

Wuhan, the Epicenter

Much of the literature on COVID-19 mentions about its origins in the central China city of Wuhan. A brief background and its political significance are necessary to understand the subject. The bourgeoning city has become a major industrial, services and supply hub today due to the reform and opening up policies since these were launched in 1978. Historically as well, Wuhan was at the forefront of the Xinhai Revolution in 1911 with its Wuchang Uprising that brought in the Warlord Era and subsequently the nationalist government under Sun Yat-Sen. Wuhan was the capital of China twice in 1927 and 1937 for a brief period owing to shifting political alliances and war. Politically as well, Wuhan has been eulogised by China's leaders. The mighty Yangtze River flowing through Wuhan was also the scene for the 73-year-old Mao Zedong's famous 15-kilometer swim[8] on July 16, 1966 (the "7.16 legend") across the breadth of the river and to his famous poem on Wuhan fish. Thus, Mao wrote:

I have just drunk the waters of Changsha
And come to eat the fish of Wuchang.
Now I am swimming across the great Yangtze,
Looking afar to the open sky of Chu.
Let the wind blow and waves beat,
Better far than idly strolling in a courtyard.
Today I am at ease.
"It was by a stream that the Master said—
'Thus do things flow away!' "
Sails move with the wind.
Tortoise and Snake are still.
Great plans are afoot:
A bridge will fly to span the north and south,
Turning a deep chasm into a thoroughfare;
Walls of stone will stand upstream to the west
To hold back Wushan's clouds and rain
Till a smooth lake rises in the narrow gorges.
The mountain goddess if she is still there
Will marvel at a world so changed.

Such public display of stamina by the then supreme leader of China was surely intended to further scale up the political activity in the country seized as it were with intense ideological and political debates and movements. Mao's macho act across the Yangtze was one of the triggers for intensifying factional political struggles in China. Wuhan also witnessed the first major insurrection on July 20, 1967 of the local military command under Chen Zaidao during the Cultural Revolution that took the central leadership by shock. After clamping down on the local command, the central leadership began curbing "mountain topism" [山头主义] – the ability of the local commanders to become autonomous from the central leadership - among the ranks. This is a dreaded word in the communist party history and politics in China, which is sought to be curbed by frequent transfers of the commanders or party secretaries.

Another of the large-scale campaigns of Mao include in the health sector[9]. Schistosomiasis (snail fever) is an endemic infectious disease in China – at one time infecting 11 million people across the Yangtze River Delta region. In the mid-50s China's leadership launched a control programme by establishing a special leading group[10]. It was launched in 1955 and in three years, after a sustained campaign in Yujiang County of Jiangxi province, it was announced that the diseases have been eliminated in the county[11]. To commemorate the event, Mao Zedong penned down two poems as "Farewell to The God of Plague" on July 1, 1958. Subsequently, a nation-wide campaign was launched that is yet to complete the mission. The two poems are as follows:

So many green streams and blue hills, but to what avail?
This tiny creature left even Hua To powerless!
Hundreds of villages choked with weeds, men wasted away;
Thousands of homes deserted, ghosts chanted mournfully.
Motionless, by earth I travel eighty thousand li a day,
Surveying the sky I see a myriad Milky Ways from afar.
Should the Cowherd ask tidings of the God of Plague,
Say the same griefs flow down the stream of time.

II

The spring wind blows amid profuse willow wands,
Six hundred million in this land all equal Yao and Shun.
Crimson rain swirls in waves under our will,
Green mountains turn to bridges at our wish.
Gleaming mattocks fall on the Five Ridges heaven-high;
Mighty arms move to rock the earth round the Triple River.
We ask the God of Plague: "Where are you bound?"
Paper barges aflame and candle-light illuminate the sky.[12]

Both of the above recent historical events – political posturing and public health related – are replicated and keep resonating in symbolic manner in the contemporary situation in China as well. Naming President Xi Jinping as the "commander" of the "people's war" against COVID-19 or repeated mention of his name as "leading" force behind tackling the COVID-19 in Wuhan and other places – all are meant to resurrect many of the historical memories, even though they expose intense political wrangling within the communist party. Eventually, Wuhan has become the epicentre of COVID-19 that spread to different parts of the world, despite its complete lockdown, though belatedly.[13]

Scholarship on Epidemics

Epidemic control and prevention methods are as much part of medicine as it is about power and societal interactions. Two streams could be identified, one by Albert Camus in his seminal work *The Plague* published in 1947 and set in the environs of Algerian town of Oran and in the backdrop of the plague epidemic. The characters in this *existentialist* work exhibit moments of isolation and psychological stress in times of quarantine but also to the elements of humanity and mutual help in addressing the epidemic[14].

A second stream is that by Michel Foucault in his seminal work on *The Birth of the Clinic* in 1963[15] where he argued that modernity and enlightenment had created an epistemological break from the medieval practices of healing towards making a human body an object of medical examination and study but also to the generation of medical terminology, identification of symptoms and methods of cure that lead to structures of power, governmentality and public health procedures. One of the effects of such origins of a different structure of power is also the enormous powers that a state is vested in terms of prevention and control, quarantine methods, but also the control over information on the epidemic itself. In an anthropological sense, there is also the classification of the epidemics as reflected in naming the viruses based on nation, race or regions. Many of the viruses, for example carry such typologies as for instance in Ebola named after the river in West Africa, Japanese encephalitis, MERS, and others. As Charles Briggs argued:

> Racialization and medicalization include control over the production, circulation, and reception of discourse. Racial and medical knowledge does not simply flow but is dependent on communicative processes structured by inequities of power and resources.[16]

Indeed, in the context of the current spread of the COVID-19 as well, stigmatisation has been reported from many parts of the world, including from China. While previously, such stigmatisation has been reported in the western hemisphere for the peoples of the eastern hemisphere, it has now spread to the rest of the world.[17]

In the context of this volume there are several ways of dissecting a topic such as COVID-19[18]. One is a scientific/medical treatment method of studying various case histories of the COVID-19 and analysing the contributing factors, medical history, and other parameters of the virus to suggest to the prevention and control measures[19]. A second is to examine the technical parameters of the COVID-19, phylogenetic sequencing, comparing to the other viruses, examining the chemical parameters and tackling the virus through generation of anti-bodies and vaccines[20]. The above two trends have garnered the lion's share of academic research in China in the last more than a decade since the outbreak of the SARS in 2003 according to the China Academic Journals database CNKI.net resources.[21] A third, that is adopted in this volume, is to look at the political relations in regard to the spread of the virus – that is locating power both at the domestic and international levels in relation to the developments in China[22]. None of the contributors to the volume are capable of conducting the first two methods of enquiry, although all available scientific and technical reports on COVID-19 are cited in the notes. On the other hand, they are all trained in Social Sciences and allied subjects and the choice of the themes in this volume are quite obvious.

Moreover, much of the literature in analysing COVID-19 in the social sciences, international relations and other subjects is concerned about the relative power variables. Here, mainstream literature can be summarised into two broad aspects, viz., traditional and non-traditional security challenges has much to ponder over. While addressing the COVID-19, clearly the state and the armed forces are in the forefront in many areas of the globe, including prominently in China – led by the Communist Party – and hence is part of the "high politics", there is also the Copenhagen School intervention of locating the subject at the interstices of politics, economics, environment, society and the military. Non-traditional security challenges, such as ethnic conflict, terrorism, energy, environmental issues, migration, health security, pandemics and others are generally considered to be in the domain of "low politics" with less or no intervention by the state and even less of that of the armed forces intervention. There has been a bourgeoning literature on the non-traditional security challenges, especially in the wake of the disintegration of the then Soviet Union and end to bipolarity. However, unlike western notions of non-traditional security challenges, in countries like China we find the active intervention of the Communist Party-State at all levels including in addressing the non-traditional security challenges. Specifically, concerning our subject matter, health security and the spread of the pandemics, it has been influencing politics, economics, society, environment and the military in many ways and affecting national and international stability issues – the key elements in the Copenhagen School's contribution in the non-traditional security aspects[23]. As Peter Chalk argued, besides taking human toll in the wake of its spread, a pandemic also has the following consequences, as they:

(1) weaken public confidence in a government's ability to respond;
(2) distort productive economic growth;
(3) destroy the underlying fabric that holds a given polity together;
(4) promote regional tension and mistrust; and
(5) strategically challenge the status-quo (if not extant ordering principles) of regional and international systems through the specter of bio-warfare (BW) and bio-terrorism (BT).[24]

To cite another author Andrew T. Price-Smith,

> ...the destruction of the populace by an ecological predator (in this case, pathogenic agents) constitutes a distinct threat to the well-being of the populace as guaranteed by the state. Since infectious disease results in far greater population mortality than typically results from war, the resurgence of older miasmas and the emergence of novel and lethal pathogens constitutes a very real threat to the security of the population of the modern state.[25]

Incidentally, COVID-19 had evoked most of the above responses at the national and international level. As COVID-19 began in China and exhibited a veritable response at the domestic and foreign policy dimensions, this volume is likewise divided into the two main sections of the domestic society, polity, economy, and others, while the external aspects explore the spread of the COVID-19 across the globe. Hence this volume is as much as an area study as it is about international relations. All the contributors tried to address the following questions: how did COVID-19 originate, what are the debates and discussions, what is its impact and how did (in the chapters on foreign policy dimensions) the bilateral relations were affected in the contagion's trail.

Thus, the first chapter locates the origins and dynamics of the spread of the COVID-19 in the backdrop of pandemics in China. It raises a few questions on when and where COVID-19 originated given the current and acute debate that is raging across the globe. It also touches upon the other controversies that soon engulfed COVID-19 – the party-state responses in addressing the issue, the inconsistencies and discrepancies in its explanation to the international community on COVID-19, its transmission, responses of the party-state, impact on the world order and other aspects. The key arguments proposed are that despite the prevalence of pandemics in China, with recent devastation caused by the SARS still fresh in memory, China was unable to stop the spread of COVID-19 both at the domestic level and abroad, creating havoc all across. Human-to-human transmissions occurred while due to internal structural constraints in the medical establishment, these were not curbed in time. However, once the pandemic was reported by Thailand and Taiwan, the party-state swung into action, albeit at high cost both in terms of internal resources mobilisation and external propaganda.

The second chapter deals with the domestic political issues in China. China's discussions on "politics in command" and "red versus expert" suggest to the pre-eminence of the political over other aspects of the society, especially on health-related aspects, although this may be changing as China entered actively the globalisation process. All major crises in China were followed by intense political activity. This has been the case during the defence minister Peng Dehuai's umbrage at Mao Zedong at the Lushan Conference in 1959, cultural revolution, death of Zhou Enlai and the movement at Tiananmen Square in 1978, Lin Biao, Gang of Four interventions, the 1989 Tiananmen Square incident when the party was vertically split between Deng Xiaoping led forces versus Premier Zhao Ziyang and others, SARS crisis of 2002-03 for Hu-Wen leadership or others. The party also witnessed intra-party wrangling as reflected in the Wang Meng- Li Lisan episodes, Zhang Guotao's role in the 1930s as well as to the Gao Gang-Rao Sushi differences with the central political leadership. Differences between Mao Zedong and Liu Shaoqi are legion. Some fell by the way side due to these political differences like Peng Dehuai and Deng Xiaoping. Post-1978 reform political leaderships as well are not immune to these differences with factional struggles becoming acute between "princelings", Communist Youth League or Zhijiang Army. It is surprising that President Xi Jinping was missing from public appearances during January 29 to February 10 period at a time when the COVID-19 was raging and important political decisions are being taken, although he clarified that he was monitoring the situation on a daily basis. President Xi eventually visited Wuhan on March 10 at a time when the virus cases in the city were receding. As the virus spread across the country, the political leadership in its 14 political bureau standing committee meetings had emphasised on safety, stability and restoration of production. Like in the past, critics pointed to several problems[26]. This is the subject matter of Jigme Yeshe Lama's chapter. This chapter looks into how the party state has responded to the pandemic that is seen to be threatening the legitimacy of the Communist Party. It also compares the steps taken by the party state in the 2003 SARS outbreak with the current COVID-19 pandemic. It is seen that the Communist Party has not learnt from past mistakes. The chapter delves into the politics and governance in the PRC under Xi Jinping, who unlike his predecessors has initiated a centralisation of authority and ushering a new mode of governance. He is seen to be taking China back to the Maoist days with the flourishing of the personality cult. The impact of this change in Chinese politics is seen in the handling of the COVID-19 which is discussed in the chapter. The outbreak also provides an opportunity to study the governance of the PRC at the grassroots, which is the primary site where the pandemic is seen to be in action. It also outlines the growing criticisms against Xi Jinping and the party state from different quarters in their handling of the COVID-19 outbreak.

The third chapter delves into the economic impact of COVID-19 on China. Priyanka Pandit reviews the impact of COVID 19 on Chinese economy. It reveals how the Chinese economy crumbled under the health induced economic crisis for a three-month period, adjusted to the new normal conditions posed by social distancing and other safety requirements, finally managing to revive its domestic demand and business activities through the government's stimulus package and other policy easing measures. While assessing China's path to economic recovery, the chapter brings forth relevant economic debates within Chinese policy circles and also points to a clear shift in Chinese policy strategy in tackling the current economic crisis. It also discusses the uneven recovery in Chinese economy and argues how the public health controls and fear of second wave continues to pose unique challenges for the Chinese leadership.

An in-depth case study analysis is provided by Tilak Jha on China's media coverage in the fourth chapter. To recall, during the SARS crisis in 2002-2003, Hu Shuli, the business editor of *Caijing* magazine, exposed the SARS incidents by aggressive investigative reportage, thus forcing the government to acknowledge the spread of the virus.[27] This chapter dealt with China's media coverage of COVID-19 pandemic. It brings into contrast the coverage between Caixin- one of the few privately-owned media outlets in China known for its reporting, and official mouthpieces People's Daily and Xinhua news agency. The chapter highlights the propaganda of the official news outlets despite contradictory facts and repetition of the patterns as during the SARS outbreak in 2003. It also does two case studies – of suppression of citizen journalism and the efforts to influence media abroad via western platforms such as Twitter which remains banned in China.

The fifth chapter is by Rajasimman Sundaraman who, in a thought-provoking analysis, examines two prevalent phenomena associated with the COVID-19 outbreak, that is of biological weapons and whether it is a deliberate act. He argued that it is not possible to clearly pinpoint the evidence regarding these two, due to a lack of concrete "investigation and credible evidence with respect to the indexpatient that led to COVID-19 outbreak centered on Wuhan". He situates the debate amidst the global preparations or interest in regard to biological weapons and geo-political considerations.

M.S. Prathibha in her chapter on the role of the armed forces of China provides concrete evidence on how they were able to provide help to the civilian authorities in prevention and control of COVID-19 at Wuhan and Hubei Province and beyond. This is aided by their on-going preparations in joint logistics and response mechanisms against COVID-19. Specifically, the concept of military operations other than war (MOOTW) came to the rescue of China's armed forces in addressing non-traditional security challenges like COVID-19.

Another related subject is the use of hi-tech gadgets in countering COVID-19. Munish Sharma's chapter is related how hi-tech items were utilised in addressing the COVID-19 pandemic in China and how the nation has showcased them in Wuhan and other places. It locates the Chinese prowess in the recently acquired technical advances in artificial intelligence, drones, supercomputing and others.[28]

Supriya Sharma explores a relatively different field when dealing with pandemics and sports which is equally, if not more, affected by the spread of the contagion as with the other sectors.. Exploring the subject at the intersections of national interests, politics, soft power, popular culture, globalisation, economy and other fields, this chapter makes a distinctive contribution to the debate on addressing COVID-19.

As sports stadia fell silent – or with some being utilized to accommodate COVID-19 patients in open theatres, this chapters provides a grim reminder to our times.

While the above section is focused mainly on the domestic dimensions of the COVID-19, the next large section has its attention on the external dimensions. With single digit casualties and less then 500 infections, Taiwan offers a significant case study and a model in addressing COVID-19. Sana Hashmi makes a detailed analysis of the two waves of COVID-19 cases in Taiwan, its aggressive contact tracing, absence of community transmission, keeping open public spaces and economy, efficiency of public management practices meshed with democratic political system have all contributed to the successful management by Taiwan, although marred by cross-Straits one-upmanship in the WHO deliberations. As an alternative and democratic model, Taiwan's tackling of COVID-19, with least collateral damages to the society or economy, offers significant policy choices for several countries. She argued that consistent efforts to shrink Taiwan's global space and poach its diplomatic allies failed. Taiwan used its success to project its soft power and push for greater international cooperation; it has been promptly helping its allies and other countries such as the United States, India, and European countries by donating masks, PPE and other medical equipment.

China-US relations have become strategic in nature in the recent times, with China becoming the 2nd largest economy in the world. Despite several cooperative measures between the two in the fields of economic, technological, people-to-people contacts, in maintaining regional stability and security aspects, differences are coming to the fore and COVID-19 spread had provided another occasion for further sharpening of such differences between the two countries. Rukmani Gupta's chapter covers the spread of COVID-19 in the United States and the nature of bilateral relations impacted by the pandemic. She argued that, in the light of the recent tariff conflict that spanned nearly two years, pandemic spread has brought forward the acrimony in the bilateral relations.

Sakshi Anand's chapter on China-Russia relations traces the spread of COVID-19 and the dichotomy of "love-hate" relations between the two. She argued that while the mortality and morbidity caused by COVID-19 has shaken the Russian healthcare and economy and generated public wrath on China, their political leadership realises that China's support is still their best bet to bail out of the situation. Beleaguered China also needs a robust Russian support to reclaim international legitimacy. This has resulted in a contradictory yet complementary scenarios between the two countries.

After the United States and Russia, one of the worst cases of COVID-19 were reported in Europe with initial global attention drawn to the appalling conditions in Italy and Spain but soon spreading to the rest of continent. Tenzin Lhadon Tsenneyar examines the spread of COVID-19 in Europe in the light of China's strategic programme of Belt and Road Initiative and other grand plans, triggers for the recently formulated "health Silk Road" and others.

Amrita Jash's chapter highlights the changing dynamics in China's ties with Japan with the spirit of bonhomie pitted against the tension caused by the pandemic. Here, the "impact of COVID-19 on Japan" is taken as the key indicator and determinant to assess the implications on Beijing's ties with Tokyo. That is, the crux of the chapter lies in examining the aspect of "stabilisation and fragility" of ties against the odds of the pandemic.

South Asia becomes important for China's COVID-19 diplomacy, as it presents a big market for Chinese medical goods as well as for its soft power diplomacy. Sriparna Pathak's chapter deals with the spread of COVID-19 in eight South Asian countries and how it was handled with the respective governments. It highlights the timeline of the emergence of the first cases in each of these eight countries, travel linkages with China, China's medical diplomacy in these countries, issues faced by these countries due to the pandemic and on the medical diplomacy received from China. Through these, an attempt is to find out how potent is China's COVID-19 diplomacy in South Asia.

Southeast Asia has also crossed more than a million cases of infections of COVID-19, with the first case reported out of China in Thailand. Ambuj Thakur analyses, with copious details, the widespread regional differences in the spread of COVID-19 and the manner in which these were addressed across by different countries. Given the long-standing territorial disputes in the South China Sea, the author examines the Southeast Asian responses to China's assertiveness in the region. He argued that the pandemic has given China the perfect opportunity to secure the space vacated by the USA in Southeast Asia through donor diplomacy as well as strong arm tactics. Even formidable regional powers like Singapore and Vietnam are treading with caution when dealing with China's new found assertiveness, thereby making it a win-win situation for the latter.

Mrittika Guha Sarkar in her chapter on Sino-Australian relations argued that the bilateral ties have downgraded substantially amidst the pandemic, particularly with Canberra leading the call for an independent investigation. This has amplified the pressure points which have been developing before the onset of the pandemic. Consequently, the chapter argues that the COVID-19 would not alter the fundamental fault lines between Australia and China but the rift might only expand as China might continue or even enhance its authoritarian and ambitious posture post the pandemic, while Australia might endure a domestic and foreign policy which would cater to its interests and protect its national security.

The next two chapters deal with the spread of COVID-19 in Latin American and African continents. From a low level of infection rate to high incidence of COVID-19 pandemic in Brazil surprised the international community. Shaheli Das in her chapter situates the spread of COVID-19 in Latin America within the context of Beijing's long-standing stakes in the region, especially as its Belt and Road Initiative has been extended to the continent. The chapter examines the impact of COVID-19 in Latin America, the kid of aid and assistance offered by China and regional responses.

Last but not the least, Abhishek Kumar Darbey's chapter analyses the China-Africa relations in the backdrop of the spread of the pandemic. He contends that China needs Africa for various reasons such as for political support at the international fora, to pursue economic interests, for uninterrupted commodity supplies, investments, for pursuing the Belt and Road Initiative objectives and expanding its military footprint in the continent. China's concern is that its ongoing projects in Africa will be affected by the pandemic resulting in heavy losses and considerable delay. While China's medical aid to African countries was welcomed, there is also the dimension of anti-Chinese feeling among the African countries, triggered partly by racist attacks on African in China.

This volume came up after over a decade of teaching traditional and non-traditional security challenges of China, with many contributors to the volume writing, publishing and lecturing as well on such topics. The contributors to this volume have all come up in the China programme at Jawaharlal Nehru University at New Delhi. They all have spent considerable time in pondering over the subjects they dealt with in this volume. In fact, all of them were selected for this volume for their passion in their designated subjects. Of course, Chinese studies in India has been mostly ideology-driven, sectarian and stuck in a time warp, giving less scope to raise and explore real issues in the field. In some ways Indian Sinology mirrors the "red versus expert" debate of China. As such it is caughtup by an Indian phenomenon – as late Air Commodore Jasjit Singh used to say – of "simple living, high thinking and no writing"!

In this context, we began a new journey, a new experiment to find answers to many questions that China has been throwing up in its seven decades of journey, specifically as a part of its rise in the last four decades. This research led to coming out with two volumes, viz., **China and the BRICS: Setting Up a Different Kitchen** in 2017 and **One Belt One Road: China's Global Outreach** in 2018. There is a wide diversity in views on China among the contributors to these volumes and the current one. No intervention has been made to alter the views of the contributors to these volumes and that's the way we wanted these to be presented. We are happy to note that these have been received well, according to our publisher the New Delhi-based Pentagon Press whom we thank for the prompt publication and distribution. Many more volumes exploring various facets of China are in the pipeline. Remote access of the JNU Library sources came in handy as India came under lockdown due to COVID-19 outbreak since late March 2020. We were thus able to access research materials necessary for this volume, including from the CNKI.

Scholars contributing to this volume monitored the COVID-19 developments and publications on a daily basis both at the China domestic level and abroad. In contributing to this volume, none of the authors received any funding from abroad or within India and that in writing the chapters only open-source information is used extensively. The moral right of each contributor over their respective chapters is asserted.

NOTES

1 Lu Xun, *Selected Works of Lu Hsun* (Beijing: Foreign Languages Press, 1960) at <https://www.marxists.org/archive/lu-xun/1922/12/03.htm>

2 For data related to the number of infections of Covid-19, besides World Health Organisation and China's National Health Commission statistics, see John Hopkins University, "COVID-19 Data Repository by the Center for Systems Science and Engineering (CSSE) at Johns Hopkins University" at <https://github.com/CSSEGISandData/COVID-19> This website also has the list of many important national health organisations reports.

3 Li Keqiang, "Premier Li's speech at the third session of the 13th NPC" *CGTN* May 22, 2020 at <https://news.cgtn.com/news/2020-05-22/Full-text-Premier-Li-s-speech-at-the-third-session-of-the-13th-NPC-QHaP1FpB8k/index.html>

4 It is said that the first major plague in North Africa, Mediterranean and Europe – the Justinianic Plague of 5th to 7th Centuries A.D. - had led to the end of the Antiquity and the beginning of the Middle Ages. The first plague was detected in 541 AD at Peluseum in Egypt's Port Said and spread to Constantinople. See William H. MacNeill, *Plagues and Peoples* (New York: Anchor Books, 1976) pp.109-111 and Elizabeth Kolbert, "Shape of Human History" *The New Yorker*, March 30, 2020 at <https://www.newyorker.com/magazine/2020/04/06/pandemics-and-the-shape-of-human-history>. MacNeill argued that with the invention of the steam ship networks across the globe in 1870s, plague through rats and fleas from Guangzhou and Hong Kong became more widespread in nature (p.138). On the contrary Mordechai and others argued that the evidence regarding transition in European orders lack substantial evidence. See Lee Mordechai, et.al. "The Justinianic Plague: An inconsequential pandemic?" *Proceedings of the National Academy of Sciences of the United States of America* (December 17, 2019) 116 (51) pp. 25546-25554 at <https://www.pnas.org/content/116/51/25546> For the introduction and impact of different epidemics in human history see Alfred Jay Bollet, *Plagues and Poxes: The Impact of Human History on Epidemic Diseases* (New York: Demos, 2004) and Joseph P. Byrne, *Encyclopedia of Pestilence, Pandemics, and Plagues* (Westport: Greenwood

Press, 2008)

5 For a general introduction to the viruses and the subject as such, see J.N. Hayes, *Epidemics and Pandemics: Their Impacts on Human History* (Santa Barbra, CA: ABC Clio, 2005); Jonathan Van-Tam and Chloe Sellwood, Ed. *Introduction to Pandemic Influenza* (Oxfordshire: CAB International 2010) and Barry Youngerman, Pandemics and Global Health (New York: Infobase Publishing, 2008).

6 On the introduction to the CoVs by SuShuo, Gary Wong, Shi Weifeng, Liu Wenjun, Bi Yuhai and George F Gao, "Epidemiology, Genetic Recombination, and Pathogenesis of Coronaviruses" *Trends in Microbiology* March 21, 2016 at <https://www.cell.com/trends/microbiology/fulltext/S0966-842X(16)00071-8?_returnURL=https%3A%2F%2Flinkinghub.elsevier.com%2 Fretrieve%2Fpii%2FS0966842X16000718%3Fshowall%3Dtrue>

7 Not directly related to China, however, the MERS-Cov has resonances in China through some of the 11,000 pilgrims from China (mainly Xinjiang and Gansu) who annually participate in the Haj pilgrimage to Mecca in Saudi Arabia. See Ma Xuezheng, Liu Fang, Liu Lijuan, Zhang Liping, Lu Mingzhu, Abuduzhayier Abudukadeer, Wang Lingbing, Tian Feng, Zhen Wei, Yang Pengfei, and Hui Kongxin, "No MERS-CoV but positive influenza viruses in returning Hajj pilgrims, China, 2013–2015" *BMC Infectious Diseases* (2017) 17:715 at <DOI 10.1186/s12879-017-2791-0>

8 Mao Zedong swam 17 times across the Yangtze between 1956 and 1966. See David Bandurski, "The Jury is Out: Mao Zedong Swam Faster Than Today's Olympic Champions" *China Media Project* May 17, 2016 at<https://medium.com/china-media-project/the-jury-is-out-mao-zedong-swam-faster-than-todays-olympic-champions-d01a38bee2f3>

9 When the PRC was established in 1949, spread of diseases has been a major concern. PRC inherited its public health management system from the Republic of China which emphasised both on traditional and modern medicine. Indeed, for many years this system continued with provisions for access to health care for all; prevention before cure; and integrate traditional and modern medicine. However, soon Mao termed the Ministry of Health as moving towards elitism in the scheme of "red versus expert" debate. One significant movement in this period is the phenomenon of "barefoot doctors" – with basic training in medicine given to personnel for six months – for imparting first aid, immunisation, family planning and others. See David Wade Chambers, *Red and Expert – A Case Study of Chinese Science in the Cultural Revolution* (Victoria: Deakin University, 1984)

10 Zhou Xiao-Nong, Eniola Michael Abe and Li Shizhu, "*Farewell to the God of plague*: China for the world disease control program" *Global Health Journal* 3 (1) (March 2019) pp.1-3 at <https://www.sciencedirect.com/science/article/pii/S2414644719300016>

11 Miriam Gross, however, argued that the successes of this control programme lay more with the urban doctors and rural educated youth than with the political campaign as such. See *Farewell to the God of Plague- Chairman Mao's Campaign to Deworm China* (Oakland: University of California Press, 2016)

12 Mao Zedong, "Farewell to The God of Plague" in *Selected Works of Mao Zedong* at <https://www.marxists.org/reference/archive/mao/selected-works/poems/poems25.htm>

13 John Sudworth, "Wuhan: City of silence: Looking for answers in the place where coronavirus started" *BBC* June 17, 2020 at <https://www.bbc.co.uk/news/extra/ewsu2giezk/city-of-silence-china-wuhan>

14 Albert Camus, *The Plague* (New York: Vintage Books, 1991)

15 Michel Foucault, The Birth of the Clinic – An Archeology of Medical Perception (New York: Vintage Books, 1973) [tr. A.M. Sheridan Smith]. One relevant passage of Foucault to the current Covid-19 epidemic is the April 29, 1776 decree that he cites as: the epidemics "are deadly and destructive at the outset only because their character, being little known, leave the doctor in uncertainty as to the choice of treatment that should be applied, and this uncertainty arises because so little has been

done to study the different treatments used, or to describe the symptoms of the different epidemics and the curative methods that have been most successful". (ibid pp. 26-27)

16 Charles L. Briggs, "Communicability, Racial Discourse, and Disease" *Annual Review of Anthropology* (2005). 34 pp.269–91 at <https://www.annualreviews.org/doi/pdf/10.1146/annurev.anthro.34.081804.120618>

17 For the impact of the "otherness" in the western society and its impact on stereotypical views see Katherine J. Roberto, Andrew F. Johnson & Beth M. Rauhaus, "Stigmatization and prejudice during the COVID-19 pandemic", *Administrative Theory & Praxis*, (June 25, 2020) DOI:10.1080/10841806.2020.1782128 at <https://www.tandfonline.com/doi/pdf/10.1080/10841806.2020.1782128?needAccess=true>

18 The literature on the subject is increasing day by day given its widespread impact. In a study conducted by several Chinese scholars of over 300 research works by February 2020, they found the professional *Lancet* and its journals have published the most articles, with others like N*ew England Journal of Medicine, The Journal of the American Medical Association* and *Nature* contributing more. Nation wise, most were published by the Chinese scientists, with the rest from the US, UK, Hong Kong, Germany, Italy, South Korea, Canada and others. See Zhang Longhao, et.al. "新型冠状病毒 (SARS-CoV-2) 全球研究现状分析" [An analysis of global research on SARS-CoV-2] 生物医学工程学杂志 [Journal of Biomedical Engineering] 37 (2) (April 2020) pp. 236-49

19 A few examples are that of the compendium of Wang Zhou Ed. *The Coronavirus Prevention Book* (Wuhan: Hubei Science and Technology Press, 2020) and Liang Tingbo, Ed. *Handbook of COVID-19 Prevention and Treatment* (Hangzhou: Zhejiang University School of Medicine, 2020)

20 See Li Shixue and Shan Ying, "新型冠状病毒肺炎研究进展述评" [Latest research advances on novel coronavirus pneumonia] 山东大学学报 (医学版) [Shandong University Journal- Health Sciences] (March 2020); Wang Yuguang et.al., "新型冠状病毒肺炎中医临床特征与辨证治疗初探" [Clinical Features and Syndrome Differentiation of Novel Coronavirus Pneumonia in Traditional Chinese Medicine] 中医杂志 (Journal of Traditional Chinese Medicine) (April 2020); Chen Jiayuan et.al "2019 新型冠状病毒基因组的生物信息学分析" [Bioinformatics analysis of the 2019 novel coronavirus genome] 生物信息学 [Chinese Journal of Bioinformatics] (January 2020); Jin Ying-Hui et.al, "" [A rapid advice guideline for the diagnosis and treatment of 2019 novel coronavirus (2019-nCoV) infected pneumonia] 解放军医学杂志 [Medical Journal of PLA], 45 (1) (January 30, 2020) pp.1-20; Shi Heshui et.al. "新型冠状病毒 (2019-nCoV) 感染的肺炎临床特征及影像学表现" [Radiological Features of Patients with 2019-nCoV Infection] 临床放射学杂志 [Journal of Clinical Radiology] 39 (1) (2020) pp. 8-11

21 For the search function "新型冠状病毒" at <http://oversea.cnki.net/kns/brief/default_result.aspx> Interestingly, Sichuan University's Huaxi Medical Institute has the largest number of articles on the subject followed by Huazhong Technological University's Tongji Medical College at Shanghai and Beijing, Wuhan and other Medical Universities journals. Subject wise, it is diseases related to respiratory systems attracted the highest attention, followed by traditional Chinese medicine, preventive and clinical medicine and others. Yearly trend wise, after the peak number of articles published on the virus in 2003, the publications jumped up in 2013-14 and 2020 with the intervening years attracting as low as 2 to 3 articles.

22 For a study of the epidemics through "critical, historical, structural, social constructionist, ecological, and political economic perspectives" with focus on marginalised sections of the society see Ananya Mukherjea Ed. *Understanding Emerging Epidemics: Social and Political Approaches* (Bingley, UK: Emerald Books, 2010)

23 The key trend-setting documents that influenced health security prognosis, policy, coordination and capacity building efforts – and to the larger securitisation of pandemics - include the US National

Intelligence Council January 2000 assessment on global infectious diseases, the September 2002 document on HIV/AIDS and the August 2003 report on SARS. See United States National Intelligence Council, "The Global Infectious Disease Threat and Its Implications for the United States" January 2000 at <https://www.dni.gov/files/documents/infectiousdiseases_2000.pdf> ; "The Next Wave of HIV/AIDS: Nigeria, Ethiopia, Russia, India, and China" September 2002 at <https://www.dni.gov/files/documents/Special%20Report_The%20Next%20Wave%20of%20HIV_AIDS.pdf>; and "SARS: Down But Still a Threat" at <https://www.dni.gov/files/documents/Special%20Report_SARS%20Down%20But%20Still%20a%20Threat.pdf> Interestingly, since the Clinton Administration's elevation of the HIV/AIDS into a national security challenges, such pandemics received wider global attention and to the securitisation process. See Roxanna Sjostedt, "Health issues and securitization - The construction of HIV/AIDS as a US national security threat" in Thierry Balzack, *Securitization Theory – How Security Problems Emerge and Dissolve* (London: Routledge, 2011) pp. 150-69

24 Peter Chalk, "Disease and the Complex Processes of Securitization in the Asia-Pacific" in Mely Caballero-Anthony, Ralf Emmers and Amitav Acharya Eds. *Non-Traditional Security in Asia-Dilemmas in Securitization* (London: Routledge, 2016) pp.112-35 (cited on p.117)

25 See Andrew T. Price-Smith, *The Health of Nations - Infectious Disease, Environmental Change, and Their Effects on National Security and Development* (Cambridge: The MIT Press, 2002) p.118

26 See Xu Zhangrun, "愤怒的人民已不再恐惧" [When fury overcomes fear] Matters February 4, 2020 at <https://matters.news/@Zhizhu_2019 > ; Josh Rudolph, "Essay by missing property tycoon Ren Zhiqiang" *The Digital Times* March 13, 2020 at https://chinadigitaltimes.net/2020/03/translation-essay-by-missing-property-tycoon-ren-zhiqiang/ *;* Xiao Qiang, "How Xi's 'controlocracy' lost control of the coronavirus" *The Japan Times* February 12, 2020 at <https://www.japantimes.co.jp/opinion/2020/02/12/commentary/world-commentary/xis-controlocracy-lost-control-coronavirus/#.XkYT46Z7nIU>

27 David Barboza, "Pushing (and Toeing) the Line in China" *The New York Times* April 18, 2005 at <https://www.nytimes.com/2005/04/18/business/worldbusiness/pushing-and-toeing-the-line-in-china.html>

28 However, at a different level, a Chinese author Sun Zhouxing raises a fundamental issue of dependence on technology and deconstructs the recent fad as well as its limitations in addressing invisible microorganisms. See Sun Zhouxing, "除了技术，我们还能指望什么？ - 由新冠疫情引发的若干技 术哲学思考" [What can we expect besides technology? - A number of technical philosophical reflections triggered by the new crown outbreak] June 22, 2020 at <http://www.aisixiang.com/data/121792-3.html>

The Domestic Dimensions

1

Origins and Dynamics of COVID-19

Srikanth Kondapalli

As COVID-19 raged across China, the epidemiological map began changing rapidly to spread the virus across the globe and bringing in its wake millions of infections and hundreds of thousands of deaths in its trail. Pertinent issues were raised domestically in China as well as at the global levels on what are the origins of this catastrophe, where did the COVID-19 erupt, how has the virus transmitted at the national and international level, how many infections and deaths it caused, what has been its impact on the socio-cultural, psychological and economic aspects, how did the party-state in China respond to provide relief measures and contain the spread of the COVID-19 and the like[1]. Its nearly six months since the COVID-19 outbreak took place at Wuhan in China, although answers to the many questions are not forthcoming satisfactorily. Many of these details have actually become controversial with the World Health Assembly demanding "independent, impartial and comprehensive" investigation into the origins of the virus and its dynamics.

This chapter thus tries to address the above issues and has the following sections – it begins by locating the overall context of the COVID-19 in China by reflecting on the spread of pandemics, and locates the arguments on the origins of the virus in Wuhan and the controversies regarding naming the virus in the background of the United States (US) leaders mentioning about this. It later explores the numbers of infections and casualties – another controversial aspect given the view about lack of transparency - transmission of the virus and issues related to resumption of economic production, clash of models of containing the virus, responsibility factor, impact on the global order and others.

It is argued here that even though a number of pandemics broke out in China and expanded outside before, however, COVID-19 spread has resulted in securitization of the issue on an unprecedented scale, given the widespread fear of the pandemic and mounting death toll, caught as it were in the midst of China's domestic political debates, nationalism as well as to the US-China strategic rivalry for influencing the regional and global orders[2]. Essentially a "low politics" issue of the non-traditional security challenges, COVID-19 has become in a short period of less than a year into "high politics" which is generally reserved for sovereignty, military and other issues. The "speech acts" of the Communist Party's politburo standing committee, President Xi Jinping, establishment of a Small Leading Group, massive mobilisation of party-state resources to counter the spread of the virus, economic meltdown, transmission to the outside world and the resultant global shocks, emerging conflict with the United States, and competition over models of development[3] – have all elevated the nature of the discourse both in China as well as globally. The persistence of conspiracy theories, the omissions and commissions of not only the Chinese leadership but also other countries' lackadaisical responses have only further enhanced the securitisation process. However, "desecuritization" of COVID-19 is possible in the near future given the massive medical relief responses to contain the contagion, natural immunity growth, development of vaccine, de-escalation in US-China relations or others.

Pandemics in China

China witnessed a number of disasters – some human-made catastrophes (人为灾难), others natural disasters (自然灾害). In addition, "Heaven-sent disasters" [天灾] is another term frequently used to denote the displeasure of the celestial beings and reflects to the cultural and historical specificity of China. It is believed by the Chinese that natural disasters and other major tragedies result in a change in political leadership – a withdrawal of the "Mandate of Heaven". The country witnessed intense political turmoil during the Great Leap Forward (that consummated over 40 million people)[4], Cultural Revolution in 1966-69, Tiananmen Square incident of 1989. China also has been home to several pandemics such as 2002-2003 SARS (that took a toll of 774 people out of confirmed cases of over 8,000)[5] and Bird Flu[6], or major natural disasters like Yangtze River floods of 1998, Tangshan Earthquake of 1976[7], Sichuan Earthquake of 2008[8]. Besides, there are also major accidents like the hi-speed railway crash at Wenzhou of 2011, scandals like HIV-AIDS blood transfusion in Henan[9], 2008 melamine milk, fake rabies vaccine by Changsheng Biotechnology company in Shandong or others. Such tragedies in China unfortunately have become the "new normal" with many following the pattern of suppression of information in order to keep "social stability", delayed responses and the like. The leadership has publicized efforts to enhance "capacity building" in addressing these national tragedies though.

Historically as well, pandemics hit China with debilitating effect on the population, health and wealth of the country[10]. The first recorded malarial infection was in China dating back to 2,700 BC.[11] Plague has also been endemic to China as with the other parts of the world. The three major plagues had a total death toll of over 200 million people across the globe.[12] The plague outbreak of 1792-93 evoked Shi Daonan, a poet at Qing Dynasty's Qianlong's court depicting the situation in his work *TianYuli* as follows:

Dead rats in the east,
Dead rats in the west!
The sight of dead rats makes one shudder,
Days after the passing of the rats, large numbers of men falter.
Under a grey sky and cloudy days,
Countless people die away.
Three men walk together, and in less than ten steps two have fallen forever!
No cries are heard when one dies in the night, for the demon of pestilence has weakened the light.
All of a sudden it all goes dark, leaving man, ghost and coffin in need of spark.
The crows caw incessantly, and the air is filled with the sounds of dogs howling.
Men look like apparitions, while the demon has robbed men's spirits.
Most men one meets in the day are ghosts, yet one wonders if one has met a human when running into another at dusk.
The ground is covered with corpses, and there is no sign of life; human bones become wind- worn over time.
There in the fields are crops to be reaped by none; and officials have no one to go to for tax.
I hope to ride the Heavenly Dragon to see the God and Goddess in Heaven, and beg them to spread their heavenly serum and milk upon the earth, so that spring will return and the dead may come to life again[13].

Based on an extensive dataset of a compilation of human plague cases recorded in local gazetteers (or *difangzhi*) between 1772 and 1964, Tamara Ben-Ari and others argued that, while the oldest evidence of plague is traced to north-eastern Hebei Province, the 1894 plague originated from Hong Kong but sourced to Dali in Yunnan Province.

After its spread through the ports to other parts of the world, it took a toll of 10 million people in China and India. They argue that the 1952-1964 period, plague prevalence shifts to Qinghai and Inner Mongolian regions.[14]

In the recent memory, the northeast of China witnessed the worst plague in 1910-11 at a time when the nation was witnessing the collapse of the Qing Dynasty and Russia and Japan were making inroads in the region through their railway lines and investments in the heavy industry. The plague killed over 60,000 people[15]. To address this situation Dr Wu Lien-The (Wu Liande) – a Malaysian medical graduate from Cambridge – was tasked to provide medical support. Dr Wu identified human-to-human transmission of the disease, made efforts to block the transmission and succeeded in tackling the situation.[16]

One of the concrete results of this episode is the institutionalisation of epidemic control first through a dedicated Manchurian Plague Prevention Service in 1912 that would become the model for subsequent interventions in the public health sector in the coming decades.[17]

No sooner than the 1910-11 plague dissipated, China was again battered by another plague. Christopher Langford argued that the 1918-1919 influenza that debilitated much of the world, specifically taking a toll of 40 to 50 million people has some origins in China[18]. According to various sources that he cited including maritime customs, trade, postal and other archival materials, the 140,000 Chinese labourers recruited by the British and the French and shipped from Qingdao, Weihai and other ports to work in France during the World War I may have carried the virus. MacPherson cites the number of cases that erupted in China – with over 46 cases of cholera epidemics erupting between 1820 and 1932, due mainly to the improvements in communications and transport facilities. In 1932, 100,000 cases were reported with 34,000 deaths.[19] The 1930s also witnessed natural calamities, with the 1931 Yangtze River floods not only claiming an estimated 2 million lives, affecting between 25 to 53 million people, but also to the spread of famines and epidemics in Wuhan and other places.[20]

Since the establishment of the People's Republic of China (PRC), the new government undertook a massive reorganisation of the health sector since 1953[21]. When the PRC was established in 1949, spread of diseases was a major concern. PRC inherited its public health management system from the Republic of China which emphasised both on traditional and modern medicine. While it continued the traditional and modern medicine mixture, new emphases include rural communes medical health system, large scale immunisation, prevention before cure, "red versus expert" and "barefoot doctor" phenomenon of basic training imparted to medical personnel for six months and sent to nook and corners of the country with focus on health education, prevention and cure of illness, immunisation, supervision of sanitary facilities, family planning and first aid. Health care centres were established at county, township and village levels and 2499 epidemic prevention centres established by 1965[22]. The apex health care system's main policy-making bodies were Scientific Committee on Medical Science in the Ministry of Health, Chinese Academy of Science and Chinese Academy of Medical Science[23]. However, soon Mao termed the Ministry of Health as moving towards elitism in the scheme of "red versus expert" debate.

By the reform programme in 1978, the health care system was restructured towards the market economy and free health care system abolished[24]. The following graphic depicts the changes in China's health care system and to the changing "guiding principles" of health care.

Graph 1.1: Changing "Guiding Principles" of Chinese Health Care System

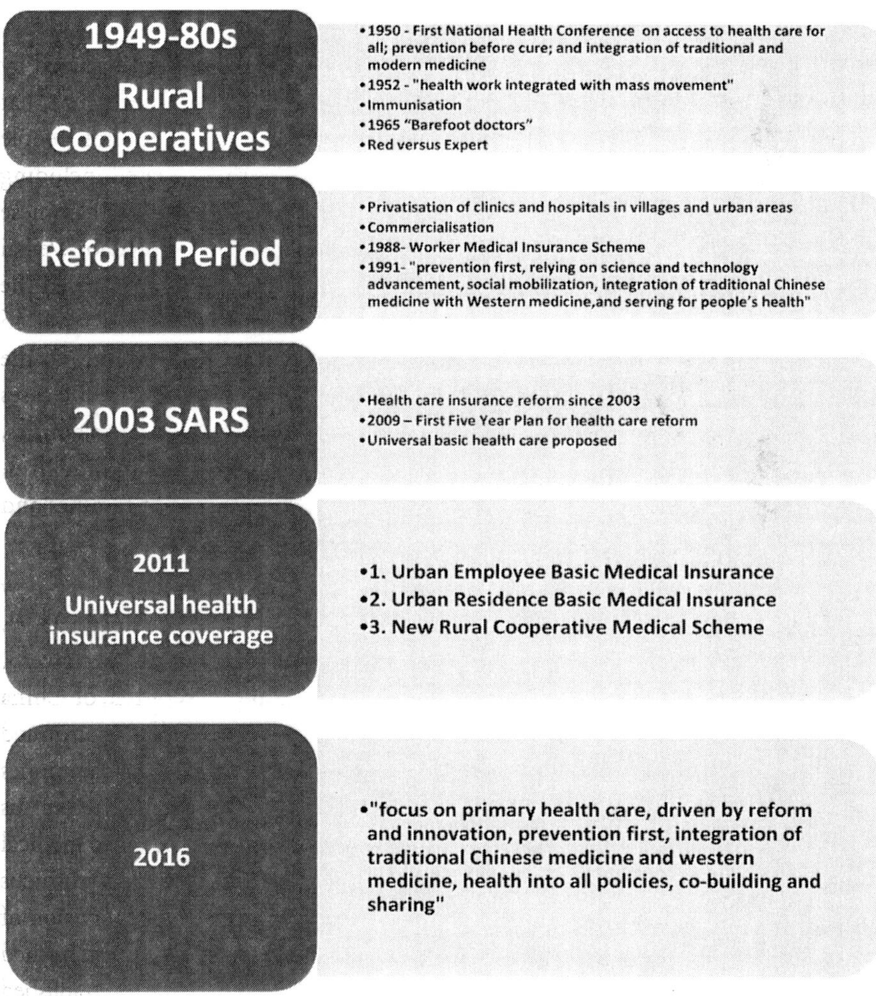

In 2018, National Health Commission was established as an apex institution after merging the previous policy making bodies. While China made progress during the reform period in the restructuring of the medical health care system, it has also been straddled with a number of problems of institutional capacity, higher health costs for the people, fast spread of diseases and epidemics and others[25]. While China has been reporting every passing year a greater number of cases of HIV-AIDS, TB, rabies, schistosomiasis, viral hepatitis and others, the number of pandemics is also increasing.

There are major plans that China is making in the health sector, though. In the recent years, the Chinese Academic of Sciences undertook a long-term blueprint till 2050 with genetically modified programmes as one of the major focus areas. Its goals in preventing and controlling infectious diseases between 2010 and 2020 is to set up early surveillance and warning centres, bio-safety labs to manage viruses and develop detection technologies; between 2020-30 "elucidate pathogen host interaction and pathogenesis as well as the mechanism of cross-species spread"; and between 2030-50 elucidate "the mechanism of virus genetic variation and individual differences in susceptibility and the mechanism of immune response and immune tolerance"[26].

Despite the above intervention of the state in public health system, epidemics continue to spread across China. The 1957 flu, dubbed as "Asian Flu" with H2N2 strain that began in China as well in two waves, spread over Taiwan, Hong Kong, India, Europe, US and other countries, killed over a million people and affecting over a million Indians.[27] Likewise of other epidemics even after the reform programme was launched since the later 1970s. For instance, even though hepatitis vaccination since 1992 has led to a decline in the faecal-oral route transmissions with high mortality rates among children and pregnant women, its variant hepatitis E emerged in the late 1990s in China.

However, the most severe challenge to the public health system of the PRC before COVID-19 remains the SARS crisis. SARS originated in the Pearl River Delta of the Guangdong-Hong Kong regions in November 2002 to July 2003 spreading fast and killing more than 700 people and infecting thousands[28]. In the initial stages, when cases were reported from Foshan in November 2002, there was no response from the central leadership and the local leadership treated this as a "medical" issue. However, as the virus spread outside – to Taiwan, Hong Kong, Southeast Asia and other countries and as global criticism grew – the central leadership swung into action after three months of the first SARS case outbreak. It was only in April 2003 – after four months – that the WHO was given permission to visit Guangdong, suggesting to its many parallels with the COVID-19 case currently.[29]

Also, Avian Influenza Viruses (AIV) have been making several rounds in China. The H1N1 influenza (also termed as Human Swine Flu or Influenza A) outbreak first in Mexico in March 2009 and spreading across the globe, received wider preparations in China[30]. Many of its subtypes like the H7N9 virus has emerged in early 2013 mainly through poultry and wild birds in the Yangtze River Delta in eastern China. In subsequent epidemic waves every year this virus spread to different parts of the country. The August 2018 outbreak of swine flu among pigs has almost debilitated the industry in China with consequences to the rise in prices of this staple diet in the country. Originally traces to Kenya in 1921 and introduced to Georgia in 2007, it spread to the rest of Europe quickly. In China, the virus was traced to a piggery farm in Shenyang in the northeast.[31] China is also a recipient of infectious diseases imported mainly from Africa and Asia. It was estimated that the imported cases of infectious diseases rose from 2 in 2005 to 11 in 2016. A total of 31,740 cases of infectious disease were imported to mainland China during 2005-2016, most of them found in Yunnan Province[32].

The section above thus suggests that despite advances in the public health care system in China, a number of diseases spread the landscape, many a time spilling over into the regional and global domains. SARS crisis in 2003 proved to be a signal of the fast spread of the virus beyond borders of China. This is the background for more enormous outbreak of COVID-19 that wreaked havoc not only in China but in over 200 countries.

What is in a name?

Worldwide, viruses are named based on the region or place of their origin, the scientist who discovered the specific virus or sometimes based on the nation in which it broke out or other political or scientific considerations. Thus, Ebola virus is based on the river name in Congo where it originated[33]; Zika virus on the Ugandan forests; Crimean-Congo hemorrhagic fever[34]; Spanish influenza, Japanese encephalitis, "Asiatic cholera" traced to the Gangetic Plains, Hantaviruses to Hantan river in South Korea[35], Middle East Respiratory Syndrome and others[36].

However, for scientific or geopolitical considerations or even for "political correctness" there has been a move to reorganise such categorisation[37]. The 1960s usage of electron microscope led to discovery of more characteristics of the viruses but also to the debates to systematically categorise them. In order to develop a comprehensive database of viruses, it was proposed in a meeting in 1991 that the International Committee on Taxonomy of Viruses develop a standard procedure in naming the viruses. In May 2015, the World Health Organization (WHO) had issued guidelines for the naming of the viruses with the aim "to minimize unnecessary negative impact of disease names on trade, travel, tourism or animal welfare, and avoid causing offence to any cultural, social, national, regional, professional or ethnic groups".[38]

Naming the virus has become controversial given the specific contextual aspects of the country involved or the status of its diaspora abroad. There are also acute power relations embedded in these terminologies, or discontinuing usage of some terminologies, specifically in the current case. Here is a rising power China which is not only authoritarian (meaning in this context restrictions placed on free flow of information) but also had a recent history of the spread of such viruses not only taking a toll domestically but also spreading it across the world. According to Ding Wang, China's outburst on labelling the virus as "Wuhan virus" is related to its authoritarian rule as well as to the voice of the ultranationalist elements in the country.[39]

For China, calling this virus as "Chinese virus" as US President tweeted on March 16 or "Wuhan virus" as the US Secretary of State Mike Pompeo mentioned, is unacceptable specifically as the leadership intends to celebrate its first centennial of the founding of the communist party in 2021 and fulfil "China dream" of a well-off society. Besides, as Wuhan is the hub of high-speed railway intersection and as a major industrial hub has implications for its foreign funded economy and tourism if "Wuhan virus" name is attached. Within Wuhan, the common saying is that the residents are pejoratively referred to abroad or in other places as "恶意毒源" [malicious poison sources] and that they should be kept apart.[40] Such distancing could have serious consequences for the economy, not to speak about the discrimination and alienation of Wuhan residents in the longer run. It also smacks of growing intolerance domestically in China about Wuhan residents. There is also the 18-month long tariff war with the US and the acute power transition debates in China with the US in the background of this renaming ceremony. Any let up with the US on this issue could have a cascading effect on China's sights of occupying the "centre stage" in global politics, as the 19th Communist Party Congress advocated. The stakes for China then are very high. Geopolitical sensitivities thus have convalesced on the COVID-19, including claims for compensation or reparations that are coming up from different quarters and actors across the globe. For according to John Lee,

> From a geopolitical perspective, COVID-19 is deeply troubling to the party because it changed the global conversation from how quickly China can construct a one thousand–bed hospital, build a dam, or commercialize self-driving cars to how the country is ruled and governed. Initial attempts to control information and suppress dissent rather than prevent a health crisis posed awkward questions about the strength and resilience of Chinese society under authoritarian institutions[41].

While the specific virus originated in Wuhan since November 2019 and the first officially reported in January 2020 and generally named it as novel Coronavirus (n-Cov), the WHO on February 11, 2020 renamed it as Coronavirus Disease-19 (COVID-19), although the International Committee on Taxonomy of Viruses retained the name SARS-Cov-2 given its similarities with the SARS virus[42]. The WHO chief stated the following for the reasons to rename the virus thus:

> ...we had to find a name that did not refer to a geographical location, an animal, an individual or group of people, and which is also pronounceable and related to the disease. Having a name matters to prevent the use of other names that can be inaccurate or stigmatizing. It also gives us a standard format to use for any future coronavirus outbreaks[43].

However, even in January scientists at the WHO, in collaboration with Chinese Academy of Sciences and various institutions at Shanghai, were still using the word "Wuhan virus" to depict the spread of the virus.[44] Besides, despite the new format of naming the viruses, all the previous names identifying viruses with regions or others are still in wide circulation globally suggesting that China's political sensitivities and pressures are being accommodated in the case of the COVID-19 case.

Geo-political considerations are also at play. While the US President Donald Trump depicted COVID-19 as "Chinese virus" on March 16, compared to his previous mention of "foreign virus", the US Secretary of State Mike Pompeo spoke about "Wuhan virus".[45] The US leaders continue to use these words in their public exchanges, suggesting that the differences with China on COVID-19 and other issues are still on the rise much to the discomfort of Chinese leaders and officials. This also explains partly to the pressure of China and the WHO in finding neutral terms for the virus. There are also racial connotations. While SARS virus was termed "Chinese virus" or "Cantonese" virus as it originated in Guangdong Province of China, the H1N1 virus is traced to Americas (mainly Canada, California and Mexico) and hence termed as "Euro-American" or "White" virus by the Chinese public health professionals. According to a study conducted by Katherine A. Mason,

> By inscribing geographical stability onto infected bodies in motion through the languages of race and genetics, my informants sought to constrain the mobility of infection and, in doing so, to contain the symbolic and material threats to China's modernity and development that flu-like infections, and the people who carried and spread them, had come to represent.[46]

Even though China's leaders have condemned the racial slant behind the "China virus" and other labels, it is ironic that China's authorities have hounded Africans from Guangzhou and other places with racial stigma[47]. Despite regretting such acts, Chinese continue to discriminate Africans and others in housing, travel and socialisation[48].

Origins and The Number Game

The number of infected patients and the tragic death of many have become controversial due to lack of credible information, fudging, or deliberate leak of misinformation regarding the spread of the disease[49]. Errors in estimates were stated to be because of the undetected cases or mild cases given the differential immunity of the individual persons. It could also be because of the slow asymptomatic transmission process and the varying incubation periods of the virus.

The following section pools from various official and other sources to depict the spread of the COVID-19 along with the numbers cited in these sources. Innumerable reports suggest COVID-19 origins at Wuhan[50]. It was reported that there were as many as 27 infected cases in Wuhan in December 2019 (some reports suggest that reports of cases were coming up as early as November).[51] The Emergency Response Law of the PRC enacted in November 2007 and International Health Regulations suggest reporting any health emergency within 24 hours– given the experience of the spread of the SARS epidemic in 2002-2003. The first case was reported on December 8 and the first patient was hospitalised on December 12, 2019.[52] These cases were traced to Huanan Seafood Market which was closed after a local ophthalmologist Li Wenliang reported about novel Coronavirus[53]. He was silenced but soon became a victim of the virus eventually[54]. On December 27, Vision Medicals, which constructed the genome structure of the new virus that has similarities with the SARS, shared the data with Wuhan officials and Chinese Academy of Medical Sciences, but fell on deaf ears. On January 2, Shi Zhengli the well-known scientist at the Wuhan Institute of Virology, reconstructed the entire genome structure of the new virus and despite the request of the World Health Organisation on January 1 for further information about the virus, China's officials have not provided the same[55]. On the contrary, the Wuhan Health Commission was in a denial mode or obfuscating the extent of viral infections as early fortnight of January coincided with the "two sessions" of Hubei Province.[56] Why was the provincial leadership or the central leadership delayed timely action in controlling the COVID-19 outbreak and spread in this crucial period is unclear. John Wong and Zheng Yongnian argued, in the case of the SARS outbreak more than a decade ago that a certain political norm crept into the communist party practice, viz., "never report a bad thing during seasons of high politics" that led to obfuscation or even curbing of the information flow at several levels.[57]

By January 3rd, the total number of infections increased to 44 with 11 in critical conditions. By January 5th these further rose to 59[58]. On January 8, researchers confirmed that the new virus was the pathogenic cause of pneumonia.[59] According to one version, the first human-to-human transmission was noted in the January 8th sequencing of the patients.[60] For the first time, only on January 11, 2020, an official bulletin was released by the Wuhan Health Commission stating that no new cases have been detected since January 3, no human-to-human transmission had taken place and that they diagnosed 41 cases of "unexplained viral pneumonia" patients mainly from the procurement section of the Huanan Seafood market[61]. They reported one death.[62] On January 11-12, China's National Health Commission informed the WHO that the outbreak was associated with the Seafood Market at Wuhan, while it shared the genetic sequence of the virus with the WHO.[63] Subsequent bulletins of the Commission did not announce any new cases till January 17, although they stated that over 700 close contacts have been tracked, while on January 14, it confirmed about a new case in Thailand originating from Wuhan on January 8[64]. The second death was reported on January 15th of a 69-year-old patient who contracted the virus on December 31, 2019 but became severe on January 4, 2020.[65]

From January 18, cases multiplied from 54 new cases to 77 and it was stated the next day that no connection to the Huanan Seafood Market was found in the fresh reported cases.[66] Since January 20 the WHO began providing a daily situation report on the number of cases.[67] It is only on January 20th that China began acknowledging in public about human-to-human transmission of the virus, despite substantial evidence to the contrary.[68] The January 21 bulletin of the National Health Commission noted the detection of cases outside of Wuhan, including faraway places like Beijing, Shanghai, Hainan, Yunnan, Jilin and Guangdong provinces as well as in Thailand, Japan and South Korea[69]. 13 provinces (and increased within days to all provinces in China and some abroad) reported new infections indicating that the migration pattern increased due to the Spring Festival rush and the rumours about an impending lockdown. On January 23rd, the Commission bulletin for the first time gave an elaborate clinical diagnosis of 17 patients who passed away succumbing to the virus. Most of them contracted the virus in December and some were being treated since then at various hospitals at Wuhan[70]. The same day Wuhan was completely locked down[71], along with 16 neighbouring cities with a ban on public gatherings, and after no new cases were reported, the authorities lifted the 76-day shutdown on April 8.[72]

The fast spread of the COVID-19 has surprised the international community. This is reflected in comparing the spread of COVID-19 with the other recent viral infections. For instance, it was stated that the MERS took about two and a half years to infect 1000 people, and SARS took roughly 4 months, while COVID-19, on the other hand, reached that figure in just 48 days, suggesting to its virulent character[73]. The estimated case fatality rate for COVID-19 is 3 percent (in comparison to about 10 percent for SARS and 40 percent for MERS).[74]

From Wuhan, COVID-19 spread to the Hubei Province (the worst hit were two cities, Huanggang and Xiangyang) followed domestically by Anhui, Guangdong, Henan, Hunan, Jiangxi and Zhejiang provinces which are the surrounding areas for the pathogen to spread. Wuhan/Hubei are connected with these areas by infrastructure and business operations. The Spring Festival rush – the annual family reunions for hundreds of millions of Chinese – further aggravated the situation by spreading the virus[75]. An estimated 3 billion trips are made in such family reunions posing grave danger in spreading the contagion.[76] However, due to community isolation the areas that are far away from Hubei province did not witness COVID-19 infections such as in Inner Mongolia, Tibet and Qinghai[77]. In later period, COVID-19 spread to Harbin city in the north-eastern Heilongjiang province with suspected infection spread from a foreigner.

It is only two days after the lockdown of Wuhan that on January 25 a small leading group was formed by the central leadership of the communist party. In the November 1, 2007 Emergency Response Law of the PRC, the Premier of the State Council is made responsible to address "emergencies"[78]. The small leading group was tasked to visit Hubei and coordinate and "to treat infected patients, speed up the augmentation of medical personnel, and coordinate civilian and military medical resources".[79] Premier Li Keqiang was named the head of this group (who visited Wuhan on January 27[80]) and chaired 30 meetings of this group, with other members including Vice Premier Sun Chunlan[81] (who is in charge of the health sector). On January 28, meeting the visiting WHO chief, President Xi stated that "The epidemic is a devil. We will not let it hide"[82]. President Xi Jinping addressed the armed forces stating the situation is "grim and complicated".[83] Two hospitals to cure patients were being constructed at Wuhan. The top party leadership at the Hubei provincial level has been replaced with those closer to President Xi Jinping's political faction. At the February 3rd meeting of the Politburo Standing Committee, Xi directed that China needs to tell its stories on addressing the COVID-19, thus triggering a war of narratives with the US and promotion of China Model. On February 10, Xi Jinping – termed by the official media as the "commander of the people's war against the epidemic" – for the first time appeared in public and inspected a local epidemic prevention and control centre where he praised the morale, spirit and determination of health workers. As the number of infections increased, the Communist Party organised 14 apex Politburo Standing Committee meetings from January till May as the table below indicates. At the February 12th meeting, Xi stated that "positive changes" occurred in tackling the COVID-19 cases due to "hard-won progress made by all sides". The meeting suggested the restoration of production and easing the burden of tax and fees. The following points were made:

- raise the hospital admission capacity to leave no one unattended to in cities with a large number of fever patients;
- reduce the infection rate by strengthening the prevention and control in communities and cutting off transmission routes;
- improve treatment for patients, especially those in severe condition, by pooling strengths in medical resources and technology;
- provide more medical resources including hospital beds and medical workers in Hubei Province, especially the city of Wuhan, which remains the top priority region;
- implement the support of 19 provincial-level regions to different areas of Hubei;
- step up health monitoring of returning personnel in regions with large population inflows[84].

Later at the February 26 meeting, all politburo standing committee members made cash donations, while Xi termed the situation in Wuhan and Hubei as "complicated and grave" and asked the party and government committees at all levels to coordinate efforts and pool resources from across the country. It also stated that as a "responsible major country", China should involve in efforts to promote international cooperation on epidemic response and directed "to continue to work closely with the World Health Organization, keep in close contact with relevant countries to share experience and coordinate measures on prevention and control, strengthen public diplomacy and communication of China's efforts, and work with other countries to uphold regional and global public health security".[85] Thus China began talking about international cooperation as a major thrust area, as COVID-19 began spreading abroad and negative public opinion across the globe began emerging. However, it took a month, on March 10, for President Xi to visit Wuhan, the epicentre of the COVID-19, even though he stated that he was monitoring the COVID-19 related work on daily basis[86].

Table 1.1: Communist Party's Politburo Standing Committee Meetings on COVID-19

January 7	prevention and control of the epidemic
January 25	to win the battle to contain the virus with "confidence and solidarity, a science-based approach and targeted measures"; A Small Leading Group to be formed. Delegation to Hubei
February 3	principle of early detection, reporting, quarantine and treatment be strictly observed
February 12	COVID-19 at "most crucial stage"; cross-region joint prevention and control and society-wide efforts to contain the virus
February 19	COVID-19 prevention and control, and promoting economic and social development
February 26	National epidemic control turning for the better
March 4	Focus on economic and social development
March 18	to stop inbound cases and measures to protect the health of Chinese citizens overseas
March 25	virus control and economic focus
April 8	need to stay alert against potential risks
April 15	virus control and economic measures
April 29	China had won a vital battle and achieved a major strategic success in the nationwide control efforts.
May 6	on the rehabilitation and psychological counselling of patients in recovery
May 14	Covid 19 control in key areas and key places to prevent its resurgence; prevention of inbound infection

Source: State Council Information Office of the PRC, "Fighting COVID-19: China in Action" June 2020

While all these events were happening, the WHO, which withheld advisories on COVID-19 spread due to lack of evidence from China, declared finally on January 30 as "public health emergency of international concern" after the virus spread to over 24 countries[87]. Delayed responses in China also led to many a country evacuating their nationals from China despite the WHO advisories to the contrary on February 4th as these acts could "cause stigma and fear". However, foreign minister Wang Yi questioned on February 14 the actions of other countries in addressing the spread of the virus, thus:

> In our view, the enhanced inspection measures taken by some countries are reasonable, while other countries have overreacted, which has caused unnecessary panic and is not consistent with WHO recommendations.... Everybody can see that the measures taken by these countries go far beyond the recommendations of the WHO. For example, measures have been taken to comprehensively stop people-to-people exchanges. In addition, not only have people in Wuhan been evacuated, but also people in regions where the epidemic is not severe. We do not interfere with the decisions of other countries. However, when these measures are taken, we must look at whether they are truly beneficial to a joint response to the epidemic.[88]

Apart from Thailand, Japan and other countries where transmission of the virus from Wuhan took place, the earliest cases of infections in Italy, Iran and Spain were traced to January-February period, mostly to either Chinese tourists from Wuhan or to the tourists who travelled to Wuhan and returned or those who were infected on *Diamond Princess* cruise ship[89]. After a week of travel in Italy, two Chinese tested positive at Rome on January 30, while on February 3 a group of 56 Italian tourists from Wuhan arrived at Rome and among whom one tested positive on February 6.[90] On February 20, the first case of COVID-19 was reported in Lodi in north-western Italy. A majority of cases were reported in Italy from three regions-Lombardy, Veneto and Emilia-Romagna.[91] Later the virus spread to most parts of the world.

China's authorities had released data on the number of infections and death due to the spread of the COVID-19. However, despite a number of data sets release, there are questions raised on transparency in the collection of data and accuracy and veracity of such numbers. Also, a change in the methodology of the definition of the confirmed cases led to a huge increase in the overall numbers of infections.[92] Adoption of new techniques to diagnose the patients with computed tomography (CT) scan also enhanced the detection capability of the COVID-19.[93] In April, Wuhan authorities stated that in order to protect the "credibility of the government" they increased the number of COVID-19 cases by as many as 50 percent to the previous data with the number of deaths increased from 2,579 to 3,869[94]. Another discrepancy in the numbers was suggested by *Foreign Policy Journal.* According to the data tracker procured from China's National University of Defence Technology at Changsha by the *Foreign Policy* journal, covering over 230 cities in China, the data sets consists of as many as 640,000 rows with location, confirmed and recovered cases, deaths and other details aggregated from various sources[95]. According to the estimates of Derek Scissors, there could be as many as 2.9 million cases in China.[96] The Rand Corporation, in a report on the subject, argued that the number of infectious cases could be as high as 37 percent of the Chinese official figures, i.e., instead of the official figures of 503 infections reported on January 22, it should be about 18,700 cases.[97]

A number of scientists have provided different model-based studies to suggest that the number of infected patients in Wuhan far outnumber the officially acknowledged figures. They also suggested that travel from Wuhan to the rest of China and the world has created the pandemic on gigantic proportions[98]. Many of such studies have also suggested that an earlier implementation of quarantine procedures could have reduced the misery of the public and death and destruction.[99]

According to a study conducted by Lauren Gardner of the Centre for Systems Science and Engineering of Johns Hopkins University, based on airport networks metapopulation model, the number of infections in China are nearly five times the figures quoted by the Chinese side at 58,000 as against the official count of 12,000 by January 31, 2020. They estimated that infections already were numerous in November 2019 and by December hundreds were infected. The movement of the infected to rest of China and the world has led to the spread of the pandemic by January 31[100]. Wuhan international airport serves over 19 million passengers a year of which more than 3,000 travel to international destinations every day. A monthly average of 520,000 travellers from Wuhan to other destinations are recorded.[101] On the other hand, Joseph T. Wu and others at University of Hong Kong estimated that 75,815 infected patients in Wuhan by January 25[102].

With increasing criticism from several quarters, the WHO has finally sent a delegation of 25 members drawn from the US, China, Russia, Germany, Japan and other countries, excluding India, Italy, Spain, Brazil or other worse affected areas, from February 16-24 to various parts of China but for only one final day to restricted members visit to Wuhan[103]. They found the virus has 96 percent similarities with bat SARS-coronavirus strains – suggesting bats as the reservoir for COVID-19. The WHO report stated that China followed three steps to contain the COVID-19, viz., in the early stages, "preventing the exportation of cases from Wuhan and other priority areas of Hubei Province, and preventing the importation of cases by other provinces"; in the 2nd stage, of "reduce the intensity of the epidemic and to slow down the increase in cases" and in the 3rd stage "reducing clusters of cases, thoroughly controlling the epidemic, and striking a balance between epidemic prevention and control, sustainable economic and social development, the unified command, standardized guidance, and scientific evidence-based policy implementation.". However, the most problematic of the above is with the early stage where the WHO stated that China had prevented cases from going out of Wuhan. This is contrary to all the available information and in fact an estimated 5 million people fanned out of Wuhan into Hubei province or across the globe as the first cases in Thailand, Japan, Italy and others attests to.

Transmission of COVID-19

In order to curb the transmission of the COVID-19 or during the previous Ebola crisis, a number of measures were suggested including scanning and identification, diagnosis and management of the cases, aggressive tracking of contacts, infection prevention and control measures in isolated hospitals, travel advisories, awareness campaigns, taking the temperature of incoming tourists at points of entry, quarantining and others. However, some felt that the latter measures are not adequate due to asymptomatic transmission cases. Hence it was suggested that the proven methods of reverse transcription polymerase chain reaction (RT-PCR) be followed.[104] However, despite these measures, the transmission of the COVID-19 took place to distant lands with disastrous consequences.

In order to understand such transmission dynamics of epidemics, there are a number of models which were utilised by several Chinese scholars to understand the spread of the COVID-19 and implement control measures and on how to restore production networks[105]. Over a hundred years ago W.O. Kermack and A.G. MacKendrick followed a SIR compartmental model to track epidemic transmission. A number of variations have been developed subsequently.[106] These models are useful for prediction of the spread of the virus as well as for policy prescriptions[107]. According to Tian Liang, et.al., over five million people working in Wuhan or recently travelled to Wuhan have exited the city spreading the virus to far flung areas. According to their study, the spread of the virus had exhibited the following pattern:

> In the first week after the lockdown, the number of newly confirmed cases continued to grow at approximately 0.3 per day. This was followed by a crossover phase that lasted two to three weeks, during which provincial and local governments took stringent tracking, isolation and quarantine measures. In this phase, the growth rate slowed down and eventually turned negative upon reaching the much-desired inflection point. In the phase of final descent, the reduction of daily confirmed cases again took a universal form of exponential decay at a rate of 0.32 per day, i.e., a tenfold reduction in the number of newly confirmed cases per week.[108]

According to another study, based on China's social networking sites WeChat (with 1.13 billion users) and QQ (with 808 million active users), COVID-19 was transported to 369 cities before Wuhan was shutdown[109]. By following the Lewy flight which is characteristic of human mobility, Bnaya Gross, et.al argued that restriction on movement of people and imposition of quarantine procedures have proved to stall the progress of the COVID-19 spread in China[110]. In another study of 70 genomes of virus strains from China and other places between 24 December 24, 2019 and February 3,2020, a group of scholars – Li Xingguang and others suggested that COVID-19 did not originate from pangolins but was due to human-to-human transmission.[111] By applying the classical susceptible exposed infectious recovered (SEIR) model[112], Peng and others argued that the epidemic has spread no later than January 1st; that the protection rate in Wuhan is lower till at least February 9th due mostly to the mixing of the susceptible to the infectious cases and that the infectious cases spreading to rest of China is far higher in numbers before January 20th. [113]

In another modified model – the C-SEIR model proposed by Chen Baoquan and others of Center on Frontiers of Computing Studies at Peking University - two new quarantined groups in SEIR were added: the quarantined suspected infection group (P), and the quarantined diagnosed infection group (Q) as follows. According to them while no measures were undertaken by Wuhan before January 23rd, leading to the spread of infections, but after aggressive quarantine measures were implemented the cases have come down.[114]

Zhou Yimin and others adopted yet another variation of the SEIR model given the new factors of indirect infections and suspected cases (i.e. with symptom but not been confirmed in time), medical treatment (through the two large hospitals built quickly at Wuhan) and traffic blockade and residential isolation. This is termed as YJ-SEIR model that utilised entropy and fuzzy comprehensive evaluation pattern[115].

However, as SEIR model is based on several assumptions and parameters, another model was applied to study the transmission dynamics. Hu Zixin and others from Shanghai and Houston based on the modified stacked auto-encoder (MAE) model and utilising artificial intelligence methods for real-time forecasting data collected from January 11 to February 27, 2020, argued that COVID-19 epidemic would be over by April 2020[116].

Three more studies are worth noting here. GaoQijun and others examined 213 patients at Jingmen Hospital in Hubei province. Their study indicated to the impact of those who visited or travelled or who came in contact from people from Wuhan recently and to the highly contagiousness of COVID-19.[117] Another study of Changsha city by Wang Guyi and others found that of the 242 patients examined, those with a short stay in Wuhan had a higher risk of being severe than those without Wuhan exposure.[118]

Models to Study Resumption of Production

One of the major concerns of China and the rest of the world is the impact COVID-19 has on the economic front as well[119]. Reeling, as it were, under the global slowdown since the Asian Financial Crisis of 1997 and Global Financial Crisis of 2008, every country has restoration of production as one of the main considerations. While the above transmission models analysed the spread of the COVID-19 to different parts of China and provided policy prescriptions on when such epidemic will come to an end, China's scholars also developed models for the restoration of business and enterprises for the restarting of economic development. These models are helpful in the identification of potential risks for the large-scale work resumption in the factories/businesses. When COVID-19 spread across the country, China's authorities have shut down factories and other work places to break the chain of contagion. It extended the Spring Festival holidays from a week to ten days and on February 8, the State Council emphasises on safety of workers and public health, although in the next two days partial onsite production activities in medical equipment manufacturing, energy, grain, transportation and logistics were encouraged[120]. By March, however, it was reported that over 90 percent of the State-Owned Enterprises are back in the production network, although small and medium enterprises constitute the bulk of the GDP of the country.[121]

In general, COVID-19 spread resulted in a slump in the GDP figures due to disruptions in demand, mobility, transport, trade sectors, production slump, spike in unemployment, blocking of supply chains due to lock down and the Shanghai Stock Exchange plunging 8 percent on February 3, with its fallout reflected in global domains as well.[122]

Disruptions in manufacturing, service sector, transportation and trade affected the production networks due to general shutdown. While wholesale prices are said to be relatively constant, the actual retail prices have shot up due to hoarding, selling at speculative prices and the like creating huge economic discomfort to the people.[123]

Specifically given the preventive quarantine measures implemented on a large scale like shut down of whole cities or provinces, stopping of all transportation networks, and others, an "evaluation for the potential outbreak risk" (EPOR) model was adopted. Based on source of infection, transmission route and susceptible population, Zhou Yimin and others developed the EPOR model[124]. The factors affecting the EPOR in factory resumption during an epidemic are mentioned in the table below based on Zhou Yimin's estimates.

Table 1.2: The EPOR of the Work Resumption during Epidemic

Self-protection	*Company prevention*	*Protection supervision level*	*Production management level*	*Internal and external outbreak threat*	*Environmental impact*
Wear disposable surgical masks; Wear KN95 masks; Separate eating; Wash hands; Wear KN95 masksand goggles; Wear Protective clothes.	Quarantine measure; Epidemic prevention; Monitoring measure; Off-peak commuting; Perfect disinfection; Harmless treatment.	Perfecting epidemic prevention supervision system; Perfecting of quarantine supervision system.	Density of workersat workplace; Worker communication frequency; Plant sector density; Management awareness of prevention and control.	Severity of the outside; External isolation strength; Epidemic trend.	Traffic condition; River abundance density; Bad weather; Mobility of contaminated objects.

Relief Measures

China has defended its response on complete shutdown of Wuhan and other places of infection since January 23. The Chinese government adopted a five-level response to counter the spread of the COVID-19 as follows:

1. regional isolation measures in Wuhan by shut down on January 23rd,
2. concentrates on the temporary isolation and
3. rescue hospital construction – Leishenshan and Huoshenshan
4. organizes the medical staff of all Provinces from China to support Wuhan in improving their treatment capacity so as to rapidly digest the backlog of suspected cases and
5. reduce the number of viral infections by blocking community transmissions and introducing mobile phone applications like "Shen I" and "Health Code."[125]

The general response was that of closing borders, restricting travel, tracing close contacts and quarantining, so that the growth rate of newly confirmed cases will gradually transition from a constant positive value to lower values and eventually become negative. As mentioned over 40,000 medical personnel were sent from different provinces to Wuhan for medical cure. China adopted transitional and modern medical treatment of the patients in the absence of the development of a vaccine. As the virus spread, the variations in responses are also visible. For instance, while the central directives are being sent to the provinces where the COVID-19 was spreading, there were also several regional variations in responding to the virus. Thus, for instance the Zhejiang University School of Medicine suggested to "四抗二平衡" [four anti and two balances] approach, viz., antivirus, anti-shock, anti-hyoxemia, anti-secondary infection, and balance in maintaining of water, electrolyte and acid base; and microecological balance. Implementation of this approach was said to have effectively addressed the spread of the virus in Zhejiang Province.[126]

Responses in Addressing COVID-19

When the virus erupted in Wuhan, China's government stated that this is a novel Coronavirus and that they were still studying the genome. It was stated that every year around the Spring time there is generally a spike in flu cases and the medical establishment is geared towards addressing such cases. However, the Huanan Seafood Market was cleaned up quickly, leaving no evidence regarding how the virus spread either from animals to humans or human-to-human or if there is any deliberate human release of the virus into the market. This has led to several conspiracy theories[127] and to several omissions and commissions of the powers that be. Subsequently, as the virus spread, people were hospitalised at various places in Wuhan. As rumours of impending lockdown continued, an estimated 5 million people travelled across Hubei Province to domestic destinations or abroad, coinciding as it were with the annual Spring Festival which generally witnesses 300 to 400 million people reaching their hometowns from their places of work and to be with their families. Eventually, to stop the exodus, China imposed travel restrictions and shutdown of the residential complexes. Social mobility was curbed with the intention of breaking the chain of infections across the board. Simultaneously, two major hospitals were built to provide health care to the affected. House-to-house temperature checks were carried out in Wuhan and other places. Monitoring infectious cases, facial recognition under face mask, monitoring mobile phone conversations, purchases, and use of big data across regions was attempted.[128]

What later came to be known as "China model" of tackling COVID-19 included large-scale and intrusive measures affecting millions of residents. Swift implementation of orders, high efficiency and restoration of "face" were the elements in this approach.[129] According to Zheng Guichu,

> It is the Chinese political system that has rallied, harnessed and guided people to contain the spread of the virus. It is the efficiency, responsiveness and transparency of the Chinese political system, its merits and advantages, that have been and will be central and crucial to the final victory in the combat. Socialism with Chinese characteristics is the choice of the Chinese people.[130]

Another, a renowned scholar Zhang Weiwei, who heads a centre to publicise "China model", likewise argued that

> China's political system is oriented toward substantive democracy. The government is responsible for the entire nation with almost unlimited liabilities. The Communist Party of China, prioritizing people's lives and security, is highly capable of nationwide mobilization and coordination. The strong sense of unity and solidarity among the Chinese people makes it easy for them to come together to fight against national emergencies. By practicing self-quarantine and refraining from public gatherings, they showed great self-discipline when confronted with the epidemic.[131]

Zheng and Zhang, of course did not go into why the party-state did not respond effectively between November 2019 to January 23 or the treatment to the whistle-blowers or discrepancies in number of casualties. Nor did they go into the enormous difficulties that migrant workers faced in Wuhan and Hubei Province. It is also not clear how the whole effort can be termed as "victory" with over 4,000 deaths estimated in official figures and millions of people displaced and disturbed across China, not to mention about the different parts of the world where the virus spread from Wuhan before January 23rd.

Comparison with other countries 'approaches to counter COVID-19 also situates China's position on this issue. Of course, the national conditions are different and responsive mechanisms are varied in nature. As Cai Fang, vice president of Chinese Academy of Social Sciences argued," Every country has its own epidemiological curve and forms part of the global epidemiological curve." Cai further suggests the twin-goals of China's model here is prevention and control and economic recovery efforts.[132]

While China's propaganda insists on its efficient handling of the COVID-19 as highlighted in the white paper on the subject, there are more efficient and least intrusive ways with which other countries have addressed the issue. As the authors in this volume have argued, Japan was able to restrict the number of infections as well as deaths and spread of COVID-19. Taiwan is another model of isolating the infected persons from the beginning. Despite widespread infections caused by "patient 31", the South Korean model reflected to aggressive testing and prevention. While disastrous at the beginning of the spread of the virus, partly traced to social habits, lax governmental responses or due to "hug a Chinese" campaign of Florence mayor, once the restrictive measures, shutdown on all social mobility, not as harsh as in China but allowing for people to go to work or buy essentials, the number of infections came down.[133] However, all models have limitations given the eruption of a 2nd wave of infections across the globe, including in Wuhan.

Responsibility Issues

A human tragedy and disaster of the scale of COVID-19 was unforeseen in the recent human history with death and destruction everywhere. Naturally, questions about the responsibility for the spread of COVID-19 has arisen with the US, Australia and nearly 120 countries at World Health Assembly taking the lead in questioning China[134], while the latter has been stating that it did not know the intensity of the virus, that it has been transparent and now has been involved in international cooperation to mitigate the negative fallout of the COVID-19. Moreover, China's leaders and officials time and again contended that the virus has no borders.

In international relations the issue of responsibility is significant and involves the United Nations (UN) bodies, international law, arbitration and others. The European Union has proposed "Responsibility to protect" on many global issues. China and other countries (like Russia, India and others) have argued in the UN about the sanctity of the UN Charter, specifically on the "non-interference" principle.

During the US intervention in Iraq, Kosovo, Afghanistan, Libya, Syria and other countries, China and others have articulated the view that such interventions are violative of the UN Charter related to sovereignty principle of the member states of the UN. A number of UN Security Council proposals were vetoed by China and Russia in the last few decades based on the view that the territorial integrity and sovereignty principles of member states are violated in the course of "regime change", unilateralism and counter-terror campaigns across the world. Since the 1990s, it also took the form of opposing the spread of "coloured revolutions" in the Eurasian region by China and Russia and this has also been the subject matter of the veto exercise against human rights violations during the "saffron revolution" in Myanmar. The influence of the Western non-governmental organisations in spreading such "coloured revolutions" was frowned upon. Thus sovereignty, territorial integrity, non-interference policies have been highlighted by China (and other countries). This is reflected in China blocking Taiwan's role in WHO and other related issues.

Indeed, sensitivity on the issue of sovereignty issues has been the hallmark of the international relations since the Westphalian Treaty was signed. Clearly, lines have been drawn on the internal and external sovereignty aspects across the world, codified and practiced for centuries during the course of inter-state interactions. For sure many of these were violated by several countries. Yet, China and other countries have advocated such principles in international relations even though they have also been accused at one time or the other of violating of the very same principles.

The spread of non-traditional security challenges, specifically pandemics, has complicated the sovereignty principles, although the role and responsibility of the state has never been completely jettisoned on such issues. While it has been broadly agreed that in the practice of international relations, nations would undertake responsibility for their subjects, flowing from the internal sovereignty principles, this aspect has become controversial and contentious. For instance, the spread of terrorism across the borders from one state to the other – often at the behest of a state – the responsibility of that state seen as sponsoring terrorism increasingly came under international scrutiny and concerted action.

Thus, the UN Security Council committees on counter-terrorism, including the 1267, 1373 and 1540, have taken measures to penalise and make accountable those state and non-state actors for spreading various forms of terrorism. There are also several other legislations and norms that were evolved by countries and international institutions to hold responsible persons who are involved in crime and other activities. The principle here is to take responsibility for the actions of one's own citizens in as much as a state holds its international sovereignty claims.

In the case of the pandemics like the spread of bird flu, SARS or currently COVID-19, the responsibility of a state for the movement and actions of its infected citizens, intentional or unintentional, is quite evident[135]. The moral responsibility and accountability of a state in this regard is also evident. On the contrary, the saying that pandemics have no borders[136] (and by implication the concerned state is not responsible for any damage and destruction) – as some Chinese leaders, officials and others have argued *ad nauseum*[137] – has also been questioned. In the words of Christopher Caldwell,

> This virus happens to travel on people. If people can be made to respect borders, viruses will 'respect' them too, in the sense that they will not cross them. If this is true of households, then it is true of nations.[138]

While China had objected to various countries evacuating their citizens from Wuhan in its early days of spread in January and the restrictions placed on incoming persons traveling from Wuhan, however, it had imposed the same conditions for the entry of foreigners into China after the COVID-19 cases within China kept dropping. This is on the suspicion that new infectious cases are being imported from abroad.

Also, China had earlier stated that it is a "responsible big country" and had moved away from Robert B. Zoellick, the then US Deputy Secretary of State's suggestion for being a "responsible stakeholder" in the international and regional orders[139]. At the Politburo Standing Committee meeting on February 26, as a "responsible major country" [负责任的大国] China should involve in efforts to promote international cooperation on epidemic response and directed "to continue to work closely with the World Health Organization, keep in close contact with relevant countries to share experience and coordinate measures on prevention and control, strengthen public diplomacy and communication of China's efforts, and work with other countries to uphold regional and global public health security".[140] Flowing from this was the announcement of President Xi at the World Health Assembly of contributing in future $2 billion in medical assistance to the affected developing countries and conducting investigation after the infections recede[141]. China's white paper on Covid-9 mentioned that "China had sent 29 medical expert teams to 27 countries, and offered assistance to 150 countries and 4 international organizations [and] exported to 200 countries 70.6 billion masks, 340 million protective suits, 115 million pairs of goggles, 96,700 ventilators, 225 million test kits, and 40.29 million infrared thermometers."[142] However, many a country has complained about the poor quality of some of the equipment supplied, besides the limited nature of quantum of such assistance to other countries in the light of the enormity of the disaster originating in Wuhan.

Summary and Conclusions

The above brief analysis of the origin and dynamics of the COVID-19 suggests that COVID-19 spread in Wuhan, Hubei and the rest of China and the world was accompanied by intense debate all across, an intense conflict between the US and China on narratives that hinged on power transition, "decoupling" and "great power competition", thus triggering the securitisation of COVID-19 to an unprecedented levels. The all-round trail of death and destruction in the wake of COVID-19 spread in China and across the world led to the subject becoming "securitised" extensively. Widespread and unprecedented focus on the COVID-19, its origins and transmission have further elevated the subject. In the light of the international criticism led by the US, Australia and nearly 120 countries in the World Health Assembly, China has gone to the other extreme of cautiousness to the extent of denial of information, curbs on whistle-blowers and restrictions on the media and medical fraternity. While China's white paper of June 7 on COVID-19 sought to project a picture of being swift, timely, open and transparent, centralised and efficient, well-coordinated, the picture is more nuanced in nature.

On the other hand, there are several inconsistencies and contradictions in China's handling of the COVID-19. One of the most glaring omissions is that of November to January 23rd period when proper detection and prevention of the COVID-19 cases could have saved not only China but the rest of the world's travails. Various modelling studies by Chinese scholars and others cited above suggested that if the cases were detected and controlled in early and in a timely manner, millions could have been saved of COVID-19 infections. Addressing the COVID-19 cases was further complicated by deliberate allowing of political events such as provincial mega meetings and public feasting that only increased the spread of the virus in Wuhan. The quick action of the authorities in erasing of evidence at Huanan Seafood Market has led to the loss of crucial information on COVID-19. Official denial of human-to-human transmission of COVID-19, and endorsed by the WHO, in the initial stages has led to incorrect assessment and spread of the virus.

China suggested that it had exhibited efficiency of the party- state machinery in addressing the COVID-19. Enormous resources of the party-state were mobilised from different provinces such as medical staff, equipment and others to treat patients in Wuhan and other places. Party units at various localities have been directed to contribute their set of quotas for this prevention and control work. However, a less intrusive, efficient and effective model in addressing COVID-19 is also exhibited by South Korea, Taiwan, Japan and after initial shocks even in Italy and Spain.

China has taken umbrage at the attacks on Chinese citizen abroad for racism.

Indeed, many Chinese descent people were targeted in Europe, Australia, the US and other countries. However, this argument in the initial stages of COVID-19 appeared to be more diversionary as China itself had exhibited internal racism among its own people in Wuhan, in addition to racial comments and attacks on Africans living in China.

Another dimension is that as early as February 26, China took the decision to activate international cooperation on COVID-19. This is in a way the scientific community's effort to share crucial experience with the outside, but could as well be an opportunity to spread China's influence abroad specifically at a time, "democratic" model in the West appeared to be slackening in addressing increasing COVID-19 infections. Xi's G20 address, Eurasian virtual meeting of the medical officials or WHA address are related to these, although its "mask diplomacy" and substandard medical equipment supplies were criticised. However, soon China was caught up with the "wolf warrior diplomatic" practice, resulting in the US criticism on "Chinese virus". This contributed to the further securitisation of the issue. Here was an important opportunity for both the US and China and the larger international community to address the pressing global public health crisis, but lost due to the increasing acrimony between them. There could have been efforts at joint R&D in vaccine development, sharing crucial diagnostic experience to mitigate the situation. Some efforts indeed were made. However, this was a major lost opportunity for multilateral cooperation on COVID-19 due to China-US rivalry – and reflects to a clear emergence of "wolf warrior diplomacy" that has taken precedence over "keeping a low profile" in China.

Also, COVID-19 spread across the globe, and its impact in a very short period has led to a debate on its impact on the world order, thus further contributing to the securitisation debate. The debate was partly triggered by American strategic expert Henry Kissinger who said that COVID-19 had ushered in a new order.[143] One of the major lacunae is the ineffectiveness of the multilateral processes to provide relief to those nations affected by COVID-19. The UN Security Council was tasked to address pressing security issues of the world. Yet there has been no positive and effective momentum in this regard and its meeting in April, hijacked as it were with the naming of the virus. The WHO remained only advisory in nature and clearly with funding cuts from member states like the US which accused it of following China's advice, even such functions are going to be affected. The other institutions such as G-7, G-20, IMF and World Bank or Asian Development Bank as well did not make much difference, although the Bretton Woods institutions have put on hold the debt payments from developing countries. The G-7 foreign ministerial meeting on March 25 failed to come out with a statement, divided as it were by the name of the virus again. Much of this paralysis in the current international institutions is traced to the emerging "decoupling" or "great power competition" between the two largest economies in the world, the United States and China[144]. With active recriminations against each other increasing, many an international body proved to be ineffective in tackling COVID-19. This suggests to the need for new but more effective multilateral responses from the international community.

The spread of the virus and its impact on the economy touched a majority of nations, thus magnifying the securitisation of COVID-19. Even as the economic growth rates for most countries has been slashed by the International Monetary Fund and other credit rating agencies (to mostly negative for most of the world, except for China at 1.7 percent and India at 1.2 percent for 2020), dwindling exports and imports due to lack of demand caused by general lockdown in many countries (with the World Trade Organisation estimating double-digit decline in trade), disruption in supply chain, curbs on travel and tourism, energy prices fluctuations and others have caused near economic depression conditions. Global debt has surpassed over $2.5 trillion according to the IMF estimates, with Japan, China, India and other countries topping the list. Individual countries have announced monetary and fiscal stimulus packages but these appear to be inadequate to address the global decline. Unemployment in formal and informal sectors is staring at many countries due to COVID-19 lockdown. There has also been 40 percent decline in foreign direct investments globally. If the aggregate demand and supply issues are not addressed at the global level, if the US-China competition is not addressed quickly, and if the 2nd and 3rd waves of COVID-19 infections increase, humanity is expected to face major economic problems in the near future. 2020 is estimated to lose over $8.5 trillion in goods and services production, a gap that could hardly be filled up even in rebound conditions. These suggests to the need for intensifying macro-economic coordination efforts and new multilateral solutions. Of course, many countries tried to utilise S&T innovation, big data, artificial intelligence, cloud computing and others to tackle the COVID-19 crisis but that also calls for new business models[145].

In relation to China, many scholars see the post-COVID-19 world order as providing opportunities and challenges, specifically in international cooperation efforts[146]. Wang Jisi, a leading American expert, argued that since President Trump took over, the bilateral relations have been affected in many fields, with COVID-19 further intensifying strategic rivalry between the two accelerating the decline in relations between the two. As a result, the decoupling in economy and technology is becoming a reality.[147] Yuan Peng, President of the China Institute of Contemporary International Relations, a large think tank whose research output (of nearly 90 percent) is directly fed for the party-state, suggested that COVID-19 spread is akin to the outbreak of a world war in the sense of the breakdown in order, economic decline, shifting focus towards Asia Pacific and leading to an intense "strategic game" between the US and China.[148]

Yan Xuetong argued that while the international system is prone to several setbacks as well as inter-state conflicts, and despite the "decoupling" with the US, it is likely to strengthen globalisation process. Yan suggested that COVID-19 does not have the capacity, like the World War II, to change the international pattern.[149] Zhang Yuyan suggested that the impact of the COVID-19 on the global pattern is mainly in the globalisation process, with more protectionist trends on the rise.[150] On the other hand, Yang Jiemian termed the current situation as a "qualitative inflection point" [回头看] in the emerging balance of power in the international system with reduction in the US power and enhancement in China's influence in World Bank and the IMF, Climate Change, WHO etc. However, Yang argued that process of change will be slow[151]. Cui Hongjian of China Institute of International Studies is circumspect in that COVID-19 has brought about a kind of stalemate and the future depended on changes in "boosting or watershed" [助推器还是分水岭] elements[152]. Writing in *Global Times* Li Haidong argued that the spread of the epidemic will in global economic crisis, leading to a remodelling of the current international relations. Li suggested that those countries which have high health safety measures and environmental protection mechanisms will become the leader of the new form of globalisation in the post-COVID-19 order. The effective addressing of the epidemic control would also translate into "legitimacy of international behaviour" [国际关系行为正当性], favouring China.[153] For Wang Yiwei, due to the superiority of the Chinese system and its efficient response mechanism, it is not only prepared to construct a "health silk road" but also prepared for positioning in the international system by enhancing its RMB circulation as well as overcoming the US threats to relocate its industries from China.[154]

In China's political system, terms such as "中国责任论", [China responsibility theory], "中国道歉论" [China apology theory] and "中国赔偿论" [China compensation theory] are sensitive issues not only related to the rise of China but also to its interactions with the external world. Equations with the United States, which have been strained of late, but also with that of the other 120 countries at the World Health Assembly meeting which demanded "independent, impartial and comprehensive" investigation into the origins of the COVID-19 could pose serious problems for China in the coming days and months. In order to overcome these problems, China set out to issue the position paper on COVID-19 on June 7, 2020 but is still concerned as possibly for the first time China, which used to argue for a "victimhood" in the aftermath of the Opium Wars in the 19th century, now has much to explain to the international community with COVID-19 destruction in the nooks and corners of the world[155]. Yao Yang, however, argued that in the light of the spread of the COVID-19, China has to rationally respond to various court cases on compensation claims, or debts of developing countries. However, China need not worry about any attempts at "decoupling" of the trade value chain and manufacturing capacity.[156]

Finally, despite the optimism among China's officials and scholars, one of the iconic projects that China had undertaken in the last 7 years and enshrined in the party constitution in 2017, the Belt[157] and Road Initiative, is facing innumerable problems due to overall economic decline, restrictions on labour mobility, reduced flow of capital and travel restrictions on Chinese nationals by more than 130 countries, despite China's outward thrust as seen in the PBSC meeting of February 26, 2020 and June 18 foreign ministerial meeting to express solidarity with BRI countries.

Thus, the stakes for China as a result of COVID-19 are high. Its leadership had undertaken a massive political campaign to paint a picture of being efficient in addressing the issue. However, there are several gaping holes in the official story. Nevertheless, any receding of the COVID-19 in the short to medium term, immunity building on a large scale or vaccine development and other developments could desecuritise the issue in the medium to long term perspective.

NOTES

1 China released a white paper on June 7, 2020 on the subject. See for the official version of China at the State Council Information Office of the People's Republic of China, "Fighting COVID-19: China in Action" *Xinhua* June 7, 2020 at <http://www.xinhuanet.com/english/2020-06/07/c_139120424.htm> The white paper stated that to "fight and win" Covid-19, China has to resort to "resolute battle to prevent and control its spread" by employing "extensive, stringent, and thorough containment measures". China's response was "open, transparent, and responsible manner and in accordance with the law" that resulted in "a decisive victory was secured in the battle to defend Hubei Province and its capital city of Wuhan".

2 See Ole Wæver, 'Securitization and Desecuritization', in Ronnie D. Lipschutz (ed.), *On Security* (New York: Columbia University Press, 1995), pp. 46–86; Barry Buzan, Ole Waever and Jaap de Wilde, *Security: A New Framework for Analysis* (Boulder, CO: Lynne Rienner, 1998), Ken Booth, *Theory of World Security* (Cambridge: Cambridge University Press, 2007) and Thierry Balzack, *Securitization Theory – How Security Problems Emerge and Dissolve* (London: Routledge, 2011)

3 Zhou Zelong elevated the discourse by suggesting that the Communist Party's "socialism with Chinese characteristics" had led to the effective prevention and control of the Covid-19 – indicating, as the party has begun, an ideological showcasing of superiority over the western or other models. Zhou enumerated four reasons – centralised leadership and response, strength, speed and intensity. See "从抗击新冠肺炎疫情看中国特色社会主义制度的显著优势" [Observing the significant advantages of the socialist system with Chinese characteristics from the fight against Covid-19] 理论建设 No. 1 (2020) pp. 5-10

4 Yang Jisheng, a former Xinhua news agency reporter wrote a book on the subject, *Mubei* (Tombstone)

[*Tombstone -The Great Chinese Famine, 1958-1962* (Farrar, Straus and Giroux, 2012) Edited by Edward Friedman, Guo Jian, and Stacy Mosher] in 2008 that estimated the death of over 35 million people. One of the most authoritative works on this period is that of Frank Dikotter, *Mao's Great Famine: The history of China's most devastating catastrophe, 1958-1962* (London: Bloomsbury, 2010).

5 See Huang Yanzhong, "The SARS Epidemic and Its Aftermath In China: A Political Perspective" *National Academy of Sciences* 2004 at <https://www.ncbi.nlm.nih.gov/books/NBK92479/> Huang argued here that "A deeply ingrained authoritarian impulse to maintain secrecy, in conjunction with a performance-based legitimacy and an obsession with development and stability during political succession, contributed to China's initial failure to publicize the outbreak. Meanwhile, an upwardly directed system of accountability, a fragmented bureaucracy, and an oligarchic political structure hampered any effective government response to the outbreak"

6 H7N9 virus emerged in China in 2013 killing over 600 people and millions of poultry across the globe. Since 2019, no reports of the spread of this virus reported.

7 See Qian Gang, *The Great China Earthquake* (Beijing: Foreign Languages Press, 1989). It killed 242,769 people besides injuring 164, 851, measuring 7.8 on the Richter scale on July 28th early morning. Tangshan earthquake coincided with the passing away of the first generation of political leadership including Mao Zedong, Zhou Enlai and Zhu De.

8 The Sichuan Earthquake on May 12, measuring 8 on Richter scale, killed 87,587 people, besides injuring 374,643 and 5 million left homeless. See "Each lesson counts" *China Daily* May 14, 2008 at <https://www.chinadaily.com.cn/opinion/2008-05/14/content_6683437.htm>. Sorace suggests that such natural disasters were followed by stepped up communist party propaganda as the saviour of the people, repression of whistle-blowers and the like. See Christian P. Sorace, *Shaken Authority – China's Communist Party and the 2008 Sichuan Earthquake* (Ithaca: Cornell University Press, 2017) pp. 4-5

9 Wu Zunyou, Ed. *HIV/AIDS in China - Beyond the Numbers* (Singapore: Springer, 2017); Sandra Teresa Hyde, *Eating Spring Rice - The Cultural Politics of AIDS in Southwest China* (Berkeley, LA: University of California Press, 2007) and Gu Jing and Neil Renwick, "China's Fight against HIV/AIDS" *Journal of Contemporary China* 17 (54) (February 2008): 85–106.

10 See Robert Peckham, *Epidemics in Modern Asia* (Cambridge: Cambridge University Press, 2016); Barry Youngerman, Pandemics and Global Health (New York: Infobase Publishing, 2008) and William H. MacNeill, *Plagues and Peoples* (New York: Anchor Books, 1976).

11 See Paul Kupperberg, *The Influenza Pandemic of 1918-1919* (New York: Chelsea House, 2008) p.44

12 Apart from the Athenian Plague of 430 BC, three major pandemics have hit the human civilisation. The first pandemic, the Justinianic Plague between 541 AD to 750 AD devastated West Asia, North Africa and Europe. The second, "Black Death" from 1347 to 1665 killed over 25 million people and the third, originating in Yunnan, spreading to Beihai, Taiwan, Guangdong and Hong Kong, resulted in over 2 million deaths. This is based on Xu Lei, Liu Qiyong, Leif Chr. Stige, Tamara Ben Ari, Fang Xiye, Wang Shuchun, Chan,Kung-Sik, Nils Chr. Stenseth and Zhang Zhibin, "Nonlinear effect of climate on plague during the third pandemic in China" *Proceedings of the National Academy of Sciences of the United States of America*, 108 (25) (June 21, 2011), pp. 10214-10219 at <http://www.pnas.org/cgi/doi/10.1073/pnas. 1019486108> See also Carol Benedict, "Bubonic Plague in Nineteenth-Century China" *Modern China*, 14 (2) April, 1988, pp. 107-155 and "The Plague in China" *Scientific American* 71 (9) September 1, 1894, p. 140 at <https://www.jstor.org/stable/10.2307/26114667> Interestingly, the Black Death was traced to Hubei Province, the current epicentre of Covid-19, with over 5 million casualties then, spreading to Persia through the Silk

Road and Europe. Coincidentally, today, Qom in Iran witnessed massive Covid-19 infections as with several Italian and Spanish cities. For this link see Parag Khanna, "Covid-19 Is Traveling Along the New Silk Road" February 28, 2020 at <https://www.wired.com/story/covid-19-is-traveling-along-the-new-silk-road/> These have implications to China's current Belt and Road Initiative as well.

13 Shi Daonan's poem cited by Tang Jinling, Yan Fei and Li Liming "History and Development of Public Health" chapter 2 at Li Liming and Jiang Qingwu Eds. *Introduction to Public Health in China* (Singapore: Springer, 2019) (cited on p.14). They point to an interesting historical fact of "sick houses". Citing the records of *Biography of Narendra-yaœas* of 557 AD, an Indian monk Narendra-yaœas built a "sick house" for lepers at Xiangquan Temple in Henan. (ibid p. 18)

14 Tamara Ben-Ari, Simon Neerinckx, Lydiane Agier, Bernard Cazelles, Xu Lei, Zhang Zhibin, Fang Xiye, Wang Shuchun, Liu Qiyong and Nils C. Stenseth, "Identification of Chinese plague foci from long-term epidemiological data" *Proceedings of the National Academy of Sciences of the United States of America*, 109 (21) (May 22, 2012), pp. 8196-8201 at <http://www.pnas.org/cgi/doi/10.1073/pnas.1110585109 >

15 William C. Summers, *The Great Manchurian Plague of 1910-1911: The Geopolitics of an Epidemic Disease* (Yale: Yale University Press, 2012) and William H. MacNeill, *Plagues and Peoples* (New York: Anchor Books, 1976) p.138. MacNeill points out to the crucial element of international cooperation in addressing the plague between 1891-1893 in Egypt. (ibid pp.245-246

16 Dr Wu wrote "Plague Fighter: The Autobiography of a Modern Chinese Physician" after his return to Malaysia. See Ma Zhongliang and Li Yanli, "Dr. Wu Lien Teh, plague fighter and father of the Chinese public health system" *Protein Cell* (March 2016) 7(3): 157–158. at <https://www.ncbi.nlm.nih.gov/pmc/articles/PMC4791421/>

17 See Kerrie L. MacPherson, "Invisible borders - Hong Kong, China and the imperatives of public health" in Milton J. Lewis and Kerrie L. MacPherson Eds. *Public Health in Asia and the Pacific - Historical and comparative perspectives* (London: Routledge, 2008) pp. 10-54 (p.26)

18 Christopher Langford, "Did the 1918–19 Influenza Pandemic Originate in China?" *Population and Development Review* 31(3): 473–505 (September 2005) pp. 473-505. Incidentally, Langford also cites evidence from Hankou port (at the current day Wuhan and the epicentre of Covid-19) that deaths occurred due to pneumonia influenza (Ibid pp. 496 and 499). See also Wataru Iijima, "Spanish influenza in China, 1918–20 - A preliminary probe "*in* Howard Phillips and David Killingray Eds. *The Spanish Influenza Pandemic of 1918–19* (London: Routledge, 2003) chapter 7 pp. 101 - 09. More on the subject by Mark Honigsbaum, *Living with Enza - The Forgotten Story of Britain and the Great Flu Pandemic of 1918* (London: Macmillan, 2009) and Alfred W. Crosby, *America's Forgotten Pandemic - The Influenza of 1918* (Cambridge: Cambridge University Press, 2003) p.9

19 MacPherson, 2008 p.31

20 Chris Courtney, *The Nature of Disaster in China: The 1931 Yangzi River Flood* (Cambridge: Cambridge University Press, 201)

21 Li and Jiang argue that what distinguishes China's public health system with others is the focus on social justice and patriotic health campaigns. They define China's public health (by the 2003 definition) as: "public health is to prevent disease and promote health through organized efforts of the whole society in improving environment and sanitation conditions, preventing and controlling of infectious and other diseases, developing good personal hygiene and healthy lifestyles, and providing healthcare services." See Li Liming and Jiang Qingwu Eds. *Introduction to Public Health in China* (Singapore: Springer, 2019) pp.2 and 10

22 See Tang Jinling, Yan Fei and Li Liming in Li and Jiang, Eds. 2019 p. 23

23 Huang Yanzhong argued that in terms of rise in life expectancy, 1949-80 period had shown substantial increase (of 33 years) compared to the reform period later (5 years). See Huang Yanzhong, *Governing Health in Contemporary China* (London: Routledge; 2013) p.1

24 Tu Jiong, *Health Care Transformation in Contemporary China - Moral Experience in a Socialist Neoliberal Polity* (Singapore: Springer, 2019); Md. Nazrul Islam, Ed. *Public Health Challenges in Contemporary China – An Interdisciplinary Perspective* (Heidelberg: Springer, 2016)

25 Tang, Yan and Li outline the achievements in the public health system of China with the following statistics:

"the number of health professionals per 1000 people rose from 0.93 in 1949 to 4.15 in 2009, while the number of beds in healthcare facilities per 1000 people grew from 0.18 in 1950 to 3.8 in 2011. By 2011, there were a total of 37,000 township hospitals in 33,000 townships, 660,000 village clinics in 590,000 administrative villages, 7776 community health centers, and 25,000 community health stations in 7110 communities. There were also 1.53 village health workers per 1000 rural residents." (Tang, Yan and Li in Li and Jiang Eds. 2019 p.28).

26 Chen Kaixian, Lin Qishui and Wu Jiarui, *Science & Technology on Public Health in China: A Roadmap to 2050* (Beijing: Science Press, 2010) pp. 39-40. Further, it stated that China will "establish infectious cDNA clones, reverse genetic system, as well as the rapid, high titerpseudotyped virus packaging system for avian influenza virus, SARS corona virus, Japanese encephalitis virus and West Nile virus" (p.41)

27 See Han Rubo, "The Forgotten Flu - The H2N2 pandemic of 1957 offers striking parallels for today" April 23, 2020 at <https://www.theworldofchinese.com/2020/04/the-forgotten-flu/> and Jeffrey N. Sfakianos, *Avian Flu* (New York: Chelsea House, 2006) p.11

28 See Arthur Kleinman, James L. Watson, Eds. *SARS in China: Prelude to pandemic*? (Stanford, Calif.: Stanford University Press, 2006); John H. Powers and Xiao Xiaosui, *The Social Construction of SARS - Studies of a health communication crisis* (Amsterdam: John Benjamins Publishing Company, 2008) and Grace O.M. Lee and Malcolm Warner, *The Political Economy of the SARS Epidemic- The impact on human resources in East Asia* (London: Routledge, 2008)

29 John Wong and ZhengYongnian argue that, in general, China's political leadership intervention on a crisis depended on the dynamic, the negative costs and other factors. See John Wong and ZhengYongnian Eds. *The SARS Epidemic: Challenges to China's Crisis Management* (New Jersey: World Scientific, 2004) pp.49-50. See also Zhong Nanshan and Zeng Guangqiao, "Management and prevention of SARS in China" in Angela R. McLean et.al eds. *SARS: A Case Study in Emerging Infections* (Oxford: Oxford University Press, 2005) pp. 31-34

30 See Xue Lan and Zeng Guang, *A Comprehensive Evaluation on Emergency Response in China -The Case of Pandemic Influenza (H1N1) 2009* (Singapore: Springer, 2019). Interestingly, these authors argue that "According to the cost–benefit analysis conducted by the evaluation team, from April 25, 2009 through to December 31, 2009, for every one RMB spent on Influenza A (H1N1) prevention and control, there was a yield of about 7.99– 11.55 RMB, suggesting that the country's prevention and control effort was cost-effective." p.xviii

31 Ge Shengqiang, Li Jinming, Fan Xiaoxu, Liu Fuxiao, Li Lin, Wang Qinghua, RenWeijie, Bao Jingyue, Liu Chunju, Wang Hua, Liu Yutian, Zhang Yongqiang, Xu Tiangang, Wu Xiaodong and Wang Zhiliang "Molecular Characterization of African Swine Fever Virus, China, 2018" Emerging Infectious Diseases [www.cdc.gov/eid] Vol. 24, No. 11, (November 2018) at <https://doi.org/10.3201/eid2411.181274>

32 Wang Yali, Wang Xuan, Liu Xiaobo, Ren Ruiqi, Zhou Lei, Li Chao, Tu Wenxiao, Ni Daxin, Li

Qun, Feng Zijian, and Zhang Yanping, "Epidemiology of Imported Infectious Diseases, China, 2005-2016" *Emerging Infectious Diseases.* Jan 2019, Vol. 25 Issue 1, pp.33-41

33 Tara C Smith, *Ebola* (Philadelphia: Chelsea House Publishers, 2006)

34 Sarah Zhang, "A Virus with a Deadly Boring Name" *The Atlantic* January 31, 2020 at <https://www.theatlantic.com/science/archive/2020/01/the-virus-that-still-has-no-name/605893/>

35 Mari Webel, "*Naming the new coronavirus – why taking Wuhan out of the picture matters*" February 19, 2020 at <https://theconversation.com/naming-the-new-coronavirus-why-taking-wuhan-out-of-the-picture-matters-131738>

36 R. Prasad, "How WHO names a new disease" *The Hindu*, February 12, 2020 at <https://www.thehindu.com/sci-tech/health/explainer-how-who-names-a-new-disease/article30801776.ece>

37 See Kai Kupferschmidt, "Discovered a disease? WHO has new rules for avoiding offensive names" *Science* May 11, 2015 at <https://www.sciencemag.org/news/2015/05/discovered-disease-who-has-new-rules-avoiding-offensive-names#>

38 "WHO, "World Health Organization Best Practices for the Naming of New Human Infectious Diseases" May 2015 at <https://apps.who.int/iris/bitstream/handle/10665/163636/WHO_HSE_FOS_15.1_eng.pdf;jsessionid=1A52572D066F031228EE8713301C028E?sequence=1>

39 Ding argued that Hong Kong people do not consider the "Hong Kong Foot" (Athletes Foot disease) as derogatory or discriminatory in nature due to their freedom and openness. See Ding Wang, ""Wuhan Virus" not a Discriminatory Term" *Hong Kong Economic Journal* (March 26, 2020) April 1, 2020 at <https://www.asiaglobalonline.hku.hk/asia-global-voices/wuhan-virus-not-discriminatory-term>

40 See Fang Fang, "Day 4 Wuhan Diary, January 26, 2020" at <https://www.badiucao.com/post/wuhandiary-day4-2020-1-26>

41 John Lee, "Combating China's COVID-19 Propaganda Offensive to Undermine the United States on the Global Stage" *Hudson Institute Policy Brief* March 2020 at < https://www.hudson.org/research/15853-combating-china-s-covid-19-propaganda-offensive-to-undermine-the-united-states-on-the-global-stage>

42 Coronaviridae Study Group of the International Committee on Taxonomy of Viruses, "The species *Severe acute respiratory syndrome-related coronavirus*: classifying 2019-nCoV and naming it SARS-CoV-2" *Nature Microbiology* 5, pp.536–544(March 2, 2020) at <https://www.nature.com/articles/s41564-020-0695-z#citeas>

43 "WHO Director-General's remarks at the media briefing on 2019-nCoV on 11 February 2020" February 11, 2020 at <https://www.who.int/dg/speeches/detail/who-director-general-s-remarks-at-the-media-briefing-on-2019-ncov-on-11-february-2020> See also Mary Hui, "Why won't the WHO call the coronavirus by its name, SARS-CoV-2?" *Quartz* March 18, 2020 at <https://qz.com/1820422/coronavirus-why-wont-who-use-the-name-sars-cov-2/>

44 Victor Corman et.al, "Diagnostic detection of Wuhan coronavirus 2019 by real-time RTPCR" January 13, 2020 at <https://www.who.int/docs/default-source/coronaviruse/wuhan-virus-assay-v1991527e5122341d99287a1b17c111902.pdf?sfvrsn=d381fc88_2>

45 Jane Li, "The US and China are in an increasingly nasty war of words over the coronavirus" *Quartz* March 17, 2020 at <https://qz.com/1819704/us-and-china-in-a-nasty-war-of-words-over-coronavirus/>. President Trump repeated three days later by suggesting efforts to "defeat the Chinese virus". See Anne Gearan, "Trump takes direct aim at China as known U.S. infections double and criticism mounts" *Washington Post* March 19, 2020 at <https://www.washingtonpost.com/politics/trump-takes-direct-aim-at-china-as-known-us-infections-double-and-criticism-mounts/2020/03/19/6df10828-6a06-11ea-abef-020f086a3fab_story.html>

46 Katherine A. Mason, "H1N1 Is Not a Chinese Virus: The Racialization of People and Viruses in

Post-SARS China" *Studies in Comparative International Development* (2015) 50:500–518 at <DOI 10.1007/s12116-015-9198-y>

47 Li Hangwei, "*Mistreatment of Africans in Guangzhou threatens China's coronavirus diplomacy*" *The Conversation* April 17, 2020 at <https://theconversation.com/mistreatment-of-africans-in-guangzhou-threatens-chinas-coronavirus-diplomacy-136348>

48 Felix Tih, "China: 260+ Nigerians evacuated over virus, racism" May 31, 2020 at <https://www.aa.com.tr/en/africa/china-260-nigerians-evacuated-over-virus-racism/1859494 >

49 Most of the estimates of course omit death due to "other reasons" such as suicides due to the unbearable circumstances of lockdown or lack of testing or medicines or by other illnesses. For instance, see the account of Fang Fang, "Wuhan Diary" *Badiucao blog* at <https://www.badiucao.com/blog>

50 According to a study of satellite images of differential in the number of vehicles at Wuhan hospitals and data related to symptoms of cough and diarrhoea, it was suggested that Wuhan hospitals may have been diagnosing such cases well before the outbreak in November. See Kaitlyn Folmer and Josh Margolin, "Satellite data suggests coronavirus may have hit China earlier: Researchers" June 8, 2020 at <https://abcnews.go.com/International/satellite-data-suggests-coronavirus-hit-china-earlier-researchers/story?id=71123270 >. However, on March 26, hundred scholars from China wrote a letter to the American audience in the light of US-China relations deteriorating on the issue. They stated: "At this stage of the pandemic, the exact source and origin of COVID-19 remain undetermined, but these questions are unimportant and finger pointing is demeaning and hurtful to everyone. In the end we will all respect the final determination of scientists". See "An Open Letter to the people of the United States from 100 Chinese Scholars" March 26, 2020 reprinted at *China Daily* April 3, 2010 at <https://www.chinadaily.com.cn/a/202004/03/WS5e86e3cea310128217284457.html>

51 According to Qiu and Xiao, the first case was reported on November 29th. See Qiu Tianyi, and Xiao Han, "Revealing the influence of national public health policies for the outbreak of the SARS-CoV-2 epidemic in Wuhan, China through status dynamic modeling" March 12, 2020 at <https://www.medrxiv.org/content/10.1101/2020.03.10.20032995v1.full.pdf>. See also Zhou Yimin, Chen Zuguo, Wu Xiangdong, Tian Zengwu, Cheng Liang and Ye Lingjian, "The Outbreak Evaluation of COVID-19 in Wuhan District of China" accessed at <https://arxiv.org/pdf/2002.09640.pdf> According to a 15-page research report prepared by western countries, excerpts of which were published in Australia's The Saturday Telegraph, on December 6 human-to-human transmission occurred from a person linked to the Seafood Market. See Sharri Markson, "Coronavirus NSW: Dossier lays out case against China bat virus program" *The Daily Telegraph* May 2, 2020 at <https://www.dailytelegraph.com.au/coronavirus/bombshell-dossier-lays-out-case-against-chinese-bat-virus-program/news-story/55add857058731c9c71c0e96ad17da60> For bioweapon dimensions of the Covid-19 see Brian Owens, "Mystery surrounds ouster of Chinese researchers from Canadian laboratory" July 19, 2020 at <https://www.sciencemag.org/news/2019/07/mystery-surrounds-ouster-chinese-researchers-canadian-laboratory>

52 Jia Lin, Li Kewen, Jiang Yu, Guo Xin and Zhao Ting, "Prediction and analysis of Coronavirus Disease 2019" March 11, 2020 at <https://arxiv.org/ftp/arxiv/papers/2003/2003.05447.pdf> These authors suggest to a pattern of local outbreak stage, community transmission and large-scale transmission in Hubei Province as well as in China and the rest of the world.

53 However, Roach and Shan argued that the first doctor to identify the virus was Zhang Jixian on December 27- i.e. three days before Li's findings. Zhang alerted the Wuhan Health Commission on December 29 about the virus. See Stephen S. Roach and Shan Weijian, "The Fable of the Chinese Whistleblower" *Project Syndicate* May 18, 2020 at <https://www.project-syndicate.org/commentary/trump-charges-against-china-covid19-alternative-facts-by-stephen-s-roach-and-weijian-shan-2020-

05> However, the other evidence suggest that the WHO did not receive the whole genome of the virus, that is crucial to alert the international community in the intensity of the disaster in waiting.

54 Before he himself contracted the virus, Li examined seven patients and alerted to the new virulent virus strain to his medical colleagues. However, the local police reprimanded him and sought false undertaking. Finally, after he passed away China's Supreme Court exonerated him. See Peter J. McDonnell, "Li Wenliang: Ophthalmologist hero" *Ophthalmology Times* February 15, 2020 at <https://www.cnn.com/2020/02/07/asia/china-doctor-deathcensorship-intl-hnk/index.html> and "China exonerates doctor reprimanded for warning of virus" *Associated Press* March 20, 2020 at <https://apnews.com/6f2e666485e9abae4bb112251eca77be>

55 This is based on *The Associated Press* investigative reports on internal debates and documents of the World Health Organisation and other sources at "China delayed releasing coronavirus info, frustrating WHO" *Associated Press* June 3, 2020 at < https://apnews.com/3c061794970661042b18d5aeaaed9fae> This report suggest to internal wrangling and cover-up within China's National Health Commission and other administrative bodies that led to delays in alerting the WHO with required information. This report also identified the genome sequencing done by Zhang Yongzhen of Shanghai Public Clinical Health Center on January 5, Wuhan University team on January 7, the Thailand medical officials' investigation from January 8 of a suspected Covid-19 case from Wuhan and notified the WHO on January 13. Finally, on January 20, renowned scientist Zhong Nanshan publicly declared the human transmission of the virus.

56 President Xi was conspicuous in not mentioning about the Covid-19 during his Spring Festival eve speech on December 31, 2019 at Beijing, giving legitimacy perhaps for lower level cadres at Wuhan to participate in the celebrations. See Chris Buckley and Steven Lee Myers, "Where's Xi? China's Leader Commands Coronavirus Fight from Safe Heights" *The New York Times* February 8, 2020 at <https://www.nytimes.com/2020/02/08/world/asia/xi-coronavirus-china.html> See also Li Xiangyu, Li Mingzi, Peng Danni and Du Wei, "The Regret of Wuhan: How China Missed the Critical Window for Controlling the Coronavirus Outbreak" *China News Weekly* February 10, 2020 at <https://chinachange.org/2020/02/09/the-regret-of-wuhan-how-china-missed-the-critical-window-for-controlling-the-coronavirus-outbreak/> and Yu Xinyan, "My Hometown is being ravaged by the Coronavirus" *The Atlantic* February 5, 2020 accessed at <https://www.theatlantic.com/ideas/archive/2020/02/watching-coronavirus-take-over-wuhan-my-hometown/606106/ >

57 Wong and Zheng op.cit., p. 49

58 Robyn Ralph, Jocelyne Lew, Tiansheng Zeng, Magie Francis, Bei Xue, Melissa Roux, Ali Toloue Ostadgavahi, Salvatore Rubino, Nicholas J Dawe, Mohammed N Al-Ahdal, David J Kelvin, Christopher D Richardson, Jason Kindrachuk, Darryl Falzarano and Alyson A Kelvin, "2019-nCoV (Wuhan virus), a novel Coronavirus: human-to-human transmission, travel-related cases, and vaccine readiness" *The Journal of Infection in Developing Countries* 14(1) (2020) pp.3-17 at <doi:10.3855/jidc.12425>

59 Wang Hairong, "An All-out War" *Beijing Review* February 13, 2020 at <http://www.bjreview.com>

60 Robyn Ralph et.al, 2020 *op.cit.*, p.4 This report also suggest that 14 hospital doctors and workers were also infected with the virus. Rui Zhang and others argued that Wuhan authorities have artificially created hospital outpatient cross-infection and additional close contacts, thus spreading the virus further. See Rui Zhang, Li Miaowen, and Zhao Kexin, "Impact of Wuhan's Epidemic Prevention Policy on the Outbreak of COVID-19 in Wuhan, China" February 29, 2020 at <http://dx.doi.org/10.2139/ssrn.3548759 >

61 Huanan Seafood Market is the largest wholesale wild animal and sea food market in Central China

with over 50 square km of retail area and over 1000 tenants. Soon after cases were detected, China's authorities cleaned up the place, thus destroying all evidence about Covid-19.

62 "武汉市卫生健康委关于不明原因的病毒性肺炎情况通报" [Wuhan Municipal Health Commission on Unexplained Viral Pneumonia] January 2020 at <http://www.nhc.gov.cn/xcs/yqtb/202001/1beb46f061704372b7ca41ef3e682229.shtml>

63 Wen Qing, "Concerted Efforts" *Beijing Review* February 13, 2020 at < http://www.bjreview.com> According to another report, China informed the WHO on January 5 of 59 cases of pneumonia that occurred in Wuhan between December 12-19, 2019. See Stan Deresinski, "Pneumonia Outbreak in China" January 17, 2020 at < www.reliasmedia.com/articles/145676-pneumonia-outbreak-in-china>

64 "武汉市卫生健康委员会关于新型冠状病毒感染的肺炎情况通报" [Wuhan Municipal Health Commission on Pneumonia Infected by New Coronavirus] January 14, 2020 at <http://www.nhc.gov.cn/xcs/yqtb/202001/1ca9c31eb92e4310b028243598e544b9.shtml>

65 "武汉市卫生健康委员会关于新型冠状病毒感染的肺炎情况通报" [Wuhan Municipal Health Commission on Pneumonia Infected by New Coronavirus] January 16, 2020 at <http://www.nhc.gov.cn/xcs/yqtb/202001/2f222cfb607e4952a705ac34c420c057.shtml>

66 "武汉市卫生健康委员会关于新型冠状病毒感染的肺炎情况通报" [Wuhan Municipal Health Commission on Pneumonia Infected by New Coronavirus] January 20, 2020 at <http://www.nhc.gov.cn/xcs/yqtb/202001/a5f1aec0660f4cd3a70518b6258fd15f.shtml>At the provincial level the local Wuhan government did not postpone the conduct and celebrations for the "two sessions" (Provincial People's Congress and the advisory body meetings) and in fact went ahead with the public feasting of over 40,000 people on the Spring Festival eve thus aggravating the human-to-human transmission of the virus to spread further. Wuhan Mayor Zhao Xianwang justified by stating that the health commission's notices so far did not indicate to any looming danger. Moreover, another Spring Festival gala celebration were held on January 21 with the participation provincial party chief Jiang Chaoliang and governor Wang Xiaodong.

67 WHO, "Situation Report-1" January 21, 2020 at <https://www.who.int/docs/default-source/coronaviruse/situation-reports/20200121-sitrep-1-2019-ncov.pdf?sfvrsn=20a99c10_4> The WHO stated that its office in Beijing was informed of the new virus on December 31, 2019. On January 10 and 11, the China National Health Commission informed the WHO that Wuhan's Huanan Seafood Market is associated with the outbreak of this virus.

68 The inconsistency in the official version of human-to-human transmission is evident also in the following admission. According to Zhang Yuntao, President of China National Biotech Group Company, which is testing one of the three Covid-19 vaccines in China, "Before we received the approval for the vaccine to be on clinical trial on April 12, we worked hard day and night for 98 days. Our work has gone through several stages". According to this admission of 98 days, the work for developing the vaccine began on January 5, 2020. However, China's official discourse acknowledging that the human-to-human transmission began was on January 20th. See "中国首个新冠灭活疫苗：受试者最多打 3 针，量产后年产能 1 亿剂以上" [China's first Novel Coronavirus inactivated vaccine: subjects will receive up to 3 injections, and the annual production capacity will exceed 100 million doses after mass production] April 2020 accessed at <https://new.qq.com/omn/20200415/20200415A0T6E900.html>

69 "1 月 21 日新型冠状病毒感染的肺炎疫情情况" [Epidemic situation of pneumonia infected with new coronavirus on January 21] January 21, 2020 at <http://www.nhc.gov.cn/xcs/yqtb/202001/930c021cdd1f46dc832fc27e0cc465c8.shtml>

70 "1 月 23 日新型冠状病毒感染的肺炎疫情情况" [Epidemic situation of pneumonia infected with new

coronavirus on January 23] January 23, 2020 at <http://www.nhc.gov.cn/xcs/yqtb/202001/5d19a4f6d3154b9fae328918ed2e3c8a.shtml>

71 Lawrence Gostin of Georgetown University Law Center, termed China's measures of complete lockdown as "astounding, unprecedented, and medieval". China's imposing surveillance system imposed innumerable restrictions on the people. See Jon Cohen and Kai Kupferschmidt, "The coronavirus seems unstoppable. What should the world do now?" *Science* February 25, 2020 at <https://www.sciencemag.org/news/2020/02/coronavirus-seems-unstoppable-what-should-world-do-now>

72 "Sustaining containment of COVID-19 in China" *The Lancet Editorial* April 8, 2020 at <https://www.thelancet.com/pdfs/journals/lancet/PIIS0140-6736(20)30864-3.pdf> However, on May 10th, five new cases were reported in Wuhan, suggesting to a 2nd wave of outbreak of Covid-19. See Christian Shepherd et.al, "Wuhan reports first new coronavirus cases since end of lockdown" *Financial Times* May 11, 2020 at <https://www.ft.com/content/fbb9a1bb-9656-4023-aa97-01ff1dae4403> Later since June 12, 79 cases were reported in Beijing in the 2nd wave. South Korea, despite its intensive testing and isolation procedures, also reported a 2nd wave – suggesting that "herd immunity" has not yet been arrived at.

73 This is based on Maged N. Kamel Boulos and Estella M. Geraghty, "Geographical tracking and mapping of coronavirus disease COVID 19/severe acute respiratory syndrome coronavirus 2 (SARS CoV 2) epidemic and associated events around the world: how 21st century GIS technologies are supporting the global fight against outbreaks and epidemics" *International Journal of Health Geographics* (2020) 19:8 at <https://doi.org/10.1186/s12942-020-00202-8>

74 Chen J. (2020). "Pathogenicity and Transmissibility of 2019-nCoV—A Quick Overview and Comparison with Other Emerging Viruses". *Microbes and Infection*, <https://doi.org/10.1016/j.micinf.2020.01.004>

75 Ye Jiachen, Hu Qitong, Ji Peng, and Marc Barthelemy, "The effect of interurban movements on the spatial distribution of population in China" March 16, 2020 at < https://arxiv.org/pdf/2003.07276.pdf>

76 Wang Hairong, "An All-out War" *Beijing Review* February 13, 2020 at <http://www.bjreview.com>

77 Hu Zixin et.al. "Artificial Intelligence Forecasting of Covid-19 in China" March 1, 2020 accessed at <https://arxiv.org/ftp/arxiv/papers/2002/2002.07112.pdf>

78 However, it also states that the county/local unit where the disaster took place, is made the immediate responsible unit to tackle such crisis. See "Emergency Response Law of the People's Republic of China" November 1, 2007 at <http://english.mee.gov.cn/Resources/laws/envir_elatedlaws/201705/t20170514_414040.shtml> Article 3 of this law states that "emergencies include natural disasters, calamitous accidents, public health accidents and public security incidents, which occur abruptly and cause or may potentially cause serious social harm and for which measures for handling emergencies need to be adopted". On why the local units in Wuhan did not alert the next administrative level in November 2019 to January 2020 period when the virus spread is not clear. This is despite Li Wenliang's alert about the new and virulent pathogen and his reprimand by the local authorities.

79 See "CPC leadership meets to discuss novel coronavirus prevention, control" *International Department of the CC of CPC* at <http://www.idcpc.org.cn/english/events/202001/t20200127_137500.html >

80 During the visit, Li stated that "we must fight resolutely to win the battle against the epidemic". See "Chinese premier in Wuhan, demands all-out efforts in epidemic prevention, control" *Xinhua* January 27, 2020 at <http://www.xinhuanet.com/english/2020-01/27/c_138737735.htm> Premier Li also ordered replenishment of doctors and nurses from other provinces and nearly 42,000 personnel

were rushed to Wuhan later. See "Premier Li visits medical staff in Wuhan" January 28, 2020 at <http://english.www.gov.cn/premier/news/202001/28/content_WS5e2f871ec6d019625c60408e.html> and "So Long, Farewell" *Beijing Review* March 26, 2020 at < http://www.bjreview.com >

81 Sun served in Fujian and Tianjin as party secretary. She reshuffled the health organisations in China by establishing National Health Commission in March 27, 2018 which is to cover "comprehensive, lifecycle" issues of health in China.

82 "Xi Jinping meets with visiting World Health Organization (WHO) Director-General Tedros Adhanom Ghebreyesus" January 29, 2020 at <https://www.fmprc.gov.cn/mfa_eng/zxxx_662805/t1737014.shtml >

83 "Unremitting efforts" *Beijing Review* March 5, 2020 at <http://www.bjreview.com>

84 "Xi chairs leadership meeting on epidemic control, noting "positive changes"" *Xinhua* February 12, 2020 at <http://www.xinhuanet.com/english/2020-02/12/c_138778351.htm>

85 "General Secretary Xi Jinping Chairs Politburo Standing Committee Meeting to Assess Epidemic Situation and Work out Priorities for Epidemic Control" February 27 2020 at <https://www.fmprc.gov.cn/mfa_eng/topics_665678/kjgzbdfyyq/t1750018.shtml>

86 "Xi Jinping: Speech at a Meeting to Plan for Coordinated Efforts to Curb the COVID-19 Outbreak and Promote Economic and Social Development" March 16, 2020 at <http://en.theorychina.org/top_2475/202003/t20200316_368508.shtml>

87 WHO. Coronavirus. February 5, 2020 at <https://www.Who.Int/news-room/detail/30-01-2020-statement-on-thesecond-meeting-of-the-international-health-regulations-(2005)-emergency-committee-regarding-theoutbreak-of-novel-coronavirus-(2019-ncov)>

88 See Wang Yi's interview at "One World One Fight" Interview with Alessandra Galloni of *Reuters* at Berlin on February 14, 2020 reprinted at *Beijing Review* February 27, 2020 at <http://www.bjreview.com>

89 Nishiura analysed 199 symptomatic cases out of 3711 persons onboard the Diamond Princess and found that movement restrictions from February 5 resulted in the reduction in infections. The first identified passenger with infection was on January 19 when he began coughing but was disembarked at Hong Kong on January 25. See Hiroshi Nishiura, "Backcalculating the Incidence of Infection with COVID-19 on the Diamond Princess" *Journal of Clinical Medicine 2020, 9*(3), 657 https://doi.org/10.3390/jcm9030657 at <https://www.mdpi.com/2077-0383/9/3/657>

90 RossellaPorcheddu, Caterina Serra, David Kelvin, Nikki Kelvin, Salvatore Rubino, "Similarity in Case Fatality Rates (CFR) of COVID-19/SARS-COV-2 in Italy and China" February 29, 2020 *The Journal of Infection in Developing Countries* (2020) 14(2) pp125-128. doi:10.3855/jidc.12600

91 Diego Giuliani, Maria Michela Dickson, Giuseppe Espa, and Flavio Santi, "Modelling and predicting the spatio-temporal spread of Coronavirus disease 2019 (COVID-19) in Italy" March 23, 2020 at <https://arxiv.org/pdf/2003.06664>

92 Yi-Cheng Chen, Ping-En Lu, and Cheng-Shang Chang, "A Time-dependent SIR model for COVID-19 with Undetectable Infected Persons" at <http://gibbs1.ee.nthu.edu.tw/A_TIME_DEPENDENT_SIR_MODEL_FOR_COVID_19.PDF>

93 See Reuters report at "China's Hubei sees surge in COVID-19 deaths with switch to CT scan diagnoses" *The Japan Times* February 13, 2020 at < https://www.japantimes.co.jp/news/2020/02/13/asia-pacific/science-health-asia-pacific/chinas-hubei-province-sees-surge-coronavirus-deaths-switch-new-methodology/#.Xruy9uR7nIW>

94 Amy Qin, "China Raises Coronavirus Death Toll by 50% in Wuhan" *New York Times* April 17, 2020 at <https://www.nytimes.com/2020/04/17/world/asia/china-wuhan-coronavirus-death-toll.html>

95 Isaac Stone Fish and Maria Krol Sinclair, "Leaked Chinese Virus Database Covers 230 Cities, 640,000 Updates" *Foreign Policy* May 12, 2020 at <https://foreignpolicy.com/2020/05/12/leaked-chinese-coronavirus-database-number-cases/> However, they did not provide an alternative list of numbers.

96 Derek Scissors, "Estimating the true number of China's COVID-19 cases" *American Enterprise Institute* April 7, 2020 at <https://www.aei.org/research-products/report/estimating-the-true-number-of-chinas-covid-19-cases/>

97 Christopher A. Mouton, Russell Hanson, Adam R. Grissom and John P. Godges, "COVID-19 Air Traffic Visualization- COVID-19 Cases in China Were Likely 37 Times Higher Than Reported in January 2020" RAND Corporation, 2020 at <https://www.rand.org/pubs/research_reports/RRA248-3.html> They estimate one million travelers from China to Japan and Thailand each, about 750,000 to South Korea, 500,000 to the United States, and 400,000 to Taiwan, in addition to others who have already went to these and other countries from December to January 22nd.

98 For a review of these case studies, see Jomar F. Rabajante, "Insights from early mathematical models of 2019-nCoV acute respiratory disease (COVID- 19) dynamics" (February 2020) accessed at <https://www.researchgate.net/publication/339252235_Insights_from_early_mathematical_models_of_2019-nCoV_acute_respiratory_disease_COVID-19_dynamics>

99 Liu Zhihua, Pierre Magal, Ousmane Seydi and Glenn F. Webb, "Predicting the cumulative number of cases for the COVID-19 epidemic in China from early data" February 28, 2020 at <https://www.medrxiv.org/content/10.1101/2020.03.11.20034314v1.full.pdf> p.9

100 Lauren Gardner, 2020. "Modeling the Spreading Risk of 2019-nCoV" *Center for Systems Science and Engineering, Johns Hopkins University* January 31, 2020 accessed at <https://systems.jhu.edu/research/public-health/ncov-model-2>

101 Derek Scissors, "Estimating the true number of China's COVID-19 cases" *American Enterprise Institute* April 7, 2020 at <https://www.aei.org/research-products/report/estimating-the-true-number-of-chinas-covid-19-cases/>

102 As cited by Jomar F. Rabajante. Another study by Reed and others suggested to the number of infected patients at 190,000 in Wuhan by February 4, while Ming and other scholars estimated such cases to be about 88,075 by January 31.

103 WHO, "Report of the WHO-China Joint Mission on Coronavirus Disease 2019 (COVID-19)" February 16-24, 2020 at <https://www.who.int/docs/default-source/coronaviruse/who-china-joint-mission-on-covid-19-final-report.pdf>

104 See George M. Bwire and Linda S. Paulo, "Coronavirus disease-2019: is fever an adequate screening for the returning travelers?" *Tropical Medicine and Health* (2020) 48:14 at <https://doi.org/10.1186/s41182-020-00201-2>

105 For a general introduction to the subject see Marc Souris, *Epidemiology and Geography – Principles, Methods and Tools of Spatial Analysis* (London: Wiley, 2019)

106 Francesco Casella, "Can the COVID-19 epidemic be managed on the basis of daily data?" March 17, 2020 at < https://arxiv.org/abs/2003.06967>

107 It was stated that the spread of the viruses was effectively studied through such methods. Successful studies of measles in Cornwall, 1969-1970, cholera in London in 1849 and tuberculosis and bronchitis in Wales, 1959-1963 were cited. See Diego Giuliani, Maria Michela Dickson, Giuseppe Espa, and Flavio Santi, "Modelling and predicting the spatio-temporal spread of Coronavirus disease 2019 (COVID-19) in Italy" March 23, 2020 at <https://arxiv.org/pdf/2003.06664>

108 Tian Liang, Li Xuefei, Qi Fei, Tang Qian-Yuan, Tang Viola, Liu Jiang, Cheng Xingye, Li Xuanxuan, Shi Yingchen Liu Haiguang and Tang Lei-Han, "Pre-symptomatic Transmission in the Evolution of the COVID-19 Pandemic" April 2, 2020 at <https://arxiv.org/vc/arxiv/papers/2003/2003.07353v1.pdf>

109 Du Zhanwei, Wang Lin, Simon Cauchemez, Xu Xiaoke, Wang Xianwen, Benjamin J. Cowling and Lauren Ancel Meyers, "Risk for Transportation of Coronavirus Disease from Wuhan to Other Cities in China" *Emerging Infectious Diseases* [www.cdc.gov/eid] Vol. 26, No. 5, May 2020 at <https://doi.org/10.3201/eid2605.200146>

110 Bnaya Gross, Zheng Zhiguo, Liu Shiyan, Chen Xiaoqi, Alon Sela, Li Jianxin, Li Daqing and Shlomo Havlin, "Spatio-temporal propagation of COVID-19 epidemics" April 5, 2020 at <https://arxiv.org/pdf/2003.08382v1.pdf>

111 Li Xingguang, Zai Junjie, Zhao Qiang, Nie Qing, Li Yi, Brian T. Foley and Antoine Chaillon, "Evolutionary history, potential intermediate animal host, and cross species analyses of SARS CoV 2" *Journal of Medical Virology* February 2020 at <https://onlinelibrary.wiley.com/doi/pdf/10.1002/jmv.25731?casa_token=nlPJyUTxLcsAAAAA:h04K3tkBPsz8pHoYiyaMmoimXdxgi02QT70NlCcjyPg1fDuPdhlMhtOIet0cV_Glyciozv_-9GczNAU>

112 SEIR is defined as:

- *Susceptible population* (S-type), referring to those who have no disease but lack of immune ability and are easy to be infected after contact with the infected ones;
- *Exposed* (E-type), referring to the people who have been exposed to the infection but with no obvious symptom in incubation period;
- *Infective* (I-type), referring to the infected people who can transmit virus to the members of S-type and turning them to the E-type or I-type members;
- *Recovered* (R-type), referring the people who are isolated or have immunity from the disease and they can be changed to S-type again if the immune period is limited.

See Zhou Yimin et.al., "The Outbreak Evaluation of COVID-19 in Wuhan District of China" accessed at <https://arxiv.org/pdf/2002.09640.pdf>

113 PengLiangrong Yang Wuyue, Zhang Dongyan, Zhuge Changjing, Liu Hong and Zhou Pei-Yuan, "Epidemic analysis of COVID-19 in China by dynamical modeling" February 18, 2020 p.4 at <https://doi.org/10.1101/2020.02.16.20023465 >

114 Chen Baoquan, Shi Mingyi, Ni Xingyu, Ruan Liangwang, Jiang Hongda, Yao Heyuan, Wang Mengdi, Song Zhenghua, Zhou Qiang and Ge Tong, "Visual Data Analysis and Simulation Prediction for COVID-19" March 2, 2020 accessed at <https://arxiv.org/ftp/arxiv/papers/2002/2002.07096.pdf>

115 Zhou Yimin et.al., "The Outbreak Evaluation of COVID-19 in Wuhan District of China" accessed at <https://arxiv.org/pdf/2002.09640.pdf>

116 Hu Zixin, Ge Qiyang, Li Shudi, Jin Li and Xiong Momiao, "Artificial Intelligence Forecasting of Covid-19 in China" March 1, 2020 accessed at < https://arxiv.org/ftp/arxiv/papers/2002/2002.07112.pdf>

117 Gao Qijun, Hu Yingfu, Dai Zhiguo, Xiao Feng, Wang Jing and Wu Jing, "The epidemiological characteristics of 2019 novel coronavirus diseases (COVID-19) in Jingmen, China" *The Lancet* March 6, 2020 at <https://papers.ssrn.com>

118 Wang Guyi, Wu Chenfang, Zhang Quan, Wu Fang, Yu Bo, Lv Jianlei, Li Yiming, Li Tiao, Wu Chao, Wu Guobao, Zhong Yanjun, "Epidemiological and Clinical Features of Corona Virus Disease 2019 (COVID-19) in Changsha, China" *The Lancet Infectious Diseases* March 10, 2020 at <https://papers.ssrn.com>

119 On the economic situation see, Ning Jizhe, "The Value of China's Economic Growth in the First Half of 2019" *Qiushi* November 14, 2019 at <http://english.qstheory.cn/2019-11/14/c_1125227698.htm> Research group of China's Minsheng Bank, "新冠肺炎疫情对我国经济金融的影响分析及政策建议" [Analysis on the impact of novel coronavirus epidemic on China's economic and financial situation and policy suggestions] 华北金融 [North China Finance] 2 (517) (2020) pp. 1-9; Zhang

Hongyu et.al, " "张红宇等：高度重视新冠疫情对农业农村经济的影响 - 妥善应对精准施策千方百计保供增收" [Attach great importance to the impact of novel Coronavirus epidemic on the agricultural and rural economy-Respond appropriately, implement precise policies, do everything possible to ensure supply and increase revenue] February 18, 2020 at <http://www.aisixiang.com/data/120244.html>; Tu Guangshao et.al. "新冠疫情的全球蔓延对中国经济影响分析" [Analysis of the impact of the global spread of novel Coronavirus epidemic on China's economy] March 15, 2020 at <http://www.aisixiang.com/data/120444.html>; Huang Qifan, "新冠疫情蔓延下全球产业链重构的三点思考" [Three thoughts on the reconstruction of the global industrial chain under the spread of novel Coronavirus epidemic] April 2, 2020 at <http://www.aisixiang.com/data/120703.html>; He Xuefeng, "从新冠疫情认识中国农民退路的重要性" [Understanding the importance of China's peasants retreat from 'novel Coronavirus epidemic] April 23, 2020 at <http://www.aisixiang.com/data/120978.html> Lin Yifu, "新冠疫情对全球经济的冲击及中国的应对" [The impact of novel Coronavirus epidemic on the global economy and China's response] May 6, 2020 at <http://www.aisixiang.com/data/121176.html>

120 See the statement on February 11 of National Development Reform Council Secretary General Cong Liang in this regard at Zhang Shasha, "Opportunity in Adversity" *Beijing Review* February 20, 2020 at <http://www.bjreview.com>

121 Lo Kinling, "China says over 90 per cent of state firms back in business after manufacturing index hits all-time low" *South China Morning Post* March 1, 2020 at <https://www.scmp.com/economy/china-economy/article/3053073/coronavirus-china-says-90-cent-state-firms-back-business>

122 The Caixin General Manufacturing Purchasing Managers Index (PMI) slumped to the worst 40.3 points in February when Wuhan and the neighbouring Hubei Province were locked down to contain the Covid-19 outbreak. While the PMI rebounded to 50.1 points in March, it again slipped to 49.4 points in April suggesting that as the domestic and global demand is weak, China's growth rates are likely to slip drastically in the coming months. In the first quarter of this year, China's economy fell by 6.8 percent. It is estimated by the International Monetary Fund that if all things go well, China may scrape through with 1.2 percent in growth for the whole of 2020. See "China's April factory activity unexpectedly dips as export orders collapse - Caixin PMI" *Reuters* April 30, 2020 at < https://www.reuters.com/article/china-economy-pmi-factory-caixin/chinas-april-factory-activity-unexpectedly-dips-as-export-orders-collapse-caixin-pmi-idUSZUN000A1Q>. See also Claudiu Tiberiu Albulescu, "Coronavirus and financial volatility: 40 days of fasting and fear" March 8, 2020 at <https://hal.archives-ouvertes.fr/hal-02501814/document>

123 Celebrated writer Fang Fang notes in her Wuhan Diary on the 35th day (i.e. February 26, 2020) that the popular search engine Baidu noted to the search frequencies of people in Wuhan as follows: "Bread: search peak up 260% above normal. Mustard: search peak 343% higher. Steamed roll (*mantou*): search peak 376% higher. Grocery shopping: search peak up 382%. Chest tightness: search peak 491% above average Fever: search peak increased 422% from average. Pneumonia symptoms search peak up 1093%. Fear: search peak up 183% from average. Funeral home: search peak up 212%." See "Day35 Wuhan Diary" at <https://www.badiucao.com/post/day35-wuhan-diary>

124 Zhou Yimin et.al., "The Outbreak Evaluation of COVID-19 in Wuhan District of China" accessed at <https://arxiv.org/pdf/2002.09640.pdf>

125 See Zhou Yimin et.al., "The Outbreak Evaluation of COVID-19 in Wuhan District of China" accessed at <https://arxiv.org/pdf/2002.09640.pdf>

126 See Xu Kaijin et.al., "Management of corona virus disease-19 (COVID-19): the Zhejiang Experience" 浙江大学学报（医学版）[*Journal of Zhejiang University (Medical Sciences)*] February 22, 2020 at <http://kns.cnki.net/kcms/detail/33.1248.R.20200222.1417.002.html>

127 Several have argued that Covid-19 is not natural but human-made or even a bio-weapon programme based on circumstantial and other sources. Some have traced the Wuhan Institute of Virology scientists like Shi Zhengli's collaborative efforts with the US, Australia and others led to the new experiments in changing the genome in the laboratory. However, China has been either silent or has denied such reports. There was also an effort to destroy evidence such as the clean-up of the Huanan Seafood Market or restrictions on scientists' publications. See Sharri Markson, "Coronavirus NSW: Dossier lays out case against China bat virus program" *The Daily Telegraph* May 2, 2020 at <https://www.dailytelegraph.com.au/coronavirus/bombshell-dossier-lays-out-case-against-chinese-bat-virus-program/news-story/55add857058731c9c71c0e96ad17da60> ; David Nikel, "Norway Scientist Claims Report Proves Coronavirus Was Lab-Made" *Forbes* June 7, 2020 at <https://www.forbes.com/sites/davidnikel/2020/06/07/norway-scientist-claims-report-proves-coronavirus-was-lab-made/#674ebf9e121d>Ricardo Barrios, "Virulent Rhetoric: Chinese State Claims of US Biological Warfare from the Korean War to COVID-19" April 1, 2020 at <https://www.ccpwatch.org/single-post/2020/04/01/Virulent-Rhetoric-Chinese-State-Claims-of-US-Biological-Warfare-from-the-Korean-War-to-COVID-19>and "China clamping down on coronavirus research, deleted pages suggest" *The Guardian* April 11, 2020 at <https://www.theguardian.com/world/2020/apr/11/china-clamping-down-on-coronavirus-research-deleted-pages-suggest>

128 "Stability Control: The CCP Uses the Police' Big Data System to Identify Infection Suspects" *China Scope* June 2, 2020 at <http://chinascope.org/archives/23485?doing_wp_cron=1591272277.8469920158386230468750>

129 Apart from the considerable discomfort to the majority of the population, distress among migrants, hospital facilities, medicine or equipment, as Fang Fang Diary outlined, there are also scandals that hit Wuhan. For instance, it was reported that the Hubei Province branch of the Red Cross came under criticism for not reaching out to the Covid-19 victims but transferring the donations worth $387 million to the Wuhan city government Gao Rui, "State-backed charity in Wuhan under fire over coronavirus donations" *South China Morning Post* February 14, 2020 at <https://www.scmp.com/news/china/society/article/3050545/state-backed-charity-wuhan-under-fire-over-coronavirus-donations>

130 Zheng Guichu, "Meeting Governance Challenges" *Beijing Review* March 5, 2020 at <http://www.bjreview.com>

131 Zhang Weiwei, "A fitting Response" *Beijing Review* March 19, 2020 p.17 at <http://www.bjreview.com>

132 Cai Fang, "Containing the virus and restarting the Chinese economy" *East Asia Forum* April 12, 2020 at <https://www.eastasiaforum.org/2020/04/12/containing-the-virus-and-restarting-the-chinese-economy/>

133 Francesco Casella, "Can the COVID-19 epidemic be managed on the basis of daily data?" March 17, 2020 at < https://arxiv.org/abs/2003.06967>

134 James Hsu a former professor of physics at National Cheng Kung University argued that China should take responsibility for the outbreak of the virus, "The evil nature of an oppressive CCP government has caused this epidemic to spread quickly and afar. Due to the lack of transparency and the unreliable statistics from the Chinese government, the sudden onset of COVID-19 in many countries has caught governments off guard. Now the damage has been done and many countries are still struggling to flatten the curve, so as not to overburden their healthcare systems". See James Hsu, "CCP, Xi must be held responsible" *Taipei Times* April 23, 2020 at <https://www.taipeitimes.com/News/editorials/archives/2020/04/23/2003735123>

135 International relations expert Yan Xuetong makes an interesting observation here that in the

international system of sovereign norms, only sovereign state can be considered as epidemic prevention unit and that differential nationally determined epidemic prevention policies will inevitably lead to conflict. See Yu Xiaoqing, "疫情会永久性改变世界秩序吗?" [Will the epidemic permanently change the world order?] 澎湃新闻 April 29, 2020 at <https://www.thepaper.cn/newsDetail_forward_7194686>

136 J Benjamin Hurlbut, "A science that knows no country: Pandemic preparedness, global risk, sovereign science" *Big Data & Society* (July–December 2017) pp.1–14 at <https://journals.sagepub.com/doi/pdf/10.1177/2053951717742417> Here the focus is on scientific access/denial to H5N1 flu virus and genomic data.

137 President Xi, during his phone call to German Chancellor, on March 25 stated for instance that "Viruses know no borders and are a common challenge faced by humanity". Foreign ministry spokesman Zhao Lijian said China's efforts "will stand the test of the time." Huang Jin from China University of Political Science and Law in Beijing said: "Blaming China and holding the country accountable for the outbreak has no legal support, because the current international laws provide no basis for holding a state responsible for a pandemic". Other legal experts in China observed that China had fulfilled international obligations. See Cao Yin, "Experts say it's groundless to hold China accountable for COVID-19" *China Daily* June 4, 2020 at <http://www.chinadaily.com.cn/a/202006/04/WS5ed832f8a310a8b24115ab5a.html>

138 Christopher Caldwell, "Sovereignty rules – The virus don't- respect -borders slogan is dead wrong" *Spectator* April 14, 2020 at < https://spectator.us/sovereignty-rules/>

139 See Robert B. Zoellick, "Whither China: From Membership to Responsibility?" September 21, 2005 at <https://2001-2009.state.gov/s/d/former/zoellick/rem/53682.htm> and Jia Qingguo, "China's diplomatic response to COVID-19" *East Asian Forum* May 17, 2020 at <https://www.eastasiaforum.org/2020/05/17/chinas-diplomatic-response-to-covid-19/> Jia here argued that China had provided aid to the Covid-19 affected countries.

140 "General Secretary Xi Jinping Chairs Politburo Standing Committee Meeting to Assess Epidemic Situation and Work out Priorities for Epidemic Control" February 27 2020 at <https://www.fmprc.gov.cn/mfa_eng/topics_665678/kjgzbdfyyq/t1750018.shtml>

141 See "Xi Jinpingÿ Fighting COVID-19 Through Solidarity and Cooperation Building a Global Community of Health for All" May 19, 2020 at <http://en.theorychina.org/top_2475/202005/t20200519_368638.shtml>. For the argument that China is a "responsible country" in HIV-AIDS cooperation see Chan Lai-Ha, *China Engages Global Health Governance - Responsible Stakeholder or System-Transformer?* (New York: Palgrave Macmillan, 2011)

142 In addition, several public diplomacy efforts were made by China and its agencies across the world to convey its position. See Zhang Hui, "全球公共卫生治理中的公共外交浅析-基于中国新型冠状病毒肺炎疫情防控案例" [Public Diplomacy in Global Public Health Governance – With China's Prevention and Control of the COVID-19 as the Case] 公共外交季刊 [R No 1 (2020) pp. 40-45

143 "The Coronavirus Pandemic Will Forever Alter the World Order" *Wall Street Journal* April 3, 2020 at <https://www.wsj.com/articles/the-coronavirus-pandemic-will-forever-alter-the-world-order-11585953005> See also Kurt Campbell and Rush Doshi, "The Coronavirus Could Reshape Global Order - China Is Maneuvering for International Leadership as the United States Falters" *Foreign Affairs* March 18, 2020 at <https://www.foreignaffairs.com/articles/china/2020-03-18/coronavirus-could-reshape-global-order> and Thomas L. Friedman, "Our New Historical Divide: B.C. and A.C. – the World Before Corona and the World After" *New York Times* May 17, 2020 at <https://www.nytimes.com/2020/03/17/opinion/coronavirus-trends.html>

144 Zhang Yuyuan argued that the previous "one superpower, many major powers" [一超多强格局] has undergone transformation. One of the effects of globalisation is the large scale of trade that flourished

but also China became its main beneficiary. With nationalism and protectionist trends in the US, Covid-19 adds to the uncertainty in this trade supply chains. Zhang argued that the existing multilateral institutions would be transformed. See Zhang Yuyuan, "新冠疫情与国际关系" [Novel Coronavirus epidemic situation and global pattern] 世界经济与政治 April 2020 at < http://www.doc88.com/p-14459450304223.html>

145 Yoichi Funabashi, "Time to build the post-pandemic world order" *The Japan Times* June 9, 2020 at <https://www.japantimes.co.jp/opinion/2020/06/09/commentary/world-commentary/time-build-post-pandemic-world-order/#.XuHD8OR7nIV>

146 See Zhang Guihong, "新冠病毒疫情考验中国应急外交" [Novel Coronavirus epidemic tests China's emergency diplomacy] 环球时报 [Global Times] February 3, 2020

147 Wang Jisi, "新冠疫情下的中美关系" [Sino-US relations under the novel Coronavirus epidemic] April 8, 2020 at <http://www.aisixiang.com/data/120783.html>

148 Yuan Peng, "新冠疫情与百年变局" [The new Coronavirus pandemic and the Centennial Change] June 17, 2020 at <http://www.aisixiang.com/data/121742.html>

149 See Yu Xiaoqing, "疫情会永久性改变世界秩序吗?" [Will the epidemic permanently change the world order?] 澎湃新闻 April 29, 2020 at <https://www.thepaper.cn/newsDetail_forward_7194686> Yan suggested that the US leadership handling of the epidemic has costed it its leading role in the world. Song Xiaoling, "阎学通：新冠疫情不会对世界格局产生根本影响" [Yan Xuetong: Covid-19 will not have a fundamental impact on the international pattern] 世界和平论坛 at <http://www.sss.tsinghua.edu.cn/publish/sss/8393/2020/20200411211002811944109/20200411211002811944109_.html>

150 Zhang Yuyan, "新冠疫情与世界格局" [The Coronavirus Pandemic and international pattern] 世界经济与政治 No 4 (2020) May 18, 2020 at <http://www.aisixiang.com/data/121342.html>

151 Yang Jiemian, "大疫背景下的国际战略格局变动" [Changes in the international strategic landscape in the context of the epidemic] March 30, 2020 at < http://www.siis.org.cn/Research/Info/4910 >

152 Cui Hongjian, "疫情对世界格局变化的双重作用" [The dual effect of the epidemic situation on global pattern change] 国际问题研究 April 30, 2020 at <http://www.ciis.org.cn/gyzz/2020-06/08/content_41178069.htm>

153 Li Haidong, "疫情深刻改变国际关系格局" [The epidemic profoundly changes the pattern of international relations] 环球时报 March 31, 2020 at <https://opinion.huanqiu.com/article/3xdewES5D3V >

154 Wang Yiwei, "新冠肺炎疫情如何影响国际格局？专家解读 7 大方面，两项直接关系中国" [How does the novel Coronavirus epidemic affect global landscape – Expert interpretation of 7 major aspects, two directly related to China] ˉst April 1, 2020 at <https://www.jfdaily.com/wx/detail.do?id=232181>

155 Fu Xinmiao, "新冠疫情两条最重要的时间线" [The two most significant timelines of the novel Coronavirus] April 14, 2020 at <http://www.aisixiang.com/data/120851.html>

156 Yao Yang, "新冠疫情之后的中国与世界关系" [Post-new Coronavirus pandemic and China's and global relations] May 24, 2020 at <http://www.aisixiang.com/data/121446.html>

157 Former Australian Prime Minister Kevin Rudd argued that regardless of how China handles the Covid-19, Xi's rule and legacy will continue to influence the body polity of China as he had laid down systemic rules and procedures all over the country. See Kevin Rudd, "The Coronavirus and Xi Jinping's Worldview" *Project Syndicate* February 8, 2020 at <https://www.project-syndicate.org/commentary/coronavirus-will-not-change-xi-jinping-china-governance-by-kevin-rudd-2020-02>

2

COVID-19 and China's Politics: Governance Issues

Jigme Yeshe Lama

This chapter deals with the political aspect of the COVID-19 outbreak that started from Wuhan, the capital city of Hubei province in the People's Republic of China (PRC). At the outset, we need to elaborate on the term "political", which entails everything and affects all; however, in this chapter it will specifically delve into the domain of domestic politics in the PRC in the aftermath of the COVID-19 outbreak in Wuhan. The outbreak of the virus and its subsequent handling can also be understood in terms of governance, the role of the Communist Party of China (CPC) and the pervasive struggle for power within the party hierarchy.[1] These are the core elements in the politics of China. The PRC has been under the governance of the CPC since 1949, when the communists won the decisive victory in the civil war against Chiang Kai-Shek's Kuomintang (KMT), who retreated to the island of Taiwan. The CPC has been playing the "leading role" in the state and society and therefore claims the right to command the government, the media, the legal system and the military in the interest of preserving the Chinese socialist system.[2] The party is seen to be at various levels of the state – provincial, municipal, county and township, with party members serving as officials in local government organisations. Thus, in the PRC the head of the party who is also the party secretary, at any level of administration, is the real "boss" in local political and policy matters.[3] This centralisation of power in China has taken a personality turn with the ascension of Xi Jinping in 2018 when changes were made to the country's constitution abolishing presidential term limits, which earlier were for two terms. How this issue affects the handling of the outbreak of the virus becomes interesting and will be investigated in this chapter.

The PRC is a party state where the institutions of the party and state are intimately intertwined. This intertwining of the two generally means domination by the CPC over all organs of the state, which is seen to have accelerated further during the period of the previous general secretary Hu Jintao. He stated that there was a need to enhance the governing capacity of the ruling party, which meant that party officials, especially young rising stars at various levels of the leadership, had to serve in important positions within both the party and the government.[4] Much of this lies in the rationality that through participating in governance, a degree of technocracy can be brought amongst the party cadres, which is much essential for modernising the party. This can also be attested to the economic reforms in China that has provided the impetus for deepening of governance in the CPC and also raised a governance mentality among its cadres. Also seen is the manner in which many party cadres, whose performance in governance and administrative positions has become important for their career advancements. Cheng Li writes how since the reform era of the 1970s, the rank of a provincial level party secretary has been the most important political credential for a top leadership position.

The earlier revolutionary background is seen to be giving way to distinguished services in the provinces. While it can be stated that the revolutionary era cadres are all a thing of the past, at present it is one's handling of the provinces that matters for the promotions of the CPC cadres. This was seen in the context of Jiang Zemin, who was promoted to the position of General Secretary of the CPC in 1989 from the post of party secretary of Shanghai where he had been credited with the successful handling of pro-democracy demonstrations. Hu Jintao had served as party secretary in both Guizhou and Tibet before being promoted to the Standing Committee in 1992.[5] It was his handling of the demonstrations in Lhasa, Tibet Autonomous Region in 1988-89 that shot him to the centre stage. The current party secretary Xi Jinping has served as governor of both Fujian and Zhejiang province and as party secretary of both Zhejiang and Shanghai. We see a large representation of leaders with provincial experience in the Politburo and its Standing Committee, which reflects the growing power and influence of the politicians who run the country's thirty one province level administrative units. Through this there is a check on local power bases, since there is a promotion of provincial leaders to positions in Beijing and a frequent reshuffling of provincial leaders.[6]

The performance of party members in various capacities at different levels of government becomes a barometer for understanding politics in China. Thus, the handling or mishandling of health crises by local authorities, as seen in the COVID-19 outbreak in the city of Wuhan is a good way of understanding politics in the PRC especially at the lower levels. The political processes of the lower administrative levels of the PRC have also received much highlight due to the economic reforms undertaken by the party state since 1978. This led to a degree of economic autonomisation exercised by the provinces, cities and lower levels. A large number of administrative divisions at the lower levels are seen to be attracting investments or investing in other countries. This is important as the party state is seen to be garnering legitimacy from the people through raising economic growth, for which a healthy population is much needed. Hence, in this context, the prevention and control of epidemics has assumed much importance for the states, which has increased with the modern state as its legitimacy is hinged on economic growth that is tied to the health of the population. This somewhat reflects on the ideas of Foucault who had analysed the modern state as a pastoral state, which fosters life, through which it exercises sovereignty. For China, the health and well-being of its population assumes significance as it is through "performance legitimacy" that the party state is seen to be exercising authority, making the tackling of epidemics extremely important from the viewpoint of governance. The PRC has in the past faced an outbreak of a number of infectious diseases, whether it is the SARS (Severe Acute Respiratory Syndrome) that started in 2002 from Foshan in Guangdong province or the Avian (H7N9) flu of 2013 and the Swine (H1N1) flu. This implies that governance in China has experience in dealing with epidemics. The next section of the chapter will study the handling of SARS by the Chinese state, offering us an insight into governance and politics in the PRC.

The SARS mis/handling by the party state

The SARS that started from 2002 from the southern province of Guangdong infected 5300 people and killed 349, was seen as a major socio-political crisis for the Chinese leadership since the 1989 Tiananmen crackdown.[7] It is also in 1989 that the Chinese state had constituted a Law on Prevention and Treatment of Infectious Diseases, which provides an outline regarding prevention, control and elimination of the occurrence and epidemic of infectious diseases and to ensure the health of the people. The law divides the infectious diseases in three classes and elaborates on the various mechanisms that will be implemented to tackle the disease. However, the law is seen to be stressing on a need for a centralised approach towards disease control, granting lesser autonomy to the lower administrative levels. This issue is seen to have led to the political establishment – not sharing information to the lower levels and to the general public, which in turn led to further problems during the SARS outbreak. However, soon the Chinese government launched a crusade against SARS, effectively bringing the disease under control in late June and eliminating all known cases by mid-August.[8] This was done through a dissemination of information to the wider public and taking the appropriate steps to curb the spread of the disease. This would imply that the party state would have adopted a similar approach to the current COVID-19 outbreak in Wuhan, which as will be understood did not happen.

Minxin Pei and others have mentioned how the CPC is seen to be committing the same mistakes with regard to the handling of the COVID-19 outbreak as it had done during the outbreak of the SARS epidemic as even now the party state is seen to be withholding information.[9] We see similarities in the PRC's response to the COVID-19 outbreak in 2020 and the SARS outbreak in 2002.[10] The outbreak of SARS and the handling of it by the Chinese government provide an understanding of the state of public health infrastructure of China. It is seen to be raising questions about the capacity and dynamics of the Chinese political structure and its ability to address future outbreaks. The government had bungled initially but then it was able to contain the spread of SARS in a relatively short period of time, which does reveal the government's capacity to avert such calamities. It can be said that the formal institutional structure and bureaucratic capacity accounted for the initial denial and inaction, the institutional forces unleashed from the terrain of state-society relations led to dramatic changes in the form and content of government policy towards SARS. This was done through mass mobilisation that brought the disease under control. However, it was seen that the prevention and control programs was termed as being troubled by problems in agenda setting, policy making and implementation, which in turn can be attributed to the Chinese political system.[11]

This was seen with the investigative report of the initial outbreak of SARS prepared by a team of health experts from the Ministry of Health, PRC that was marked as "top secret" and thus classified as a state secret, the reporting of which would lead to persecution for leaking state secrets. Hence the public were kept uninformed about the disease, which led to much confusion, anxieties and speculation. This led to informal messages and information about SARS spreading through local internet sites that obviously leads to more panic and uncertainty. It was only on 11 February 2003 that the provincial health officials finally broke the silence by holding press conferences but also downplaying the risk of the illness, which when conveyed to the public led to them losing vigilance about the disease. There was also a news blackout which continued during the run-up to the National People's Congress (NPC) annual session held in the month of March, which marked the beginning of a new government following the selection of new leaders to the Politburo Standing Committee in November 2002. The holding of the NPC was given precedence over handling the SARS with majority of the leaders preoccupied with the legislature that no explicit directive was given from above even though the then Health Minister Zhang Wenkang, brought the disease to the attention of Wang Zhongyu, the secretary general of the State Council and also to Li Lanqing, the vice premier in charge of public health and education.[12] This is seen to be stemming from the fact that in the hierarchy of ministries within the PRC, the Ministry of Health is somewhat given a lower status than the other portfolios. Furthermore, this can also be explained through the idea of a "fragmented authoritarianism" model of the Chinese political system. Under this, authority below the peak of the Chinese system is fragmented and disjointed, leading to a bogged down policy process which is characterised by extensive bargaining. Thus, we need to understand how in China there is truly a disjointed and fragmented bureaucracy within an authoritarian political structure that has led to policy immobility, which can only be overcome through the intervention of upper level power holders who have the authority to aggregate conflicting interests. This has in turn led to a shirking of responsibilities by the lower levels to the upper levels, which has created policy paralysis. This can further increase with the lower level officials distorting the flow of information as any negative information would also reduce their chances for a promotion and thus, we see the lower officials not presenting the full picture to their bosses.

Moreover, in the PRC there are no checks and balances offered by the civil society, which makes the lower administrative officials hide their mistakes from the upper levels. For instance, during the SARS outbreak, Beijing municipal authorities had withheld the actual SARS situation in the city from the party centre for a long period, which led to the central leaders misjudging the situation.[13] This reveals to a certain extent the degree of daily negotiations on the 'political' level that occurs in an authoritarian one-party state like China, where the popular narrative is that of a singular entity controlling everything in the state. On the other hand, through analyzing the Chinese state's responses from different levels tackling the outbreak of SARS or COVID-19, we do see what anthropologists have termed as the "everyday practices of the state".[14] The "everyday practices of the state" entails the daily proceduralism and the banal activities that the state undertakes through a number of means, which in turn becomes the most important mode of exercising power.

It is within these micro-politics of the state that we can observe modes of subversions and dissensions within the state, something that is also visible in the context of China, where within the CPC we have jockeying for power and divisions. This has remained a hallmark since the pre revolutionary period. Within the CPC, we see a division between two factions, firstly, the 'princelings' whose parents or relatives have a revolutionary legacy and secondly, the former members of the Communist

Youth League. The current general secretary and President of China Xi Jinping is a princeling, whose father Xi Zhongxun was a former revolutionary as well as an important figure during the economic reforms in China. Both factions are seen to be vying for power and influence within the party hierarchy. Lately, it has been seen that under Xi Jinping, the influence of the former youth league members have decreased, through shrinking the Youth League's central leadership, placing it under firmer party control and returning it to its grassroots to try to win over the country's young people.[15] This aspect of the state is also seen to be visible when the officials and bureaucrats are seen to be inactive towards certain issues or giving precedence to other issues. This was present during the SARS outbreak when the officials of the provincial government gave importance to local economic development that would have been paralysed with a publicisation of the SARS epidemic to the general public, causing socio-economic instability.[16] Something similar is seen in the party state's handling of the recent outbreak of COVID-19 in Wuhan, Hubei province, whereby the party state is seen to have not learnt from its past experiences with the SARS epidemic.

Party State and COVID-19: No Lessons Learnt

Technically the party state, with regard to the COVID-19 outbreak could have simply followed the steps that it had undertaken while tackling the earlier SARS epidemic, which however has not happened. While differences in the outbreak pattern and other trajectory of both diseases can be seen, which is obvious, yet there has not been much of a change in the responses at present from the Chinese state towards the COVID-19 outbreak. Specifically with the outbreak of COVID-19, the micro-politics of the party state is visible that in this context is seen to be assuming the form of misgovernance and corruption, as in Wuhan, an unregulated local market, maximized profit by dealing in exotic animals and cutting corners on health regulations, produced a novel coronavirus.[17] After the outbreak, a text-book method adopted by the communist party, where the first step that was taken was to quash the news of the outbreak and force the whistleblowers to retract and to engage in Maoist criticisms was adopted.[18] The local authorities had summoned Dr. Li Wenliang, who had shared information about the outbreak of the virus on social media and had compelled him to sign a statement that his warning constituted "illegal behavior".[19] Instead of openly confronting the growing crisis the local party officials are seen to be instituting a blanket of secrecy and confidentiality on the matter with an urge to avoid public alarm and embarrassment. There was a further muzzling of doctors and others who had raised red flags. As a precautionary measure, they had closed the food market where the spread of virus was believed to have started, but didn't broadly curb the wildlife trade.[20] These micro measures from the state stems from the fact that in China there is a strong tendency to indulge in a systemic cover-up of scandals and deficiencies that may reflect poorly upon the party's leadership, instead of doing what is necessary to respond.[21] Minxin Pei writes about how the CPC has indulged in this modus operandi for long especially while dealing with crises, which if peered through the micro-politics of the state reveals the fact that the lower level officials are seen to be hiding facts, so as to prevent a blemish on their career prospects. The first case of the COVID-19 outbreak was reported on 8 December 2019, which however was brought forth only several weeks later to the public domain. In the official report, it was claimed that the virus was not transmitted among humans and also that no healthcare workers had been infected. This narrative was continued on 5 January 2020, even though 59 cases had been confirmed by then. On 11 January 2020, the first death due to COVID-19 occurred in China, yet the official narrative remained the same as before. On the other hand, the authorities as alluded earlier, initiated a process of censoring the public sphere with regard to any references about the outbreak. Also the security agencies started harassing people for "spreading rumors" about the disease. Much of these had undermined initial containment efforts.

According to Minxin Pei, this is linked to the survival of the one-party state as its survival depends on secrecy, media suppression and constraints on civil liberties.[22] However, we do see these repressive policies leading to outbursts from the population which will be elaborated in the next section. Prior to this, it needs to be understood why the local government in China is seen to be indulging in this process of censorship and secrecy when it comes to handling problems. One way of analyzing this is through the lens of a rise in power of Xi Jinping, who is consolidating authority, similar to Mao Zedong and also displaying autocratic tendencies. This leads to a rise in fear among the lower rung officials who will not want to draw negative attention towards them.

The centralization of power, inherent in the Chinese system and one that has accentuated further with the ascension of Xi, leads to a stronger top down approach with regard to authorization, something that has been argued by the local officials from Wuhan, as with the outbreak of the COVID-19 they have mentioned about not receiving authorization from Beijing to spread "sensitive information".[23] With the initial spread of the virus, the local authorities insisted that it could be controlled and treatable. Instead, they questioned eight people who posted on social media about the virus, saying that they were spreading rumours.[24] The authorities also did not cancel a gathering on 19 January 2020 by the Baibuting neighbourhood in which 40,000 families had gathered to celebrate the Chinese New Year and also failed to act until scores of migrant workers left Wuhan to return home for the Chinese Lunar New Year festivities.[25] Much of these activities would reflect an atmosphere of normalcy, which the authorities would have liked to maintain. Even though a number of deaths had been recorded and the COVID-19 outbreak was in full swing, the officials gave the go-ahead for tens of thousands to attend the annual feast, which is prepared by the families themselves, with each contributing and sharing dishes.[26] The misjudgement of the situation by the local authorities can also be gauged from the fact that on the day it broke the news of the epidemic to the world, it also announced that it was distributing 200,000 free tickets to residents for festival activities during the Lunar New Year holiday.[27]

The central government initially backed Wuhan's officials. Wang Guangfa, a prominent government respiratory expert, told the state broadcaster China Central Television on January 10 that the Wuhan pneumonia was "under control" and mostly a "mild condition".[28] The local government and especially the then mayor of Wuhan, Zhou Xianwang, who was termed to have neither the expertise nor the willingness to follow health experts' advice, was of the opinion that an escalation in disease prevention may hurt the local economy and social stability. The mayor's superiors, which included the party secretary of Wuhan, Ma Guoqiang as well as the party secretary of Hubei, Jiang Chaoliang were all seen to be following the same modus operandi that is was to act only when told, to refrain from asking questions and speculate – an art in Chinese politics about what their superiors were thinking.[30] Thus, they did not take any precautionary measures to curb the virus. Under them, the joint session of their respective legislatures and advisory bodies were held during this period when the flu was spreading. Also, the local authorities gave permission to a gala to usher in the Year of the Golden Rat on 21 January 2020, which reveals them downplaying the outbreak.[31] This is further explained by Jude Blanchette, of how there is a natural inclination for party officials at all levels to bury negative information and censor dissenting views irrespective of who's in charge in Beijing. Moreover, under Xi, the inclination to suppress has become endemic that has led to a prolonged period of inaction leading to the virus to spread.[32] As stated earlier, under Xi there has been a stronger inclination towards centralization in decision making, which was also visible with the local government in Wuhan, whereby it's former mayor Jiang Chaoliang stated that the local government was obliged to seek permission before fully disclosing information about the virus.[33] Thus, the role of Xi and the Politburo of the CPC becomes important, which will be briefly discussed. All official narratives paint Xi Jinping as the commander of the people's war against the epidemic.[34] He had assumed full command over the control efforts from the beginning of the outbreak. He chaired 14 meetings of the

Standing Committee of the Political Bureau of the Central Committee of the Communist Party of China (CPCCC), four meetings of the Political Bureau, meetings of the Central Commission for Law- based Governance, Central Cyberspace Affairs Commission, Central Commission for Further Reform, and Central Commission for Foreign Affairs, and a meeting with prominent non-CPC figures. At these meetings, he heard briefings about epidemic prevention and control work and made decisions on overall plans for strengthening control efforts and international cooperation.[35] These narratives denote the work done by the party state through the agency of Xi in handling the disease.

The initial handling of the outbreak of the virus in Wuhan, which comprised of the lockdown of Hubei as well as other measures, can be termed as a mode to secure people's confidence in the strength of the CPC's capacity to govern. Let us elaborate a bit on the governance in the PRC, which is denoted as one that has tackled the epidemic well. In an article written by He Lei, a Lieutenant General of the PLA and a deputy to the 13th NPC and former Vice President of the Academy of Military Sciences, PLA wrote about the manner in which the COVID-19 situation has been tackled by the Chinese people and the PRC through the CPC's centralized and unified leadership. Clearly the institutional advantage of socialism with Chinese characteristics has manifested itself in the form of the CPC's centralized and unified leadership. The author stresses how this is the core of China's anti epidemic spirit. More interestingly the fight against the pandemic is termed as being highly scientific and under the leadership of Xi Jinping.[36] The evoking of a 'scientific' approach here as well as in other state narratives is important as it can be understood as adhering to modern principles of governance and public administration which is based on rationality and scientific ideas. This notion assumes significance as we will observe in the later sections, how the CPC is seen to be giving much credence to its governance system for tackling the COVID-19 outbreak in China, which can be a model of governance for others. However, a paralysis and a lack of transparency at all levels of government particularly during the early stages of the COVID-19 outbreak reveal a gap between official rhetoric and reality on the ground. The earlier experiences learnt from SARS in 2003 that took the form of sharing transparent information was not learned by the PRC's response to COVID-19.[37] The governing authorities in Hubei and the city of Wuhan as mentioned earlier were seen to be misjudging the spread of the virus as well as according to their narrative, were awaiting orders from Beijing. Still what is important is how the officials in Wuhan are seen to be committing a series of errors at all levels, which was much visible as most of these mistakes were perpetrated in press conferences.

The governor of Hubei, Wang Xiaodong held a press conference without a mask, in violation of the provincial capital Wuhan's own rules mandating masks in public spaces. On the other hand, the mayor of Wuhan had worn his mask incorrectly by having it inside out, which was seen as a major sign of incompetence by the public. He had also quoted wrong figures with regard to Hubei's annual mask production – giving three revisions to his answer from 10.8 billion to 1.8 billion to 1.08 million.[38]

'All the King's Men and all the king's horses'

The mishandling by officials at all levels in Hubei of the COVID-19 outbreak that led to a massive rise in public anger somewhat led to the central authorities purging the highest officials of the party state in the province and replacing them with individuals who are deemed as being close to Xi Jinping. The highest official in a province or any administrative structure is the party secretary, a post that was held by Jiang Chaoliang in Hubei, and he was replaced by the mayor of Shanghai, Ying Yong. Even the party secretary of the city of Wuhan, Ma Guoqiang lost his job. He was replaced by Wang Zhonglin, the party secretary of the city of Jinan in the eastern province of Shandong.[39] Most of these new officials have been termed as being close to Xi Jinping and are considered as hardliners as seen through their backgrounds. For instance, Ying Yong's background is in public security, the law courts and the feared discipline inspection commission. He earned Xi Jinping's trust while serving as a police chief and discipline inspector in the coastal province of Zhejiang, when Xi was the party boss from 2002-07.[40] The removal of the earlier authorities and the sending of Ying Yong and Wang Zhonglin to Hubei signify the central government's determinations to fix Hubei and be accountable to the people. Further politico- administrative steps that were taken by Beijing comprised of the removal of two top health officials, Zhang Jin and Liu Yingzi from the province. Liu was the director of the health commission, while the former was the communist party secretary of Hubei's health commission. It is seen that the top leadership from Beijing was sending in trusted people to run Hubei so as to turn around the situation. The top leadership had also sent a top team from the nation's anti-corruption agency, the National Supervisory Commission, to investigate how the police dealt with Li Wenliang, the doctor who had leaked out the news regarding the outbreak and had sadly contracted the disease. They had also deputed the chief of the party's top law enforcement body, the Central Political and Legal Affairs Commission, Chen Yixin in handling the outbreak.[41] He is deemed as a protégé of Xi Jinping, and has been appointed as a deputy head of the national team overseeing the handling of the outbreak in Hubei, headed by Vice-Premier Sun Chunlan.[42]

Xi Jinping expected him to bring frontline discipline and social stability in

Hubei. According to independent political economist Hu Xingdou, Chen's appointment came "at a time of government dysfunction and social disorder". "It will help improve the situation, by [Chen] directly telling local officials what to do and watching them do it".[43] He was part of Vice Premier, Sun Chunlan's team that included a number of health officials. What is important is that Chen Yixin in 2018 was a former party secretary of Wuhan and was also Hubei province's deputy party secretary.[44] This means that he has experience of governance in the province as well as in Wuhan and during his tenure he had sharply criticised officials who were slack, and those who could not bring about reforms to cut red tape and spur investment. He has stressed on the need to step up containment measures to prevent the further spread of the disease. He specifically pointed out the need for officials not to relax in Wuhan despite signs of progress. Indicating the need for stricter controls at special facilities and a need for the security apparatus to increase vigilance in the region, Chen Yixin is seen to be following a traditional security centric approach of the party state while dealing with issues. This directive is also seen to have emerged from errors committed by the officials from Wuhan Women's prison, where officials had been sacked after a former inmate infected with coronavirus was able to leave the locked down city and reach Beijing upon her release.[45] However, whether all the king's men can deliver or not is another issue again as the newly appointed party secretary of Wuhan Wang Zhonglin on 24 February 2020 eased the one-month old lockdown on the city of 11 million as he speculated that this was President Xi Jinping's thinking. However, this unilateral decision was seen to be contradictory to Xi's thinking and hence Wuhan was lockdown again. The same party secretary had also on 6 March 2020 chided the local residents to be grateful to President Xi and the party, after people had expressed their displeasure to Politburo member and Vice Premier Sun Chunlan regarding activities of governance, which for them were mostly fake and an eyewash. Wang Zhonglin had further stated on the need for the people to be educated, which led to further social media outrage.

The actions of the new party secretary in Wuhan can be understood as an important aspect of Chinese politics, since governance in many cases is seen to be replaced with the need to please the boss rather than pleasing the people. Much of this can be further linked to the strong prevalence of guanxi or patronage based on connections. In Chinese politics, performance counts, but ultimately promotions hinge on loyalty and patronage. On the other hand, Sun Chunlan stressed on the need to end bureaucratism and formalism and called for a thorough investigation into the episode. There were also calls for officials to confront the problems. On 10 March 2020, President Xi visited Wuhan to express the gratitude of the party to the people as they were leading from the forefront. A tendency towards centralization is witnessed with Xi stressing on the need for the State Council Inter Agency Task Force sent to Wuhan, to strengthen its guidance and oversight.[46] Thus, Xi Jinping is seen to be reinforcing the strength of the CPC CC in tackling the epidemic and thus justifying the centralized command system implemented by the CPC CC. The role and responsibilities of Xi has been strongly accentuated that has led to the defeat of the COVID-19 virus, which was possible due to the governance efforts of the party state that is based on a centralized and efficient command system under the leadership of Xi Jinping.[47] This provides us with a glimpse of everyday politics in China, especially at the grassroot level, reflecting degrees of negotiations indulged in by the local officials. It also reflects the manner in which through public pressure, seen mostly in the form of social media criticisms, the party state interacts with the public. Still, the COVID-19 outbreak has led to laying bare the fundamental weaknesses of Xi's rule.[48] The COVID-19 outbreak has added an additional source of stress and unpredictability to the regime's mounting challenges. Before Xi, the Chinese style of governance was adaptive and decentralized that which could termed as "directed improvisation". However, this has changed as Xi has tightened political control. There is a strong feeling that his grip on power was slipping and the mishandling of the COVID-19 virus has further dented his image.[49] This is much witnessed with the series of strong criticisms launched against Xi Jinping on social media, which will be elaborated in the next section and forms an important, rather subversive aspect of understanding Chinese politics.

The Emperor's New Clothes

There is a popular tale of an emperor who was so arrogant and oblivious to the truth that he strutted naked before his subjects, who were too scared to tell him the truth. This is exactly how Ren Zhiqiang has described Xi in a scathing criticism written by him in an online article. Before delving into his criticism, a bit of information regarding Ren becomes important, who is a communist party member having a history of criticizing Xi Jinping's policies especially those that have curtailed the media in China. He is a former head of the state-run real estate conglomerate Huayuan Group. His parents were former high officials in the CPC. Thus, somewhat making him a princeling, similar to Xi Jinping. The latest criticism from him was on the leadership's mishandling of the virus outbreak that led to his investigation by the party's disciplinary watchdog body that on 7 April 2020 termed him as undergoing a "review and monitoring investigation". This article is seen to be critical of the party state's attempts at hiding true figures and distorting reality.[50] Although his article does not mention the top leadership by name, he is not only critical ofthe initial cover-up of the virus outbreak, but also the way in which Beijing is now promoting its success in handling it. Furthermore, the article is also critical of Xi's rise to power as that has led to centralization and the lack of accountability.

Interestingly, the COVID–19 outbreak, which started in China and is now a global crisis, is termed by him as a "crisis of governance" within the CPC. It is precisely the lack of freedom of press and speech that had prevented the outbreak from being tackled earlier, causing the situation to worsen.[51] This somehow fits into the arguments made earlier in the chapter regarding governance in the PRC especially under Xi Jinping, which has become more personality driven and thus fraught with much errors as has been displayed with the mishandling of the COVID-19 outbreak. Ren Zhiqiang is seen to be criticizing a speech given by Xi Jinping on 23 February 2020 that was teleconferenced to cadres nationwide extolling the achievements of the party with regard to handling of the outbreak. However, for Ren, the speech was hollow as it did not clarify the cause of the outbreak and further the information was much suppressed from the public. He states that this epidemic shows that the party defends its own interests, the government officials defend their own interests and the monarch only defends the status and interests of the core. In his criticism, Ren Zhiqiang mentions how such a system leads to only obeying of the ruler's orders with no regard for the people. There is a further concealment of the cause of the outbreak of the virus, instead of letting information flow, which has also stemmed from the fact that the Chinese system is one that prohibits the freedom of press and speech. In his article, Ren links the lack of freedom of speech to an increase in a lacuna in governance, which was seen with the COVID-19 outbreak. Towards the end of his critical piece, he connects everything to Xi Jinping's autocratic tendencies, whereby his style of governance is like that of a clown, standing naked and insisting on continuing being emperor.[52]

Xu Zhangrun, a former faculty of Tsinghua university in the past had criticised Xi and the party for which he had been censured and reprimanded. However, it had not deterred him from criticising Xi and the Chinese state on their handling of the COVID-19 outbreak. This is seen with him writing an online essay titled "When Fury Overcomes Fear" in which he is seen to be criticising the new governance style that has come about under Xi, which is seen to have been unable to respond effectively to the outbreak that has led to much harm upon the common people. For Xu, the cause of the problem at present is as he calls it the Axle (that is Xi Jinping) and the cabal that surrounds him. He elaborates that as there was the imposition of bans on the reporting of accurate information about the virus, it further led to deception being employed at every level of government, which had taken the form of bureaucrats shrugging off responsibility for the unfolding crisis while continuing to seek the approbation of their superiors. This led to the crucial window of opportunity that was available to deal with the outbreak shut to them. Professor Xu terms the epidemic as revealing the rotten core of Chinese governance that has been negatively affected by what he terms as "organisational discombobulation", resulting from a monopolisation of power by Xi Jinping.[53] This is the argument that this chapter also puts forward, where Xi's centralisation of power, has led to fallout on governance. There has been a structural and systemic crisis in governance as the party state is seen to be concentrating on its narrow interests and not on its citizens. According to the Professor the fault lies with the self-aggrandising attitude of Xi Jinping, which in turn has led to the exacerbation of the viral outbreak. Xu also mentions that the mishandling of the viral outbreak has led to massive rage against the leadership that has been much expressed online. He believes that with the centralisation of power by Xi, this has led to the officials indulging in a "self-indulgent behaviour of the 'core leader' whose favour is constantly sought through their adulation for the peerless achievements of the system". Hence under such a system the officials are seen to be not caring for the people, in whose name the governance of the PRC is meant for.[54] This is also elaborated earlier where the COVID-19 outbreak in China and its accentuation can be linked to the mishandling by officials and thus this is seen as a crisis of governance in China under Xi.

The arguments outlined by Xu Zhangrun regarding the party state aggrandising the authority of Xi is strengthened through the release of a book compiled by the state media writing congratulatory paeans on China's leadership on handling the virus outbreak, whereby Xi Jinping is given plaudits for his sense of mission and outstanding leadership.[55] The book is titled "A Battle against Epidemics: China combating COVID-19 in 2020", which paints a portrait of leadership resolve in the face of a major challenge. The book is published by the Central Propaganda Department, the Information Office of the State Council and the China Intercontinental Communication Centre, which all are essentially a single party. Through this publication there is an attempt to show the resolve of the CPC and especially it tries to collectively reflect Xi Jinping's commitment to the people, his sense of mission, his far-reaching strategic vision and outstanding leadership as the leader of a major power. Much of this narrative can be termed as attempting to counter the under-current of popular anger on Chinese social media. The official media is seen to be highlighting the idea that the country and the leadership has been successful thus revealing the superiority of the leadership of the CPC and the system of socialism with Chinese characteristics. One way of understanding this publication is seeing it from the centralisation of governance under Xi that makes it necessary for the ruling narrative to be constantly self-congratulatory.[56] However, the COVID-19 mis/handling by the CPC is seen to have raised criticisms against the party state and especially an increase in opposition to Xi Jinping.

Challenges to the Emperor

The outbreak of the COVID-19 in Wuhan, Hubei and its spread to other cities in China has negatively affected economic growth, which still remains a primary source of legitimacy for CPC. Furthermore, with the global spread of COVID-19 it has dented the image of China. Thus, Xi Jinping is seen to be facing two challenges, which are the revival of China's economy and the return of the work force to the production lines and offices in the world's second largest economy. Plus the handling of diplomatic work when feelings everywhere are running high against China remains a priority.[57] There has been an increase in criticisms against Xi's style of governance especially regarding the mis/handling of the COVID-19. Furthermore, voices of dissent are seen to be on the rise from intellectuals, journalists, whistle-blowers and other members of the nascent civil society in China, who have been insisting from day one that Xi and the CPC needed to be forthcoming about the outbreak that would have obviously lowered the spread of the virus.[58] Civil society members that included the Tsinghua university professor Xu Zhangrun and a dozen odd intellectuals have published a web based appeal stating the "freedom of expression starts today", whereby they also demanded for a proper treatment of victims of the pandemic and an establishment of a Dr. Li Wenliang Day and a National Freedom of Expression Day.[59]

Strong criticisms were levied against Xi and the mishandling of the COVID-19 by the constitutional expert Xu Zhiyong, who simply asked Xi to "step aside" and strongly stressed on how the leadership lacked conscience and also human nature. Much of the critics are seen to be stressing on how under Xi there is an authoritarian regime that has covered up the pandemic, including the death of Li Wenliang. A similar narrative is seen in the criticism levied by the constitutional scholar Zhang Xuezhong, who published a letter calling on members of the NPC to draft a new constitution. According to him, this was the need of the hour as the spread of the COVID-19 in the country had illustrated the flaws in the country's current constitution. He remarked the need for constitutional reforms, freedom of expression as well as the release of political detainees, which was widely circulated in China after it was posted on WeChat.[60] Willy Wo Lap Lam writes about how a narrative in the social media was over Xi Jinping's visit to Wuhan on 10th March 2020, albeit to encourage and cheer up the medical workers as well as ordinary Wuhan residents, which however turned into a "no-show" as during his visit, thousands of People's Armed Police Force (PAPF) and municipal police had been deployed to protect Xi who remained at a safe distance from the very people whom he was supposed to meet.[61] The growing discontent against Xi Jinping and the CPC can be traced from the 19th Party Congress as there was the abolition of term limits on appointments to China's apex post, with criticisms being levied by party cadres and atleast one former member of the CPC's 350 odd member powerful Central Committee (CC).[62] The voices against Xi Jinping have risen with the outbreak and the mishandling of the COVID-19 by the administration in China, with criticisms emerging inside the party and former party members. This was seen with a major criticism in the form of two letters posted on 2nd March and 23rd February 2020 to Xi Jinping by Zhao Shilin, a retired professor of Minzu University, Beijing and former member of the CPC CC, where he targeted the system of governance in China under Xi especially in his mishandling of the COVID-19 outbreak. Earlier Xi Jinping had remarked that the battle against COVID-19 was a grand test of the capacity of the nation's system of governance. To this, Zhao Shilin had remarked that Xi has failed miserably.[63]

The former professor and ex-CPC CC member stated that the major reason for this failure was stringent security, focusing solely on ensuring the party's image and pre-eminence and the centralisation of authority. These had led to or had prevented the cadres from doing their jobs and showing initiative. He further emphasised on the need for a systemic political reform that will implement the socialist core values of freedom, democracy, equality and rule of law as well as guaranteeing political rights of citizens, like freedom of speech. In his second letter, he reiterated that there should be more than one voice in a healthy society to demand free speech.[64] There are also signs of discontent from within the party, whereby reports have emerged of children of high-level veteran party cadres calling for an urgent meeting to discuss Xi Jinping's replacement. They had proposed an emergency leadership group led by either Vice President Wang Qishan or Politburo Standing Committee member Wang Yang.[65] As it is much the case with Chinese politics, the idea of internal opposition within the CPC is much shrouded in mystery and is thus based on speculations. While external opposition as reiterated above is seen to be growing, the responses from the regime are also an indicator of the rise in challenges to its authority.

Xi Jinping and the party state are seen to be hitting out at China's nascent civil society, who have been risking their personal safety and have been sounding the alarm to the public regarding the outbreak. However, much of the whistle-blowers have also disappeared and in the name of curtailing public gatherings, meetings of institutions of civil society such as both the legally recognised and the underground churches have been suppressed.[66] The feeling of fear in the consciousness of the leadership especially Xi Jinping is seen to be understood through the usage of the phrase "Stability is the big picture" by the party state in its official discourses. Furthermore, a new Small Leading Group, titled the "Safe China Construction

Coordinating Small Group" has been formed, chaired by China's law and order supremo, Guo Shengkun and which consists of the ministers of both Public and State Security, the President of the Supreme Court, the Procurator General, the senior leadership of the police and the PLA, and the new Justice Minister. The main priority of this group is "to prevent and crack down on activities that endanger the political security of the country".[67] Under this, a number of purges and removal of officials within the party hierarchy has taken place, such as the Vice Minister of Public Security, Sun Lijun who had been handpicked to tackle the pandemic in Wuhan was removed for allegedly violating "party discipline and law". Another official, Fu Zhenghua who was Sun's colleague in the Ministry of Public Security had also been removed. Much of these removals took place in the aftermath of a high-level security review that was held in the third week of April 2020 on the need for greater security monitoring of top leaders.[68]

The party state is also seen to be on an overdrive to muffle voices raised against its handling of the COVID-19 epidemic, with the detaining of numerous whistle-blowers and critics, many of whom have simply disappeared. More than 5100 people were arrested for sharing information in the first weeks of the outbreak, dissidents were labelled as sick so that the government could place them in medical quarantine, also health apps used by some millions of people to show that they are clear of coronavirus are being used to monitor people's movements and further tighten control.[69] The party state has also targeted those who were compiling a digital record of the coronavirus outbreak on Github, a software development website owned by Microsoft. Cai Wei and his partner who had participated in this project was arrested by Beijing police on 19 April 2020, both were accused of "picking quarrels and provoking trouble", a commonly used charge against dissidents in China. The arrests were linked to the Github project, named "Terminus 2049", in which both had participated, with the project preserving censored news stories, videos and articles from individuals shared on social media apps like WeChat since January 2018. The purpose of the project was to encourage the public to resist the state sponsored censorship. During the outbreak, the project shifted its focus to storing articles on the state's mishandling of the epidemic, and it remained one of the few major foreign websites that could be accessed in China. Along with the couple associated with GitHub, a number of journalists have also disappeared which includes the citizen journalists Chen Qiushi and Fan Bin whose whereabouts are still unknown, while Li Zehua, a former employee of the state broadcaster, recently resurfaced after being detained and placed under quarantine by the police.[70] The party state's draconian policies of mass arrests in the aftermath of the COVID-19 outbreak should be understood in terms of an undercurrent of dissent among the

Chinese population that was visible due to the leaders shaken by a nationwide outcry which saw the hash tag #wewantfreedomofspeech shared two million times in the space of hours.[71] A large portion of these criticisms have been directed towards the governance system that is present in the PRC, especially under the leadership of Xi Jinping.

The Governance of the Emperor

Even though there are glaring instances of a lacunae in the governance system under Xi Jinping, which led to the mishandling of the COVID-19 outbreak, the party state in its most recent pronouncements have given full credence to the governance based on the model of the "centralised command system" under Xi for challenging the COVID-19 crisis. While it is clear that the COVID-19 epidemic is the most extensive and challenging public health emergency that China has encountered since the founding of the PRC, as stated by Premier Li Keqiang in his government work report delivered to the third session of the 13th NPC that was held in May 2020. Yet the work report proclaims that under the strong leadership of Xi Jinping as its core, and through the hard work and sacrifice of the Chinese people, the PRC has won major strategic achievements against the epidemic.[72] Premier Li mentions about how the central leading groups for COVID-19 made timely decisions and plans, thus providing the much needed guidance and supervision to all local authorities and government departments who have fulfilled their respective duties. He terms that the epicentre of the COVID-19, the city of Wuhan has been defended and the party has achieved a decisive victory.[73] The Premier himself had headed the Central Leading Group for Novel Coronavirus Prevention and Control and had chaired more than 30 meetings regarding COVID-19 control and economic resumption.[74] Accolades for the present governance system under Xi Jinping has also been sounded in the recent white paper on China's struggle against the COVID-19, titled "Fighting COVID-19: China in Action" that stresses on the CPC's victory against the COVID-19, commending on Xi Jinping's command and his resolute steps to defeat the virus.

While the white paper does mention about how the role of the people was important, it remarks that the CPC leadership is the most reliable shelter against storms and it has been the party under the leadership of Xi, which could fight against the COVID-19 outbreak.[75] Interestingly, the paper terms the COVID-19 epidemic as a 'shared memory' of the 1.4 billion Chinese people and will be remembered by the Chinese people.[76] While the idea of a 'shared memory' in the white paper can be termed as being rhetorical, it needs to be understood that "memories" of the population is an important space of contestation with the modern nation state attempting to mould them into a "memory", a unitary, homogenous discourse that fits into the format of the state. Even with regard to the COVID-19 outbreak and its mishandling by the CPC, the ruling elite is seen to be attempting to mould the consciousness of the larger population, which is done through creating a singular narrative regarding the viral outbreak, one that portrays the CPC in a positive light. This is done through censoring other narratives and criticisms that have emerged from the civil society and other sections of the Chinese population. The need to have monopoly over the 'memory' is important as it eventually forms the basis for gaining legitimacy by the modern state.

The white paper thus creates a memory of how the COVID-19 outbreak has been defeated due to the governance system in PRC, which as elaborated earlier is based on a centralised command under the leadership of the CPC CC with Xi Jinping as its core, whereby China has placed an efficient system under which the central authorities exercise overall command, while local authorities and all sectors follow the leadership and instructions of the central authorities, perform their respective duties and cooperate with each other. This is termed as a highly efficient system that is responsible for the victory against the virus.[77] Even in the 14th May 2020 meeting of the Politburo of the CPC, the role of Xi Jinping was strongly commended who in turn stressed on the need to see the serious and complex situation overseas and the still daunting task of preventing domestic resurgence. More importantly, Xi urged the need to prevent rebounds in key regions and key sites especially in Heilongjiang province, Jilin province and other regions with clusters of local infections.[78] In tackling the virus, the centralised command governance system will be obviously deployed as the party state is seen to be highlighting its governance model as the perfect tool of the state in defeating epidemics and thus exercising 'biopower'.

A discourse that is seen to be emerging from the Chinese party state with regard to the COVID-19 outbreak and its handling is the notion of a superiority of their governance system in tackling epidemics and other emergencies. According to Lieutenant General He Lei, a former Vice-President of the Academy of Military Sciences, PLA and a deputy to the 13th NPC, the CPC's efficient governance is also highlighted through a rapid deployment of resources as seen with the sending of 340 medical teams and more than 42,000 medical personnel nationwide to provide emergency assistance to Hubei. Furthermore, in a mere ten days, makeshift hospitals including the Huoshenshan and the Leishenshan hospitals were set up in Hubei. Also, there was the adoption of a "counterpart assistance" strategy, pairing 19 donor provinces with counterpart cities affected by COVID-19 in Hubei. All of these highlight the advantage of centralised leadership of the CPC, which has also accelerated the scientific efficiency in their governance.[79]

Conclusion

This chapter is a humble attempt in understanding politics and governance of PRC specifically in the aftermath of the COVID-19 outbreak. The epidemic originated from the city of Wuhan, Hubei province and emerged as a serious challenge to Xi Jinping and the party state, with Xi's leadership somewhat at stake. From 2018 onwards, Xi had centralised power and changed the status quo in Chinese politics, bringing about a 'cult of personality' and forgoing the earlier model of 'collective leadership'. Thus, the mis/handling of the COVID-19 in China is much blamed on the new 'governance style' of Xi Jinping, something that was remarked by Xi himself – who stated that the battle against COVID-19 was a grand test of the capacity of China's system of governance.[80] As the chapter has elaborated, much of the criticisms by intellectuals or party members such as Ren Zhiqiang with regard to COVID-19 outbreak, has specifically pointed out flaws in governance under Xi Jinping. Furthermore, as the chapter tries to outline, the outbreak of an epidemic and its handling by the state is an important way of understanding governance and the political process of any country, which is visible in the context of the COVID-19 mishandling by the party state in the PRC. With state legitimacy in China dependent on economic growth, the health of the population who are drivers of economic process gains importance. Hence, as the chapter outlines, the state's responses to the epidemic becomes in itself a mode of legitimisation of/by the party state. Thus, the criticism against the CPC of mishandling the outbreak does dent its legitimacy, which is a direct challenge to Xi Jinping's leadership. More importantly as is outlined in the chapter, the party state failed to learn from its past experiences regarding SARS that had affected China a decade back, which has not escaped from the citizen's memories. Hence, the mishandling of the current epidemic by the party state has increased criticisms and discontent against it, which according to Willy Wo Lap Lam has also led to an "emancipation of the civil society" which has definitely caught the attention of the public as the pandemic is seen to be affecting everyone.[81]

Thus, hiding of facts and lack of transparency will lead to the weakening of the party state and the mishandling of COVID-19 is an opportunity for civil society elements and right lawyers in China to demand for accountability and transparency from the state.[82] While this heralds change in politics in the PRC, it should also be noted that the COVID-19 outbreak has been used as an opportunity by the CPC to stifle voices against the administration.[83] The present situation is deemed by the ruling elites as one of which the 'political security' of China has been threatened and thus there is a need to strengthen the coercive apparatus of the state and prevent any further dissension.[84] Earlier any challenge to the party state was faced by the collective leadership especially if it came from within, which under Xi Jinping is quite different.[85] Much of this stems from Xi Jinping centralising power and authority in China. As Kevin Rudd writes no matter how bad the coronavirus epidemic gets, the crisis will not change the manner in which China is governed under Xi as since 2012, he has strengthened the CPC's hold on power and developed a comprehensive national agenda from which all including domestic crisis management must follow.[86] Finally the party state is seen to be championing its model of governance based on a centralised leadership system as the best form of governance in tackling public health emergencies such as the COVID-19, which should be adopted by other countries to gain legitimacy from its population.

NOTES

1 A plethora of writings are available for a better understanding of governance, politics and power in Communist China, of which a few are: Bo Zhiyue, *China's Elite Politics: Governance and Democratisation* (World Scientific, 2010); Cheng Li (ed), *China's Changing Political Landscape: Prospects for Democracy*, (Brookings Institution Press, 2008); Tony Saich, *Governance and Politics of China*, (New York: Palgrave, 2001); Chris Ogden, *Handbook of China's Governance and Domestic Politics* (Routledge, 2013); Hongyi Lai, *China's Governance Model: Flexibility and Durability of pragmatic Authoritarianism* (Routledge, 2016); Teresa Wright, *Accepting Authoritarianism-State Society Relations in China's Reform Period* (Stanford: Stanford University Press, 2010); David Shambaugh, *China's Communist Party: Atrophy and Adaptation* (University of California Press, 2008); Roderick MacFarquhar, *China in Political Transition* (Singapore: East Asian Institute, 2003); Peter Hay Gries and Stanley Rosen (eds), *State and Society in 21st Century China: Crisis, Contention and Legitimation (Asia's Transformations)*, (Routledge, 2004).

2 Cheng Li, "China's Communist Party State: The Structure of Power" in William A. Joseph edited *Politics in China: An Introduction* (New York: Oxford University Press, 2014) pp 193.

3 Ibid.

4 Ibid, p. 196.

5 Ibid, p. 197.

6 Ibid, p. 198.

7 Yanzhong Huang, "The SARS epidemic and its aftermath in China: A political perspective" in Stacey Knobler et al edited *Learning from SARS* (Washington DC: National Academies Press, 2004)

8 Ibid.

9 Minxin Pei, "How China's coronavirus crisis, like the SARS epidemic, was worsened by the Communist Party's penchant for secrecy", *South China Morning Post*, January 29, 2020 at https://www.scmp.com/comment/opinion/article/3047999/how-chinas-coronavirus-crisis-sars-epidemic-was-worsened-communist.

10 Jennifer Hsu, "Xi Jinping emerges stronger from the Covid-19 outbreak", *The Interpreter*, April 6, 2020 at https://www.lowyinstitute.org/the-interpreter/xi-jinping-emerges-stronger-COVID-19-outbreak

11 Yanzhong Huang, 2004.

12 Ibid.

13 Ibid.

14 Aradhana Sharma and Akhil Gupta (eds), *The Anthropology of the State: A Reader* (Malden, MA: Wiley Blackwell, 2005), p. 11.

15 Chris Buckley and Stephen Lee Myers, "As New Coronavirus spread, China's old habits delayed fight", *The New York Times*, February 1, 2020 at https://www.nytimes.com/2020/02/01/world/asia/china-coronavirus.html
16 Yanzhong Huang, 2004.
17 Andrews Mertha, "COVID-19 reveals how China's internal politics now affects the whole world", *The Washington Post*, March 6, 2020 at https://www.washingtonpost.com/politics/2020/03/06/COVID-19-reveals-how-chinas-internal-politics-now-affect-whole-world/
18 Ibid.
19 Chris Buckley and Stephen Lee Myers.
20 Chris Buckley and Stephen Lee Myers.
21 Minxin Pei.
22 Minxin Pei.
23 Andrews Mertha, "COVID-19 reveals how China's internal politics now affects the whole world", *The Washington Post*, March 6, 2020 at https://www.washingtonpost.com/politics/2020/03/06/COVID-19-reveals-how-chinas-internal-politics-now-affect-whole-world/
24 Li Yuan, "China silences critics over deadly virus outbreak", *The New York Times*, January 22, 2020 at https://www.nytimes.com/2020/01/22/health/virus-corona.html
25 Andrews Mertha.
26 Huang Kristin, "Coronavirus: 10 new cases confirmed, 30 more suspected in Wuhan after thousands attend lunar New Year banquet", *South China Morning Post*, February 5, 2020 at https://www.scmp.com/news/china/society/article/3049173/coronavirus-10-new-cases-confirmed-30-more-suspected-wuhan-after
27 Li Yuan, "China silences critics over deadly virus outbreak", *The New York Times*, January 22, 2020 at https://www.nytimes.com/2020/01/22/health/virus-corona.html
28 Ibid.
29 National Post, "The true cost of China's coronavirus cover-up: How state censorship let the outbreak spread", *National Post*, February 7, 2020 at https://nationalpost.com/news/the-true-cost-of-chinas-coronavirus-cover-up-how-state-censorship-let-the-outbreak-spread
30 Benjamin Kang Lim, "Rocky ride for Wuhan's new party secretary", *The Strait Times*, March 23, 2020 at https://www.straitstimes.com/authors/benjamin-lim-kang
31 Ibid
32 National Post, "The true cost of China's coronavirus cover-up: How state censorship let the outbreak spread", *National Post*, February 7, 2020 at https://nationalpost.com/news/the-true-cost-of-chinas-coronavirus-cover-up-how-state-censorship-let-the-outbreak-spread
33 Rebecca Ratcliffe and Michael Standaert, "China coronavirus: Mayor of Wuhan admits mistakes", *The Guardian*, January 27, 2020 at https://www.theguardian.com/science/2020/jan/27/china-coronavirus-who-to-hold-special-meeting-in-beijing-as-death-toll-jumps
34 Global Times, "Xi vows to win people's war against novel coronavirus", *Global Times*, February 10, 2020 at https://www.globaltimes.cn/content/1179056.shtml
35 Xinhua, "Xinhua Headlines: China publishes white paper on COVID-19 fight", *Xinhua*, June 7, 2020 at http://www.xinhuanet.com/english/2020-06/07/c_139121660.htm
36 He Lei, "Institutional advantage helps China fight COVID-19", *Global Times*, May 18, 2020 at https://www.globaltimes.cn/content/1188714.shtml
37 Jennifer Hsu
38 AFP, "Outrage as Chinese officials in Wuhan fail to properly wear masks", *New Strait Times*, January 27, 2020 at https://www.nst.com.my/world/world/2020/01/560199/outrage-chinese-officials-wuhan-fail-properly-wear-masks
39 William Zheng, "Coronavirus : Beijing purges Communist party heads in Hubei over 'botched'

outbreak response in provincial capital of Wuhan", *South China Morning Post*, February 13, 2020 at https://www.scmp.com/news/china/politics/article/3050372/coronavirus-beijings-purge-over-virus-takes-down-top-communist

40 The Economist, "Xi Jinping sends in the hard man to deal with the Wuhan virus", *The Economist*, February 13, 2020 at https://www.economist.com/china/2020/02/13/xi-jinping-sends-in-the-hard-men-to-deal-with-the-wuhan-virus

41 *The Economist*, Ibid.

42 Jane Cai, "Beijing pins hope on 'guy with the emperor's sword' to restore order in Coronavirus-hit Hubei", *The South China Morning Post*, February 12, 2020 at https://www.scmp.com/news/china/politics/article/3050087/beijing-pins-hopes-guy-emperors-sword-restore-order-coronavirus

43 Ibid.

44 Ibid.

45 Lau Mimi, "No time to relax in Wuhan's coronavirus battle, top Chinese law enforcer says", *The South China Morning Post*, March 8, 2020 at https://www.scmp.com/news/china/politics/article/3074102/no-time-relax-wuhans-coronavirus-battle-top-chinese-law

46 Ministry of Foreign Affairs of the PRC, "General Secretary Xi Jinping chairs Politburo Standing Committee Meeting", *Ministry of Foreign Affairs of the PRC*, May 15, 2020 at https://www.fmprc.gov.cn/mfa_eng/topics_665678/kjgzbdfyyq/t1779619.shtml

47 CGTN, "How China's top-down command system helped contain COVID-19?", *Businesswire*, June 10, 2020 at https://www.businesswire.com/news/home/20200610005922/en/CGTN-Chinas-Top-down-Command-System-Helped-COVID-19

48 Yuen Yuen Ang, "Is Political Change coming to China", *Project Syndicate*, February 14, 2020 at https://www.project-syndicate.org/commentary/china-coronavirus-xi-hold-on-power-by-yuen-yuen-ang-2020-02

49 Yuen Yuen Ang

50 Associated Press, "China investigates communist party member critical of President Xi Jinping over coronavirus outbreak", *The New Indian Express*, April, 8 2020 at https://www.newindianexpress.com/world/2020/apr/08/china-investigates-communist-party-member-critical-of-president-xi-jinping-over-coronavirus-outbreak-2127343.html

51 William Zheng, "Chinese coronavirus critic Ren Zhiqiang under investigation, Communist party disciplinary committee says", *South China Morning Post*, April 7, 2020 at https://www.scmp.com/news/china/politics/article/3078858/chinese-critic-ren-zhiqiang-under-investigation-communist-party

52 Josh Rudolph, "Translation: Essay by missing property tycoon Ren Zhiqiang", *China Digital Times*, March 13, 2020 at https://chinadigitaltimes.net/2020/03/translation-essay-by-missing-property-tycoon-ren-zhiqiang/

53 Xu Zhangrun, "Viral Alarm: When Fury overcomes Fear" translated and annotated by Geremie R. Barme in *China File*, February 10, 2020 at https://www.chinafile.com/reporting-opinion/viewpoint/viral-alarm-when-fury-overcomes-fear

54 Xu Zhangrun

55 Hilton Yip, "Make no mistake, this is Xi Jinping's coronavirus", *Hong Kong Free Press*, March 8, 2020 at https://hongkongfp.com/2020/03/08/make-no-mistake-xi-jinpings-coronavirus/

56 David Bandruski, "A Fairy Tale Ending", *China Media Project*, February 27, 2020 at https://chinamediaproject.org/2020/02/27/a-fairytale-ending/

57 Vijay Gokhale, "Xi Jinping: A matter of State Security", *Observer Research Foundation*, May 7, 2020 at https://www.orfonline.org/expert-speak/xi-jinping-a-matter-of-state-security-65774/

58 Willy Wo-Lap Lam, "The Coronavirus Pandemic and the spread of the Chinese civil society", *The*

Jamestown Foundation, April 1, 2020 at https://jamestown.org/program/the-coronavirus-pandemic-and-the-rise-of-chinese-civil-society/

59 Willy Wo-Lap Lam.

60 Al Jazeera, "China legal scholar briefly detained after coronavirus criticism", *Al Jazeera*, May 12, 2020 at https://www.aljazeera.com/news/2020/05/china-legal-scholar-briefly-detained-coronavirus-criticism-200512045430550.html

61 *Al Jazeera*

62 Jayadeva Ranade, "Its getting worse for Xi Jinping", *The Tribune*, March 28, 2020 at https://www.tribuneindia.com/news/comment/its-getting-worse-for-xi-jinping-62050

63 Ibid.

64 Ibid.

65 Ibid.

66 Willy Wo-Lap Lam.

67 Vijay Gokhale.

68 Ibid.

69 ANI, "Why is China silent over disappearances of COVID-19 whistleblowers?", *Times of India*, April 20, 2020 at https://timesofindia.indiatimes.com/world/china/why-is-china-silent-over-disappearances-of-COVID-19-whistleblowers/articleshow/75248500.cms

70 Li Jane, "Chinese internet users who uploaded coronavirus memories to Github have been arrested", *Quartz*, April 27, 2020 at https://qz.com/1846277/china-arrests-users-behind-github-coronavirus-memories-page/

71 ANI

72 CGTN, "Full text: Premier Li's speech at the third session of the 13th NPC", *CGTN*, May 22, 2020 at https://news.cgtn.com/news/2020-05-22/Full-text-Premier-Li-s-speech-at-the-third-session-of-the-13th-NPC-QHaP1FpB8k/index.html

73 Ibid

74 CGTN, "How China's top-down command system helped contain COVID-19?", *Businesswire*, June 10, 2020 at https://www.businesswire.com/news/home/20200610005922/en/CGTN-Chinas-Top-down-Command-System-Helped-COVID-19

75 Xinhua, "Xinhua Headlines: China publishes white paper on COVID-19 fight", *Xinhua*, June 7, 2020 at http://www.xinhuanet.com/english/2020-06/07/c_139121660.htm

76 Ibid.

77 Ibid.

78 Ministry of Foreign Affairs of the PRC, "General Secretary Xi Jinping chairs Politburo Standing Committee Meeting", *Ministry of Foreign Affairs of the PRC*, May 15, 2020 at https://www.fmprc.gov.cn/mfa_eng/topics_665678/kjgzbdfyyq/t1779619.shtml

79 He Lei, "Institutional advantage helps China fight COVID-19", *Global Times*, May 18, 2020 at https://www.globaltimes.cn/content/1188714.shtml

80 Jayadeva Ranade, "Its getting worse for Xi Jinping", *The Tribune*, March 28, 2020 at https://www.tribuneindia.com/news/comment/its-getting-worse-for-xi-jinping-62050

81 Willy Wo-Lap Lam

82 Willy Wo-Lap Lam

83 Willy Wo-Lap Lam

84 Vijay Gokhale

85 Vijay Gokhale

86 Kevin Rudd, "The Coronavirus and Xi Jinping's Worldview", *Project Syndicate*, February 8, 2020 at https://www.project-syndicate.org/commentary/coronavirus-will-not-change-xi-jinping-china-governance-by-kevin-rudd-2020-02 accessed on June 6, 2020.

3

From Crisis to Recovery: China's Economy during COVID-19

Priyanka Pandit

After facing economic headwinds for some years, the China's leadership had hoped for an economic rebound in the first half of 2020.[1] At the Central Economic Work Conference (CEWC) held in December last year, optimism ran high among the Chinese economists who projected around 6 percent growth rate for this year.[2] Although International Monetary Fund claimed that the Chinese economy has begun to stabilise since September last year with improved economic performance across several sectors. These expectations however came crashing following the large-scale socio-economic disruptions caused by the Coronavirus (COVID-19) outbreak, first identified in Wuhan city of central China's Hubei Province.

The sudden outbreak of the virus had an unprecedented impact on the economic and social development in Hubei province. The province with over 56 million population and a vibrant industrial base was completely shut down for over two months since January 23 this year. Ranked 8th among all provinces in China, Hubei has been the largest comprehensive transportation hub with strong regional advantages, including good transport and communication infrastructures.[3] Its capital city Wuhan, suffered the worst economic setback, being the region's political, economic, and commercial centre (See figure 3.1). China's GDP plummeted to 6.8 per cent in the first quarter of 2020, the worst hit since the Cultural Revolution of 1976.[4] Adding to the economic volatility is the measures taken by the Chinese leadership to contain and control the spread of the virus through unprecedented quarantine, shutting down of businesses and factories, travel bans and social distancing economically affected sixteen cities in China, whose overall contribution was about two-thirds of China's economic output.[5]

China's slowing growth rates following the virus outbreak led to widespread speculations both within and outside China. Will China lose its prominence in the global economy and what will be its implications for other economies in the world are some of the key questions widely deliberated upon and discussed both at scholarly and policy circles. Speculations grew in the run upto the "two sessions" which is the annual meeting of the National People's Congress (NPC) and Chinese People's Political Consultative Conference (CPPCC), not only setting the tone for the 14th five-year plan (2021-2025) but also providing direction to the Chinese economy.[6] Usually scheduled for March, this year's "Two Sessions" got delayed due to coronavirus pandemic and were held from 21 May to 22 May.[7] The dropping of hard growth targets by the Chinese leadership generated further debates about the state of Chinese economy and the challenges facing the regime from the economic fallout of the pandemic.

COVID-19 and Economic Policy Debate in China

The Chinese economy has been undergoing significant structural shifts since 2014.[8] Its economic growth continued to slow through 2014, falling to 6.9 percent in 2015. The new normal model of growth as the Chinese government refers, has its origins in the 2008 global financial crisis. The financial crisis, which began in the subprime market of the United States (US) soon swept across the Atlantic to Europe and to the emerging economies in Asia. As global demand slumped, Chinese exports suffered major setbacks.

Figure 3.1: China's Economic Growth

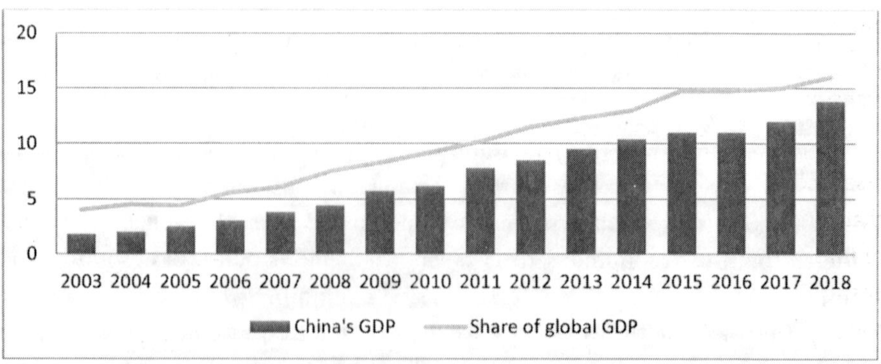

Source: World Bank, OECD (https://theconversation.com/the-growing-impact-of-coronavirus-on-the-global-economy-132030)

To mitigate the negative effects, the Chinese government quickly implemented a large-scale stimulus package of 4 trillion yuan, about $586 billion at that time.[9] The stimulus package, although stabilised the economy to a large extent by injecting enough liquidity, it however resulted into the problem of overcapacity which lasted for many years. The overcapacity was not only in labour-intensive traditional industries such as steel and cement, but also in so-called high value-added emerging industries including new energy sectors.[10] The problem also prompted Chinese policymakers to push for markets overseas, and as a result Belt and Road Initiative was developed, which amongst many, promises new markets for Chinese goods and investments. The stimulus also led to excessive liquidity, creating a huge bubble in the real estate market, rising debt in the governments, mostly at the local level. The new normal model therefore was a structural corrective measure taken by the Chinese leadership to bring the economy back on track.[11] Discussions then were mostly focussed on the nature of China's economic reforms which would ensure more stable and sustainable economic development. Two prominent schools of thought emerged on this issue: one belonging to Professor Justin Lin Yifu and the other led by Professor Zhang Weiying, both from the Peking University.[12]

According to Prof Lin, technological innovation is key to modern economic growth and development. In his view, a country heavily dependent on cheap labour and manufacturing will eventually enter the middle-income trap when it loses its competitiveness in manufacturing production, thereby getting stuck at the lower end of the global value chain.[13] Lin argues that growth economists, development economists, and economic historians have paid little attention to the technological catching up that has happened in developing countries. Drawing from his theories of new structural economics, he points to the role governments can play in technological upgrading and help economies avoid middle income trap by consciously investing in technological innovation. Industrial policies like subsidies, tax breaks, financial and non-financial incentives and protections, he argues, are important in facilitating industrial technological innovation and capability building during structural transformation.[14]

Weiying Zhang, however carried opposing views. Although he believes that resource allocation is key to economic efficiency, he does not agree with Lin's idea that government or smart industrial policies would facilitate innovation.[15] A proponent of market economy, he emphasises on the power of the markets and how they can ensure stable economic growths. In his opinion, entrepreneurs have played a crucial role in bringing about China's rapid economic growth over the last three decades and that further economic growth would depend on entrepreneurial innovation.[16] His ideas of technological innovation are drawn from free market western approach to technological development in which free reins are given to entrepreneurs for resource allocation and privatisation is promoted. For Zhang, all government regulations like anti-monopoly law, subsidies to state-owned enterprises and other industrial polices obstruct innovation, and China should rethink its policies to avoid middle-income trap.

The debate however took a different turn with US President Trump launching a trade war against China. The economic slowdown grew more pronounced since June last year, and analysts debated whether the economic slowing is the continuing symptoms of the underlying structural issues in Chinese economy or effect of tariffs imposed on Chinese goods by Washington. Discussions intensified ahead of China's annual Central Economic Work Conference and influential policy advisors debated whether the Chinese leadership should defend their growth rates or streamline their focus on economic stability and not be obsessed with growth numbers. Prof. Yu Yongding, former central bank advisor and Yao Jingyuan, advisor to China's State Council argued in favour of maintaining a 6 percent growth rate in 2020 and warned the leadership to not let the economic growth rate break the 6 per cent threshold.[17] In their view, 2020 being a crucial year in terms of completion of five-year plan and for achieving the longstanding goal of a "modestly prosperous" nation, had to maintain a growth rate of 6 percent. Economists like Gao Shanwen, on the other hand, was critical of the 6 percent growth rate and argued for a more sustainable model of growth, not fixated on targets.[18] A joint report by Renmin University of China and the China Chengxin Credit Ratings Group also echoed similar views. The report pointed to achieving modest growth rates which would ensure stable employment across China.[19]

While the Chinese President Xi claimed victory in its fight with the pandemic in the first week of March this year, it did not however signal that the Chinese economy was well under control. Not only were the structural issues facing Chinese economy exacerbated due to pandemic, the fear of contagion and other government measures had brought the economic activities to an almost standstill. Misperceptions and speculations mushroomed around the effects of pandemic on China's economy. The Chinese officials described the Western criticism of China's economy a "Western conspiracy" who wished "ill" for China and wanted it to collapse.

The other issue that witnessed a lot of deliberations within Chinese policy-circles was around the stimulus package of the government in response to the slowdown.[20] The other related aspect that also became a point of debate was policy easing measures which includes larger government spending, rate cuts, tax reliefs that Beijing pledged to increase support for the economy. The intervention is reminiscent of the 4 trillion RMB stimulus introduced by Beijing after the 2008 financial crisis.[21] Beijing had learnt tough lessons from its ultra-loose fiscal package and it has since dominated economic debate. Most of the economists in China were opposed to issuing a large stimulus and cautioned the policy makers from setting 6 percent growth targets for this year. In their opinion, the ambitious goal of somewhere around 6 percent would demand a flood of stimulus, which may lead to inflationary pressures. The People's Bank of China (PBC) policy adviser and former Deutsche Bank AG economist Ma Jun argued that a target of 6 percent would be most likely unachievable and not solve issues like unemployment which has seen a sharp increase since the COVID pandemic.[22] Sharing Ma's view, Zhang Bin, the director of the Global Macroeconomics Institute at the state-affiliated think-tank the Chinese Academy of Social Sciences, suggested for not setting targets for this year as this would lessen the pressure on both local and central governments. Describing the current economic uncertainty facing China, he called for greater urgency measures than 2008. Echoing similar concerns was Justin Yifu Lin, who argued that COVID-19 is different from the global financial crisis (effects felt mostly at the demand side) in which both demand and supply side are impacted at the same time. To his opinion, the Chinese government who mainly relied on monetary and fiscal policies to support infrastructure investment to stabilise the economy and generate employment in the aftermath of financial crisis, the current pandemic however requires new support measures particularly for the small- and medium-sized enterprises as well as boosting household consumption to weather this health induced economic and financial breakdown. In his view, the Chinese government should take advantage of its favourable fiscal and monetary policy space to stabilise the financial system, increase credits to help enterprises, invest in new infrastructure and provide necessary support for families adversely affected by the pandemic.[23] These measures will not only expand domestic demand, maintain social stability but also eliminate the bottleneck of future economic growth. He is hopeful that like it has since 2008, China will continue to drive world's economic recovery and growth as it emerges from the coronavirus crisis.[24]

Thus, the overall mood among the Chinese economists have been positive vis-a-vis economic recovery in the post-Covid phase. Although China's GDP shrank to 6.8 per cent in the first quarter of 2020, the worst year-on-year fall ever recorded since Cultural Revolution, the Chinese economists and policy makers hope that China will soon pick up its economic momentum and drive global economic growth. The western economists however do not fully agree with this picture. They can infact be divided into two blocs; one set arguing the breakdown of global supply chains (GVCs) due to disruptions in Chinese economy and portends a de-globalised world. According to IMF's fiscal tracker, China's COVID-19 support packages (including spending, loans and guarantees) is very less compared to that provided by Germany, Japan and the US.[25] Beijing's stimulus amounted to only 2.5 per cent of its gross domestic product by April, compared to 34 per cent for Germany, 20.5 per cent for Japan and 11.1 per cent for the US. For example, Hao Zhou, an economist at Commerzbank in Singapore argues that China's economic recovery will be both uneven and complicated in the short to medium term.[26] In his view, the second wave of corona virus in china will further delay the picking up of domestic consumption, thereby undermining the Chinese narrative of recovery. The World Bank Chief economist Aaditya Mattoo also argues that the pandemic could cause China's growth to slow down to 2.3 percent from 6.1 percent and push more than 11 million people in East Asia into poverty.[27] Few economists however argue that the setback in Chinese economy is temporary and it will soon be on its path to recovery. They also believe that the global economic revival is contingent on how fast the Chinese economy recovers and a decoupling from China in the global value chains will both very costly and onerous task. Economists like Dani Rodrick, Michael Spence, Amitendu Palit argue that although alternatives to China are being talked about in the discussion on GVCs, that is easier said than done.[28] In their opinion, China is deeply integrated into the global manufacturing supply chains owing to its distinct broad-based manufacturing capacities and that any diversification of supply networks in the post-Covid period will not reduce China's overall significance in GVCs (refer to figure 3.2) Also, in recent years China has moved up the GVC ladder through technological innovation. The development of AI-powered technologies in manufacturing and services has received a further boost under the "Made in China 2025" policy, and robots in Chinese manufacturing production are being

Figure 3.2: China's integration in the global economy (% of world)

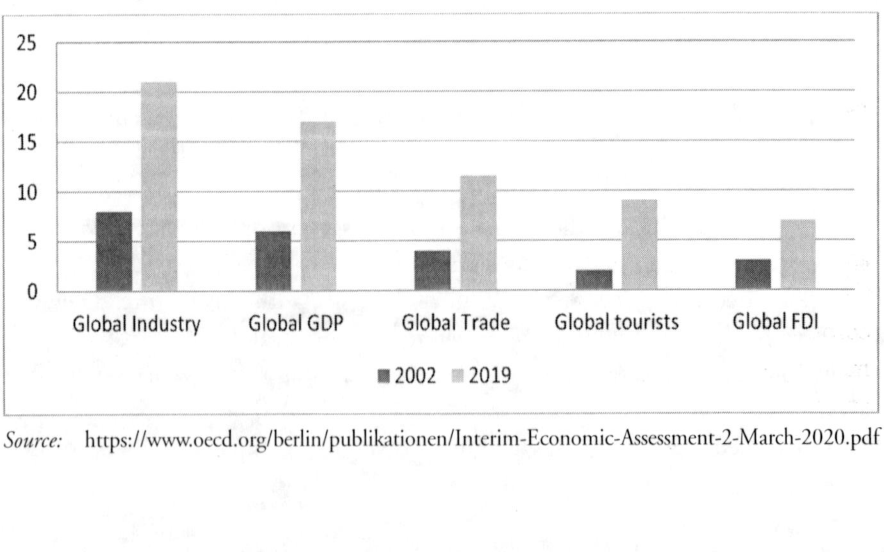

Source: https://www.oecd.org/berlin/publikationen/Interim-Economic-Assessment-2-March-2020.pdf

rapidly deployed following the coronavirus outbreak. In other words, through the adoption of automation and digital technologies as well as adapting it as per the customer preferences, China will continue to remain an attractive regional/global manufacturing hub in the post-Covid world.

The Initial Months of the Outbreak

In the early stages of the outbreak, the Chinese economic activity severely suffered. Not only the domestic production slowed, the overseas activities and outbound investments, too came almost to a standstill. The enforced shutdown which started during the Lunar New Year, considered to be usually the busiest time for most services businesses led to a noticeable downturn as the virus began spreading quickly.[29] But the economic impact was nowhere as devastating as in Hubei province, which, despite much help from the rest of China, suffered heavily while helping to slow down the spread of the disease across the nation (see figure 3.3).[30]

Figure 3.3: Impact of the Coronavirus on Wuhan's economy sector-wise

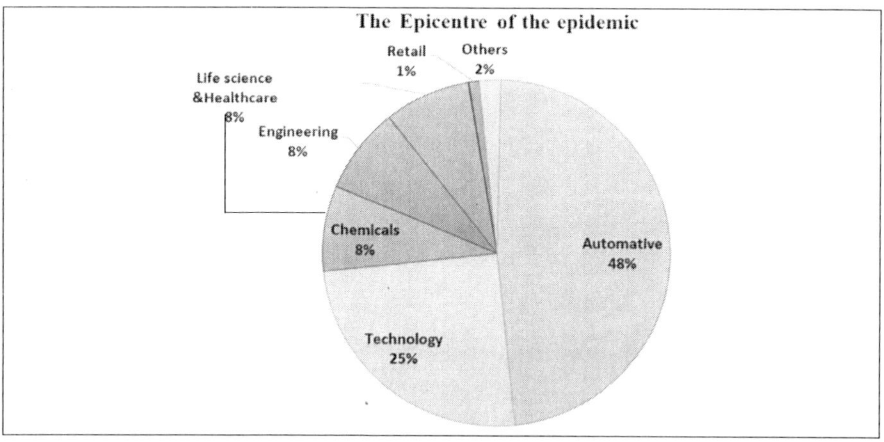

Source: Pictet Asset Management, Resilience360 DHL (https://www.am.pictet/en/uk/global-articles/2020/monthly-market-views/emerging-markets/corona-virus-impact-on-emerging-markets)

The coronavirus has proved to be a lot more damaging than the SARS of 2003 and the measures adopted to contain the spread have turned out to be worst for the Chinese economy (See figure 3.4). Economists predicted that the loss from the coronavirus is going to be four times larger than caused by SARS.[31] One of the major reasons is the structural shift that Chinese economy underwent from being an export dependent economy to the one led by consumption and services.

According to the National Bureau of Statistics, China's value-added industrial output fell by whopping 13.5 percent in the first two months of 2020, and manufacturing industry plunged to an all-time low by 15.7 percent in February.[32]

Figure 3.4: Economic Indicators across China's businesses as the coronavirus spread Year-over-year change (Jan-Feb 2020)

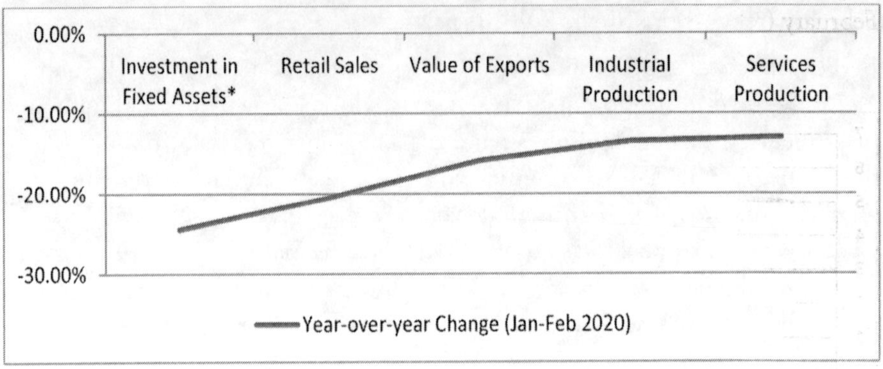

Source: https://www.visualcapitalist.com/covid-19-economic-impact/

What started as a series of sudden stops in economic activity, quickly cascaded through the economy and morphed into a full-blown shock simultaneously impeding supply and demand-as visible in the very weak January-February readings of industrial production and retail sales (refer figure 3.5).[33] The fixed asset investment in the first quarter fell 16 per cent compared to last year, while total retail sales of consumer goods fell by 16 per cent in March.[34] The output from the State-Owned Enterprises (SOEs) and overseas-funded enterprises went down by 7.9 percent and 21.4 percent, respectively.[35]

Figure 3.5: Historic Drop in Industrial Production and Retail Sales

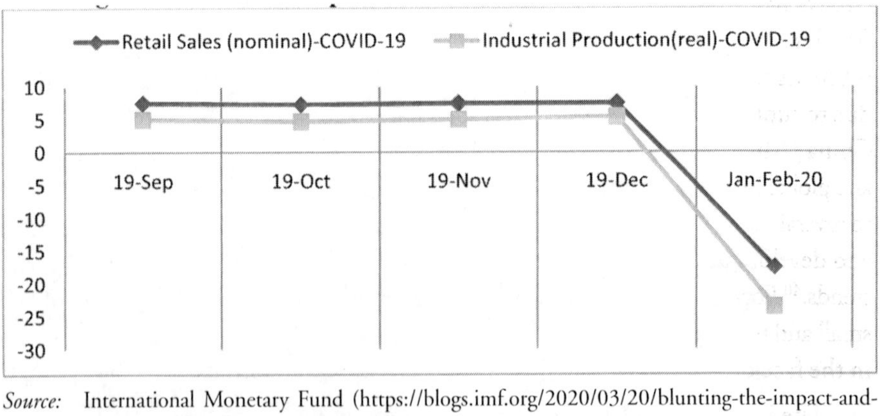

Source: International Monetary Fund (https://blogs.imf.org/2020/03/20/blunting-the-impact-and-hard-choices-early-lessons-from-china/)

While exports were held back as the factories and transport remained shut to contain the coronavirus, the demand for particular type of imports grew, such as the medical-related supplies and raw materials to produce masks and latex for hospital beds, medical equipment and pharmaceuticals. There was also a rapid drop in employment index with urban unemployment surging to 6.2 percent at the end of February (refer to figure 3.6).[36]

Figure 3.6: Unemployment Spikes

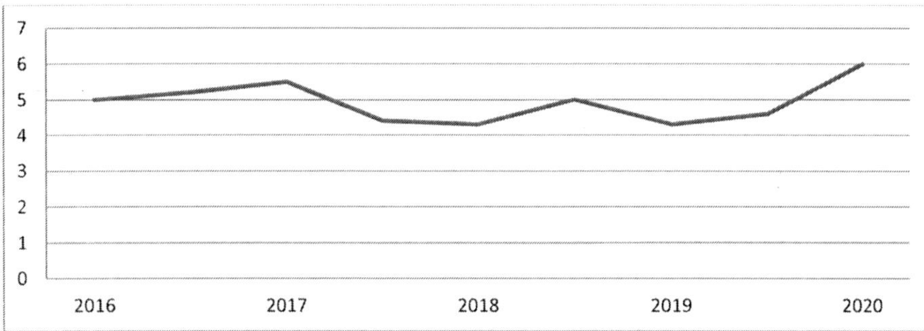

Source: National Bureau of Statistics, China and Bloomberg (https://www.bloombergquint.com/business/five-charts-show-the-economic-risks-that-china-is-now-facing)

The rising debts in Chinese economy had been a source of worry since the past year. According to research by the Renmin University, China, efforts to counter trade war pressures had pushed China's debt to 248.8 percent of GDP at the end of March 2019.[37] Adding to the domestic debt burden, has been the pressure exerted by China's BRI partners, especially the weak ones, to restore debts, arising from its $1 trillion Belt and Road transcontinental trade and infrastructure initiative. This was further aggravated during the initial stages of virus outbreak when China recorded trade deficit of US $7.1 billion in the January-February period, its first since 2012.[38] Besides, the impact of quarantine measures taken by the governments in many countries were felt in the supply networks too. The global value chains were disrupted due to supply shortages of raw materials, components and major sub-systems from China.[39] In fact, the slowdown in Chinese economy sent shock waves to the regional and global supply networks, triggering the possibility of huge financial losses. According to several estimates, the pandemic would worsen the debt situations in both developed and developing economies, evident in the decline in consumption and investment trends.[40] For instance, given the huge levels of debt in Chinese businesses, particularly small and medium sized enterprises (SMEs), they were at the high risks of bankruptcy in the face of languishing commercial activities.[41]

The impact of the virus has also been felt in China's financial markets. As the virus began to spread globally, Beijing found it difficult to secure funds abroad to pay for its imports and US dollar debt. The yuan fell below 7 to the US dollar level in March this year and the Chinese policy makers feared further depreciation pressure on the yuan, unmanageable debts in Chinese enterprises and investors, leading to even more selling of the yuan and potentially creating a negative debt spiral.[42] The financial support from the Chinese banking system was also limited and they only offered about ¥254 billion in loans related to the containment efforts in February, this year.[43] Faced with the pandemic stress, the Chinese banks tried their best to control the rise in non-performing or bad loans during the first quarter.

Is the Worst Crisis Over?

The Chinese President Xi Jinping took a celebratory "victory lap" on 10 March by visiting the epicentre of virus in Wuhan, the capital of Hubei province.[44] His visit indicated that the worst of the outbreak was over, and that China has successfully contained the virus as compared to the major Western nations. By late March, the Chinese health authority declared that the number of new domestically transmitted cases fell to zero and all other new cases were found in recent returnees from abroad to China.[45] But these official assurances fell short and the fear of contagion continued to dampen outdoor business activities. Moreover, the slump in global economy began to affect Chinese economy directly. As the Chinese economy began restarting slowly, countries across the world were struggling to contain the virus. The global economy faced a slump both in demand and supply of goods. With shops shut and businesses stalled in Europe, US and other parts of the world, the demand for Chinese exports declined sharply and existing orders were even cancelled.[46] Likewise, exports from the ASEAN countries too are badly hit due to contraction of demand in the Chinese markets.[47] Thus, the prospects for economic recovery remained uncertain despite the government's financial package.

The Chinese government's travel ban and other outdoor activities affected consumption, business activities and led to cut down in imports.[48] In the post-lockdown period, the effects of prolonged containment efforts continued to withhold full economic recovery. Factories were still struggling to return to full capacity given the shortages of labour and essential parts. Despite restoration of transportation, the labour force remains trapped in villages.[49] The migrant workers are facing difficulties to return to their workplaces, due to the checkpoints put in place by the local governments requiring them to show certificates of clearances from their employees.[50] As a result, 80 percent of the small businesses who cannot issue the certificates remain closed due to lack of labour force. Also, these companies lack enough protective gears for their employees that have been made mandatory as part of the virus prevention requirements.[51] After the laxity displayed by the Wuhan local authorities due to which the virus remained undetected in the beginning, thereby infecting many, the local government officials in other regions became more alert in ensuring checks to prevent any export of risks through free movement of people.

Notwithstanding the challenges facing the economy, the period exhibited early stages of recovery both in terms of movement of people, goods, production, and business confidence. While scientists in China cautioned it about the second wave of infections, business in China began to pick up slowly with varying recovery dynamics across sectors (See figure 3.7).[52] The leading sectors or the high performing sectors included software and services particularly the ones dealing in healthcare equipment and services, which recovered early than other sectors.[53] The low performing industries included the bulk of sectors that recovered more slowly but reached prior levels within a few weeks. The hardest hits were the transportation, retail and energy, which remained down for long and showed minimal signs of recovery.[54] As the production slowed and the flow of goods and people came to a halt, China's demand for energy products such as crude oil and liquified natural gas (LNG), plummeted. These pressures on the energy demand exacerbated the oil supply glut that had materialized at the end of 2019. As per the report by the Organization of the Petroleum Exporting Countries (OPEC) in April 2020: China witnessed largest ever monthly decline in petroleum demand in February 2020.[55]

The sectors which picked up early conducted themselves in a different way. From an interactive mode of business activities, they shifted to online e-commerce, smaller stores and technology led solutions which ensured the health safety and social distancing norm. By carrying out these adaption, they were able to re-open supply chains in a highly flexible manner. This resulted in recovery of more than 50 percent just few weeks after the lockdown relaxation. Some of them also set up a crisis task force that met daily to review procedures and issued top-down guidance for the whole chain. They leveraged its internal information platform, an app called *Huatong*, to make sure employees and franchisees were armed with timely information. This allowed franchisees to adapt central guidance to their own local situations, in terms of disease conditions and local public health measures.[56]

Some Chinese companies came up with innovative ideas to support their employees. For example, China's largest kitchenware manufacturer Supor issued very specific operational guidelines and procedures for its employees about how to limit exposures and maintain social distancing while dining in canteens as well as contingency plans for tricky situations.[57] Additionally, the company made arrangements for health checks of the employees and their families from the early stages of the outbreak and also procured protective gears for them. These timely innovations made the company well prepared for an early resumption of work, and even reopening some production lines in the second week of February. Although the number of unemployed soared during the outbreak, some Chinese enterprises decided to relocate and re-allocate their labour force in a creative way. Instead of layoffs, they reallocated their employees in new activities and even outsourced them to other companies providing essential services.[58] Some of them also operated through social media platforms, such as WeChat, the popular Chinese social media app, to communicate and coordinate with the employees. These companies not only leveraged digital tools to influence customers, but also virtually engaged them in online sales.[59]

Figure 3.7: COVID-19 recovery dynamics differ across sectors in China

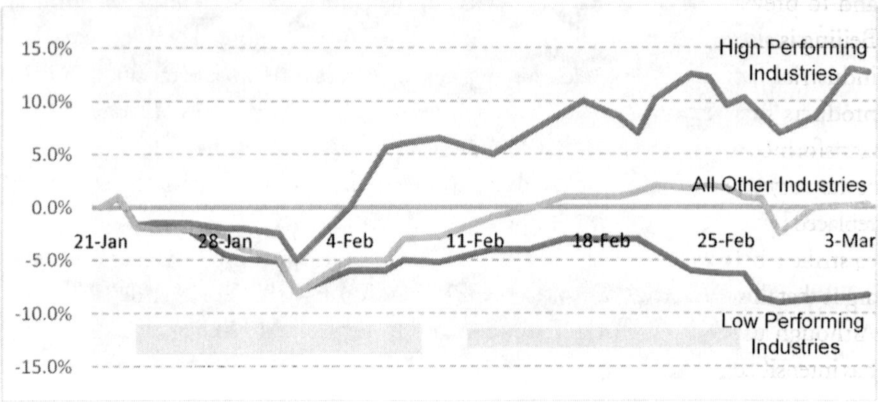

Source: https://hbr.org/2020/03/how-chinese-companies-have-responded-to-coronavirus

However, these early signs of recovery were absent in China's overseas investments and regional infrastructure projects.[60] In fact the Chinese government turned its focus "inwards" to mitigate the effects of prolonged containment on domestic economy.[61] In the early April, the priority of the leadership was to normalise domestic economic activities and to stabilise the financial situation. This prompted delays and disruptions of the ongoing projects and in turn casting a long shadow of uncertainty on China's Belt and Road Initiative (BRI).[62] The travel restrictions as part of quarantine measures imposed by the host countries also prevented Chinese workforce from reaching the project sites and to resume work. Besides, the Chinese workers residing in these countries faced stigmas and were branded as the carriers of coronavirus by the locals. Despite assurances by the Chinese President Xi about zero new cases of COVID-19 in mainland China, host countries remained extremely wary of future outbreaks.[63] In Malaysia, for example, the Chinese workers hailing from Wuhan were not allowed to return to the East Coast Railway Link project even after obtaining clearances from the Chinese health officials.[64]

The Prognosis

As China's economic recovery has been slower than expected, the question that looms big is whether China will be able to restore its prominence in the global economy in the post-COVID period. Although many expect that China's stimulus package of $500bn would boost the sagging demand and lead to a surge in infrastructure investments, the Chinese government on the other hand, has clearly outlined its "six priorities": employment, basic livelihood, companies, food and energy security, stable supply chains and smooth operation of government, and vows to utilise the stimulus in these areas.[65] Additionally, the central bank has announced some policy easing measures along with injecting some liquidity to shore up investor confidence and to prevent the Chinese companies, especially SMEs from going bankrupt.[66] Beijing is also paying attention to building new infrastructures such as data centres, industrial facilities powered by artificial intelligence and cold-chain logistics for products such as frozen goods, all of which could secure China's position in the transformed GVCs over the next decade.[67] The transformation of the GVCs pertain to its very nature in which countries' traditional comparative advantages will be replaced by technological competitiveness. With firms adopting technological solutions to strike a balance between social distancing norms and economic activities, many argue that this will lead to reshoring in GVCs, particularly automation-driven reshoring.[68] Although use of automation in manufacturing is not new, the current pandemic has intensified the need given the change in customer preferences for digital technology over interactive economic activities and the spurt in inward-looking government policies.

Stimulus, however, as economists argue may not work in the long term for the fact that COVID-19 affects both the demand and supply side networks.[69] On the contrary, the tricky trade-offs arising from these policy measures are likely to burden the financial system further by pushing up fiscal deficit and debt-to-GDP ratio. What is requires is to develop a well-structured and carefully targeted spending plan which does not let the unemployment to rise and ensures liquidity in SMEs so that they can stay afloat.[70] Further efforts would also require carrying out structural reforms including rural reforms and financial sector. Also, a reckless shift to automation will have a disastrous impact on China's labour market which has already seen the worst in the first two months of the outbreak. However, there are some data which depict hopes for the Chinese economy. Compared to the major developed and developing countries, China's manufacturing and non-manufacturing PMI (Purchasing Managers Index) numbers have shown amelioration in the month of June (refer figure 3.8). This is an indication that factory activity has picked up and in fact done better than what the market analysts predicted. The non-manufacturing data (services sector) from the government also displayed improvement in June. Services which accounted for more than half of China's employment in 2019, play a very important role in Chinese economy as they offer a good source of employment opportunities for the jobless migrant workers.[71]

Figure 3.8: China Official PMI Data

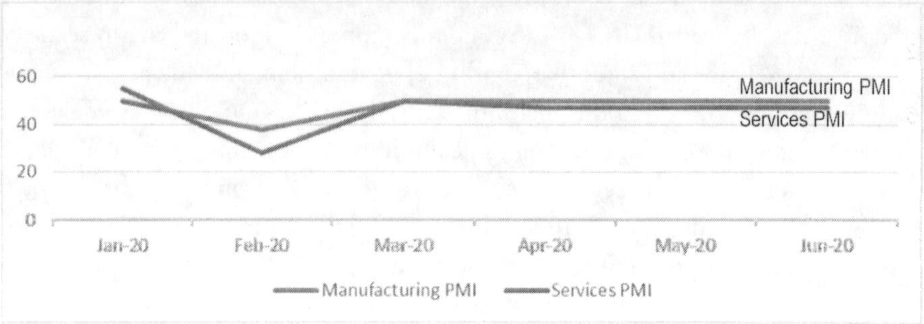

Source: NBS China

However, concerns remain over the agricultural sector as food production and transportation disruptions affect China's food security.[72] Other services which are hesitantly picking up include restaurants, tourism and sports where infection risks are high. As the fears of a second wave of infections grasped China with recent outbreak in Beijing, the consumer confidence is yet to fully resume.[73] With regard to the tourism sector which constitutes an important part of China's tertiary industry, some provinces plan to boost local tourism with initiatives such as longer weekends, cash coupons and lower ticket prices.[74] Other provinces are even deliberating stimulus packages in the coming weeks.

In sum, the COVID-19 outbreak poses a unique challenge for the Chinese policy makers. While the Chinese leadership takes pride in its extraordinary measures to control and contain the pandemic, the economic fallout has been unprecedented for Beijing. Neither a stimulus package nor supporting measures are enough, these interventions need to be regularly monitored by the Chinese leadership. Along with these doses of supporting measures, a clear guidance on standards and protocols for businesses to re-open, adapt and access new markets as well as to enhance SMEs entrepreneurial potential and spur processes of collaboration need to be outlined. To ensure a more sustainable and resilient economic recovery, the Chinese government should also strengthen social safety nets by improving public health systems, effective advance warning system, a common information base, large medical research, vaccine development budgets, co-ordinated strategies for fighting emergencies etc. And it also remains to be seen whether Beijing has drawn the obvious lesson from the pandemic, that flow of information from the below is crucial for an early detection of crisis, of any kind.

NOTES

1 "China's economy to rebound in first half of 2020: J.P. Morgan economist", *Xinhua*, December 9, 2020 at <http://www.xinhuanet.com/english/2019-12/09/c_138617547.htm>

2 Houze Soung, "In Year-End Economic Confab, Beijing Will Look to Reorder Priorities", *Macro Polo*, 11 December 2019 at https://macropolo.org/china-central-economic-work-conference-2020/

3 "Economic Profile of China's Hubei", *Canadian Trade Commissioner*, 2016 at <https://www.tradecommissioner.gc.ca/china-chine/market-facts-faits-sur-le-marche/112025.aspx?lang=eng>

4 "Coronavirus-Hit Chinese Economy Shrinks By 6.8 Pct In First Quarter Of 2020, Worst Since 1976", *Outlook*, 17 April 2020 at <https://www.outlookindia.com/website/story/world-news-coronavirus-hit-chinese-economy-shrinks-by-68-pct-in-first-quarter-of-2020-worst-since-1976/350911>

5 Amy Gunia, "As Wuhan Coronavirus Drags on Chinese Markets, the World Economy Braces for a Slowdown", *Time,* 31 January 2020 at <https://time.com/5775027/wuhan-coronavirus-global-economy/>

6 B.R Deepak, "China's Two Sessions in the time of Covid", *Sunday Guardian*, 23 May 2020 at <https://www.sundayguardianlive.com/opinion/chinas-two-sessions-time-covid>

7 K J M Verma, "China to hold annual parliament session from May 22", *Outlook*, 2020 at <https://www.outlookindia.com/newsscroll/china-to-hold-annual-parliament-session-from-may-22/1818035>

8 Song Ligang, Zhou Yixiao, and Luke Hurst, *The Chinese Economic Transformation* (ANU Press: 2019).

9 Wang Yong, "China's economic challenges: Grappling with a 'New Normal'", *Global Asia* 2014, 9(4), 15 at <https://www.globalasia.org/v9no4/cover/chinas-economic-challenges-grappling-with-a-new-normal_wang-yong>

10 Ibid.

11 Chen Anping & Nicolaas Groenewold, "China's 'New Normal': Is the growth slowdown demand-or supply-driven?," *China Economic Review*, 2019, 58, https://doi.org/10.1016/j.chieco.2018.07.009 at <https://www.sciencedirect.com/science/article/abs/pii/S1043951X18300993>

12 "China's industrial policy: Plan v market", *The Economist,* 5 November 2016 at <https://www.economist.com/finance-and-economics/2016/11/05/plan-v-market>

13 Zhang Jing & Chen Jian, Introduction to China's new normal economy, *Journal of Chinese Economic and Business Studies* 2017, 15(1), 2, DOI: 10.1080/14765284.2017.1289454 at <https://www.tandfonline.com/doi/full/10.1080/14765284.2017.1289454>

14 Justin Lin Yifu, "Industrial policies for avoiding the middle-income trap: a new structural economics perspective", *Journal of Chinese Economic and Business Studies* 2017, 15(1), 5&6 https://doi.org/10.1080/14765284.2017.1287539 at <https://www.tandfonline.com/doi/abs/10.1080/14765284.2017.1287539>

15 Zhang Weiying "China's future growth depends on innovation entrepreneurs", *Journal of Chinese Economic and Business Studies,* 2017, 15(1), 19 & 20 https://doi.org/10.1080/14765284.2017.1287540 at <https://www.tandfonline.com/doi/abs/10.1080/14765284.2017. 1287540?src=recsys&journalCode=rcea20>

16 Ibid.

17 Kevin Yao, "REFILE-China urged to lower 2020 growth target as trade war bites", *Reuters,* 27 November 2019 at <https://www.reuters.com/article/china-economy-growth/refile-china-urged-to-lower-2020-growth-target-as-trade-war-bites-idUSL4N2872HV>

18 Sidney Leng, "China could struggle to keep growth above 4 per cent over next decade, warns prominent economist", *South China Morning Post,* 28 November 2020 at <https://www.scmp.com/economy/china-economy/article/3039786/china-could-struggle-keep-growth-above-4-cent-over-next>

19 Ibid.

20 Frank Tang, "Coronavirus: China should not rely on massive stimulus to overcome 'unprecedented' economic slowdown", *South China Morning Post,* 12 March 2020, at <https://www.scmp.com/economy/china-economy/article/3074932/coronavirus-china-should-not-rely-massive-stimulus-overcome>

21 Shen Jianguang "2008 lessons learned, China in better position to embrace 3.6 trillion yuan new stimulus", *CGTN,* 6 April 2020, at <https://news.cgtn.com/news/2020-06-04/2008-lessons-learned-China-better-meets-3-6-trln-yuan-new-stimulus—R3dTPKISFq/index.html>

22 "China Debates Slashing Economic Growth Target Amid Virus Reality", *Bloomberg,* 2020 at <https://www.bloombergquint.com/global-economics/china-debates-slashing-economic-growth-target-amid-virus-reality>

23 Justin LinYifu, "China will drive global economic recovery", *Financial Review,* 18 May 2020 at <https://www.afr.com/policy/economy/china-will-drive-global-economic-recovery-20200515-p54thv>

24 Ibid.

25 ShenJianguang, "China's stimulus sceptics need not fear side-effects this time", *Financial Times,* 31 May 2020 at <https://www.ft.com/content/304d0fe3-6456-41e5-a765-29483cc02262>

26 "Does Beijing's Covid outbreak threaten China's recovery?", *Financial Times,* 21 June 2020 at <https://www.ft.com/content/fd682c9c-7dbc-4dcc-bffe-509a10c96a6f>

27 "World Bank warns China's growth could screech to a halt", *The Economic Times,* 31 March 2020 at <https://economictimes.indiatimes.com/news/international/business/world-bank-warns-chinas-growth-could-screech-to-a-halt/articleshow/74905037.cms?from=mdr>

28 Dani Rodrick, "China as Economic Bogeyman", Project Syndicate, 2020 at <https://www.project-syndicate.org/commentary/west-should-stop-criticizing-china-industrial-policy-by-dani-rodrik-2020-07>

Amitendu Palit, "Indo-Pacific supply chains: A feasible idea?", *Financial Express*, 2020 at <https://www.financialexpress.com/opinion/indo-pacific-supply-chains-a-feasible-idea/1993860/> ; Michael Spence, "Can China's Economy Withstand the Coronavirus?", Project Syndicate, 2020 at <https://www.project-syndicate.org/commentary/china-economy-coronavirus-resilience-by-michael-spence-2020-02?barrier=accesspaylog>

29 Vivek Mishra, "Chinese economy clobbered by coronavirus but set to recover soon - Reuters poll", *Reuters,* 2020 at <https://in.reuters.com/article/china-health-economy-poll/chinese-economy-clobbered-by-coronavirus-but-set-to-recover-soon-reuters-poll-idINKBN20807K>

30 Hegle Berger, Kenneth Kang, and Chayong Rhee, "Blunting the Impact and Hard Choices: Early Lessons from China", *IMF Blogs*, 20 March 2020 at <https://blogs.imf.org/2020/03/20/blunting-the-impact-and-hard-choices-early-lessons-from-china/>

31 Manoj Joshi, "The economic fallout of Covid-19", *Raisina Debates*, ORF, 2020 at <https://www.orfonline.org/expert-speak/the-economic-fallout-of-covid-19-61526/>

32 Press Release, "Industrial Production Operation in the First Two Months of 2020", *National Bureau of Statistics of China*, 2020 at <http://www.stats.gov.cn/english/PressRelease/202003/t20200317_1732640.html>

33 Hegle Berger, Kenneth Kang, and Chayong Rhee, "Blunting the Impact and Hard Choices: Early Lessons from China", *IMF Blogs*, 20 March 2020 at <https://blogs.imf.org/2020/03/20/blunting-the-impact-and-hard-choices-early-lessons-from-china/>

34 Thomas Hale, "China's economy shrinks for first time in four decades", *Financial Times,* 16 April 2020 at <https://www.ft.com/content/8f941520-67ad-471a-815a-d6ba649d22ed>

35 Priyanka Pandit, "How Does COVID-19 Affect China's Economic Juggernaut?", *ICWA Viewpoint,* 01 April 2020 at <https://www.icwa.in/show_content.php?lang=1&level=3&ls_id=4665&lid=3510>

36 Ibid.

37 Charlie Campbell "'How Can I Get Through This?' The Impact of Coronavirus on China's Economy Is Only Just Beginning", *Time,* 21 April 2020 at <https://time.com/5824599/china-coronavirus-covid19-economy/>

38 Manoj Joshi "The economic fallout of Covid-19", *Raisina Debates*, ORF, 18 February 2020 at <https://www.orfonline.org/expert-speak/the-economic-fallout-of-covid-19-61526/>

39 Franscisco Betti, Jun Ni Shien-Ming Wu, "How China can rebuild global supply chain resilience after COVID-19", *World Economic Forum 2020,* at <https://www.weforum.org/agenda/2020/03/coronavirus-and-global-supply-chains/>

40 Jayati Ghosh, "The COVID-19 Debt Deluge", *Project Syndicate* 2020, at <https://www.project-syndicate.org/commentary/coronavirus-debt-crisis-by-jayati-ghosh-2020-03?a_la=english&a_d=5e6f43f7daa89412a008d424&a_m=&a_a=click&a_s=&a_p=%2Ftopic%2Fthe-covid-19-crisis&a_li=coronavirus-debt-crisis-by-jayati-ghosh-2020-03&a_pa=topic-commentaries&a_ps=&a_ms=&a_r=>; Raghuram Rajan, "The Pandemic Stress Test", *Project Syndicate,* 2020, at <https://www.project-syndicate.org/commentary/covid19-economic-weaknesses-by-raghuram-rajan-2020-03?a_la=english&a_d=5e6b98c139cf2352ac701109&a_m=&a_a=click&a_s=&a_p=%2Ftopic%2Fthe-covid-19-crisis&a_li=covid19-economic-weaknesses-by-raghuram-rajan-2020-03&a_pa=topic-commentaries&a_ps=&a_ms=&a_r= >; Kenneth Rogoff, "That 1970s Feeling", *Project Syndicate,* 2020 at <https://www.project-syndicate.org/commentary/next-global-recession-hits-the-supply-side-by-kenneth-rogoff-2020-03>

41 Priyanka Pandit, "How Does COVID-19 Affect China's Economic Juggernaut?", *ICWA Viewpoint,* 01 April 2020 at https://www.icwa.in/show_content.php?lang=1&level=3&ls_id=4665&lid=3510

42 "China Yuan falls on Trump's new tariffs threat", *The New Indian Express,* 1 May 2020 at <https://www.livemint.com/market/stock-market-news/china-s-yuan-falls-below-sensitive-level-of-7-to-us-dollar-1564978556725.html>

43 Ibid.

44 Huang Yukon, "China's economic growth now depends on the West", *East AsiaForum* 24 March 2020 at <https://www.eastasiaforum.org/2020/03/24/chinas-economic-growth-now-depends-on-the-west/>

45 The New Indian Express "COVID-19: China reports zero increase in domestically-transmitted coronavirus cases", at <https://www.newindianexpress.com/world/2020/mar/26/covid-19-china-reports-zero-increase-in-domestically-transmitted-coronavirus-cases-2121745.html>

46 D Weinland & X Liu "Chinese economy suffers record blow from coronavirus", *Financial Times,* 16 March 2020 at <https://www.ft.com/content/318ae26c-6733-11ea-800d-da70cff6e4d3>

47 Priyanka Pandit, "How Does COVID-19 Affect China's Economic Juggernaut?", *ICWA Viewpoint,* 01 April 2020 at <https://www.icwa.in/show_content.php?lang=1&level=3&ls_id=4665&lid=3510>

48 Jayati Ghosh, Raghuram Rajan and Kenneth Rogoff, Project Syndicate 2020.

49 Sun Yu, "China's stranded workers drag down coronavirus-stricken economy", *Financial Times,*

March 4, 2020 at <https://www.ft.com/content/43d05790-5d10-11ea-b0ab-339c2307bcd4>

50 Ibid.

51 "How China's old habits kept the world in the dark even as killer epidemic grew", *The Economic Times,* February 3 2020 at <https://economictimes.indiatimes.com/news/international/world-news/how-chinas-old-habits-kept-the-world-in-the-dark-even-as-killer-epidemic-grew/articleshow/73864203.cms?from=mdr>

52 Martin Reeves et al. "How Chinese Companies Have Responded to Coronavirus", *Harvard Business Review,* 10 March 2020 at <https://hbr.org/2020/03/how-chinese-companies-have-responded-to-coronavirus>

53 David Aikman & Alan Chan, "Five ways Chinese companies are responding to coronavirus", *World Economic Forum* 20 February 2020 at <https://www.weforum.org/agenda/2020/02/coronavirus-chinese-companies-response/>

54 Tan Weizhen "Here are the Chinese industries likely to be hit hardest by the coronavirus outbreak", *CNBC* 20 February 2020, at <https://www.cnbc.com/2020/02/20/here-are-the-chinese-industries-likely-to-be-hit-hardest-by-coronavirus.html>

55 Kaj Malsen and Suzanna Stephens, "Cascading Economic Impacts of the COVID-19 Outbreak in China", U.S. *China Economic and Security Review Commission*, 21 April 2020 at <https://www.uscc.gov/sites/default/files/2020-04/Cascading_Economic_Impacts_of_the_Novel_Coronavirus_April_21_2020.pdf>

56 Martin Reeves et al. "How Chinese Companies Have Responded to Coronavirus", *Harvard Business Review,* 10 March 2020 at <https://hbr.org/2020/03/how-chinese-companies-have-responded-to-coronavirus>

57 Stephen Onyekwelu, "Chinese response to coronavirus holds lessons for Nigerian CEOs", *Business Day,* 18 March 2020 at https://businessday.ng/coronavirus/article/chinese-firms-response-to-coronavirus-holds-lessons-for-nigerian-ceos/

58 Martin Reeves et al. "How Chinese Companies Have Responded to Coronavirus", *Harvard Business Review,* 10 March 2020 at https://hbr.org/2020/03/how-chinese-companies-have-responded-to-coronavirus

59 Guan Mingyu et.al, "How consumer companies in China are preparing for the next normal: A virtual roundtable", *McKinsey* 2020 at https://www.mckinsey.com/featured-insights/asia-pacific/how-consumer-companies-in-china-are-preparing-for-the-next-normal-a-virtual-roundtable#

60 Chan Kung and Wei Hongxu, "Will COVID-19 Halt China's 'Going out' Economic Strategy?", *The Diplomat,* March 14 2020 at <https://thediplomat.com/2020/03/will-covid-19-halt-chinas-going-out-economic-strategy/>

61 "China's belt and road plan is getting lashed by coronavirus", *The Economic Times,* 6 March 2020 at <https://economictimes.indiatimes.com/news/international/business/chinas-belt-and-road-plan-is-getting-lashed-by-coronavirus/articleshow/74499725.cms?from=mdr>

62 "China Reports Zero Rise In Domestic Coronavirus Cases", *NDTV,* 23 March 2020 at <https://www.ndtv.com/world-news/china-reports-zero-rise-in-domestic-coronavirus-cases-2199060>

63 Ibid.

64 Laura He, "Coronavirus devastates China's economy and the 'nightmare' is not over", *CNN Business,* 16 March 2010 at https://edition.cnn.com/2020/03/16/economy/china-economy-coronavirus/index.html; "China takes major steps to prop up coronavirus-hit economy", *Reuters* 20 February 2020 at <https://www.reuters.com/article/us-china-health-policy-factbox/china-takes-major-steps-to-prop-up-coronavirus-hit-economy-idUSKBN20E101>

65 ShenJianguang, "China's 'six priorities' and fiscal stimulus will spearhead its COVID-19 recovery",

World Economic Forum 8 June 2020 at <https://www.weforum.org/agenda/2020/06/china-stimulus-covid19-economic-recovery/>

66 Kaushik Basu, "Epidemics and Economic Policy", *Project Syndicate* 2020 at <https://www.project-syndicate.org/commentary/covid19-coronavirus-economic-policy-response-by-kaushik-basu-2020-03>; M L El-Erian "The Race Between Economics and COVID-19", *Project Syndicate*, March 26 2020 at: <https://www.project-syndicate.org/commentary/covid19-will-change-economics-three-ways-by-mohamed-a-el-erian-2020-03>; Stephen S Roach, "When China Sneezes", *Project Syndicate* 2020, at <https://www.project-syndicate.org/commentary/china-coronavirus-shock-prospects-for-global-recession-by-stephen-s-roach-2020-02>

67 Jianguang Shen 8 June 2020

68 Priyanka Pandit "As Global Value Chains Shift, Will China Lose Its Dominance?", *The Diplomat*, 11 June 2020 at <https://thediplomat.com/2020/06/as-global-value-chains-shift-will-china-lose-its-dominance/>

69 Yu Shi "Stimulus no panacea for economic woes", *China Daily*, 20 March 2020 at<http://global.chinadaily.com.cn/a/202003/20/WS5e73fb72a3101282172809 25.html>

70 Asit Ranjan Mishra, "Stimulus is a solution, but be wary of fiscal deficit, says IMF's Gita Gopinath", *Livemint* 10 April 2020 at <https://www.livemint.com/news/india/more-than-stimulus-virus-affected-countries-need-proactive-fiscal-policies-imf-s-gita-gopinath-11586441168288.html>

71 Sidney Leng "China's unemployment risks surge as service providers bear the brunt of coronavirus outbreak", *South China Morning Post*, 31 January 2020 at <https://www.scmp.com/economy/china-economy/article/3048396/chinas-unemployment-risks-surge-service-providers-bear-brunt>

72 Gao Jingyu & Kong Xinyu "China's Economy Recovering; Global COVID-19 Efforts Needed", *Asian Infrastructure Investment Bank* 10 April 2020 at <https://www.aiib.org/en/news-events/media-center/blog/2020/China-Economy-Recovering-Global-COVID-19-Efforts-Needed.html>

73 "China's new strategy to tame second-wave virus outbreaks", *Medical Express* 9 July 2020 at <https://medicalxpress.com/news/2020-07-china-strategy-second-wave-virus-outbreaks.html>

74 Gao Jingyu& Kong Xinyu 10 April 2020

4

China's Media and COVID-19: A Content Analysis of Caixin, Xinhua and People's Daily

Tilak Jha

1. Introduction

This is not the first time China has faced a virus-created health crisis. Over the past two decades, two of the three zoonotic coronavirus outbreaks – namely the Severe Acute Respiratory Syndrome (SARS-CoV) in 2003 and Severe Acute Diarrhoea Syndrome Coronavirus (SADS-CoV) in 2012 - began in China. Both caused worldwide pandemic and claimed thousands of human or animal lives. A paper authored by a scientist of the Wuhan Institute of Virology predicted in January 2019 the high likelihood of a SARS or Middle East Respiratory Syndrome (MERS)-like coronavirus outbreaks in China.[1] Ironically, the same research centre has been accused by the US President Donald Trump to be the reason behind the massive global damage caused by the COVID-19 outbreak.[2] More importantly though, Chinese state media's response to the COVID-19 has come under severe criticism from several quarters. There are concerns about whether Chinese state media[3], massively abetted the spread of the COVID-19 by repeating the mistakes of trying to cover up the news of the seriousness of the disease, as it did during the SARS crisis in 2003.[4] This paper discusses whether, despite the evidence and experience of 2003 that news related to contagious disease are best left uncensored, Chinese media – especially official media – failed to rise to the occasion. This paper does a comparison of the coverage of COVID-19 issue by the Communist Party of China (CPC) mouthpiece the *People's Daily* (PD) and one of China's most reputed private news platforms –

Caixin. It will also bring into perspective the lessons from SARS coverage in 2003. The paper also takes into account the coverage of the English-language Tweets of *Caixin* and the *People's Daily* on COVID-19 during this period. By drawing upon the contrast, this paper tests how much substance is there in the charges that China and its media did substantially cover up coronavirus outbreak coverage, at least in the initial days.

2. Why *Caixin* and the PD

Some of the most detailed reports on COVID-19 have come from private mainland China-based media platform - particularly Caixin group. Hu Shuli founded the hard-hitting business journalism platform *Caijing* in 1998 with the support of several US-educated Chinese businessmen and reform minded officials in the Communist Party of China. Under Hu, *Caijing* was credited with blowing open the official cover-up of SARS in 2003, among others (*Caijing* 2004).[56] *Caijing* was said to have to have led the reporting of SARS beginning as early as February that year by starting to report about the disease in Hong Kong. It was well before the government and the official media acknowledged the scale of the danger. *Caijing* published investigative reports detailing "large-scale SARS infection incidents in hospitals..."[7]

Hu left *Caijing* after differences with the owners to co-found a similar investigative reporting platform – *Caixin*, in 2009. Under Hu, the winner of the 2014 Ramon Magsaysay award, *Caixin* has been one of the very few mainland China-based publications which has uncovered many stories on corporate and government corruption. Hu's *Caixin* is said to be surviving even under Xi Jinping's increasing control over media in China - which some say is witnessing its worst time since the days of Tiananmen Square 'incident' until Arab Spring.[8] This has been possible because of her connections including friendship with China's vice president Wang Qishan and lineage from a line of Communist Party intellectuals.[9]

The Renmin Ribao or its English version the *People's Daily* (PD)[10] on the other hand is the official mouthpiece of the CPC Central Committee and is seen as articulating its viewpoint since it began publishing on 15 June 1948. Though, there are other party media outlets, the PD is by far the "most official political daily newspaper" of the CPC. The PD is considered to be a ministerial-level media outlet along with the official *Xinhua* news agency and stands at the top of the CPC Propaganda Department (CPCPD) hierarchy.[11] The CCPPD vets the editorial of major Beijing newspapers. However, when it comes to the PD, the CPCPD also drafts the editorial in some cases. Same stands true for and main stories of *Xinhua*.[12]

The PD is a must-read for CPC cadres and government officials and is seen as the voice of the Chinese party-state. The importance of the newspaper can be gauged from the fact that nearly all the top leaders of China go to "inspect" the *People's Daily* on a chosen occasion and give a call to stick to the party's ideology.[13] It is the symbol of the mass media-led propaganda which has been accorded a prime status by the CPC leadership since its early years.[14]

In its own words, the PD over past six decades "has adhered to the correct direction from the party, and has actively and timely promoted its theory, line, principles and policies, and the central major decisions and plans…" both in China and abroad, to facilitate the CPC to "unite and lead the people across the country to a great victory in the revolution, construction and reform".[15] The PD is not known for breaking exclusive stories or showing how journalism is done. Its reputation is of being the flag bearer of the CPCCC and the guide of the public opinion in China. The paper is seen as authoritative statement of Chinese government policies and views government on various issues and it usually carries news about top Chinese leaders on the front page.[16] However, its editorials have been representative of "typical public discourse in China representing the Communist ideology of China" and its coverage often reflects the pushes and pulls inside the party and its leadership.[17]

This study examines the contrast in the coverage of coronavirus crisis by *Caixin* on one hand and the *People's Daily* and official news agency *Xinhua* on the other. The paper also takes into account the coverage of the English-language Tweets of *Caixin* and PD on COVID-19 during this period. By drawing upon the contrast, the paper tests how much substance is there in the charges that China and its media did substantially cover up coronavirus outbreak coverage in the initial days.

3. How PD and Chinese media in general covered COVID-19

Official Chinese media is known to follow the party-stateline. The founding principles of modern China says that media should fundamentally be the party's "ears, eyes, throat, and tongue".[18] Under current President Xi Jinping, although, it is de facto required to follow more of the leader himself.[19] That's increasingly true for China's top legislative and consultative bodies – the National People's Congress (NPC) and the Chinese People's Political Consultative Conference (CPPCC) – as well. At this year's NPC and CPPCC shortened annual session held in May, the NPC passed crucial regulations on privacy[20], biosecurity, first-ever draft civil code[21] and national security legislation for Hong Kong – all bearing Xi's mark on it and widely supported by the official Chinese media led by *Xinhua* and the PD. Repeating the leader's line, CPPCC Chairman Wang Yang called in his work report on 21 May for "preventing and controlling the virus, resuming work and production, stabilising public expectations and strengthening law-based governance".[22] In his address to the 13th NPC on 22 May, Premier Li Keqiang also praised the contribution of media personnel, among others. Li also declared a "decisive victory" against coronavirus in Hubei, though he conceded headwinds due to the infectious disease.[23]

The NPC still faced unexpected headwinds. On the eve of the high-profile annual session, Tsinghua University Professor Xu Zhangrun wrote a long commentary urging the country's leadership "to rethink its handling of the epidemic and apologise for its mistakes". Another Shanghai-based scholar Zhang Xuezhong wrote an open letter to NPC deputies in which he criticised China's handling of the pandemic and the country's political system. Liang Yanping, a Hubei University professor was also banned from teaching after she voiced support for Fang Fang - the award-winning documenter of life under lockdown in Wuhan.[24]

However, rather than questioning, arguing, debating and investigating the government and local administration's multiple failures in containing the coronavirus outbreak, Xi himself has been the core of the Chinese media narrative over the issue. State media has hailed Xi as the leading figure in China's battle against coronavirus while putting the blame of any mishandling on provincial officials.

The official media's narrative, led by *Xinhua* and the PD, has also continued to evolve as per the state's rhetoric on Xi. However, the PD stood a step ahead of all other official publications. To be specific, during the coronavirus crisis, the PD top stories often constituted a special propaganda series called "The General Secretary Came to My Home (总书记来过我的家)". The paper did not write anything about the coronavirus crisis until Xi Jinping gave his "important directions (重要指示)" on 20 January. Xi's written instructions on 20 January to openly report the coronavirus-related cases and prioritise the health and safety of people was reported prominently by the PD on 21 January.[25] Nevertheless, even after that, the coronavirus did not make it to the front page of the PD until on 26 January when the CPC Politburo Standing Committee (PSC) held a meeting on the issue. Over the next weeks either, only the subsequent PSC meetings and Xi's inspection tours, directives and speeches – including about the glorious achievements of Xi on the front of prosperity – made it to the PD's front page.

For nearly all other Chinese newspapers, the pandemic coverage started around late January with reporting about how Xi was leading the efforts to contain the outbreak. Xi's 20 January instructions were reported prominently by the wider Chinese media. Similar was the reporting on Xi's call for "scientific controls" during a top party meeting on 25 January. "If we maintain our confidence and work together with scientific controls and targeted measures, winning the battle of prevention and control against the epidemic will happen", Xi was quoted as saying. On 27 January, Xi instructed party members to "let the party flag fly high at the front line of the battleground" against COVID-19 and asked them to "keep in mind that the people's interests are the highest priority in the current arduous battle."

Since early February, official media highlighted Xi's push at the CPC Politburo Standing Committee (PSC) meetings for "law-based epidemic prevention and control" in which he warned against official cover-ups or negligence, illegal wildlife trade, rumours or resisting quarantine. The Chinese leader also called for tighter controls over public opinion and media[26] and the official media highlighted on 2 February that the CPC members were a "vanguard" against COVID-19.[27]

Meanwhile, Wuhan doctor Li Wenliang – who had tried to warn his colleagues about the virus in December - died from the virus on 7 February. His death sparked a social media outcry according to international media, a fact which remained largely unnoticed in the Chinese media. In a rare admission, the 16 February edition of party journal *Qiushi* revealed that Xi had acknowledged public discontent over the party-state's initial handling of the outbreak in his 5 February speech. Xi reportedly said that "the masses are dissatisfied".[28]

On 10 February, after his first public inspection of COVID-19, Xi called for a "people's war against novel coronavirus".[29] "Close attention must be paid to employment and large-scale layoffs should be avoided", Xi said and added... "minimize the impact of the epidemic on the economy and reach goals and tasks of economic and social development this year," *Xinhua* quoted on 11 February.[30] Following end of the extended Lunar New Year holidays on 10 February for regions outside Hubei, Chinese media joined Xi's message to resume work and production. At a meeting on 23 February, Xi pledged further policy support for businesses hit hard by the outbreak. The Chinese president called to "prevent economic growth from slipping out of the reasonable range" while noting that the virus would have an "unavoidable" and "considerable impact on the economy and society".[31]

On 11 February, all Chinese newspapers led by Xinhua, CPC mouthpiece PD and official broadcaster China Central Television (CCTV) showed Xi wearing mask and inspecting a hospital in Beijing. Party papers called him the "commander of the people's war against coronavirus" and underlined announcements made by him. Xinhua added (11 February 2020): "Under Xi's leadership, China has carried out national mobilization, across-the-board deployment and swift responses, adopted the most comprehensive and rigorous prevention and control measures and launched a people's war against the epidemic."

National broadcaster CCTV also released a series of video clips titled "General Secretary directs this people's war". They all have Xi in focus and are based on his directions, speeches and activities since the coroanvirus outbreak. The videos credit the Chinese leader for everything from deployment of medics and troops in Wuhan to punishment of hundreds of local officials for "disciplinary violations".[32]

On the other hand, official papers brushed aside criticism of Xi's "disappearance" during the outbreak. It took the Chinese media nearly a month after Xi's first instructions on combating the epidemic on 20 January, to reveal that he had given directives earlier than previously reported. Subsequently, timelines by *Xinhua*, *Renmin Ribao* (*People's Daily*) and other state media reported how Xi took "personal command" of the country's response to the outbreak from 7 January. The fact being original reports on those days made no mention of Xi's earlier instructions. Chinese media is yet to explain why Xi's instructions on containing the outbreak on 7 January did not make it to their reports at the time.

There was also little or no reporting of public petition by some academics in favour of free speech by the Chinese state media led by *Xinhua* and PD.[33] Rather, they highlighted replacement, firing and disciplining of officials in Wuhan and Hubei. Nationalist *Global Times*[34] – a bureau-level Beijing-based tabloid – reported replacement of party bosses in Hubei and Wuhan on 13 February and blamed the "city authorities' neglect of duty...they were slow to take measures in the face of the epidemic outbreak."[35]

Not that these are things which the Chinese media does not do on a regular basis. However, there seems to be a clear case of media changing goalposts to boost the successes of the state and the leader while ignoring the fault lines, as *Caixin*'s coverage would unveil. A key example would be the treatment of whistle-blower Dr. Li Wenliang from Wuhan. Dr Li was silenced by the local police in late December even as the labs had confirmed by then that the illnesses were indeed related to coronavirus. However, for weeks, the state and the local media did no mention of him. Once it started mentioning him in the first weeks of February, he was hardly given any importance beyond the party's "hero rhetoric" of hailing medics, soldiers, grassroot officials and community workers.

Chinese state media also helped glamorise the party's recruitment drive in late February by attracting front-line workers to tackle COVID-19 outbreak. "The move will encourage frontline personnel to win the battle with firm faith, tenacity and confidence", *Xinhua* quoted a circular issued by the Organization Department of the Central Committee of the CPC (CPCCC) on 26 February.[36]

Soon after authorities declared that the peak of the epidemic was over, around mid-March, official party papers began claiming victory over COVID-19. "After an intense battle against COVID-19, the peak of the epidemic in China is over. It is time for China to gear up to help other countries and help themselves resume a normal life," a *Xinhua* commentary declared on 14 March[37]. It added: "China always shares solutions with others. It published guidelines on COVID-19 diagnosis, treatment, prevention and control and shared them with more than 100 countries..." The papers wasted no time in comparing and praising China's response against COVID-19 compared to the steps taken by other countries.

In general, Chinese media has followed the official line in highlighting its success in controlling the pandemic. Chinese media has criticised foreign criticism of Beijing's handling of the coronavirus crisis domestically and what critics call its 'ruthless' pursuit of long-term foreign policy goals amid the pandemic.[38] State media also came heavily against charges of Chinese "predatory investments" and below standard medical supplies.[39] It has also rejected allegations of suppression of information and termed such charges as "politicising" and "stigmatising". Rather, in a series of articles, the PD[40,41] said that it was for other virus-hit nations to learn from China how to contain the spread of COVID-19. The trend continues.

4. *Caixin*'s coverage of COVID-19

Caixin's coverage of China's coronavirus crisis has been a sharp contrast compared to the PD. In *Caixin*'s English-language edition - oriented more towards audience from outside China - the first report on coronavirus was published at most on 6 January. The *Bloomberg* copy[42] published by *Caixin* talked about the widening of Pneumonia outbreak in China's Wuhan. On 9 January, *Caixin* published two stories citing CCTV and the World Health Organisation (WHO) which for the first time mentioned about the possibility of the new infections being caused due to "an emerging type of coronavirus".[43] Since, then one after another factual copies kept coming on *Caixin* – not always investigative, break through stories, not far away from the official media's line but enough which gave the indication of the extent of the crisis. To be fair, even Hu's *Caixin* cannot be expected to replicate 2003 SARS coverage in Xi's China. Yet, at least by 20-21 January - the time when PD started covering the issues – *Caixin*'s coverage had laid it threadbare.

A *Caixin* copy on 21 January[44] about capital market crash noted Xi weighing in on the outbreak and "urging a redoubling of control and prevention efforts to ensure a stable and peaceful Spring Festival." The WHO was yet to declare the coronavirus a global health emergency even towards the end of January, however, *Caixin*'s headlines were telling. On 25 January, *Caixin* published the first "Reporter's Notebook" – sort of investigative story about overwhelmed hospitals. On 29 January, one more *Caixin* report[45] questioned the inevitable: "Was there a cover-up?" The content of the subhead made it amply evident, that there indeed was a cover up.

On the following days, *Caixin* almost regularly published stories both in its English and Chinese editions which can be called journalistic. This included one on 31 January which talked about the Weibo post of Zhejiang University professor Wang Liming. Wang, who has nearly half a million followers on Weibo wrote: "I'm beyond furious...This is the first time that I've found unmistakable evidence that human-to-human transmission of the new coronavirus has been intentionally hidden". His post went viral and was deleted, *Caixin* mentioned. From 3 February onwards, *Caixin* also published a four-part in-depth report about: "How Wuhan lost the fight to contain the coronavirus".[46]

In brief, when the party-affiliated newspapers kept pliantly toeing the state line without asking the right questions, *Caixin* poked some big hole in the official rhetoric. One of the most remarkable of them came on 29 February 2020. The *Caixin* investigative article published with inputs of eight journalists[47] noted that the new coronavirus was sequenced in Chinese labs "weeks before officials publicly identified it as the cause of a mysterious viral pneumonia cluster in Wuhan". It said: "Test results from multiple labs in December suggested there was an outbreak of a new virus. However, the results failed to trigger a response that could have prepared the public, despite being fed into an infectious disease control system that was designed to alert China's top health officials about outbreaks."

The article noted: "As early as December 27, a Guangzhou-based genomics company had sequenced most of the virus from fluid samples from the lung of a 65-year old deliveryman who worked at the seafood market where many of the first cases emerged. The results showed an alarming similarity to the deadly SARS coronavirus." And yet when Dr. Li Wenliang expressed alarm online on 30 December, he was reprimanded by the local police for "spreading rumours". On 31 December, China notified the WHO about an "unidentified infectious disease" even as several private firm including industry leader BGI had confirmed by then that it was a "previously unseen coronavirus".

Rather than acknowledging the findings, the "gene sequencing companies received an order from Hubei's health commission to stop testing and destroy all samples..." On 3 January, the country's top health authority, the National Health Commission "ordered institutions not to publish any information related to the unknown disease and ordered labs to transfer any samples they had to designated testing institutions, or to destroy them." The order did not specify the designated institutions, *Caixin* added.

Almost a week later on 9 January 2020, Beijing finally announced that a "novel coronavirus was behind Wuhan's viral pneumonia outbreak" even as it downplayed that the virus could transmit from humam-to-human. It took another 12 days and almost a month since the private firm Vision Medicals also concluded it being a new coronavirus that China confirmed it transmitted between humans.

The above sequence of events shows there is little doubt that whether the Wuhan lab was the source of infection or not, China did play hide and seek in keeping the public and the world informed about the extent of the danger COVID-19 posed and *Caixin* played a crucial role in it. As mentioned earlier, *Caixin* is not immune to China's politics and it does have to balance it coverage. As on 12 April, a *Caixin* article noted that China's government was paternalistic and likely to impose "one-size-fits-all measures at considerable human cost". However, it also underlined the advantages of the model by encouraging the communities to respond to the challenges posed by COVID-19, among others, and advised against "ideological bigotry".[48] In China's journalism landscape of today, even to call this much consistently is a feat.

4.1 State media and Caixin on Economy post COVID-19

After reports of GDP and per capita disposable falling by 6.8 per cent and 3.9 per cent respectively year-on-year in January to March quarter came, on 23 April, *Caixin* underlined growing pressure on China to bring it back on track. It noted "collapse in China's economic growth caused by the COVID-19 pandemic" and the difficulties in recovery. The article said that despite the government taking several measures to spur economic activity, "millions of small businesses and households are battling to survive, and unemployment, especially among migrant workers, has remained elevated." It warned quoting economists that the "traditional stimulus measures" such as lending bank and infrastructure spending "may not be sufficient this time around". It added: "Many analysts expect GDP will continue to shrink in the second quarter, albeit at a narrower pace...."[49]

The same week, the *People's Daily*'s (English edition) economy or opinion section gave no indication of China's economic troubles in any of the three dozen odd stories published. A Xinhua factual report copy on 22 April[50] discussed the decision to give targeted assistance to small businesses and the State Council promise "to enhance support to those living in poverty, living on minimum subsistence allowances or unemployed..." Another Xinhua copy claimed that Beijing was "bent not broken" despite GDP contraction and that China was "powering ahead in returning to work and resuming business and production."

5. Case study: Suppression of citizen journalists

Chinese citizen journalists who reported about gaps in coronavirus management in Wuhan and elsewhere have faced repercussions. International media reported about at least three citizen journalists who – after their independent reporting of the ground realities - went missing. Twenty-five years old Li Zehua went missing in Wuhan after he posted a video on YouTube on 20 February showing porters being hired for transporting corpses of people who likely died of coronavirus. He also posted live video footage of police raiding his home afterwards.[51] Li was released only after weeks of what appears to be a forced quarantine on 23 April.[52]

Two other citizen journalists, former rights lawyer Chen Qiushi and Wuhan businessman Fang Bin met similar fate for posting reports about overcrowded hospitals. When Fang posted a video of dead bodies stuck up in a minibus outside a hostel. However, he was reportedly released soon, apparently due to the global attention he got.[53]

In line with media's restrained role in China, on 4 February, the CPC's Propaganda Department announced sending 300 journalists to ensure that the rhetoric regarding the control and prevention of COVID-19 remains under its control.[54] The CPCPD objective was in line with a key CPC meeting on 3 February chaired by Xi himself. The meeting called for strengthening control over online media and, publicising and showcasing front line workers' fight against coronavirus and the unity of the Chinese people under the leadership of the party.[55] What is also important to point here is that the English version of the same meeting published by *Xinhua* itself had no such details.[56]

Chinese author Fang Fang's online diary with details of Wuhan people's sufferings during the new coronavirus and criticism of the government's mishandling of the crisis also deserves mention. Fang wrote a hard-hitting update regularly for 60 days which was followed by thousands of Chinese netizens. Her diary was published soon after as a book. She writes: "I kept wondering, since I had first heard about this virus back on December 31, how come everyone had such a lax attitude about it for the following 20 days? We should have already learned our lessons from the SARS outbreak back in 2003." She further says: "To be perfectly frank, part of the reason is that we had been too careless, and there are also objective life situations that contributed to that. But more important is the fact that we have placed too much faith in our government. We had faith that there was no way that the governmental leaders in Hubei Province would adopt such a lax and irresponsible attitude when it came to such a critical event where lives were in the balance. We also had faith that they would never hold fast to their 'political correctness' and old ways of doing business in the face of a new threat that could affect the lives of millions of people." She further said: "Deeply ingrained habitual behaviours, like reporting the good news while hiding the bad, preventing people from speaking the truth, forbidding the public from understanding the true nature of events, and expressing a disdain for individual lives have led to massive reprisals against our society, untold injuries against our people, and even terrible reprisals against those officials themselves.... It is absolutely essential that we continue to fight until those responsible are held accountable."

If none of the above was enough, China did everything in its capacity to censor content that could go against the party-state at the highest level both at the domestic and the international level. Of course, even against Fang Fang, Chinese cyber nationalists humiliated her as soon as it became know that her work were to be published abroad. Several users accused her of being a traitor and capitalising on a tragedy for fame. A few though continued to see merit in her writings. [57]

6. Case study: English Tweets by PD and *Caixin*

The English-language Tweets of PD (@PDChina) and Caixin (@caixin) – both primarily catering to the wider world and an upwardly mobile section of Chinese - present some interesting insights. To understand it, this paper did a case study of 3200 Tweets by PD and *Caixin* before 10 May 2020. The Tweets were sourced from Vicintas.io – an onlineTweet analysis platform. The *Caixin* Tweets went back to 5 November 2019 - however, 3200 PD Tweets ended up till 25 February. Clearly, @PDChina has been much more active on Twitter compared to @caixin. To assess the engagement with the readers, this study took into account only retweets as it is considered to be reflecting the highest level of engagement.

As on 10 May, PD had more than 7 million followers compared to a little above 85000 for Caixin. However, unlike PD, Caixin's Tweets usually are serious hard-core stories. The PD – which claims to be China's biggest newspaper and party mouthpiece– Tweets soft stories accompanied by a video almost on a daily basis. The analysis of the 3200 Tweets of PD shows that its most retweeted Tweet was one about a video showing a unique friendship among 11 ducks in a Chinese neighbourhood:

> "What a unique friendship! Chinese netizen shared videos showing every morning the neighbor's ducks come to his door and call for their friends, then all 11 ducks go to the river together. (https://t.co/jNfU77Aso1)"

The above Tweet was retweeted 15,384 times between 10 March and 10 May. The second highest retweeted story was about coronavirus but stood a distant second with 3581 retweets:

> "Not one is infected with #Covid_19 among the 40,000 medics from across China aiding Hubei. How do they do that? Video shows you how many layers of protection they need. https://t.co/r9bniL1lN5"

The above one and the next 11 most retweeted PD stories were about coronavirus – but none even mildly questioned coronavirus-related cover up or anything. To be fair, they all support Chinese official propaganda of the situation being well in control.

Caixin's Twitter handle on the other claims to be pursuing "Award-winning journalism from China's most respected newsroom." *Caixin*'s most retweeted story was a Tweet on 25 February about coronavirus. It was retweeted 613 times till 10 May.

> "In China's Guangdong province, 14% of recovered COVID-19 patients tested positive for the virus in later checkups, raising the question whether recovered patients can still infect others. https://t.co/Y7xdi4hccJ"

The Tweet clearly raises some questions about recovered patients in Guangdong. The next 10 most retweeted Caixin stories were all on coronavirus. Almost all of them raised valid questions – some of them difficult ones as the three below:

> "No words can adequately describe the sacrifices of the people of Wuhan. I say to the government: You need to rein in your arrogance and humbly offer thanks to your masters – in this case, the millions of people in Wuhan," writes local writer Fang Fang. https://t.co/xmnaEh1a4I.

> The only thing some Chinese plants are manufacturing is false data, a @Caixin investigation has found. https://t.co/I4wYJlQ2o0.

> "As early as Dec. 27, test results from labs suggested there was an outbreak of a highly infectious virus in Wuhan. That was more than three weeks before Chinese authorities confirmed publicly that the virus was spreading between people.#coronavirus https://t.co/wsWWaomyOA https://t.co/2Ksa42eU9q".

The above testimony sufficiently tells the priorities of PD and justify claims about China and Chinese media launching a Twitter-offensive to shape rhetoric on coronavirus.[58,59]

7. Conclusion: Comparing the official response: SARS vs COVID-19

The first SARS case was registered in China's Southern Guangdong province on 16 November 2002[60] and Beijing reported the incident to the WHO, almost after six weeks on 26 December 2003.[61]. The epidemic peaked in February 2003 and the WHO issued a global alert on 12 March 2003.[62] Even as the situation kept going

Figure 4.1: Caixin's top Tweets:

1	Tweet Id	Text	Name	Screen Nar	UTC	Created At	Favorites	Retweets	Language
2	12324391	In China's Guangdong province, 14% of recovered Covid-19 patients t	Caixin Glol	caixin	2020-02-25T22:56:	Tue Feb 25 22:56:04 +0000 2020	633	613	en
3	12295043	Biggest coronavirus study finds more than 3,000 infected Chinese me	Caixin Glol	caixin	2020-02-17T20:34:	Mon Feb 17 20:34:07 +0000 2020	478	450	en
4	12368249	When sending a #coronavirus patient to a CT scan, a doctor in Wuhar	Caixin Glol	caixin	2020-03-09T01:23:	Mon Mar 09 01:23:40 +0000 2020	1565	404	en
5	12369213	Another doctor in #Wuhan has succumbed to the #coronavirus. Zhu H	Caixin Glol	caixin	2020-03-09T07:46:	Mon Mar 09 07:46:56 +0000 2020	431	313	en
6	12261275	A key test used to confirm new #coronavirus cases is failing to catch	Caixin Glol	caixin	2020-02-08T12:56:	Sat Feb 08 12:56:06 +0000 2020	274	253	en
7	12201505	I stayed in Wuhan as the last trains pulled out, along with a few Caixi	Caixin Glol	caixin	2020-01-23T01:05:	Thu Jan 23 01:05:26 +0000 2020	458	248	en
8	12380786	"No words can adequately describe the sacrifices of the people of Wu	Caixin Glol	caixin	2020-03-12T12:25:	Thu Mar 12 12:25:29 +0000 2020	433	210	en
9	12420837	As of Sunday, Hubei province said it had zero new "confirmed cases"	Caixin Glol	caixin	2020-03-23T13:40:	Mon Mar 23 13:40:08 +0000 2020	193	178	en
10	12351846	The only thing some Chinese plants are manufacturing is false data, a	Caixin Glol	caixin	2020-03-04T12:45:	Wed Mar 04 12:45:43 +0000 2020	232	171	en
11	12435211	Some funeral houses in #Wuhan began to allow people to pick up ash	Caixin Glol	caixin	2020-03-27T12:51:	Fri Mar 27 12:51:52 +0000 2020	179	166	en
12	12333654	As early as Dec. 27, test results from labs suggested there was an ou	Caixin Glol	caixin	2020-02-28T12:17:	Fri Feb 28 12:17:01 +0000 2020	246	163	en
13	12214454	#nCoV2019 update: - Worldwide confirmed #coronavirus cases rise to	Caixin Glol	caixin	2020-01-26T14:50:	Sun Jan 26 14:50:56 +0000 2020	122	145	en
14	12017335	The quickening speed of bond defaults in China, especially among ail	Caixin Glol	caixin	2019-12-03T05:23:	Tue Dec 03 05:23:04 +0000 2019	192	140	en
15	12308612	At least five of China's prisons have confirmed a whopping 512 cases	Caixin Glol	caixin	2020-02-21T14:26:	Fri Feb 21 14:26:05 +0000 2020	107	117	en
16	12292563	The Wuhan Institute of Virology, the only P4 level biosafety laborator	Caixin Glol	caixin	2020-02-17T04:08:	Mon Feb 17 04:08:56 +0000 2020	155	107	en

Figure 4.2: PD's top Tweets

1	Tweet Id	Text	Name	Screen Nar	UTC	Created At	Favorites	Retweets	Language
2	12374317	What a unique friendship! Chinese netizen shared videos showing every morning the neighbor's ducks cor	People's D	PDChina	2020-03-10T17:	Tue Mar 1	9834	15384	en
3	12435508	Not one is infected with #Covid_19 among the 40,000 medics from across China aiding Hubei. How do the	People's D	PDChina	2020-03-27T14:	Fri Mar 27	7104	3581	en
4	12410468	After 58 days of lockdown, #Wuhan train station sees one last full-front disinfection work before it reoper	People's D	PDChina	2020-03-20T17:	Fri Mar 20	6150	2710	en
5	12388800	The novel #coronavirus may cause testicular damage and male infertility, Chinese experts found, recomm	People's D	PDChina	2020-03-14T17:	Sat Mar 14	2959	2626	en
6	12405110	"The pandemic of influenza in 2009 originated in North America, we didn't call it North American flu," @D	People's D	PDChina	2020-03-19T05:	Thu Mar 1	5573	1956	en
7	12471671	The role of mask: comparison of airflow when people wearing and not wearing mask talk and cough. (vide	People's D	PDChina	2020-04-06T14:	Mon Apr 0	2590	1673	en
8	12406422	#Wuhan police announced to revoke the reprimand order against Dr. Li Wenliang and solemnly apologize	People's D	PDChina	2020-03-19T14:	Thu Mar 1	2589	1586	en
9	12352878	Chinese scientists found the novel #coronavirus has two strains, of which the more infectious type shows	People's D	PDChina	2020-03-04T19:	Wed Mar (	2543	1426	en
10	12506652	Remember to wear a mask in public like this baby from Henan, who always puts his mask back on quickly	People's D	PDChina	2020-04-16T06:	Thu Apr 16	4676	1346	en
11	12409562	How many times of hand washing do you count as the doctor takes off the protective set? https://t.co/Tjv	People's D	PDChina	2020-03-20T11:	Fri Mar 20	2199	1272	en
12	12407171	A team of 13 Chinese medical staff arrived in #Milan, #Italy to help contain the #Covid_19 #pandemic. Th	People's D	PDChina	2020-03-19T19:	Thu Mar 1	4188	1227	en
13	12340255	Do you think it is just a girl playing with ink and a broom? No rush, watch till the end. https://t.co/Rh8Oj4	People's D	PDChina	2020-03-01T08:	Sun Mar 0	4800	1184	en
14	12362797	#BREAKING: A hotel building collapsed in Quanzhou, SE China's Fujian at around 7 pm Saturday, trapping	People's D	PDChina	2020-03-07T13:	Sat Mar 07	1428	980	en
15	12398429	#China has completed its clinical research on #Favilavir, an antiviral drug for #COVID19. The drug has sho	People's D	PDChina	2020-03-17T09:	Tue Mar 1	1648	972	en
16	12377425	#Photo_of_the_day: The last night at #Wuhan's last makeshift hospital, Doctor Jiang Wenyang is lying on	People's D	PDChina	2020-03-11T14:	Wed Mar 1	2679	902	en

out of control, it took the CPC's top decision-making body – the PSC, almost 22 weeks after the first case appeared in Guangdong, to issue directions.[63] On 20 April 2003, the PSC "warned against the covering up of SARS cases and demanded the accurate, timely, and honest reporting of the SARS situation.[64]

Renowned Chinese respiratory specialist Zhong Nanshan who has become of the face of China's war to contain coronavirus wrote a paper in 2006 on lessons from SARS. Zhong became famous in April 2003 when he confronted the official assurance that the SARS outbreak was under control. He had said: "The virus is still spreading, so how can we say it's under control?"[65] Zhong wrote in the paper[66] that a key lesson learnt from almost three SARS outbreaks in China between November 2002 and May 2004 was that: "In an emergent event, an information blackout makes absolutely no sense."

Zhong further argued: "The first case of SARS appeared in Guangdong province, China, in November 2002, but information about it was not broadcast on Central TV...until February 2003, though rumours spread via cell phones and the internet...the absence of open news was an attempt to maintain social stability. But the silence led to panic buying...Soaring prices...undermining the intended social stability. Things began to change when information, in the form of daily roundups on SARS epidemics and public education on disease prevention, reached the community." In his suggestions to better contain any similar outbreak next time, Zhong put the onus on health workers and collaboration. As *Caixin* coverage showed, China ignored both the factors during the initial days of the COVID-19 outbreak.

Critics had been more forthcoming. Jonathan Mirsky noted[67] in an article that "Communist China's long obsession with secrecy is one cause of the present SARS crisis. This passion for secrets. . .is heightened by a conviction common to all Communist countries: any disaster, natural or man-made, can reflect badly on the Party...Low-ranking officials who cannot conceal secrets will not rise through the hierarchy, and the highest officials hesitate before telling some or all of the truth." He concluded by saying Beijing has not learnt "that the truth should be told about 'negative' events". China's critics have been no less generous this time either. One western commentator wrote:[68] "The Chinese Communist Party is the most destabilizing force in the world today. It is a real threat to peace, prosperity and security around the globe."

Another fact is that coronavirus has spilled over from lab earlier. A paper (Furmanski 2014) noted that "SARS is particularly dangerous to handle in the laboratory because there is no vaccine, so all laboratory workers are susceptible.... Moreover, about 5% of SARS patients are 'super-spreaders' who pass the infection to many (over 8) secondary cases.... The existence of SARS 'super-spreaders' makes even a single laboratory infection into a potential pandemic. SARS has not naturally recurred, but there have been six separate 'escapes' from virology labs studying it: one each in Singapore and Taiwan, and in four distinct events at the same laboratory in Beijing." Following a spill over of SARS infection from Chinese National Institute of Virology (NIV), part of China's Centre for Disease Control (CDC), the WHO had expressed "serious concerns" about its biosafety procedures.[69]

Nobody will ever know what happened with COVID-19. For now, after 'successfully' 'controlling' the domestic narrative on Coronavirus outbreak inside the country, Beijing is busy influencing global opinion about China's role in it. China Foreign Ministry and embassy officials have increased their engagement over non-Chinese social media platforms such as Twitter – a service which remains banned in the country. Meanwhile, Chinese media except rare exceptions such as *Caixin* have joined hands in promoting a favourable view of China and giving more space than ever before to similar articles and opinions expressed elsewhere.

NOTES

1 Fan, Yi, Kai Zhao, Zheng-Li Shi, and Peng Zhou, "Bat Coronaviruses in China." *Viruses* 2019, 11 (3), https://doi.org/10.3390/v11030210.

2 Roland Oliphant, Nicola Smith and Henry Samuel, "The inside Story of the Wuhan Virus Laboratory Blamed by President Trump for Releasing Covid-19," *The Daily Telegraph*, May 4, 2020 at https://www.telegraph.co.uk/news/0/wuhan-virus-inside-story-laboratory-blamed-donald-trump/.

3 Following publications can be consulted on how the Chinese media has addressed pandemics or structurally how the party-state media functions in China:

i) Molter, Vanessa, and Renee DiResta, "Pandemics & Propaganda: How Chinese State Media Creates and Propagates CCP Coronavirus Narratives," *Harvard Kennedy School Misinformation Review* 2020 1 (3), https://doi.org/10.37016/mr-2020-025.

ii) Jha, Tilak, "中國改革時代的媒體與輿論." 全球政治評論 [Media and Public Opinion in China's Reform Era]: 39-52, https://gioip.nchu.edu.tw/uploads/asset/data/5c8de2e31d41c84ce8000784/%E5%85%A8%E7%90%83%E7%89% B9%E9%9B%86002-tilak_jha.pdf.

iii) Rawnsley, Gary D., and T. Rawnsley Ming-yeh, (eds.), *Routledge handbook of Chinese media*, Routledge.

iv) Shao, Guosong, Jiayin Lu, and Ye Hao, "Assessing China's Media Reform," Asian Perspective 40(1): 27-50.

v) Jinqiu, Zhao, "The SARS epidemic under China's media policy," *Media Asia* 30(4): 191-196.

vi) Verma, Raj, "China's diplomacy and changing the COVID-19 narrative", *International Journal* (2020): 0020702020930054.

vii) Xie, Baohui, *Media transparency in China: Rethinking rhetoric and reality,* Lexington Books.

viii) Stockmann, Daniela, *Media commercialization and authoritarian rule in China*, Cambridge University Press 2013, Harvard.

ix) Volland, Nicolai, *The Control of the Media in the People's Republic of China*, Ph.D. Dissertation 2003, Germany: University of Hiedelberg, http://www.ub.uni-heidelberg.de/archiv/8048.

x) Tong, Jingrong, and Sparks, Colin, "Investigative journalism in China today," *Journalism Studies* 10(3): 337-352.

4 "China Accused of Sars Cover-Up," *The Guardian*, April 9, 2003 at http://www.theguardian.com/world/2003/apr/09/sars.china.

5 ChanHo-him and Bai Tongdong, "Editor of Leading Chinese Financial Magazine 'steps Aside, Not Down'" *SCMP,* January 30, 2018 at https://www.scmp.com/news/china/policies-politics/article/2131157/chinas-top-business-magazine-editor-hu-shuli-steps.

6 Martin Furmanski, "Laboratory Escapes and 'Self-Fulfilling Prophecy' Epidemics." Scientist's Working Group on Chemical and Biologic Weapons Center for Arms Control and Non-proliferation, February 2014 at https://armscontrolcenter.org/wp-content/uploads/2016/02/Escaped-Viruses-final-2-17-14-copy.pdf.

7 Yu Sun, "Lessons from SARS Coverage," *Nieman Foundation*, December 15, 2003, at https://nieman.harvard.edu/articles/lessons-from-sars-coverage/.

8 Aris Teon, "The Deterioration of China's Media Freedom in the Xi Jinping Era" *The Greater China Journal*, February 20, 2020 at https://china-journal.org/2019/02/20/the-deterioration-of-chinas-media-freedom-in-the-xi-jinping-era/.

9 Emma Graham-Harrison and Tom Phillips, "How One Brave Woman Is Taking on Growing Might of China's Censors," *The Guardian,* March 13, 2016 at http://www.theguardian.com/world/2016/mar/13/china-censorship-economy-editor.

10 Zhao, Yuezhi, *Media, market, and democracy in China: Between the party line and the bottom line,* Vol. 148 (University of Illinois Press 1998).

11 Wang Haiyan, Colins Sparks and Huang Yu, "Measuring differences in the Chinese press: A study of People's Daily and Southern Metropolitan Daily," *Global Media and China*, 3(3): 125-140 at https://doi.org/10.1177%2F2059436418806022.

12 Shambaugh, David, "China's propaganda system: Institutions, processes and efficacy," In *Critical Readings on the Communist Party of China*, (Brill 2017: 713-751).

13 Zhang, Xiaoling, *The transformation of political communication in China: From propaganda to hegemony,* Vol. 29. (World Scientific 2011: 96).

14 Zang, Xiaowei, ed. *Understanding Chinese Society* (Routledge 2015).

15 人民日报社简介 [People's Daily Profile], *Renmin Ribao (People's Daily)* at http://www.people.com.cn/GB/50142/104580/index.html.

16 Qian Shaochang, *People's Daily and China Daily: a comparative study,* Gazette (Leiden, Netherlands) 40(1): 57-68.

17 Wu Rongquan, Karen, "Public discourse as the mirror of ideological change: a keyword study of editorials in People's Daily," In Proceedings of the Corpus Linguistics 2001 conference.

18 Young Doug, *The Party Line: How The Media Dictates Public Opinion in Modern China* (John Wiley & Sons, 2013).

19 Brady, Anne-Marie, "Plus çachange?: Media control under Xi Jinping," *Problems of Post-Communism* 2017, 64(3-4): 128-140.

20 "China drafting law on personal information protection", *Xinhua*, 14 May 2020 at http://www.xinhuanet.com/english/2020-05/14/c_139057466.htm.

21 "Xinhua Special: China adopts world's first modern-day civil code", *Xinhua*, 28 May 2020 at http://www.xinhuanet.com/english/2020-05/28/c_139095781.htm.

22 "China to introduce national security legislation for HKSAR", *Xinhua*, 22 May 2020 at http://www.xinhuanet.com/english/2020-05/22/c_139076678.htm.

23 "Full text: Premier Li's speech at the third session of the 13th NPC", *CGTN*, 22 May 2020 at

https://news.cgtn.com/news/2020-05-22/Full-text-Premier-Li-s-speech-at-the-third-session-of-the-13th-NPC-QHaP1FpB8k/index.html.

24 Zhang, Pinghui, "Chinese professor banned from teaching over Hong Kong protest comments", *SCMP* 20 June 2020 at https://www.scmp.com/news/china/politics/article/3089929/chinese-professor-banned-teaching-over-hong-kong-protest

25 习近平：要把人民群众生命安全和身体健康放在第一位坚决遏制疫情蔓延势头[Xi Jinping: Prioritise people's life and health to resolutely curb the spread of the coronavirus epidemic], *People's Daily,* 21 January 2020 at http://cpc.people.com.cn/n1/2020/0121/c64094-31557684.html.

26 习近平总书记关于新冠肺炎疫情防控工作重要论述及外方积极表态 [Xi's important statements on prevention and control of new coronavirus epidemic and foreign praise], Chinese Embassy in Mauritania, March 3, 2020 at http://mr.china-embassy.org/chn/sgzyhd/t1753876.htm.

27 "Xi Focus: Commanding China's fight against novel coronavirus outbreak" *Xinhua,* February 2, 2020 at http://www.xinhuanet.com/english/2020-02/02/c_138749978.htm.

28 *Bloomberg*, "Rare release of Chinese President Xi Jinping's speech on coronavirus puzzles top China watchers", *Strait Times*, February 18, 2020 at https://www.straitstimes.com/asia/east-asia/rare-release-of-chinese-president-xi-jinpings-speech-on-coronavirus-puzzles-top-china.

29 *Xinhua*, "Xi Focus: Xi Vows to Win People's War against Novel Coronavirus," English.news.cn, April 11, 2020 at http://www.xinhuanet.com/english/2020-02/11/c_138771934.htm.

30 "Xi vows to win people's war against novel coronavirus", *Xinhua,* February 11, 2020 at http://www.xinhuanet.com/english/2020-02/11/c_138771934.htm.

31 Orange Wang, "Coronavirus: China pledges to hit 2020 targets despite economic impact of epidemic," *SCMP,* February 24, 2020 at https://www.scmp.com/economy/china-economy/article/3052088/coronavirus-china-pledges-hit-2020-targets-despite-economic.

32 时政微视频〔3〕丨总书记指挥这场人民战争——重地之战_央视新闻客户端_央视网 [Major Battle-ground." Text and Video. General Secretary Directs This People's War] *CCTV*, March 8, 2020 at http://m.news.cctv.com/2020/03/08/ARTIAbien7wCke9VhoJ27n83200308.shtml.

33 William Zheng, "Beijing Purges Top Officials at Coronavirus Epicenter amid Public Anger," *SCMP*, February 13, 2020 at https://www.inkstonenews.com/politics/beijing-purges-top-officials-epicenter-coronavirus-outbreak-amid-public-anger/article/3050451.

34 "Govt Must Continue Efforts against NCP," *Global Times*, February 11, 2020 at https://www.globaltimes.cn/content/1179239.shtml.

35 Chen Qingqing and Zhao Yusha, "China Reshuffles Top Officials in Coronavirus Epicenter Hubei Province," *Global Times*, February 13, 2020 at https://www.globaltimes.cn/content/1179429.shtml.

36 "CPC to recruit new members at epidemic-fighting frontline", *Xinhua,* February 26, 2020 at http://www.xinhuanet.com/english/2020-02/26/c_138821713.htm.

37 "Commentary: Transitioning to a post-peak epidemic phase in China", *Xinhua,* March 14, 2020 at http://www.xinhuanet.com/english/2020-03/14/c_138877437.htm.

38 Alex Ward, "How China Is Ruthlessly Exploiting the Coronavirus Pandemic It Helped Cause," *Vox*. April 28, 2020 at https://www.vox.com/2020/4/28/21234598/coronavirus-china-xi-jinping-foreign-policy.

39 "China's Coronavirus Diplomacy Has Finally Pushed Europe Too Far," *Bloomberg*, April 22, 2020 at https://www.bloombergquint.com/politics/china-s-coronavirus-diplomacy-has-finally-pushed-europe-too-far.

40 中国持续援助发展中国家战疫 [China assists developing countries in fight against epidemic], *People's Daily*, April 6, 2020 at http://paper.people.com.cn/rmrbhwb/html/2020-04/04/content_1980094.htm.

41 病毒溯源要以科学为依据 [Efforts to trace virus should be based on science], *People's Daily*, April 23, 2020 at http://paper.people.com.cn/rmrb/html/2020-04/23/nw.D110000renmrb_20200423_4-01.htm.

42 *Bloomberg*, "China's Pneumonia Outbreak Widens to 59 Amid Hunt for Source" *Caixin*, January 6, 2020 at https://www.caixinglobal.com/2020-01-06/pneumonia-outbreak-widens-to-59-amid-hunt-for-source-101501347.html.

43 Mathew Walsh, "New Virus in SARS Family May Be Cause of China's Pneumonia Outbreak," *Caixin*, Jan 9, 2020 at https://www.caixinglobal.com/2020-01-09/new-virus-in-sars-family-may-be-cause-of-pneumonia-outbreak-101502535.html.

44 Han Wei and Wei Yan, "China's Spreading Coronavirus Sends Jitters to Capital Markets", *Caixin*, Jan 21, 2020 at https://www.caixinglobal.com/2020-01-21/chinas-spreading-coronavirus-sends-jitters-to-capital-markets-101506504.html.

45 Guo Yingzhe, "Novel Coronavirus: What We Know So Far", *Caixin*, Jan 29, 2020 at https://www.caixinglobal.com/2020-01-29/novel-coronavirus-what-we-know-so-far-101509383.html.

46 Gao Yu et. al, "In Depth: How Wuhan Lost the Fight to Contain the Coronavirus". *Caixin*, February 3, 2020 at https://www.caixinglobal.com/2020-02-03/in-depth-how-wuhan-lost-the-fight-to-contain-the-coronavirus-101510749.html,

47 Gao, Yu. et.al, "How Early Signs of a SARS-Like Virus Were Spotted, Spread, and Throttled" *Caixin*, February 29, 2020 at https://www.caixinglobal.com/2020-02-29/in-depth-how-early-signs-of-a-sars-like-virus-were-spotted-spread-and-throttled-101521745.html.

48 Song Bing, "Opinion: A Country's Culture Is Fundamental to How It Fights Covid-19" *Caixin* April 12, 2020 at https://www.caixinglobal.com/2020-04-12/a-countrys-culture-is-fundamental-to-how-it-fights-covid-19-101541609.html.

49 Guo Yingzhe, "In Depth: Pressure Grows on China to Step Up Help for Economy," *Caixin*, April 23, 2020 at https://www.caixinglobal.com/2020-04-23/in-depth-pressure-grows-on-china-to-step-up-help-for-economy-101546346.html.

50 *Xinhua*, "China to Enhance Assistance to People in Need, Small Firms," *People's Daily*, April 22, 2020 at http://en.people.cn/n3/2020/0422/c90000-9682586.html.

51 Jane, Li, "Another citizen journalist covering the coronavirus has gone missing in Wuhan", *QZ.com*, 12 February 2020 at https://qz.com/1801361/wuhan-virus-citizen-journalists-fang-bin-chen-qiushi-go-missing/.

52 Yew Lun Tian, "Chinese citizen journalist resurfaces after going missing in Wuhan", *Reuters*, 23 April 2020 at https://in.reuters.com/article/health-coronavirus-china-journalist/chinese-citizen-journalist-resurfaces-after-going-missing-in-wuhan-idINKCN225161.

53 "Coronavirus: Why have two reporters in Wuhan disappeared?" *BBC*, 14 February 2020 at https://www.bbc.com/news/world-asia-china-51486106.

54 中宣部调集 300 多名记者深入湖北和武汉进行采访 [The CPCPD to mobilise more than 300 journalists to conduct interviews in Hubei and Wuhan], *Sina News*, 4 February 2020 at https://news.sina.com.cn/c/2020-02-05/doc-iimxyqvz0328664.shtml.

55 中共中央政治局常务委员会召开会议研究加强新型冠状病毒感染的肺炎疫情防控工作中共中央总书记习近平主持会议[CPC General Secretary Xi Jinping presides over CPCCC Politburo Standing Committee meeting to study and strengthen prevention and control work of pneumonia outbreaks caused by new coronavirus infection], *Xinhua*, 2 February at http://www.xinhuanet.com/politics/leaders/2020-02/03/c_1125527334.htm.

56 "Xi chairs leadership meeting on epidemic control", *Xinhua*, 3 February 2020 at http://www.xinhuanet.com/english/2020-02/03/c_138753250.htm.

57 "Fang Fang: The Wuhan writer whose virus diary angered China", *BBC*, 18 May 2020 at https://www.bbc.com/news/world-asia-china-52712358.

58 Betsy Morris and Robert McMillan, "China Pushes Viral Messages to Shape Coronavirus Narrative", *The Wall Street Journal*, April 10, 2020 at https://www.wsj.com/articles/china-pushes-viral-messages-to-shape-coronavirus-narrative-11586516402.

59 Anna Schecter, "China launches new Twitter accounts, 90,000 tweets in COVID-19 info war," *NBCnews.com*, May 20, 2020 at https://www.nbcnews.com/news/world/china-launches-new-twitter-accounts-90-000-tweets-covid-19-n1207991.

60 WHO, "Update 10 - Data from China, countries introduce stringent control measures," March 26, 2020 at http://www10.who.int/csr/sars/archive/2003_03_26a/en/.

61 WHO, "China's latest SARS outbreak has been contained, but biosafety concerns remain – Update 7, May 18, 2004 at https://www.who.int/csr/don/2004_05_18a/en/.

62 Xu, Rui-Heng et al, "Epidemiologic clues to SARS origin in China," *Emerging infectious diseases* 2004, 10(6): 1030-7 at doi:10.3201/eid1006.030852.

63 Zhang Feng, Officials punished for SARS virus leak, Chinadaily.com.cn. July 7, 2004 at http://www.chinadaily.com.cn/english/doc/2004-07/02/content_344755.htm.

64 Jonathan Mirsky, "How the Chinese Spread SARS," *ChinaFile*, May 29, 2003 at https://www.chinafile.com/library/nyrb-china-archive/how-chinese-spread-sars.

65 Emily Feng and Amy Cheng, "They call him a hero: Dr. Zhong is the public face of China's war against coronavirus" *NPR*, April 2, 2020, at https://www.npr.org/sections/goatsandsoda/2020/04/02/825957192/dr-zhong-is-the-supreme-commander-in-china-s-war-against-coronavirus.

66 Zhong Nanshan and Guangqiao Zeng, "What We Have Learnt from SARS Epidemics in China," *BMJ*, 2006, 333 (7564): 389–91. https://doi.org/10.1136/bmj.333.7564.389.

67 Jonathan Mirsky, "How the Chinese Spread SARS," *ChinaFile*, May 29, 2003 at https://www.chinafile.com/library/nyrb-china-archive/how-chinese-spread-sars.

68 James Jay Carafano, "China's Coronavirus Lies—3 Possible Reasons for Their Propaganda Campaign", May 7, 2020, *Heritage.org* at https://www.heritage.org/asia/commentary/chinas-coronavirus-lies-3-possible-reasons-their-propaganda-campaign.

69 Zhao Xiaojian and Zhu Xiaochao, "China CDC Blamed for SARS escape", *Caijing.com.cn* Daily Update May 20, 2004 at http://english.caijing.com.cn/2004-05-20/100013918.html.

5

Deciphering the Myth: COVID-19 Out-break

Rajasimman Sundaram

Introduction

It is not for the first time that the human race is faced with a pandemic (*Coronavirus Disease 2019* – COVID-19) and has remained resilient and turned the corner in the face of far more death-dealing catastrophes in its journey to the present. In coming years COVID-19 would have passed by and will belong to the league of deadly infectious diseases [Bubonic Plague (1347-1351), Smallpox, Spanish Flu (1918-1919), Swine Flu (2009-2010), Ebola (2014-2016), MERS (2012-Present), and SARS (2002-2003)] that once intervened in our way of life. However, rarely has a pandemic been emphatically stated to be a misadventure of a nation-state – *a deliberate act.*[1] The current outbreak when viewed from a political perspective is far different from that of the SARS outbreak in China (November, 2002 – June, 2003) when an increased U.S.-China collaboration resulted on global health. In October, 2003 the U.S. Secretary of Health and Human Services Tommy Thompson visited China and signed a multiyear partnership with the Chinese Ministry of Health to develop a more robust public health infrastructure in China.[2] The U.S. Secretary of State Colin Powell stated, "It is upon such concrete forms of cooperation on issues of regional and global importance that a 21st century U.S.-China relationship will be built..."[3]

The idea of imaginable human intent behind the outbreak of *COVID-19* remains a matter of grave concern given that it will induce mistrust and insecurity within the international system on an almost near-permanent basis and also trigger a military response.[4] In fact, mistrust and lack of transparency leading to uncertainty and insecurity – *security dilemma* – is already clear and present. *The Role of Science and Technology in the context of International Security and Disarmament* was first added to the agenda of the First Committee in 1988, with India as the main sponsor. The UN secretary general's report in 2018 states – "in the biological field, scientific advances that may be relevant to a range of activities across the biological weapons development spectrum–manipulating, growing, recovering, concentrating, stabilizing, and testing – could undermine the norm against biological weapons."[5]

On 13 March, Chinese foreign ministry spokesman [Deputy Director General of the *Foreign Ministry's Information Department*] Zhao Lijian provided semi-official support to the theory that the origin of the COVID-19 may not be Wuhan (Hubei province in central China), but the United States (US).[6] Such a view was based on reports that suggest the US Army's participation in the *International Military World Games* held in Wuhan in October, 2019 to be the original cause of the pandemic.[7] Following this, on 18 March the US President stated "...but as you know, China tried to say at one point, maybe they stopped now that it was caused by American soldiers. That can't happen. It's not going to happen, not as long as I'm president...but it comes from China".[8] On 28 April, a request by the *Department of Foreign Affairs and Trade* (DFTA, Australia) on instituting an independent international investigation of the origin of the pandemic was turned down by the Chinese Ambassador to Australia Cheng Jingye on grounds of it being a 'political maneuver' and requested the Australian government to put aside ideological bias and stop political games.[9] Furthermore, while the US government incriminates China and the *World Health Organization* (WHO) for deferred information sharing on the outbreak, a report published in *The Times of Israel* on 16 April, 2020 suggests that the US intelligence community was aware of the emerging disease in the second week of November, 2019 and shared this information with two of its closest allies – Israel and NATO.[10] Apart from available actionable intelligence prior to the COVID-19 outbreak, the US was also aware of the potential outbreak of a pandemic at the level of strategic planning. The almost prophetic foreword of *The National Biodefense Strategy* (2018) states:[11]

> It is a vital interest of the United States to manage the risk of biological incidents. In today's interconnected world, biological incidents have the potential to cost thousands of American lives, cause significant anxiety, and greatly impact travel and trade.

Yet another piece of information that challenges the myth surrounding the origin of COVID-19 outbreak in central China was a *BBC NEWS* report published on 05 May that claims '...the virus may have arrived in Europe almost a monthearlier than previously thought.'[12] This claim was based on the testimony of Dr. Yves Cohen [Head of Emergency Medicine at Avicenne and Jean-Verdier hospitals near Paris] according to which- the patient, 43 years old Amirouche Hammar was admitted to hospital on 27 December with 'no' travel history to China and tested positive in retrospect examination.[13] Up until now it was believed that the first case of COVID-19 in France was confirmed on 24 January.

Likewise, the first previously known death in the US was in Seattle on 26 February and the first in California on 4 March. However, samples from the autopsies dated to 06 February and 17 February sent to the *Centers for Disease Control and Prevention* (CDC), confirm the presence of the virus and thus dent the previously accepted chain of events and timeline upon which the international political discourse is set.[14] In an interview to *BBC Hard Talk*, the Chinese Ambassador to the United Kingdom while answering the question on whether the COVID-19 outbreak originated in Wuhan (China), Liu Xiaoming stated, "...it was first discovered in Wuhan, but I can't say it originated from Wuhan. According to many information and report including BBC, it can be anywhere and everywhere...it can be in aircraft carriers and can be found even in submarines...so we cannot say it originated from China".[15]

Myth I: Links to Bio-Warfare [Defense]

It is now a well-established historical fact that China was a victim of chemical and bio-warfare at the hands of Japanese imperial army during the early decades of the 20th century and this deleterious experience has shaped People's Republic of China's (PRC) attitude towards bio-warfare in unequivocal term. In July, 2005 the Tokyo High Court acknowledged the use of biological weapons against China by Japan during the Second World War.[16] Furthermore, Chinese military opines that the US military used both biological and chemical weapons during the Korean War of 1950-53 on more than 200 occasions.[17] The use of biological weapons by the US military during the Korea War is generally held as a figment of China's politico-military leadership's imagination – *a manufactured history*. However, archival evidence now suggest that the US military planners did authorize the use of biological weapons on an experimental basis two weeks after China entered the Korean War on 27 October, 1950.[18]

In its own official admission, China has researched only *defensive* biological technology necessary for China's defense and has never researched, produced, or possessed biological weapons. In its confidence-building declarations to the Biological

Weapons Convention (BWC), China has declared several facilities as having a "national defensive biological warfare R&D program". China's bio-warfare defense program commenced officially in 1958.[19] By early 1990's the People's Liberation Army's *Anti-Biological Warfare Unit* was officially called 'Military Medical Research Institute of the Beijing Military Region' or 'Institute of MilitaryMedicine.'[20] While China is a signatory to both the *Chemical Weapons Convention* (CWC) in 1993 and BWC in 1984 pending ratification[21] it has maintained a consistent strategic policy with respect to these international disarmament mechanisms that display unique Chinese characteristics. Chinese experts believe the original BWC was a fraud and centered on the objective to exclude some nations from economic and technological exchange.[22] China's approach towards biological weapons and multilateral conventions (BWC) that seek to ban their employment in the event of war along with their research and development, production, stockpiling, and means of delivery remain consistently limited due the inherent nature of this enterprise:[23]

1) The peaceful and military use of rapidly transforming field of bio-technology is not distinguishable.
2) Research and development of offensive biological weapon is in distinguishable to that of defensive biological weapons program.
3) It is almost hopeless to contemplate a 'verification protocol' to ensure compliance without the cost to national sovereignty and security.
4) All attempts to eliminate biological weapons are inevitably tied to the peaceful and scientific efforts made in the field of bio-technology.

This associated complexity in national decision making in regard to biological weapons is not only true for Chinese policy makers but also other major powers such as Russia and the US. Amidst the initial days of COVID-19 breakout, the 2019 Meeting of States Parties to the *BWC* was held on 03-06 December where in the Chinese Ambassador Li Song stated – "...in particular, on core issues such as formulating a legally binding protocol that includes a verification regime, a certain State Party has continued to challenge the merits of the protocol and stood in the way of the negotiations, while at the same time pointing fingers at other countries' compliance of the Convention..."[24] The implementation rate for the biological weapons-related prohibitions of UN resolution 1540 which overlaps with the BWC was only 62%, compared with 74% for its chemical weapons- related prohibitions.[25] Yet another factor that determines China's overall approach towards the BWC and the pending verification protocol, is the equal importance of rights and obligation of states parties as well as the balance between the effectiveness of verification measures and protection of the legitimate security and commercial interests of States Parties.[26]

Ridiculed as a gentleman's agreement with no teeth, the BWC as an international treaty has no provisions to monitor its compliance to this day – absence of an agreed verification protocol.[27] The US walked out of an UN ad-hoc group tasked with drafting such a protocol in 2001 on grounds of the displeasure and concerns from its pharmaceutical industries.[28] The consistent US policy in this regard is that – "a legally binding protocol would not achieve meaningful or greater security. It is extraordinarily difficult to verify compliance."[29] In his statement to the 2019 Meeting of States Parties to the BWC held on 03-06 December Ambassador Robert A. Wood expressed lack of optimism in achieving a common ground with others in regard to science and technology and Article VII of the BWC.[30] The *Article VII* of the BWC stipulates that:[31]

> Each State Party to this Convention undertakes to provide or support assistance, in accordance with the United Nations Charter, to any Party to the Convention which so requests, if the Security Council decides that such Party has been exposed to danger as a result of violation of the Convention. [Article VII, BWC]

Furthermore, Articles III and IV of the BWC contradict the Article X and has been a matter of debate at the *Meeting of Experts on Strengthening National Implementation* on 05 August, 2019.[32] The resulting contradiction may not necessarily reflect the varying national positions held on this complex matter, but the nature of problem itself – *Biodefense.*

> ***Article III***
>
> Each State Party to this Convention undertakes not to transfer to any recipient whatsoever, directly or indirectly, and not in any way to assist, encourage, or induce any State, group of States or international organisations to manufacture or otherwise acquire any of the agents, toxins, weapons, equipment or means of delivery specified in Article I of the Convention. [Emphasis Added]
>
> ***Article IV***
>
> Each State Party to this Convention shall, in accordance with its constitutional processes, take any necessary measures to prohibit and prevent the development, production, stockpiling, acquisition or retention of the agents, toxins, weapons, equipment and means of delivery specified in Article I of the Convention, within the territory of such State, under its jurisdiction or under its control anywhere. [Emphasis Added]
>
> ***Article X***
>
> (1) The States Parties to this Convention undertake to facilitate, and have the right to participate in, the fullest possible exchange of equipment, materials and scientific and technological information for the use of bacteriological

> (biological) agents and toxins for peaceful purposes. Parties to the Convention in a position to do so shall also co-operate in contributing individually or together with other States or international organisations to the further development and application of scientific discoveries in the field of bacteriology (biology) for the prevention of disease, or for other peaceful purposes. [Emphasis Added]
>
> (2) This Convention shall be implemented in a manner designed to avoid hampering the economic or technological development of States Parties to the Convention or international co-operation in the field of peaceful bacteriological (biological) activities, including the international exchange of bacteriological (biological) agents and toxins and equipment for the processing, use or production of bacteriological (biological) agents and toxins for peaceful purposes in accordance with the provisions of the Convention. [Emphasis Added]

Given the inherent nature of bio-defense which is indistinguishable with its offensive aspects along with the scientific enterprise that supports it; cannot link the COVID-19 out-break to the pursuit of defensive biological warfare capabilities of a particular nation. It is perhaps on account of this above stated contradiction associated with the nature of bio-technology that China defers from the Australia Group established in 1985 with 43 members that seeks – "to ensure that exports do not contribute to the development of chemical or biological weapons".[33]

Myth II: A Deliberate Act

In the absence of investigation and credible evidence with respect to the index patient that led to COVID-19 outbreak centered on Wuhan (capital of Hubei, central China) with a population of 11-12 million, initial reports suggested the outbreak was zoonotic. However, experts such as Dr. Francis Boyle – drafter of the US Bioweapons Act [Biological Weapons Anti-Terrorism Act of 1989] and author of *Bio warfare and Terrorism* (2015) – claimed that coronavirus (2019-nCoV) was certainly an 'offensive biological warfare weapon.'[34] Supporting such a claim was a study by Indian scientists based at the *Indian Institute of Technology* and *University of Delhi* published on 30 January, 2020 which stated:

> The finding of 4 unique inserts in the 2019-nCoV, all of which have identity/similarity to amino acid residues in key structural proteins of HIV-1 is unlikely to be fortuitous in nature".[35]

In fear of not feeding into the conspiracy theories this report was voluntarily withdrawn by its authors along with the proclamation to continue further research on the topic.[36] Studies related to cross-species virus transmission opine that "...rarely, viruses gain the ability to spread efficiently within a new host that was not previously exposed or susceptible...to infect a new host, a virus must be able to efficiently infect the appropriate cells of the new host, and that process can be restricted at many different levels, including receptor binding, entry or fusion, trafficking within the cell, genome replication, and gene expression".[37] Furthermore, it takes considerable amount of time and overcome multiple biological barriers before a virus can successfullyspread efficiently between individuals of the new host. For example, HIV-1 that spread from Chimpanzees to humans initially in 1930's took almost 40 years of adaptation before becoming wide spread in-between human beings in 1970's and smallpox virus took thousands of years for host switching from primates or camels to humans.

A host of prima-facie factors indicate that the current out-break was an outcome of the worldwide human efforts at research and development of weapons related to the biological domain – intentionality of course being unanswered. Within the framework of the Sino-French Cooperation Agreement on Emerging Infectious Diseases Prevention and Control (signed in October 2004), in 2015 China inaugurated its first ever *Biosafety Level-4* (BSL-4) laboratory [the *Wuhan National Biosafety Laboratory* (Level 4) of the *Chinese Academy of Sciences*38] in Hubei province.[39] This need for a BSL-4 lab in China followed the *Severe Acute Respiratory Syndrome Coronavirus* (SARS-Cov) [2002-2003], however, the *National Development and Reform Commission* of People's Republic of China (March, 2015) states:

> According to China's "One Belt, One Road" initiative, the chance that exotic pathogens could be brought into the country has dramatically increased...our new BSL-4 facility will play an integral role in -preventing and controlling highly pathogenic microbes."[40] [Emphasis Added]

Amidst reports that the source zero of the present outbreak is un-related to the live-stock wet market in Wuhan[41] and the close proximity of the BSL-4 lab within few miles of the wet market, has led to theory of an accidental leakage of the genetically re-engineered virus from within the BSL-4 lab itself in Wuhan. While China intends to create additional 05-07 BSL-4 labs by 2025 in addition to the one in Wuhan, it developed its BSL-4 laboratory user training program only in 2017 [Dr. Han Xia, Associate Professor at Wuhan Institute of Virology, *Chinese Academy of Sciences*]. Furthermore, its know-how to operate these ultra-modern laboratories and formulate leak-proof medical protocols depends on assistance and cooperation from foreign countries [France, the US, and Australia] through its exchange programs. However, China's confidence at not just operating such facilities but also leading within this scientific field can be gauged by the fact that in order carry forward the South-South cooperation, in November, 2019 Chinese Foreign Ministry and the Chinese Academy of Sciences jointly held the 3rd Biosafety management and Technology Training Course in Wuhan Institute of Virology, to help developing countries train research personnel in the field of prevention and control of communicable diseases.[42]

In a dedicated body of research conducted by Wuhan-based virologist Dr. Shi Zhengli since 2004 concludes the presence of a natural reservoir of coronavirusesin bats in southern China and based on analyses using polymerase chain reaction, full genome sequencing, antibody tests of blood samples of Wuhan patients on 07 January, concluded 96 percent similarity to that of a coronavirus, the researchers had identified in horseshoe bats in Yunnan.[43] Dr. Shi Zhengli having cross-checked with the previous laboratory research data and records affirms that none of the sequences matched those of the viruses her team had sampled from bat caves and thereby debunking the myth of an incidental or accidental leak out of the lab.[44] With no links to the Huanan seafood market, the first case linked to the Wuhan outbreak was reported on 01 December, 2019. Dr. Li Wenliang, an ophthalmologist in Wuhan was the first to address the public regarding a potential outbreak on 03 January, 2020 by raising an alarm over Chinese social media [*We Chat*] along with few others. After initially being reprimanded by the Wuhan police for spreading false information, Dr. Li fell sick on 10 January and finally succumbed to the illness on 07 February.[45] Some reports suggest the initial lackluster response on part of the Hubei provincial government to the already known epidemic was due to its pre-occupation with the so-called "two meetings time" (两会时间) from January 6 to January 17 – the 4th Plenum of the 13th Wuhan CPPCC, the 5th Plenum of the 14th Wuhan People's Congress, the 3rd Plenum of the 12th Hubei Provincial CPPCC, and the 3rd Plenum of 13th Hubei Provincial People's Congress.[46] The Hubei province is now at the cusp of seeking herself the status of a first-tier city in China.

A study done by a group of Chinese researchers and published by *The Lancet* on 24 January stated:

> By Jan 2, 2020, 41 admitted hospital patients had been identified as having laboratory-confirmed 2019-nCoV infection... 27 (66%) of 41 patients had been exposed to Huanan seafood market.[47]

Furthermore, in his estimates of the clock and TMRCA for 2019-nCoV based on 27 genomes, Kristian Andersen, an evolutionary biologist at the *Scripps Research Institute* traces the earliest ancestor of the COVID-19 virus to 01 October, 2019.[48] According to Chinese researchers at *Fudan University*, based on nucleotide substitution rate, the most recent common ancestor (tMRCA) of 2019-nCoVs appeared about 0.253-0.594 year before the epidemic.[49] Given the initial stability of viruses scientists suspect the existence of un-noticed mini outbreak where the viruses maintain a low transmission rate before turning into a pandemic.[50] The first death caused since the outbreak occurred on 09 January involved a 61 year old man with no connection to the Huanan seafood market.[51] And as late as 18 January, it remained unknown to Wuhan municipal authorities of the human-to-human transmission.[52]

Unlike China's experience with SARS-Cov in February 2003, this time around quick-reaction on part of Chinese health agencies and government policy with respect communication and sharing of information both within and outside China has been laudable.[53] During the SARS-Cov (2002-03), while the first case was reported in the Guangdong province in southern China on 16 November, 2002 it took four months for the WHO to issue a global alert on 12 March, 2003 followed by the CDC issuing first health alert and media tele-briefing about an atypical pneumonia that was named *Severe Acute Respiratory Syndrome* (SARS) on 15 March, 2003. It was not until 24 March, 2003 that the CDC laboratory analysis suggested a new coronavirus may be the cause of SARS and CDC published a sequence of the virus believed to be responsible for the global epidemic of SARS only on 14 April, 2003. The WHO announced that the global SARS outbreak as 'contained' only on 05 July, 2003. A total of 8,096 persons worldwide with probable SARS resulted in 774 deaths – a fatality rate of 9.56 percent.[54] Despite the efficiency of world health agencies since this epidemic (SARS) having improved substantially, including that of China's, the challenged posed by the COVID-19 seems to be comparatively more dramatic than SARS. This time around compared to the SARS-Cov (2002-03) outbreak, China has been at least six times faster in obtaining the whole genome sequence of the virus as early as 07 January and shared the same with the international scientific community by the weekend of 11-12 January.[55]

A multitude of factors raise lack of credence without providing credible evidence in support of the narrative that the COVID-19 is a cross-species virus transmission. Much of this narrative is in dubiety for lack of absolute knowledge regarding the origin of COVID-2019. The second factor being the existence of China's BSL-4 laboratory within the perimeter of Wuhan city where in it can be stated beyond doubt that research and development related to bio-defense was being undertaken. However, this is not sufficient to incriminate the BSL-4 laboratory for accidental or deliberate sabotage. This is not the first time that such allegations centered on BSL-4 labs are being raised. Previously, reports suggest human action in case of Ebola and AIDS in Africa.[56] In 2018, the *Lugar Center* – BSL-3 (about 17 km from the US Vaziani airbase in the Georgian capital), has been incriminated by the Russian government for alleged breach of biological weapons convention.[57]

Foremost of the factors that falsify the narrative of cross-species virus transmission is the availability of early warnings. For example, at the Munich Security Conference (24 February, 2017), Mr. Bill Gates stated:[58]

> ...we also face a new threat that the next epidemic has a good chance of origination on a computer screen of a terrorist intent on using genetic engineering to create a synthetic version of a smallpox virus or a contagious and highly deadly strain of flu...and there is a reasonable probability of that taking place in the years ahead.

This prophecy was not just a linear extrapolation of past incidents of pandemic but based on scientific know-how. Incidentally, a joint-study conducted (2017) by the scientists of –

(1) *The Tata Institute of Fundamental Research* (India)
(2) *The National Centre for Biological Sciences* (India)
(3) *The Wuhan Institute of Virology* (China)
(4) *The Uniformed Services University of the Health Sciences* (U.S.)
(5) *The Duke-National University* (Singapore)

In the Indian state of Nagaland without the explicit permission of the government of India and claimed to be funded by the US Department of Defense Threat Reduction Agency (DTRA) was published in *PLOS Neglected Tropical Diseases* journal (2019) originally established by the *Bill and Melinda Gates Foundation.*[59]

> The study presented evidence for prior exposure of bat harvesters and two resident fruit bat species to filovirus surface glycoproteins by screening sera in a multiplexed serological assay. Antibodies reactive to two antigenically distinct filoviruses were detected in human sera and to three individual filoviruses in bats in remote Northeast India. Sera obtained from *Eonycteris spelaea* bats showed similar patterns of cross-reactivity as human samples, suggesting them as the **species responsible for the spillover**. In contrast, sera from *Rousettus leschenaultii* bats reacted to two different virus glycoproteins. The study stated that its **results indicated circulation of several filoviruses in bats and the possibility for filovirus transmission from bats to humans.**[60] [Emphasis Added]

Following the outbreak in Wuhan, an inquiry into a study conducted in Nagaland by researchers from the U.S., China and India was ordered by the government of India and a report to this effect has been submitted to the Indian Ministry of Health. Furthermore, in a written reply to questions from *The Hindu*, the U.S. CDC in Atlanta said it "did not commission this study and had not received any enquiries [from the Indian government] on it."[61] In February, 2019 a study done by Chinese researchers based at CAS Key Laboratory of Special Pathogens and Biosafety, Wuhan Institute of Virology, Chinese Academy of Sciences, Wuhan and University of Chinese Academy of Sciences, Beijing concluded that three zoonotic coronaviruses had been identified as the cause of large-scale disease outbreaks in previous two decades and their agents originated from bats, and two of them originated in China. The study further emphasized that "it is highly likely that future SARS- or MERS-like coronavirus outbreaks will originate from bats, and there is an increased probability that this will occur in China".[62]

Yet another signal of early warning was noticed at Canada's *National Microbiology Laboratory* (NML) in Winnipeg. In June, 2012 Egyptian virologist Dr. Ali Mohamed Zaki isolated and identified a previously unknown coronavirus from the lungs of 60-year-old Saudi man in Jeddah, Saudi Arabia. Having failed to nail the causative agent, Dr. Zaki referred the case to Ron Fouchier, a leading virologist at the *Erasmus Medical Center* (EMC) in Rotterdam, the Netherlands. This coronavirus sample was then acquired by Scientific Director Dr. Frank Plummer directly from Ron Fouchier and arrived at the *National Microbiology Laboratory* (NML) in Winnipeg (Canada) on 04 May, 2013. According to the WHO, three months after the hospitalization of the patient in Jeddah, a second patient with a history of travel to Saudi Arabia who had been transferred from a hospital in Qatar to a hospital in London was infected with the same virus.[63] In October, 2012 Dr. Zaki and Dr. Fouchier along with other researchers published a brief report to this effect in *The New England Journal of Medicine* and stated that:[64]

> The virus (called HCoV-EMC) replicated readily in cell culture, producing cytopathic effects of rounding, detachment, and syncytium formation. The virus represents a novel beta coronavirus species. The closest known relatives are bat coronaviruses HKU4 and HKU5. Here, the clinical data, virus isolation, and molecular identification are presented. The clinical picture was remarkably similar to that of the severe acute respiratory syndrome (SARS) outbreak in 2003 and reminds us that animal coronaviruses can cause severe disease in humans. [Emphasis Added].

The death of Dr. Frank Plummer under mysterious circumstances in Kenya on 04 February amidst the outbreak was at the forefront of research on SARS, H1N1 flu and Ebola epidemics and considered a key in the investigation of the Wuhan outbreak.[65] Yet another disturbing related fact is the case of policy breach or bio-espionage by Chinese researchers linked to the BSL-4 lab in Wuhan – Dr. Xiangguo Qiu.[66] Dr. Qiu had been studying powerful viruses, Ebola virus foremost in the NML (Canada) since 2006 and was escorted out of Canada's only BSL-4 lab *NML* at Winnipeg along with her biologist husband (Dr. Keding Cheng) and other team members from China on 05 July, 2019. Dr. Qiu was head of the *Vaccine Development and Antiviral Therapies Section* in the Special Pathogens Program at NML and was closely involved with the development of Ebola (2014-2016) vaccine along with Dr. Gary Kobinger. Since this incident occurred during diplomatic tussle between China and Canada, it remains unknown if the intent of bio-espionage it true or not.

With reasonable doubts it can be stated that the *Wuhan National Biosafety Laboratory* (Level 4) of the Chinese Academy of Sciences was conducting research & development on a novel strain of Coronavirus along with other known lethal pathogens perhaps with the intention of developing a panacea. Furthermore, this Coronavirus was possibly linked to the case that emerged in Saudi Arabia in 2012.[67]

Based on the above-mentioned factors there are three possible sources of the COVID-19 outbreak with varying degrees of probability.

Source 1	Hunan sea food wet market	Very-Low
Source 2	BSL-4 Lab in Wuhan	Low-Medium
Source 3	A source other than (1) and (2)	Very-High

Conclusion

Myth attempts to capture in terms conceivable to humans some of the indeterminate qualities of the divine unknown. Hence myth is something that is understood as – "does not tell truth, but does tell the truth"; a myth is something that "never was, but always is."[68] The myth surrounding the COVID-19 outbreak while not real has a 'reality' of its own and is subject to reinterpretation in light of emerging evidences. This 'reality' acts as a metaphor in conducting politics and other tasks, such as preparation for war and peace. A metaphor being omnipresent links the limited abilities to gain knowledge with the ultimate truth. Metaphors condition the perception and this in turn provides meaning to the unknown reality.

According to a declassified (24 February, 1977) *Department of the Army* (US) report – *US Army Activity in the US Biological Warfare Programs* – the US biological warfare (BW) programme began amidst the Second World War and was banned by President Nixon in November, 1969. However, the report states, "...because a potential BW threat still exists the US still maintains a defensive BW program in accordance with the 1969 Presidential policy statement." Furthermore, the report states that the US policy regarding BW was to first deter its use against the US and its forces, and secondly to retaliate if deterrence failed.[69] More recently, The US assistance to Saddam Hussein to employ chemical weapons (Musturd Gas and Sarin) during the Iraq-Iran War in 1988 and the US and British allegations against Russia for using a nerve agent (polonium) in March, 2018 against its former spy based in Britain make it clear that efforts at research and development of biological & chemical weapons for both defensive and offensive purposes has hardly seized despite internationally agreed conventions in place.[70] For example, Ebola outbreak is not associated to West Africa alone, historically the Ebola type of virus first broke out in Germany (Marburg Virus) followed by Reston in the US (Prof. Horace Campbell). Hence its outbreak in the Democratic Republic of Congo (DRC) was perhaps a result of human intent, given that it occurred close to an American laboratory in Uganda near DRC border.[71]

Both from the perspective of its links with bio-defense and its intent driven pursuit fails short of incriminating China for the out-break of COVID-19. Any nation has the legitimate right to defend itself against biological weapons and pursue research and development in this regard for peaceful purpose. Like all previous weapons of war, bio-weapons are at an early stage of development and will evolve in more sophisticated formats in coming decades. However, while bio-weapons will produce a whole new range of consequences unlike other known conventional and unconventional weapons of the past, their ability to alter the inherent nature of war itself will remain the same. The true nature of war is to serve itself, and it being called politics through other means will remain a constant challenge. The myth surrounding the COVID-19 outbreak leads up to a situation wherein a nation is both right and wrong at the same time in pursuing research and development of bio-weapons. This dilemma will shape strategic decision making for long, many years after the WHO declares the world to be free of COVID-19.

NOTES

1 Previously Taiwan had blamed the breakout of the 'Foot and Mouth' disease to a deliberate act of the mainland Chinese government, only for the allegation to be found inaccurate later.

2 Jennifer Bouvey, "From SARS to 2019 – Coronavirus (n CoV): US-China Collaborations on Pandemic Response", *Testimony presented before the House Foreign Affairs Sub-Committee on Asia, the Pacific, and Non-Proliferation* [The RAND Corporations], 05 February 2020 at https://www.rand.org/content/dam/rand/pubs/testimonies/CT500/CT523/RAND_CT523.pdf

3 Colin L. Powell, "Remarks at Conference on China-U.S. Relations," *US Department of State*, 05 November 2003 at https://2001-2009.state.gov/secretary/former/powell/remarks/2003/25950.htm

4 Peter Hirschberg (Eds), "Exclusive: Internal Chinese report warns Beijing faces Tiananmen-like global backlash over virus" *Reuters*, 04 May2020 at https://www.reuters.com/article/us-health-coronavirus-china-sentiment-ex/exclusive-internal-chinese-report-warns-beijing-faces-tiananmen-like-global-backlash-over-virus-idUSKBN22G19C

5 *Joint NGO Statement to Biological Weapons Convention Meeting of States Parties*, Geneva. 05 December 2018 at https://www.unog.ch/80256EDD006B8954/(httpAssets)/6E001B2E6A06E36AC125835B0051F90B/$file/MSP_2018_+joint_+NGO_+statement_FINAL.PDF

6 Vanessa Molter, Graham Webster, "Coronavirus Conspiracy Claims: What's Behind a Chinese Diplomat's COVID-19 Misdirection", *Freeman Spogli Institute for International Studies* (Stanford University), 31 March 2020 at https://fsi.stanford.edu/news/china-covid19-origin-narrative.

7 Ryan Pickrell, "Chinese Official Says US Army May Have 'Brought the Epidemic to Wuhan'", *military.com*, 12 March 2020 at https://www.military.com/daily-news/2020/03/12/chinese-official-says-us-army-may-have-brought-epidemic-wuhan.html

8 Dan Mangan, "Trump defends calling coronavirus 'Chinese virus' — 'it's not racist at all'", *CNBC*, 18 March 2020 at https://www.cnbc.com/2020/03/18/coronavirus-criticism-trump-defends-saying-chinese-virus.html

9 *Sky News*, 29 April, 2020. Also refer, James Palmer, "Chinese Diplomats Make Veiled Threats", *Foreign Policy [China Brief]*, 29 April, 2020.

10 ToI Staff, "US alerted Israel, NATO to disease outbreak in China in November — TV report", *The Times of Israel*, 16 April 2020 at https://www.timesofisrael.com/us-alerted-israel-nato-to-disease-outbreak-in-china-in-november-report/?fbclid=IwAR1q1rm42Lr9BpcMYLBOZv CNgu8 I12v5NbnlJmG9mDDhJDBMeUO_Fw0jTuI

11 The President of the United States of America, *The National Biodefense Strategy*, 2018p.i at https://www.whitehouse.gov/wp-content/uploads/2018/09/National-Biodefense-Strategy.pdf

12 "Coronavirus: France's first known case 'was in December'", *BBC News*, 05 May, 2020 at https://www.bbc.com/news/world-europe-52526554

13 A. Deslandes, V.Bertia, Y.Tandjaoui- Lambotte, ChakibAlloui, E.Carbonnelle, dJ.R. Zaharad S. Brichler Yves Cohen, "SARS-CoV-2 was already spreading in France in late December 2019", *International Journal of Antimicrobial Agents*, 03 May 2020 at https://www.sciencedirect.com/science/article/pii/S0924857920301643

14 "Coronavirus: First US Deaths Weeks Earlier Than Thought", *BBC News*, 22 April, 2020 at https://www.bbc.com/news/world-us-canada-52385558

15 *Coronavirus: Liu Xiaoming, China's UK Ambassador, on China's role in COVID-19, BBC HARDtalk*, 30 April, 2020 at https://www.youtube.com/watch?v=PNv75d0lyGg

16 "Japan high court rejects damages for Chinese germ warfare victims", *Agencia Angola Press*, 19 July, 2005 at http://www.angop.ao/angola/en_us/noticias/internacional/2005/6/29/Japan-high-court-rejects-damages-for-Chinese-germ-warfare-victims,b951b47f-83e3-4f1a-a08d-7d8877d778fd.html

17 Milton Zeitenberg, "Resolution of the Korean War Biological Warfare Allegations", *Critical Reviews in Microbiology*, 24:3, (1998) p.175 and Lu Qiang and Yang Qingzhen eds, *Wuqi yu zhansheng jishi congshu* [Weapons and Warfare Reference Series] #14: *Huaxue Wuqi Yu Zhanzheng* [Chemical Weapons and Warfare], Beijing: Guofang Gongye Chubanshe (National Defense Industry Press, 1997), p.128-35; Cited in Eric Coddy, "China's Role in the Chemical and Biological Disarmament Regimes" *The Nonproliferation Review* (Spring 2002), p.18.

18 Stephen Endicott and Edward Hagerman, "US Cold War Secrets: First Victims of Biological Warfare", *Le Monde Diplomatique*, July1999 at https://mondediplo.com/1999/07/13bioa. Also refer, Thomas Powell, "Biological Warfare in Korea: A Review of Literature" *Socialism and Democracy*, Vol.33, No: 02, (2019), 67-107.

19 Li Yimin in Liu Huaqiu ed., *Arms Control and Disarmament Handbook*, Beijing: National Defense Industry Press, December, p.363; Cited in Eric Coddy, "China's Role in the Chemical and Biological Disarmament Regimes" *The Nonproliferation Review* (Spring 2002), p.27.

20 Wong Mei, "Biological Army Unit Does Research in Bacteriological Warfare, Making Profit of 1 Million Yuan Each Year," *Ming Pao, Hong Kong Daily*, 27 December1994.

21 Refer http://disarmament.un.org/treaties/t/bwc

22 Michael D. Swaine and Alaistair I. Johnston, "China and Arms Control Institutions," in Elizabeth Economy and Michel Oksenberg, eds., *China Joins the World: Progress and Prospects*, Council on Foreign Relations: New York City, 1999, pp. 90-135

23 Li Yimin Cited in Eric Coddy, "China's Role in the Chemical and Biological Disarmament Regimes", *The Nonproliferation Review* (Spring 2002), p.27.

24 "The 2019 Meeting of States Parties to the Biological Weapons Convention", *The United Nations Office* (Geneva), 03-06 December, 2019 at https://www.unog.ch/80256EDD006B8954/(httpAssets)/55A3A7FFC6F4B3E0C12584C70028626B/$file/BWC+Eng.pdf

25 *Meeting of the States Parties to the Convention on the Prohibition of the Development, Production and Stockpiling of Bacteriological (Biological) and Toxin Weapons and on Their Destruction*, BWC/MSP/2019/MX.3/2 [The United Nations: Geneva], 01 November, 2019 at https://undocs.org/bwc/msp/2019/mx.3/2

26 "The Negotiation of a Protocol to the Biological Weapons Convention", *Permanent Mission of the People's Republic of China to the United Nation's Office at Geneva and Other International Organizations in Switzerland*, 16 April, 2004 at http://www.china-un.ch/eng/cjjk/cjjblc/cjlc/t85361.htm

27 Lynn C. Klotz, "The Biological Weapons Convention protocol should be revisited", *Bulletin of the Atomic Scientists*, 15 November2019 at https://thebulletin.org/2019/11/the-biological-weapons-convention-protocol-should-be-revisited/

28 Laura H. Kahn, "The Biological Weapons Convention: Proceeding without a verification protocol", *Bulletin of the Atomic Scientists*, 09 May, 2011 at https://thebulletin.org/2011/05/the-biological-weapons-convention-proceeding-without-a-verification-protocol/

29 *Under Secretary of State Ellen O. Tauscher Address to the Annual Meeting of the States Parties to the Biological Weapons Convention*, December 9, 2009, Geneva, Switzerland at https://geneva.usmission.gov/2009/12/09/tauscher-bwc/

30 *U.S. General Statement at the 2019 BWC Meeting of States Parties* Delivered by Ambassador Robert A. Wood U.S. Permanent Representative to the Conference on Disarmament and Special Representative for Biological and Toxin Weapons Convention Issues Geneva, December 3, 2019 at https://www.unog.ch/80256EDD006B8954/(httpAssets)/2D725C7AED52848DC12584C50055376E/$file/E.1++U.S.+General+Debate+Statement.pdf

31 *Convention on the Prohibition of the Development, Production and Stockpiling of Bacteriological (Biological) and Toxin Weapons and on Their Destruction* [United Nations Office for Disarmament Affairs] at http://disarmament.un.org/treaties/t/bwc/text.

32 *Convention on the Prohibition of the Development, Production and Stockpiling of Bacteriological (Biological) and Toxin Weapons and on Their Destruction*, United Nations Office for Disarmament (Geneva) at http://disarmament.un.org/treaties/t/bwc/text

33 See the weblink https://australiagroup.net/en/index.html

34 Professor of international law at the *University Of Illinois College Of Law.*

35 Prashant Pradhan, Ashutosh Kumar Pandey, Akhilesh Mishra, Parul Gupta, Praveen Kumar Tripathi, Manoj Balakrishnan Menon, James Gomes, Perumal Vivekanandan and Bishwajit Kundu, "Uncanny similarity of unique inserts in the 2019-nCoV spike protein to HIV-1 gp120 and Gag" *bioRxiv*, 31 January 2020. Available at http://dx.doi.org/10.1101/2020.01.30.927871doi

36 "Indian Scientists Discover Coronavirus Engineered With HIV (AIDS) Like Insertions", *GreatGameIndia*, 01 February, 2020 at https://greatgameindia.com/indian-scientists-discover-coronavirus-engineered-with-aids-like-insertions/

37 Colin R. Parrish, Edward C. Holmes, David M. Morens, Eun-Chung Park, Donald S. Burke, Charles H. Calisher, Catherine A. Laughlin, Linda J. Saif, and Peter Daszak, "Cross-Species Virus Transmission and the Emergence of New Epidemic Diseases", *Microbiology and Molecular Biology Reviews*, September 2008, 72 (3): 457-470.

38 Available at http://english.whiov.cas.cn/News/Events/201502/t20150203_135923.html

39 Han Xia, Yi Huang, Haixia Ma, Bobo Liu, Weiwei Xie, Donglin Song, and Zhiming Yuan, "Biosafety Level 4 Laboratory User Training Program, China", *Centers for Disease Control and Prevention*, 05 Vol:25, No:05, May 2019 at https://wwwnc.cdc.gov/eid/article/25/5/18-0220_article#r7

40 *National Development and Reform Commission of People's Republic of China*, "Vision and actions on jointly building Silk Road economic belt and 21st-Century maritime Silk Road" [in Chinese]. 2015 March 30 [cited 2018 Dec 5]. http://www.ndrc.gov.cn/gzdt/201503/t20150330_669162.html External Link

41 Kat Eschner, "We're still not sure where the Wuhan coronavirus really came from", *Popular Science*, 28 January2020 at https://www.popsci.com/story/health/wuhan-coronavirus-china-wet-market-wild-animal/

42 Statement by H.E. Ambassador Li Song at the 2019 Meeting of States Parties to the BWC at https://www.unog.ch/80256EDD006B8954/(httpAssets)/55A3A7FFC6F4B3E0C12584C70028626B/$file/BWC+Eng.pdf

43 Zhou, P., Yang, X., Wang, X. et al. A pneumonia outbreak associated with a new coronavirus of probable bat origin, *Nature*, 579, 270–273 (2020). https://doi.org/10.1038/s41586-020-2012-7

44 Jane Qiu, "How China's 'Bat Woman' Hunted Down Viruses from SARS to the New Coronavirus", *Scientific American*, 27 April, 2020 at https://www.scientificamerican.com/article/how-chinas-bat-woman-hunted-down-viruses-from-sars-to-the-new-coronavirus1/

45 Huo Jingnan, Emily Feng, Scott Neuman, "China to Investigate After Whistleblower Doctor Dies From Coronavirus", *NPR*, 07 February 2020 at https://www.npr.org/sections/goatsandsoda/2020/02/07/803680463/china-to-investigate-after-whistleblower-doctor-dies-from-coronavirus

46 Qiang Gang, "Questions for Hubei's Delegates", *China Media Project*, 10 February 2020 at https://chinamediaproject.org/2020/02/10/questions-for-hubeis-delegates/

47 "Clinical features of patients infected with 2019 novel coronavirus in Wuhan, China", *The Lancet*, 24 January, 2020 at https://www.thelancet.com/action/showPdf?pii=S0140-6736%2820%2930183-5

48 Kristian Andersen, "Clock and TMRCA based on 27 genomes", *Scripps Research*, 25 January 2020. Available at http://virological.org/t/clock-and-tmrca-based-on-27-genomes/347

49 Chenglong Xiong, Lufang Jiang, Yue Chen, Qingwu Jiang, "Evolution and variation of 2019-novel coronavirus", *bioRxiv*, 30 January 2020 at https://www.biorxiv.org/content/10.1101/2020.01.30.926477v1.full.pdf

50 Ralph Baric, a virologist at the University of North Carolina at Chapel Hill cited in Jane Qiu, "How China's 'Bat Woman' Hunted Down Viruses from SARS to the New Coronavirus" Scientific American, 27 April 2020 at https://www.scientificamerican.com/article/how-chinas-bat-woman-hunted-down-viruses-from-sars-to-the-new-coronavirus1/

51 "01 Dead, 41 Diagnosed with Coronavirus-related Pneumonia in Wuhan", *Job Tube Daily*, 12 January, 2020.

52 Jon Cohen, "Wuhan seafood market may not be source of novel virus spreading globally", *Science*, 26 January 2020 at https://www.sciencemag.org/news/2020/01/wuhan-seafood-market-may-not-be-source-novel-virus-spreading-globally

53 Dr. Tedros Ghebreyesus, Director-General of WHO cited in "Emerging understandings of 2019-nCoV", *The Lancet*, Vol. 395. 01 February, 2020.

54 Refer "CDC SARS Response Timeline", *Center for Disease Control and Prevention*, Available at https://www.cdc.gov/about/history/sars/timeline.htm

55 "Whole genome of novel coronavirus, 2019-nCoV, sequenced", *Institut Pasteur*, 31 January, 2020 at https://www.sciencedaily.com/releases/2020/01/200131114748.htm

56 Antonie Roger Lokongo, "Ebola: Who created this terrible virus and why?", *Pambazuka News*, 08 January 2015 at https://www.pambazuka.org/food-health/ebola-who-created-terrible-virus-and-why. Adam B. Ellick and Adam West-Brook, "Operation Infektion – Russian Disinformation: From Cold War to Kanye" *The New York Times*, 12 November 2018 at https://www.nytimes.com/2018/11/12/opinion/russia-meddling-disinformation-fake-news-elections.html

57 Ilya Tuskanov, "US Sanctions Russia Over Biolab Access While Covering Up Own Secrets Labs", *Sputnik News*, 12 August 2018. Available at https://sputniknews.com/military/201808121067142155- us-suspected-biolab-access/ ; "Russian Specialists Studying Documents on US Laboratory in Georgia - Russian MoD" *Sputnik News*, 14 September, 2018 at https://sputniknews.com/world/201809141068034581-specialists-ministry-laboratory/

58 Available at https://www.youtube.com/watch?v=6QmH3SCX0Ro

59 Pam Barker, "India to Probe Wuhan Institute of Virology; Dr. Francis Boyle – Coronavirus is a Bio Weapon [VIDEO]",*Europe Reloaded*, 04 February2020 at https://www.europereloaded.com/india-to-probe-wuhan-institute-of-virology-dr-francis-boyle-coronavirus-is-a-bio-weapon-video/

60 Pilot Dovih, Eric D. Laing, Yihui Chen, Dolyce H. W. Low, B. R. Ansil, Xinglou Yang, Zhengli Shi, Christopher C. Broder, Gavin J. D. Smith, Martin Linster, Uma Ramakrishnan, Ian H. Mendenhall, "Filovirus-reactive antibodies in humans and bats in Northeast India imply zoonotic spillover", *PLOS Neglected Tropical Disease*, 31 October 2019. Available at https://journals.plos.org/plosntds/article?id=10.1371/journal.pntd.0007733

61 Bindu Shajan Perappadan, "Study on bats and bat hunters in Nagaland to be probed", *The Hindu*, 03 February 2020 at https://www.thehindu.com/news/national/study-on-bats-and-bat-hunters-of-nagaland-come-under-the-scanner/article30722099.ece

62 Fan, Yi; Zhao, Kai; Shi, Zheng-Li; Zhou, Peng, "Bat Coronaviruses in China", *Viruses*, 11, no. 3 (2019), 210.

63 Novel coronavirus infection – updates – revised interim case definition. Geneva, *World Health Organization*, 2012 at http:// www.who.int/csr/don/2012_09_29/en/ index.html.

64 Ali Moh Zaki, M.D., Ph.D., Sander van Boheemen, M.Sc., Theo M. Bestebroer, B.Sc., Albert D.M.E. Osterhaus, D.V.M., Ph.D., and Ron A.M. Fouchier, Ph.D. (2012), "Isolation of a Novel Coronavirus from a Man with Pneumonia in Saudi Arabia", *The New England Journal of Medicine*, 17 October. p.1.

65 A year ago Dr. Plummer had chosen to participate in a surgical trial for experimental brain surgery to treat his alcoholism. "World-renowned HIV researcher Frank Plummer, 67, dies", *BBC*, 05 February, 2020 at https://www.bbc.com/news/world-us-canada-51317386

66 "Chinese Researchers Caught Stealing Coronavirus from Canadian Lab", *GreatGameIndia*, 23 July, 2019 at https://greatgameindia.com/chinese-researchers-caught-stealing-coronavirus-from-canadian-lab/

67 J.R. Nyquist, "Did China's Plan to Destroy the United States Backfire?", *The Epoch Times*, 31 January 2020 at https://www.theepochtimes.com/did-chinas-plan-to-destroy-the-united-states-backfire_3223117.html

68 McDonald, C. Lee, "Myth, politics, and Political Science", *The Western Political Quarterly*, Vol.22, No.1, 1969 pp.141150.

69 "US Army Activity in the US Biological Warfare Programs: Volume 1" (Unclassified 24 February, 1977), *National Security Archive* at https://nsarchive2.gwu.edu/NSAEBB/NSAEBB58/RNCBW_USABWP.pdf

70 Christian Caryl, "The message that Vladimir Putin sends with poison", *The Washington Post*, 09 March 2018 at https://www.washingtonpost.com/news/democracy-post/wp/2018/03/08/the-message-that-vladimir-putin-sends-with-poison/. Mark Memmot, "New Details On How U.S. 'Helped Saddam As He Gassed Iran'" *NPR*, 26 August 2013 at https://www.npr.org/sections/thetwo-way/2013/08/26/215733981/new-details-on-how-u-s-helped-saddam-as-he-gassed-iran

71 "USA and epidemic spreading in Africa", *The Standard*, 05 August, 2017 at https://www.thestandard.co.zw/2017/08/05/usa-epidemic-spreading-africa/.

6

COVID-19 and the Role of China's Armed Forces

M.S. Prathibha

The COVID-19 pandemic has brought attention to the role of the People's Liberation Army (PLA) in combating the spread of the virus. The PLA's capabilities in responding to COVID-19 show that the military reforms of 2015 in joint logistics and joint command have helped play a role in its response to the pandemic. Moreover, the Chinese leadership deliberated on a strategy that would utilise the military's resources in the same way that the PLA would deal with Military Operations Other Than War (MOOTW)[1]. Finally, the leadership was able to integrate the military response within the civilian authority at the central level, and implement direct command at the local level.

This chapter analyses the following: First, the way the PLA has helped the civilian authorities to control the spread of the pandemic. Secondly, China's military reforms, especially in joint logistics and command and its impact on the response mechanism against COVID-19. Third, the PLA's growing capabilities in MOOTW, and the future role of the PLA in combating non-traditional security threats, including pandemics.

PLA's COVID-19 Response and Coordination

The PLA Logistics Support Department (LSD) led the efforts to control the spread of COVID-19 in China. Therefore, the PLA LSD on behalf of the military pledged its support to the country's effort to fight the pandemic to achieve the goal set up by the Chinese leadership.[2] This goal was to achieve "zero infection" in the Chinese community (打胜仗、零感染) as elusive as it may be. Various military medical institutions and the armed forces involved in the fight against the pandemic pledged support to this goal, and at the same time, attempted to reduce the scope of infection among military's medical staff.[3] At the ground level in Hubei, the PLA undertook emergency operations such as supplying medical equipment and supplies. The manpower came predominantly from the medical staff of various PLA hospitals under the command of the PLA LSD. The immediate concern of the armed forces sent to Hubei was to help in the local efforts to fight the pandemic. At the central level, the PLA LSD directed the decisions regarding the scope of the operations and the role of various medical institutions during the pandemic. The Director of the PLA LSD Health Department (后勤保障部卫生局) Chen Jingyuan, who is an expert on environmental medicine and toxicology was the points man from the Logistics Department, and kept track of the city's growing need for supplies and the patient surge in hospitals. The Comprehensive Planning Bureau (中央军委后勤保障部综合计划局) selected three teams consisting of 150 personnel each from military medical universities affiliated with Ground Forces, Air Force and Navy and another 950 staff members from affiliated medical institutes under the PLA LSD.[4] These were supplemented by additional medical personnel from affiliated institutes of all the military service branches. Some of the hospitals, where the PLA LSD selected experts were from the PLA Ground Force Medical University, the PLA Navy Medical University and the PLA Air Force Military Medical University (空军军医大学, Xian), the PLA Center for Disease Control and Prevention, and the PLA Academy of Military Sciences. Moreover, to make sure that the medical staff and experts are best deployed at the frontline, the PLA also created the Army Frontline Command and Coordination Group (军队前方指挥协调组) in Wuhan, which in turn selected experts from the PLA General Hospital, and sent them to the Huashenshan Hospital in Wuhan for joint consultations.[5] At the peak of the pandemic, around 4000 medical personnel from all the military service branches, Strategic Support Force, Joint Logistics Support Force and the People's Armed Police Force were part of the medical team in Wuhan.

The Health Bureau of the PLA LSD coordinated with the National Health Commission to make sure safety procedures are followed in the course of controlling the spread of the pandemic in cities. For instance, the PLA took charge of three hospitals under its direct command after the medical teams reached Hubei province - the Wuhan Huoshenshan Hospital, the Wuhan Taikang Tongji Hospital and the Guanggu Branch of the Hubei Maternity and Child Health Care Hospital. The Army Military Medical University was in charge of two wards of Wuhan Jinyintan

Hospital, the Naval Military Medical University was responsible for the intensive care unit at the Wuhan Hankou Hospital, the Air Force Military Medical University provided critical care at the Wuhan Wuchang Hospital among others.[6] Moreover, as they had hospitals under their command, they had to make sure that the blood supplies are safely secured. This led to both the organisations issuing guidelines to the medical staff to make sure that protection procedures are followed including health conditions of the blood donors, safety protection methods in blood donation centres and treatment of medical waste.[7] Only when the infections were cured according to their satisfaction did the medical teams return from Wuhan. Experts from the Third Military Medical University also carried out investigations into COVID-19 deaths and established the pathological sample bank on the disease.[8]

To transport supplies to the local outbreak centres, the Transportation and Delivery Bureau of the CMC Logistics Support Department (中央军委后勤保障部运输投送局) gave instructions to the theatre commands to utilise their military vehicles. In Wuhan, the PLA Central Command contributed the most in terms of using their military transport to the outbreak areas. The Joint Logistics Support Force organised the transportation details and coordination from multiple locations. According to one report, provincial military districts deployed militias to the outbreak areas to carry out epidemic prevention duties such as disinfection, transportation, and distribution of propaganda material.[9]

Various military hospitals under the PLA LSD were involved in the fight against the pandemic. They played an important role in the PLA's response to the pandemic, including provision of staff with prior experience of dealing with pandemics, arranging testing kits and developing vaccines. The PLA Military Medical University (中国人民解放军陆军军医大学第二附属医院), in short the Xinqio Hospital (新桥医院) in Chongqing sent medical teams to Wuhan, comprising personnel who had prior experience in fighting SARS and EBOLA in Africa.[10] From the PLA Air Force Military Medical University Tangdu Hospital (中国人民解放军空军军医大学第二附属医院,唐都医院), the Department of Respiratory Medicine sent its staff as part of the medical team.[11]

Among the PLA organisations, the PLA Joint Logistics Support Force (JLSF), which was established in 2016 was mobilised for the first time during the pandemic and was charged with securing supplies needed to fight the pandemic. The PLA JLSF ensured that the Chinese military personnel had medical supplies for their use and helped the city of Wuhan with transport and logistics for supplying vegetables to the supermarket and shops.[12] This was part of the procedures to ensure civil-military integration that were adopted by the PLA JLSF to streamline transportation routes to the city.[13]

Impact of Reforms in Military Logistics and Response to the Pandemic

When the Chinese military reforms were announced in late 2015, the PLA Logistics Support Department was established as part of the reforms on January 10, 2016. The primary focus of the department was to establish a logistics system that will meet the requirements of the joint operations command, and centrally manage logistics support for the entire military. Once the department was established, it was given tasks such as logistics support planning, research, setting up standards, inspection and supervision. After these structural changes, the JLSF was established on September, 13, 2016 under the CMC, which followed the standards of a modern joint logistics support system.

The troops are headquartered in the Wuhan Joint Logistics Support Base and under its management, there are five joint logistics support centres (Wuxi, Guilin, Xining, Shenyang, and Zhengzhou), which provides support to the troops stationed in the region.[14] The five centressupport the five theatre commands and the movement of forces in inter-regional exercises, which also entails coordination among the theatre command logistics.[15] They fall under the jurisdiction of the Joint Logistics Department in the military districts. The reforms in military logistics are among the major achievements within the PLA not only by virtue of modern infrastructure and technology, but also because of the importance given to the role of logistics in military strategy. For instance, the leadership believes that logistics is of "vital importance to support and sustain military operations. In military strategic manoeuvring, the destruction of the enemy['s] supply lines and guarding one own supply lines is a crucial element in deciding the outcome of a war".[16] Therefore, all the military hospitals under the jurisdiction are managed by the Wuhan Joint Logistics Support Base and the five logistics centres.

The rationale behind these reforms was to make sure that as per the modern requirements for the Chinese military, the logistics supply required for the troops are adequately managed. This might also involve integrating civil-military supplies so that logistics is modern and fluid during conditions of war. The Chinese not only established this system but made sure that problems that were previously associated with logistics supply were rectified. A major rectification campaign that lasted almost half a year was carried out in the PLA Logistics Support Department in 2018, where many issues such as legal requirements, enthusiasm in providing health services for military personnel, health service guarantees, procurement problems of medical supplies, plagiarism in research, supervision and accountability, underwent scrutiny for all the military hospitals associated with the PLA LSD.[17] For instance, they conducted clean up and regulatory activities (清理整治), euphemism for weeding out corruption and ensuring accountability in their military logistics supply. One of the reasons for the rectification campaign was that to make sure that the supply lines are efficient and civilian resources are maximised, corruption levels had to be checked. During the COVID-19 pandemic, the reforms were visible as they were able to achieve civil-military integration through reforms, to aid in the logistics supply to the city of Wuhan and other outbreak centres.

As part of the reforms one such logistical change was that the PLA reformed the functioning of the military hospitals under its jurisdiction. For instance, among the PLA hospitals, the PLA General Hospital's Fifth Medical Centre played the most important role in responding to the pandemic. Under the military reforms, this hospital was formed by merging the 302 Hospital and the 307 Hospital. In fact, many of the hospitals in Beijing was merged under the PLA General Hospital and divided into eight centres. Many military hospitals in the military regions were also renamed and became part of the JLSF, such as the No. 900 Hospital of the JLSF (previously, the Fuzhou General Hospital of the Nanjing Military Region); 960th Hospital was renamed from Jinan Military Region General Hospital (by combining four hospitals together under the JLSF).[18]

A total of 20 hospitals that were listed as being reorganised under the Joint Logistics Support Force.[19] Under some hospitals in the region, they combined many of the smaller hospitals, military academies, and colleges under the newly formed hospital under the Joint LSF. The JLSF therefore, became almost like any other force structure, but at the deputy theatre level (副战区级). Similarly, the JLSF, which is under the CMC Logistics Support Department is also supposed to be responsible for maintenance and repair, and joint logistics support. As per the military reforms, the PLA is looking at joint training, joint operations, and joint support, and the JLSF satisfies these requirements. Moreover, many of the military universities were put under the jurisdiction of the Army, Navy, Air Force services (PLA Army Medical University in Chongqing, PLA Air Force Medical University in Xian, PLA Navy Medical University in Shanghai, etc), probably to make sure that the services are concentrated more on developing capabilities rather than operational matters, similar to its roles in developing capabilities rather than be in charge of the operational planning of the troops. Mostly, the reorganisation seems to be an effort to shift the priorities of the military universities from looking at profits for their functionality to focus on developing capabilities to raise the combat effectiveness, which includes military personnel training, military medicine science and technology, and health care centres.

According to Former President of the PLA Air Force Medical University, Zhou Xianzhi,

> "the nature of warfare is changing rapidly with information warfare at its core…it presents new challenges to the kind of military medical service that was available in the past… as the military missions are expanding and induction of new weapons system and expanding operational capabilities of the military personnel, the way military health support is administered is deeply changing as it has expanded from treating war wounds to improving combat effectiveness… the fields of bio-security, such as brain research, bio-materials, stem cells and proteomics research have become new frontiers of military medical technology… for instance, the Air Force Military Medical University have to keep up with the actual transformation of the PLA Air Force capabilities and mission requirements and build a military medical discipline with aerospace as the core".[20]

Similar reforms were conducted for the PLA Academy of Military Sciences (军事科学院), which played a major role in combating the pandemic. After the reforms, AMS had become an important strategic agency with its headquarters in Beijing that promotes civil-military integration, scientific collaboration with local governments, and lead all other academic and military units in scientific research. After the reforms, eight institutes such as the Academy of Military Medical Sciences (军事医学研究院), National Defense Engineering Research Institute (国防工程研究院), Army Political Work Research Institute (军队政治工作研究院), Systems Engineering Research Institute (系统工程研究院), War Research Institute (战争研究院), Chemical Defense Research Institute (防化研究院), Military Legal Research Institute (军事法制研究院), National Defense Science and Technology Innovation Research Institute (国防科技创新研究院) were placed under the PLA AMS.[21] Among these Institutes, the Academy of Military Medical Sciences (AMMS) was the principal agency involved in work concerning the pandemic. For instance, they are responsible for developing the COVID-19 vaccine in collaboration with private industries. The vaccine is already in clinical trials and remains one among many in the race for a COVID-19 vaccine. By being under the direct control of the AMS, the Institute was able to get the leadership's attention and was quickly able to mobilise its military medical researchers, and directly sending their team to Wuhan. The team led by Major General Chen Wei has shown quick results on the basis of the genome structure of the virus, which was quickly published by the Chinese scientific community.[22]

By bringing the military hospitals under the PLA LSD, both centrally as well as in the military regions, the PLA was able to streamline both food as well as medical supplies, including medical services and ensure that overall, it meets the standards of a modern logistics system. Naturally, these have come in handy when handling the pandemic, especially in the PLA's ability to combine both military and civilian resources under its command. Moreover, the military reforms of 2015 centralised many military hospitals of the PLA (for example the PLA General Hospital under the PLA Logistics Support Department) enabling the hospitals to use the 'joint operations system' for the first time to coordinate and dispatch medics to control the spread of the epidemic within the military.

MOOTW Capability and PLA Military's Response

While the pandemic has highlighted the ability of the PLA and its logistics system to respond to the crisis, there are reasons why the Chinese leadership had used its military in a much more extensive manner than other countries. The philosophy behind using the military to deal with the pandemic is connected to the Chinese leadership's focus on increasing the PLA's capability in handling non-traditional security threats. The military tasks of the PLA were therefore enhanced, and besides the prevalence of a political ideology behind the use of the PLA for domestic operations, it also meant that non-traditional security threats and their mitigation could be used to raise its military preparedness.

Therefore, China gave importance to non-traditional security threats for two fundamental reasons. First, the non-traditional security threats such as terrorism, natural disasters, piracy, nuclear security, and epidemics had an adverse effect on domestic stability, and required more sustained efforts from its military. Secondly, the operations related to non-traditional security offered the PLA military an avenue to train its forces, and raise its combat readiness. Therefore, the PLA called it Military Operations Other Than War (MOOTW) that allowed its military to conduct operations without engaging in military conflicts.

Though the MOOTW philosophy is an American concept, the Chinese have incorporated it into their military strategy, as they saw their global interests grew beyond its territorial boundaries. Within its boundaries, the military capability was used during natural disasters such as the Wenchuan earthquake among others. In particular, during the Wenchuan earthquake, around 146, 000 PLA and Armed Police Force personnel were deployed and engaged in disaster prevention and mitigation, flood control, flood relief, earthquake relief, safety protection, forest fire prevention and other coordinated actions. First brought into the Chinese military lexicon and taken seriously as a concept during Hu Jintao's time, the PLA has continuously improved its MOOTW capabilities, and called to contribute within the ambit of "diversified military missions". The defining period for these operations seemed to be 2008, when the military seemed to have assisted in the peacetime operations to aid the successful completion of the Olympics.

Since 2008, the Chinese military and People's Armed Police Force have been involved in MOOTW operations as per the instructions of the CMC

(军队非战争军事行动能力建设规划 – MOOTW Military Capability Building Plan)[23] in operations such as counter-terrorism, stability maintenance, disaster relief, security duties, safeguarding rights and interests, international peacekeeping, international rescue, etc. Moreover, the MOOTW operations research wing was established to conduct in-depth theoretical research on the kind of operations that could be envisaged for the PLA, improving the rapid response capability of the forces, involvement in MOOTW exercises as well as teaching MOOTW operations research to graduate students.[24] Mostly, the PLA concentrated on improving its emergency operations capability, such as command, emergency regulations, emergency construction of disaster relief equipment and materials, and fundamentally, a joint system that can carry forward decisions taken at the CMC level down to the troop level.

The MOOTW capability has been precisely developed because it is an important tool for projecting the power of the military in a non-war situation, and to be conducted during peacetime to deal with non-traditional challenges to the state that have increased as a result of the changing nature of security threats and the military's capability to shape the strategic situation.[25] In other words, MOOTW has become important not only for establishing stability, but also for protecting national interests. Moreover, from the Chinese perspective, one needs to be vigilant as MOOTW operations could transform in to war operations if MOOTW operations are insufficient to achieve strategic objectives in a situation, especially when political and diplomatic solutions have failed to bring peace.[26]

While many use non-traditional security threats and MOOTW interchangeably, from Chinese perspective, there are differences between the two concepts. For instance, while non-traditional security threats encompass a wide range of security threats, MOOTW cannot be used as the nomenclature for all non-traditional security threats.[27] For instance, MOOTW could be applied to non-traditional security threats such as natural disasters, epidemics, social unrest, riots etc, but not transnational crime, international drug smuggling, non-proliferation issues, which would require diplomatic, political and other means to resolve it.[28]

When China was developing the MOOTW capabilities, especially after 2008, it realised that the requirements for MOOTW were distinct from traditional military operations, even though the core military capabilities for bothwere common. For instance, for the military to develop MOOTW capability, they would have todevelop special military capabilities, such as engineering repair and construction forces, personnel trained in rescue operations, road and bridge repair capabilities, quick infrastructure construction, professional units for clearing of explosives, and research into special engineering equipment (useful in earthquakes, and natural disasters), targeted training in search and rescue, facility repairs, and all other diversified emergency responses.[29] Over the years, these capabilities were improved and a more integrated command system that could ensure a information network for sharing resources between different agencies has also been improved.

MOOTW operations are also one of the ways in which the PLA is using its militia of various categories to respond to rescue missions, thereby each category forming professional rescue teams such as water conservation, and fire rescue, and are divided into professional rescue and auxiliary rescue teams.[30] One of the most important requirements for the functioning of the MOOTW operations is the civil-military integration. In the Chinese view, for emergency and rescue operations, the military would have to work together with local forces, therefore requiring it to establish links to the ground mechanism during emergencies, and the integration of military and civilian practices.[31] Thus, local cooperation is essential for a successful MOOTW operations as they provide background support to the military, such as joint emergency operations as well as data and intelligence sharing.

However, the Chinese leadership considers MOOTW as an extension of military tasks, not the primary one, and therefore does not want the PLA to make it as an fundamental priority as it would weaken the development of core military capabilities that are focused on winning wars. Probably, the reason why the PLA prefers to include militias and the Police Armed Police Force (PAPF) is so that they can contribute significantly to MOOTW operations, and build the capabilities as they would understand local conditions better. One of the responsibilities within MOOTW is to ensure that important targets or those prone to terrorist attacks are safeguarded during disasters, therefore the PLA incorporated these protection measures into the command system of the MOOTW operations.[32] Some of these targets would include information networks, power grids, nuclear power plants, energy bases, transportation hubs, water conservation facilities, etc.

After the military reforms of 2015, the capabilities in MOOTW were also given more importance.Since the MOOTW capabilities in engineering, nuclear, bio-chemical and medical services had increased substantially, many other capabilities required to make the MOOTW system more efficient were given priority. These included emergency response mechanisms, accurate information using satellite reconnaissance, updating information database in real-time, communication coordination between emergency departments and local governments, elimination of risks in safety, equipment and materials preparation, and diversified use of different rescue teams such as the local command teams, technical guidance teams, professional rescue units, dangerous machinery squads, and comprehensive support units.[33] Post-reforms, capabilities in MOOTW have been focused on increasing coordination between the military and local forces, finding solutions to the practical difficulties that arise when attempting to plan MOOTW operations such as the unexpectedness of the situation, diversified tasks, high dispersion, etc.[34]

Therefore, the developments in MOOTW capabilities have certainly helped in dealing with COVID-19, as epidemic prevention also forms a major part of it.

Conclusion

Overall, the PLA has established itself as a force that can deal with certain non-traditional security threats and make effective use of MOOTW capability. The effect of both military reforms and the modernisation of MOOTW capabilities has ensured that the PLA's response mechanism is fast, especially when supported by a highly centralised agency at the CMC level. In the context of the pandemic, the PLA moved into action immediately after the Chinese leadership established the Joint Control and Prevention Mechanism, which placed about 32 agencies under its wing and had become the central agency with its full support.This made it easier for the PLA Logistics Support Department to establish command and coordinate emergency operations with the help of its regional military logistics departments.

NOTES

1 For the burgeoning literature on MOOTW see United States Joint Chiefs of Staff, "Joint Doctrine for Military Operations Other Than War" *Joint Pub 3-07* at https://www.bits.de/NRANEU/others/jp-doctrine/jp3_07.pdf; United States Air Force, "Military Operations Other Than War" *Air Force Doctrine Document 2-3* October 5, 1996 at https://www.globalsecurity.org/military/library/policy/usaf/afdd/2-3/afdd2-3.pdf; PRC Ministry of National Defense, "Military Operations Other than War" at http://eng.mod.gov.cn/Database/MOOTW/index.htm#; "MOOTW" *China Military* at http://eng.chinamil.com.cn/china-military/node_83137.htm; *Fan Gaoyue and James Char, "Introduction to China's Military Operations Other Than War"* S. Rajaratnam School of International Studies Policy Report February 2019 at https://www.rsis.edu.sg/wp-content/uploads/2019/02/PR190225_Introduction-to-Chinas-Military-Operations-Other-than-War.pdf ; Cynthia Watson, "The Chinese Armed Forces and Non-Traditional Missions: A Growing Tool of Statecraft", *China Brief,* 9(4), February 20, 2009; Ministry of Defence, "Operation Sadbhavana" *Press Information Bureau* March 15, 2013 at https://pib.gov.in/newsite/feacontent.aspx?relid=93711; R. Atkinson, "Medicine in Military Operations Other Than War (MOOTW)" *Orthopaedic Proceedings* 84-B (III) February 21, 2018 at https://online.boneandjoint.org.uk/doi/abs/10.1302/0301-620X.84BSUPP_III.0840220e; and William H. Wilst et.al, "The Role of Public Health in the Prevention of War: Rationale and Competencies" *American Journal of Public Health*104(6),June 2014;: e34–e47 at https://www.ncbi.nlm.nih.gov/pmc/articles/PMC4062030/

2 Xinhua, "Transcripts of the Press Conference of Army's Support to Local Fight Against Covid-19" (军队支援地方抗击新冠肺炎疫情新闻发布会文字实录), *Xinhua* March 2, 2020, at http://www.xinhuanet.com/mil/2020-03/02/c_1210497902.htm

3 Sun Xingwei, Gao Ying, "Adhere to Scientific Treatment and Strive Well for Self-Protection, Strive To Achieve "Winning the Battle of Zero Infection", (坚持科学施治搞好自身防护，力争实现"打胜仗、零感染"), *PLA Daily*, January 30, 2020, at http://www.mod.gov.cn/topnews/2020-01/30/content_4859243.htm

4 "Central Military Commission: The Army Sent Three Batches of More Than 4000 Medical Personnel to Support Wuhan" (中央军委：部队共派出 3 批次 4000 多名医务人员支援武汉), *People's Weekly*, 2020 (5), at http://paper.people.com.cn/rmzk/html/2020-04/02/content_1979854.htm

5 Sun Xingwei, "Army Frontline Command and Coordination Group Organised Experts To Go To Huoshenshan Hospital for Consulatation" (军队前方指挥协调组组织专家赴火神山医院会诊), *PLA Daily*, February 15, 2020, at http://www.xinhuanet.com/mil/2020-02/15/c_1210475215.htm

6 Yue Jinsong and Tang Shunan, "The PLA's War on the Spectrum of Epidemic in Wuhan" (解放军武汉战"疫"谱), *Qiushi*, 9 March 2020, at http://www.qstheory.cn/laigao/ycjx/2020-03/09/c_1125686658.htm

7 National Health Commission of the State Council and Health Bureau of the PLA Logistics Support Department Notice Regarding the Guarantee of Safe Supply of Blood During the Period of New COVID-19 Epidemic (国家卫生健康委员会办公厅中央军委后勤保障部卫生局关于做好新型冠状病毒肺炎疫情期间血液安全供应保障工作的通知), *State Health Medical Letter 2020*, No. 113, February 5, 2020, at http://www.gov.cn/zhengce/zhengceku/2020-02/11/content_5477191.htm

8 "Chinese Academy of Sciences' Academician and Professor of Army Medical University Bian Xiuwu Leads the Team in Establishing the World's First COVID-19 Pathology Sample Bank" (中科院院士、陆军军医大学教授卞修武带领团队建立全世界首个新冠肺炎病理样本库), *Chongqing Daily*, April 6, 2020, at http://cq.gov.cn/zwxx/jrcq/202004/t20200406_6976517.html

9 Jun Weimin, "Remembering the trust of the People and the Party, Fighting Hard on the Epidemic on the Front line Battle - The PLA Resolutely Implements Xi Jinping's Important Instructions and Fully Committed to Epidemic Prevention and Control" (牢记党和人民重托奋战在防控疫情斗争第一线——人民军队坚决落实习主席重要指示全力投入疫情防控纪实), *Qiushi*, 2020 (5): 1 March, at http://www.qstheory.cn/dukan/qs/2020-03/01/c_1125641785.htm

10 Three Medical Teams from PLA Army Military Medical University Expedition, Epidemic Veterans Once Again Went to the Battlefield" (陆军军医大学三位医疗队员出征 "防疫老兵"再赴战场), *Sina Military*, 27 January, 2020, at https://mil.news.sina.com.cn/2020-01-27/doc-iihnzhha4873686.shtml

11 "Air Force Medical University Tangdu Hospital Department of Respiratory Medicine's 'Two Places and Three Lines', Fully Prepared to Fight Pandemic" (空军军医大学唐都医院呼吸内科"两地三线"全力战疫), *Zhongguo Xinwenwang*, http://www.shx.chinanews.com/news/2020/0415/77935.html

12 Zhao Lei, "PLA Support Force Joins Disease Fight", *China Daily*, February 7, 2020, at http://eng.chinamil.com.cn/view/2020-02/07/content_9735244.htm

13 Wang Xin and Zhang Yanhong, "First Batch of Anti-Epidemic Materials of Joint Logistics Support Force Arrive in Wuhan" (联勤保障部队首批防疫物资抵汉), *Hubei Daily*, January 27, 2020, at https://www.hubei.gov.cn/hbfb/bmdt/202001/t20200127_2015316.shtml

14 Wang Jun, "Experts Explain in Detail the Relationship Between CMC Joint Logistics Support Force and CMC Logistics Support Department" (专家详解军委联勤保障部队与军委后勤保障部是何种关系), *The Paper*, November 27, 2016, at https://www.thepaper.cn/newsDetail_forward_1569162

15 Kevin McCauley, "China's Military Reforms and Modernisation: Implications for the United States", Testimony Before the US-China Economic and Security Review Commission, 15 February 2018, at https://www.uscc.gov/sites/default/files/McCauley_Written%20Testimony.pdf

16 Zhang Zhihao, "President Encourages PLA Logistics Force", *China Daily*, October 21, 2019, at https://www.chinadaily.com.cn/a/201910/21/WS5dace947a310cf3e3557184c.html

17 Zhou Na, "PLA Logistics Support Department Health Bureau Deployed Clean-Up and Remediation Activities in Military Health Care and Industry" (中央军委后勤保障部卫生局部署军队医疗卫生行业领域清理整治活动), *Zhongguo Junwang*, April 14, 2018, at http://www.81.cn/jwzb/2018-04/12/content_8002342.htm

18 Yue Huairang and Zhang Jiaran, "Information About Military Hospital Reform Has Been Successively Disclosed: Four Hospitals Have Been Jointly Organised as No. 960 Hospital of the PLA"

(军队医院改革信息陆续披露：4所医院共组解放军第960医院), *The Paper*, May 11, 2018, at https://www.thepaper.cn/newsDetail_forward_2602017

19 These hospitals in general come under the 900 series, such as the No. 900 Hospital (previously Fuzhou General Hospital), No. 901, No. 902, No. 903, No. 904, No 905, No. 910, No. 920, No. 924, No. 928, No. 940, No.960, No. 967, No. 968, No. 980, No. 982, No. 983, No. 988, No. 990 etc. See, Li Xingpeng, "There are New Developments in Military Reforms, Recently 20 Military Hospitals Have Been Listed Together" (军改又有新动态 近20所部队医院密集挂牌), *Medical Think Tank*, November 1, 2019, at http://med.china.com.cn/content/pid/52668/tid/1014

20 Cai Pengcheng, Wang Yu, "New Round of Military Reforms: Why Was Three Military Medical Universities Given New Names" (新一轮军改，三所军医大学为啥被赋予新名称), *Zhongguo Junwang Zonghe*, October, 3, 2018, at http://www.81.cn/jwgz/2018-03/10/content_7967390_4.htm

21 Wang Jun, "The Eight Affiliated Research Institutes Under the Newly Formed PLA Academy of Military Sciences are Unveiled", (新组建的军事科学院下属八个研究院全部亮相), *The Paper*, September 9, 2017, at https://www.thepaper.cn/newsDetail_forward_1789598

22 Josephine Ma, "China's Military Becomes World's First To Use Experimental Coronavirus Vaccine", *South China Morning Post*, June 29, 2020, at https://www.scmp.com/news/china/science/article/3091093/chinese-military-approves-use-experimental-coronavirus-vaccine

23 "National Defense and Army Building Achievements: Loyal Writings of the MOOTW Operations", (国防和军队建设成就：在非战争军事行动中书写忠诚), *Xinhua*, October 25, 2012, at http://mil.cnr.cn/ztl/cehua/10/201210/t20121025_511221356.html

24 "Great Military Practice in Peacetime, Summary of Military and People's Armed Police Force MOOTW Operations Since 2008" (和平年代的伟大军事实践——全军和武警部队２００８年以来遂行非战争军事行动任务综述), *Xinhua*, September 4, 2011, at http://www.gov.cn/jrzg/2011-09/04/content_1939920.htm

25 Xin Fudong, "The Aspects of 'War' in Non-War " (非战之"战"面面观), *PLA Daily*, December 1, 2016, at http://www.mod.gov.cn/intl/2016-01/12/content_4636253.htm

26 Xin Fudong Ibid.

27 Sun Zhenwu, Wang Dawei, and Sun Fengcheng, "Non-Traditional Security Threats and MOOTW Operations", (非传统安全威胁与非战争军事行动), National Party Congress, October 19, 2010, at http://www.npc.gov.cn/zgrdw/huiyi/lfzt/ybyjgfxza/2010-08/19/content_1588539.htm

28 Sun Zhenwu et.al., Ibid

29 Ding Haiming, "Voice of Representatives: Military Observations of MOOTW Operations" (代表心声：非战争军事行动的"军事观察"), *PLA Daily*, March 9, 2009, at http://www.npc.gov.cn/zgrdw//npc/xinwen/dbgz/dbzs/2009-03/09/content_1489927.htm

30 Zhou Jiarong and Bi Junchang, "Laying a Solid Foundation for the Mission of MOOTW Operations" (打牢遂行非战争军事行动任务的基础), *Guofang Bao*, May 17, 2010, at http://www.mod.gov.cn/gflt/2010-05/17/content_4157034.htm

31 Wang Yuren, "MOOTW Operations: The Engine of Integrated Civil-Military Development" (非战争军事行动军民融合式发展的引擎), *PLA Daily*, December 20, 2012, at http://theory.people.com.cn/n/2012/1220/c136458-19956943.html

32 Wu Hongqiang and Wu Mengyuan, "Protection of Important Targets in MOOTW Operations" (非战争军事行动中重要目标的防护), Guangzhou Municipal People's Government, June 22, 2010, at http://www.gzccad.gov.cn/gzsrmfb/llyj/201006/575602a773644291aa303cd6152e5162.shtml

33 Shi Honghui, "Make MOOTW Operations More Efficient" (让非战争军事行动更高效), *PLA Daily*, October 25, 2018, at http://www.mod.gov.cn/jmsd/2018-10/25/content_4827747.htm

34 Wu Min, Ge Zhixiang and Liu Luhui, "Representative Liu Yongjun: Make MOOTW Operations Scientific and Efficient" (刘勇军代表：让非战争军事行动科学高效), *PLA Daily*, March 14, 2019, at http://www.xinhuanet.com/2019-03/14/c_1210081567.htm

7

China's 'Hi-Tech' Response to COVID-19

Munish Sharma

Introduction

The global response to contain and quell the COVID-19 pandemic witnessed a flux of tailor-made technology solutions – right from the diagnostic testing of SARS-COV-2 infection to the modeling-based prediction and containment of the outbreak, and from the mitigation of acute risks to the 'hot pursuit' of a vaccine. This is the first time humanity has witnessed a health emergency of such severity and global expanse. The pandemic triggered an unprecedented exigency for digital healthcare and epidemiology applications such as data collection, statistical analysis, data visualization, computer modeling, community engagement, monitoring, and supply chain management. With rapid improvement in computational power, refined algorithms, and large data sets comprising of methodically collected medical and epidemiological data, the battle against COVID-19 has been supported by technology to a great extent. Integrating data and activities, geographic information systems and satellite imagery have aided governments in visualization, response and transportation planning, and continuity of operations.[1] Unmanned aerial vehicles (UAVs) were put in use to transport supplies and material, disinfect public areas, and surveillance and policing, minimizing human interactions. World's fastest supercomputers, 'Summit' for instance, ran colossal computations for epidemiology, bioinformatics, and molecular modeling to screen compounds for a new drug and vaccine against the disease thus accelerating research and cutting down time.[2] Advanced simulations, powered by Artificial Intelligence (AI) forecasted the trends of the spread and evaluated the effectiveness of the enforced containment measures. At another pertinent end, smartphone apps provided instant access to medical specialists, while chatbots helped with virtual screening and triage. Digital training resources were also of great help for healthcare professionals.[3] Some of the applications developed to combat COVID-19 were already time-tested, while most of them were built at a 'war-footing', that too under severe travel restrictions.

With the spread of the pandemic to every corner of the world, advances in emerging technologies of the sorts of Artificial Intelligence, Big Data Analytics, Autonomous Vehicles, 5G, Internet of Things, and Virtual Reality were leveraged to develop applications as diverse as fusing geospatial data with real-time information for situational awareness, predictive modeling, genomic sequencing, contact tracing, logistics planning and supply chain optimization for essential or relief goods, decision support for medical diagnosis, telemedicine, surveillance and monitoring in congested public areas, smart medical devices, drug development, and even in training and stress management. The list can go on. Interestingly, the same set of technologies have been in the spotlight owing to the unfolding competition between the United States (US) and China in the technology sphere. The latter, of late, has made significant advances in this space, vying for global technology leadership. China, the first epicenter and therefore the first respondent to the COVID-19 health emergency, capitalized the prowess it has gradually built in emerging technologies[4] with profound support and funding from the government. State-led policy measures over the last five years, 'Made in China 2025' in 2015, the 'Next Generation AI Development Plan' and the 'Three-Year Action Plan for Promoting the Development of a New Generation Artificial Intelligence Industry (2018-2020)' in 2017 have laid the foundation and directed the efforts of the research institutions and the industry towards integration of information technology and AI with manufacturing, healthcare, agriculture, transportations and other sectors, with the vision of global leadership in manufacturing and AI technology and applications. An extensive use of AI, Big Data, Robotics and Autonomous Vehicles improved efficiency in the various functions of epidemic monitoring, virus tracking, prevention, control and treatment, and resource allocation.[5] The development of these solutions could be hastened, but not the expertise in underlying technology. It takes years of conjoint efforts to reach a pedestal. China was ahead of others temporally and that rendered a lead time to build 'hi-tech' technology applications, setting the examples for others. China, on top of that, left no stone unturned in 'showcasing' its ability to build innovative solutions at the cutting-edge of technology.

Emerging technologies and COVID-19

The global response to COVID-19 could be deemed as one of the most technologically advanced responses ever to a pandemic. The World Health Organization (WHO) recognized the expansive role of technology and social media, first time in the human history at this scale, to keep people safe, productive and connected when the circumstances actually required them to be physically apart.[6] The circumstances even brought corporate rivals together in the quest of technology and medical solutions. Smartphone manufacturers Google and Apple came together to enable interoperability between Android and iOS devices and the use of Bluetooth technology for contact tracing, eventually helping governments and health agencies reduce the spread of the virus, of course, with due credence to privacy and security.[7] Two of the world's largest vaccine manufactures, GlaxoSmithKline and Sanofi joined their forces to reduce the development time for vaccine against COVID-19.[8] Most fascinating amongst all is the innovative technology solutions built using emerging technologies.

At the first place, it was an AI powered infectious disease outbreak risk software built by a Canadian start-up BlueDot[9] which identified a cluster of 'unusual pneumonia' in Wuhan on 30 December 2019, nine days before the WHO actually confirmed the discovery of a novel coronavirus which was later named as SARS-COV-2. The firm consolidates and analyzes data from a myriad of sources such as healthcare organizations of the sorts of Center for Disease Control (CDC) or the WHO, news reports, movement of travelers on commercial flights, livestock health reports, and climate data from satellites from all across the world, round the clock.[10] AI assists the human expertise at BlueDot to make accurate predictions, that too well in time.

Finding applications in solving both social and medical issues thrown open by COVID-19, a whole lot of AI based applications have moved from experimental phase to real-world implementation primarily in biotechnology and pharmaceuticals, medical diagnosis and epidemiological research modeling.[11] In biotechnology and pharmaceuticals, AI has been of immense help in estimating the protein structure of SARS-CoV-2 using computational models, identification of existing drugs which could be repurposed, find new compounds, and other characteristics of the virus. For medical diagnosis, AI has been leveraged for imaging, such as Computed Tomography (CT) and X-Ray scans, prognosis and predictions of treatment outcomes. AI in epidemiological research modeling has led to enhanced understanding of evolution of the pandemic and its effect on different demographic and geographic regions and socio-economic conditions leading to improved public policy responses.

In the battle against COVID-19, one of the most prevalent uses of AI was seen in diagnostic assistance technology, where algorithms helped radiologists in identifying abnormalities and their severity in chest X-Rays and CT scans within seconds as compared to around 15 minutes[12] in the case of a manual diagnosis, helping with both diagnosis and prognosis of the disease.[13] For instance, the 'Chest X-Ray AI Image Support Decision Tool' developed by Vuno was developed and trained to identify nodules, pneumothorax, effusions, and interstitial opacity in chest X-ray images and produce the diagnosis in just three seconds.[14] Accurate and fast diagnosis not just reduces the burden on radiologists and relieves pressure off the resource-constrained healthcare system in the pandemic-affected geographies, but also limits the spread. In addition to diagnostics, AI found wide-ranging applications in epidemiological analysis and the pharmaceutical industry which were running against time to identify risk prone areas, identify drug candidates, develop new drugs and vaccines, and predict the spread of the contagion and the disease.

AI-based predictive modeling played a pivotal role in accurate and timely understanding of the severity and geographical spread of the contagion. A better picture with forecasts and predictions helped public health agencies with data inputs to raise early warnings, allocate medical resources, and augment their planning and preparedness for the pandemic. Using machine learning to train neural networks researchers enhanced the existing Susceptible-Exposed-Infectious-Removed (SEIR) model in epidemiology, which is widely used to predict the spread of a disease by grouping people as susceptible, exposed, infected, or recovered, to predict the impact of quarantine measures.[15] The COVID-19 pandemic has generated large swathes of datasets which will further train AI- based models for future prediction of the epidemics.

Another key application of AI during COVID-19 was to accelerate both the processes of discovering new drugs as well as identifying existing drugs which could be repurposed to treat the disease. Discovering novel drug candidates is a time consuming, complex and an expensive process, and it takes years to secure regulatory approvals.[16] Repurposing drugs requires careful and rational examination, which is also a slow process but the safety of already-approved drugs is well established. AI has helped in the pursuit of both these options for COVID-19. Researchers from South Korea and the US used machine learning to identify *atazanavir*, while a UK AI startup, Benevolent AI, and Imperial College identified *Baricitinib*, a drug approved for rheumatoid arthritis. Evaluating multiple scenarios with a multitude of parameters, AI in the drug design process has reduced time span from several months to just a few days.[17] With the use of AI, Insilico Medicine synthesized novel molecules with the potential to bind a specific SARS-CoV-2 protein, while Innoplexus identified the most promising ones from millions of generated candidate molecules.[18]

This endeavour has benefited tremendously from supercomputing,[19] an existing and well-known technology, putting enormous computing power at the disposal of entities involved in the research to computationally identify molecular candidates for drugs against COVID-19 before they could be tested experimentally. The simulations generally use computers for drug docking calculations and molecular dynamics simulations to rapidly zero in on the most promising molecules as drug candidates. Out of thousands of compounds just a handful are to be shortlisted. While a comprehensive simulation model of a SARS-CoV-2 drug target protein may take months on a typical computer cluster, it takes just a day on Summit – world's most powerful supercomputer.[20] Supercomputing resources were also pooled together and provided free to the research institutions. One of such voluntary initiatives is the COVID-19 High-Performance Computing Consortium bringing together the resources available with the federal government, industry, and academia in the US. Moreover, it was Cloud Computing that made access to these supercomputers possible, amidst mobility constraints due to COVID-19 health emergency.

The mobility constrains also led to a huge increase in demand for the delivery of groceries, medical supplies, essentials and food, while running acutely short of human resources in supply chain and delivery infrastructures due to social distancing protocols in place. Robots and unmanned and autonomous vehicles, both on the ground and in the air, came handy in maintaining continuity of essential services and supplies.[21] Robots were deployed to disinfect surfaces in hospitals and public areas. UAVs were delivering medical supplies in hospitals and essential goods, especially in isolated zones. They were also pressed into service for surveillance and patrolling, and the agricultural ones were repurposed to spray disinfectants. Autonomous (self-driving) vehicles, empowered by AI, made contactless deliveries possible, effectively without human intervention.

In the entire discourse on COVID-19 the reference to China's case is quite frequent, not just as the origin of the virus outbreak but also with regard to its technology-enabled response which has set examples for other countries to follow or to ape. Technologies which were earlier in the experimental phase, or merely pilot runs, found wide adoption in the fight against COVID-19. Amongst all, AI stands apart. China's response, whether in modeling diagnosis or transportation and logistics, had a fine share of AI-enabled applications. Swift development of these applications did not happen overnight. Sustained investment in research and development for years bore fruit for China.

China's response to COVID-19: the technology factor

Artificial Intelligence has been a priority technology area for the Chinese political leadership. The State Council has issued several policy measures for the development of AI-related technologies. The 'National Medium- and Long-Term Plan for the Development of Science and Technology (2006-2020)' of the State Council essentially laid the foundation for R&D in AI, prioritizing the development of intelligent sensors, intelligent robots, and virtual reality as one of the 'frontier technologies'.[22] Intelligent sensors included image and natural language comprehension and biometric identification, while intelligent robots were meant for service and dangerous operation. The 'Made in China 2025' plan,[23] first mentioned by Premier Li Keqiang in the 2015 Government Work Report, has also laid down the approach to integrate information technology into China's manufacturing sector envisioning a leadership position among the world's manufacturing powers.[24] Information technology and controlled machine tools and robots are amongst the ten key sectors, basically paving the way for intelligent control systems, intelligent process controls, supply chain optimization in the manufacturing sector, and the wide-scale industrialization of intelligent vehicles, machinery, robots, and appliances. The plan also envisaged an increasing role for industrial robots in automobile, machinery, electronics industry, and service robots in medical treatment, domestic services, education and entertainment.

The State Council rolled out the 'Next Generation AI Development Plan' in July 2017, setting the vision for China as a hub for global AI innovation and a leader in AI technology and applications by 2030.[25] To further reinforce this plan and implement the 'Made in China 2025' plan, the Ministry of Industry and Information Technology issued the 'Three-Year Action Plan for Promoting the Development of a New Generation Artificial Intelligence Industry (2018-2020)' in December 2017.[26] It laid down the guidelines for the integration of AI with areas as diverse as healthcare, transportation, agriculture, finance, logistics, sensors and smart manufacturing.

In a nutshell, aggressive planning and recalibration of the goals indicate leadership's vision of AI as a driving force behind the upcoming industrial transformation and therefore China's next-generation of socioeconomic development. Concomitant to the elevated interests and investments in AI research, scientific publications by the Chinese researchers have also increased in volume.[27]

Chinese technology giants like Alibaba[28], Baidu[29] and Tancent[30] have also built research capacity and made significant advances in areas like voice recognition, Natural Language Processing, machine learning, computer vision, autonomous robotic systems, and computational biology. All in all, the groundwork was essentially in place after years of state-led aggressive planning and intervention in technology research and development and the industrial policy. With the government scrambling to subdue the COVID-19 induced crisis, China's technology companies, from tech-giants to the young start-ups, stepped up to solve time-critical real-world problems but in a much 'intelligent' way.

As scientists and researchers were reeling against time to discover the characteristics of the corona virus in their quest to find a drug or a vaccine against COVID-19, their abilities have been augmented to a large extent with the wide-spread use of AI, which was already making breakthroughs in bio technology and pharmaceuticals industry. AI had also made inroads to the healthcare sector, and by the time of the outbreak of COVID-19 it had time-tested and fairly advanced applications in medical-imaging and radiological diagnosis. Baidu Research, one of the frontrunners in AI R&D globally, open-sourced its Linearfold algorithm available to research institutions and entities engaged in epidemic prevention and gene testing, helping them reduce the time taken to predict the secondary structure for the COVID-19 RNA sequence from 55 minutes with traditional RNA folding algorithms to just 27 seconds.[31] Genome Sequencing for Coronavirus Diagnostic Solution, an AI-powered platform jointly developed by the Zhejiang Provincial Center for Disease Control and Prevention, Alibaba DAMO Academy (the research arm of Alibaba), and Matridx Biotechnology, allows swift and accurate viral genetic data screening and protein structure analysis and report generation for COVID-19 samples.[32] The technology actually solves issues with Polymerase chain reaction method.[33]

With the rapid increase in the numbers of infected people, chest CT scan was identified as a handy diagnostic tool for pneumonia, and AI augmented human assessment of the scans.[34] Alibaba's Cloud-based CT Image Analytics Solutions takes 20 seconds to prepare and transmit the diagnosis. It can compute the proportion of lesions and affected volume ratio to the entire lungs.[35] AI-based solution 'InferRead CT Lung COVID-19' developed by a start-up Infervision, is capable of not just detecting the infection but also measuring the density, morphology and volume of lesions in 50 seconds.[36] Baidu's open-source deep learning platform, PaddlePaddle was also available for other companies, and a medical data analysis company, LinkingMed used it to build an open-source AI model for pneumonia CT image analysis, providing quantitative assessment like number, volume, and proportion of pneumonic lesions for diagnosis within a minute.[37] Another prognostic prediction algorithm developed by the Huazhong University of Science and Technology was used to predict the likelihood of a COVID-19 infected patient to develop acute respiratory distress syndrome.[38] The developers made these technology platforms, and especially the insights from the early stages of the outbreak, available to healthcare agencies, hospitals, medical practitioners, and researchers in other parts of the world as well. Alibaba's

'Free Computational and AI Platforms to Help Research, Analyze and Combat COVID-19 Program' supports disease control centers and genome research institutions worldwide for the research analysis and prevention of COVID-19.[39] It allowed free access to its High Performance Computing and AI platform for researchers on life sciences applications aiding in CT imaging diagnostics and the drugs and vaccines discovery through Computational-Driven-Drug-Design (CDDD) and AI-Driven-Drug-Design (AIDDD) for COVID-19.[40]

Robots and autonomous vehicles were a common feature in the Chinese measures for COVID-19 prevention and medical care. They were deployed in large numbers for spraying disinfectants, patrolling and surveillance, delivering food or supplies in hospitals and quarantine wards, and performing initial screening to reduce human interface. By early February, the Ministry of Industry and Information Technology had called for enhanced industrial cooperation to contribute to the discovery, awareness and control of COVID-19.[41] Some of the Chinese companies had already deployed robots and autonomous vehicles by then. Autonomous vehicles, such as a self-driving van developed by Unity Drive Innovation, a Shenzhen-based startup, were used as "contactless" alternative to regular deliveries as early as February 2020.[42] UNIDO's Investment and Technology Promotion Office and the White Rhino Auto company partnered to bring unmanned distribution vehicles to Wuhan's Guanggu Field Hospital in mid-February.[43] CloudMinds donated robots to several medical facilities in China, including the Wuhan Wuchang Field Hospital which is dubbed as 'Smart Field Hospital', helping medical staff in consultations, disinfection, cleaning and medicine delivery. The robots are capable of autonomous navigation and avoiding obstacles.[44]

Keenon's delivery robots across 100 hospitals helped with transportation of medical supplies and others tasks reducing the workload of medical staff.[45] Baidu also partnered with Neolix to deliver food and supplies using Apollo autonomous vehicle.[46] UVD Robots deployed disinfection robots in about 2,000 hospitals, while Xenex Corp covered around 500 hospitals and even exporting to other countries in the need of such robots.[47] A number of providers, including JD.com and Meituan Dianping, have used autonomous delivery vehicles for contactless delivery services distributing medical supplies to hospitals as well as vegetables and groceries to those in need.[48] The autonomous delivery vehicle developed by JD.com has been on road-trials since 2016, but its large-scale deployment had been restricted to various technological and legal constraints. The company also deployed UAV for deliveries.[49]

With around 1,353 UAV manufacturers in China, they were an obvious choice for a number of logistics operations in the isolated areas, containment zones and hospitals, such as delivery of emergency supplies, aerial patrols, aerial thermal imaging, and spraying disinfectant.[50] Da Jiang Innovations, one of the leading manufacturers of commercial UAVs,[51] deployed UAVs for most of these operations, working closely with the authorities.[52] Antwork, a delivery start-up, deployed UAV transport services to carry medical samples and quarantine material in hospitals.[53] These remotely piloted devices are easy to operate, inexpensive to procure and they can be mobilized quickly. Robots and UAVs have effectively relieved pressure off medical, paramedical, sanitation and support staff.

Beyond its direct use in medical research, diagnosis and hospitals, AI has also supported the surveillance activities as part of disease containment measures. Facial recognition systems are nothing new to the Chinese citizens, in fact they are very much part of the daily life now. The banks and the airports use them for authentication, few outlets use them for payments, and the law enforcement uses it for surveillance. China's facial recognition system also encompasses the nation-wide network of millions of CCTV cameras. The same was used to identify non-compliant individuals and restrict the movement of people, for instance, allowing only low-risk individuals to ply on the roads. Chinese companies, such as SenseTime and Hanwang Technology, augmented the existing technology to recognize faces even with masks on them with 95 percent accuracy, which otherwise without masks is 99.5 percent.[54] Facial recognition systems reduce physical contact with a device or a human being and the entire process is not time consuming either.[55] With social distancing protocols in place and restrictions on physical contact in the aftermath of COVID-19 pandemic, facial recognition is slated to be the preferred medium for authentication, even though it has known implications for privacy of the individuals.

Early rollout of 5G services has also helped Chinese companies in provisioning the above-mentioned technologies. In fact, some of the use-cases which were in experimental phase have matured enough to be integrated with clinical practices. 5G, as compared to 4G, offers higher data speed and enable massive device connectivity at extremely low latency, unravelling use-cases such as telemedicine and autonomous vehicles. In China, 5G enabled high-definition online consultation services, therefore helping hospitals with remote diagnosis on COVID-19 pneumonia when the availability of experts was severely constrained.[56] A CT and X-ray coordination solution built by Beijing Jincheng Medical Technology Co Ltd used 5G to transmit images to doctors outside the Hubei province for diagnosis and patient data for telemedicine.[57] Huawei also built a 5G network at Huoshenshan Hospital in Wuhan,[58] facilitating a whole gamut of 'intelligence' devices and services at the hospital. Moreover, the extensive use of autonomous vehicles in China, as discussed above, relied heavily on 5G services. The same enabled both, low-latency controls of UAVs and robots, and the transmission of real-time high-definition images. The whole idea of deploying autonomous vehicles for an array of tasks could see the light of the day because of 5G services in place.

Conclusion

The COVID-19 pandemic has certainly cleared the way for emerging technologies, especially AI, to a much wider adoption in public health and medicine. China – the first epicentre of the pandemic – has set an example in the use of these technologies, some of which were still in experimental phase before the pandemic, finding wide references in the technology literature and acceptance in other parts of the world. The vision of global leadership in technology innovation and development is explicit from China's long term plans for emerging/frontier technologies, being realized through dedicated three-year action plans. AI has received unparalleled attention of the political leadership in China, propelling public and private investments in the research and development of applications. When the pressing need to subdue the pandemic arose, Chinese companies were quick in churning out AI-based technology solutions for everything from clinical diagnosis to drug discovery, and logistics to surveillance. In a way, policy interventions and facilitation on part of the government had already prepared the ground for Chinese companies to make the giant leap forward. The pandemic was more of an impetus to put the technology at test, and China left no stone unturned in 'demonstrating' its prowess.

The 'Made in China 2025' strategic plan is also destined to gain from this crisis with industries turning to broader integration of information technology into in their manufacturing processes, replacing human intervention. With profound support of the government, Chinese companies will try their best to grab this opportunity by transforming the domestic manufacturing base as well as supplying technology to other countries in the process of implementing the same. The COVID-19 crisis also saw Chinese companies supplying robots and UAVs to other countries, but the most striking of all is the offering of their super computing resources and AI solutions in support of the global life sciences research. This also indicates that China is well integrated with the global research in advanced technology, fostering collaborations and even providing critical-resources at the need of the hour. The Chinese technology giants are, or aspire to be, at the forefront of all the technology domains the government has listed to be the priority areas, and this endeavour is supported in no small measure by the 'army' of start-ups.

However, along with access to technology it is equally important to possess the ability to scale up technology as and when the situation demands. The example of a nation-wide facial detection system stands as a testimonial to China's ability to scale up technology and ensure implementation. The dreadful effects of COVID-19-like extremely contagious diseases on the public health and economy at large are also likely to legitimize the existing mass surveillance program in China and elsewhere, even calling in for more intrusive provisions to forecast and prevent any such breakout in the future. The Chinese government is going to walk a tightrope to ensure that intrusive surveillance measures are not imposed on 1.4 billion Chinese citizens in the pretext of public health risks.

NOTES

1 Esri, "COVID-19", at https://www.esri.com/en-us/covid-19/overview

2 Dario Gil, "IBM helps bring supercomputers into the global fight against COVID-19", at https://newsroom.ibm.com/IBM-helps-bring-supercomputers-into-the-global-fight-against-COVID-19

3 "Tech's role in tracking, testing, treating COVID-19", *Mobihealthnews*, May 01, 2020, at https://www.mobihealthnews.com/news/roundup-techs-role-tracking-testing-treating-COVID-19

4 For more details on emerging technologies and China, see Richard P. Suttmeier, "A new Techno-nationalism? China and the development of technical standards", *Communications of the ACM*, Vol. 48, No. 4, 2005; EY, "China is poised to win the 5G race", 2018; Kai-Fu Lee, *AI Superpowers: China, Silicon Valley, and the New World Order*, Boston: Houghton Mifflin Harcourt, 2018; Huw Roberts et al., "The Chinese Approach to Artificial Intelligence: An Analysis of Policy and Regulation, September 1, 2019; "The AI powered state: China's approach to public sector innovation", Analysis and Policy Observatory, May 2020; McKinsey Global Institute, "Artificial Intelligence: Implications for China", April 2017; "Big Data for Development in China", UNDP China Working Paper, November 2014; Jun Zhu et al., "The future of artificial intelligence in China", *Communications of the ACM*, November 2018, Vol. 61 No. 11, pp. 44-45; Yue Liu et al., "An Overview of Big Data Industry in China", *China Communications*, vol. 11, no. 12, pp. 1-10, December. 2014; Lv Xiaozhan and Zhou Ping, "A comparative study on big data research in China and the USA", Proceedings of the 23rd International Conference on Science and Technology Indicators (2018), Centre for Science and Technology Studies, Leiden University; Munish Sharma, "Decrypting China's Quantum Leap," *The China Journal*, no. 80 (July 2018): 24-45.

5 Qi Xiaoxia "How next-generation information technologies tackled COVID-19 in China", *World Economic Forum*, April 08, 2020, at https://www.weforum.org/agenda/2020/04/how-next-generation-information-technologies-tackled-COVID-19-in-china/

6 World Health Organization, "ITU-WHO Joint Statement: Unleashing information technology to defeat COVID-19", April 20, 2020, at https://www.who.int/news-room/detail/20-04-2020-itu-who-joint-statement-unleashing-information-technology-to-defeat-COVID-19

7 Apple, "Apple and Google partner on COVID-19 contact tracing technology", April 10, 2020, at https://www.apple.com/in/newsroom/2020/04/apple-and-google-partner-on-COVID-19-contact-tracing-technology/

8 Natalie Huet, "Coronavirus vaccine: Pharma giants GSK and Sanofi team up to find COVID-19 solution", *Euronews*, April 14, 2020, at https://www.euronews.com/2020/04/14/coronavirus-vaccine-pharma-giants-gsk-and-sanofi-team-up-to-find-COVID-19-solution, accessed on May 02, 2020.

9 Bluedot, at https://bluedot.global/

10 Ben Dickson, "How AI Is Helping in the Fight against COVID-19", *PC Magazine*, April 08, 2020, at https://in.pcmag.com/artificial-intelligence-2/135748/how-ai-is-helping-in-the-fight-against-COVID-19

11 Joseph Bullock et al, "Mapping the landscape of Artificial Intelligence applications against COVID-19", April 24, 2020, at https://arxiv.org/pdf/2003.11336.pdf.

12 "A European Initiative for Automated diagnosis and quantitative analysis of COVID-19 on imaging", at https://imagingcovid19ai.eu/

13 The Lancet, "COVID-19 and artificial intelligence: protecting health-care workers and curbing the spread", Volume 2, April 2020, at https://www.thelancet.com/pdfs/journals/landig/PIIS2589-7500(20)30054-6.pdf, see also Ory Six, "Dignosing COVID-19 using AI-based medical image analyses", *Quantib*, March 20, 2020, at https://www.quantib.com/blog/diagnosing-COVID-19-using- ai-based-medical-image-analyses See also Delft Imaging, "Triage for COVID-19 Using Artificial Intelligence on Chest X-rays", at https://www.delft.care/cad4covid/

14 Vuno, "VUNO Med®-Chest X-ray got approval of MFDS", August 21, 2019, at https://www.vuno.co/news_detail/60, see also "COVID-19: How Korea is using innovative technology and AI to flatten the curve", *ITU News*, April 02, 2020, at https://news.itu.int/COVID-19-how-korea- is-using-innovative-technology-and-ai-to-flatten-the-curve/

15 Mary Beth Gallagher, "Model quantifies the impact of quarantine measures on COVID-19's spread", *MIT News*, April 16, 2020, at http://news.mit.edu/2020/new-model-quantifies-impact-quarantine-measures-COVID-19-spread-0416. See also Mary L. Martialay, "Machine Learning Models Predict COVID-19 Impact in Smaller Cities", *Rensselaer News*, April 17, 2020, at https://news.rpi.edu/content/2020/04/17/machine-learning-models-predict-COVID-19-impact-smaller-cities,

16 Ulrik Kristensen, "How AI is speeding development of COVID-19 therapies", *The Scientific Advisory Board*, April 01, 2020, at https://www.scienceboard.net/index.aspx?sec=sup&sub=Drug&pag=dis&ItemID=607.

17 Tata Consultancy Services, "The Race for a Cure for COVID-19", at https://www.tcs.com/company-overview/tcs-artificial-intelligence-cure-COVID-19

18 Insilico Medicine, "Insilico Medicine publishes molecular structures for the key protein target of 2019-nCoV", February 06, 2020 at https://insilico.com/ncov-sprint, See also "Insilico and Boehringer to use AI for drug targets discovery", *Pharmaceutical Technology*, April 15, 2020, at https://www.pharmaceutical-technology.com/news/insilico-medicine-boehringer-ai-deal/ ; Megan Scudellari, "Five Companies Using AI to Fight Coronavirus", *IEEE Spectrum*, March 19, 2020, at https://spectrum.ieee.org/the-human-os/artificial-intelligence/medical-ai/companies-ai-coronavirus Stratos Davlos, "How Innoplexus is discovering novel molecules for COVID-19", at https://www.innoplexus.com/blog/how-innoplexus-is-discovering-novel-molecules-for-COVID-19/

19 "AI Accelerating Drug Discovery To Fight COVID-19", *Drug Discovery Online*, April 28, 2020, at https://www.drugdiscoveryonline.com/doc/ai-accelerating-drug-discovery-to-fight-covid-0001 and "COVID-19 research news", *Science Node*, April 28, 2020, at https://sciencenode.org/feature/COVID-19%20research%20updates.php

20 Oak Ridge National Laboratory, "Drug Discovery for COVID-19", at https://www.olcf.ornl.gov/cv19-project/drug-discovery-for-COVID-19/; Argonne National Laboratory, "Argonne's COVID-19 modeling combines physics and artificial intelligence", April 27, 2020, at https://federallabs.org/news/argonnes-COVID-19-modeling-combines-physics-and-artificial-intelligence; Dario Gil, "IBM helps bring supercomputers into the global fight against COVID-19", at https://newsroom.ibm.com/IBM-helps-bring-supercomputers-into-the-global-fight-against-COVID-19

21 Tim Dawkins, "How COVID-19 could open the door for driverless deliveries", *World Economic Forum*, April 07, 2020, at https://www.weforum.org/agenda/2020/04/how-COVID-19-could-open-the-door-for-driverless-deliveries/

22 The State Council - The People's Republic of China, The National Medium- and Long-Term Program for Science and Technology Development (2006-2020) - An Outline.

23 State Council - The People's Republic of China, "Made in China 2025", July 07, 2015.

24 Li Keqiang, "Report on the Work of the Government", *Delivered at the Third Session of the 12th National People's Congress,* March 5, 2015, at http://english.www.gov.cn/archive/publications/2015/03/05/content_281475066179954.htm, accessed on May 07, 2020, also see The State Council - The People's Republic of China, "'Made in China 2025' plan issued", at http://english.www.gov.cn/policies/latest_releases/2015/05/19/content_281475110703534.htm

25 Zhang Dongmiao, "China maps out AI development plan", *Xinhua,* July 20, 2017, http://www.xinhuanet.com/english/2017-07/20/c_136459382.htm, and "Notice of the State Council on Printing and Distributing a New Generation of Artificial Intelligence Development Plan", July 08, 2017, at http://www.gov.cn/zhengce/content/2017-07/20/content_5211996.htm

26 Ministry of Industry and Information Technology, "Notice of the Ministry of Industry and Information Technology on Printing and Distributing the 'Three-year Action Plan for Promoting the Development of the New Generation Artificial Intelligence Industry (2018-2020)'", December 14, 2017, at http://www.miit.gov.cn/n1146295/n1652858/n1652930/n3757016/c5960820/content.html

27 "Scimago Journal and Country Rank", at http://www.scimagojr.com/countryrank.php?category=1702&area=1700

28 Alibaba AI Labs, "Research Focus", at https://damo.alibaba.com/labs/ai

29 Baidu Research, "Research Areas", at http://research.baidu.com/Research_Areas?id=55

30 Tencent AI Lab, "Research Areas", at https://ai.qq.com/hr/ailab.shtml

31 See n. 5.

32 Alibaba Cloud, "How Is Alibaba DAMO Academy Helping to Fight the Outbreak of the Novel Coronavirus?", March 10, 2020, at https://medium.com/datadriveninvestor/how-is-alibaba-damo-academy-helping-to-fight-the-outbreak-of-the-novel-coronavirus-eeb65648ac2,; "Alibaba Cloud offers AI, cloud services to battle COVID-19 globally", *BioSpectrum Asia,* March 19, 2020, at https://www.biospectrumasia.com/news/46/15625/alibaba-cloud-offers-ai-cloud-services-to-battle-covid- 19-globally.html

33 Alibaba Cloud, "Whole Genome Sequencing Analysis for COVID-19", https://www.alibabacloud.com/solutions/genome-sequencing

34 Xu Xiaowei et al, "Deep Learning System to Screen Coronavirus Disease 2019 Pneumonia", 2019, pp. 1–29, also see Lin Li et al, "Artificial Intelligence Distinguishes COVID-19 from Community Acquired Pneumonia on Chest CT", Radiological Society of North America, 2020.

35 Cecilia Li, "How Damo Academy's AI System Detects Coronavirus Cases", *AliZila,* March 10, 2020, at https://www.alizila.com/how-damo-academys-ai-system-detects-coronavirus-cases/

36 "Infervision Launches Solution to Fight against Coronavirus", *Imaging Technology News,* March 31, 2020, at https://www.itnonline.com/content/infervision-launches-solution-fight-against-coronavirus, accessed on May 12, 2020, also see Beth W. Orenstein, "Imaging COVID-19 – Radiology's Evolving Role in Diagnosing and Managing the Coronavirus", *Radiology Today,* Vol. 21, No. 5, p. 10, at https://www.radiologytoday.net/archive/rt0520p10.shtml

37 Baidu, "How Baidu is bringing AI to the fight against coronavirus", *MIT Technology Review,* March 11, 2020, at https://www.technologyreview.com/2020/03/11/905366/how-baidu-is-bringing-ai-to-the-fight-against-coronavirus/

38 Wim Naudé, "Artificial Intelligence against COVID-19: An Early Review", *Towards Data Science,* April 01, 2020, at https://towardsdatascience.com/artificial-intelligence-against-COVID-19-an-early- review-92a8360edaba

39 See n. 33.

40 Alibaba Cloud, "Elastic High Performance Computing Technology", at https://www.alibabacloud.com/solutions/lifesciences-ehpc and n. 32.

41 "China Focus: Robots deployed on front lines to combat coronavirus", *Xinhua*, February 07, 2020, at http://www.xinhuanet.com/english/2020-02/07/c_138763788.htm and "Xinhua Headlines: China goes high-tech in fight against coronavirus", *Xinhua*, March 14, 2020, at http://www.xinhuanet.com/english/2020-03/14/c_138877590.htm

42 Erico Guizzo, "Robot Vehicles Make Contactless Deliveries Amid Coronavirus Quarantine", *IEEE Spectrum*, April 02, 2020, at https://spectrum.ieee.org/automaton/transportation/self-driving/robot-vehicles-make-contactless-deliveries-amid-coronavirus-quarantine

43 *Charles Arthur and Ruan Shuhui, "In China, robot delivery vehicles deployed to help with COVID-19 emergency", United Nations Industrial Development Organization,* at https://www.unido.org/stories/china-robot-delivery-vehicles-deployed-help-COVID-19-emergency

44 Catherine Clifford, "Look inside the hospital in China where coronavirus patients were treated by robots", *CNBC*, March 23, 2020, at https://www.cnbc.com/2020/03/23/video-hospital-in-china-where-COVID-19-patients-treated-by-robots.html

45 "China's Autonomous Delivery Vehicles Navigate the Coronavirus Outbreak", *Synced*, March 21, 2020, at https://syncedreview.com/2020/03/21/chinas-autonomous-delivery-vehicles-navigate-the-coronavirus-outbreak/

46 Eugene Demaitre, "COVID-19 pandemic prompts more robot usage worldwide", *The Robot Report*, March 18, 2020, at https://www.therobotreport.com/COVID-19-pandemic-prompts-more-robot-usage-worldwide/

47 Veronica Combs, "Interest in autonomous vehicles and delivery drones grows during COVID-19 pandemic", *Tech Republic*, April 13, 2020, at https://www.techrepublic.com/article/mayo-clinic-uses-self-driving-shuttles-to-transport-coronavirus-tests-on-florida-campus/

48 See n. 21, also see Peng He and Zili Huang, "How Chinese companies are responding to COVID-19 mobility challenges", *World Economic Forum*, March 03, 2020, at https://www.weforum.org/agenda/2020/03/china-COVID-19-coronavirus-mobility-solutions/

49 Tracy Yang, "In-Depth Report: Drones & Robots: Deploying New Technology to Handle Crisis", *JD.com*, February 26, 2020, at https://jdcorporateblog.com/in-depth-report-drones-robots-deploying-new-technology-to-handle-crisis/

50 "China Focus: Unmanned aerial vehicles assist fight against novel coronavirus", *Xinhua*, February 10, 2020, at http://www.xinhuanet.com/english/2020-02/10/c_138770880.htm, and "China science, technology news summary", *Xinhua*, February 11, 2020, at http://www.xinhuanet.com/english/2020-02/11/c_138773756.htm, and "Coronavirus control: Drones with thermal imaging technology adopted in central China", *Xinhua*, February 16, 2020, at http://www.xinhuanet.com/english/2020-02/16/c_138788719.htm

51 Divya Joshi, "Here are the world's largest drone companies and manufacturers to watch and stocks to invest in 2020", *Business Insider*, December 21, 2019, at https://www.businessinsider.com/drone-manufacturers-companies-invest-stocks?IR=T

52 DJI Enterprise, "Innovating to Fight COVID-19: Four Ways Drones are Contributing", https://enterprise.dji.com/news/detail/fight-COVID-19-with-drones

53 Tracy Cozzens, "China fights coronavirus with delivery drones", *GPS World*, March 06, 2020, at https://www.gpsworld.com/china-fights-coronavirus-with-delivery-drones/ and Li Nianzhen, "How a Chinese drone delivery startup is capitalizing on COVID-19", *NIKKEI Asian Review*, March 21, 2020, at https://asia.nikkei.com/Business/Startups/How-a-Chinese-drone-delivery-startup-is-capitalizing-on-COVID-19

54 Charlie Wood, "A Chinese firm claims it has built facial recognition tech that identifies people wearing masks with 95% accuracy", *Business Insider*, March 18, 2020, at https://www.businessinsider.in/tech/news/a-chinese-firm-claims-it-has-built-facial-recognition-tech-that-identifies-people-wearing-masks-with-95-accuracy/articleshow/74695329.cms, and Martin Pollard, "Even mask-wearers can be ID'd, China facial recognition firm says", *Reuters*, March 09, 2020, at https://www.reuters.com/article/us-health-coronavirus-facial-recognition/even-mask-wearers-can-be-idd-china-facial-recognition-firm-says-idUSKBN20W0WL

55 Thales, "Facial recognition – fascinating and intriguing", May 06, 2020, at https://www.thalesgroup.com/en/markets/digital-identity-and-security/government/biometrics/facial-recognition

56 Zheng Guichu, "8 reflections from China's experience in fighting COVID-19", *Global Times*, March 27, 2020, at https://www.globaltimes.cn/content/1183967.shtml

57 Zhang Chunming and Guan He, "5G Applications Help China Fight against COVID-19", Research Center for Radio Management, China Academy of Information and Communications Technology, at http://www.caict.ac.cn/english/research/covid19/study/202004/P020200426371477971478.pdf

58 "Huawei builds 5G network at Wuhan Huoshenshan Hospital", *CGTN*, March 13, 2020, at https://news.cgtn.com/news/2020-03-13/Huawei-builds-5G-network-at-Wuhan-Huoshenshan-Hospital-OP6qhHRc1G/index.html

8

Sports and COVID-19: Consequences on China's Sports Diplomacy

Supriya Sharma

Introduction

Sports has long been an important tenet of bridging the tendency of fulfilling state objectives. Whenever a country is provided with an opportunity to host a sporting event, it devises strategies that would reflect that nation's interests. Hence, sports plays an eminent role in representing the substituted expressions of a nation's accomplishments simultaneously feeding to its soft power characteristic of formulating a positive international image. Sporting mega events indirectly symbolises contention between nations and sports competitions could frequently be seen to exemplify national conflict.

Not just that, sports is an institution that brings together people from different parts of the world and represents trans-national cultures and enlightens on the cross-cultural relations. A Brazilian citizen may be a huge fan of Usain Bolt who hails from Jamaica and a Jamaican citizen may be a huge fan of Lionel Messi, who is a world-renowned footballer from Argentina. People from different countries travel to nations that are hosting sports mega events to cheer their favourite athletes. Hence, Sports is a medium of building relationships beyond ethnic divides and gives out the message of mutual respect, compassion, equality of opportunity, mutual tolerance and rule of law.[1]

Sports and politics infringe on one another and therefore, they cannot be isolated.

Governments are inescapably involved with sports and are subject to state. Sports is run by ruling bodies, nationally, it is under the jurisdiction of the state and internationally, several non-governmental international bodies, for example the International Olympic Committee (IOC) come into play. These bodies set the rules, structures and rewards of the competitions.[2]

Sports as a means of foreign policy is used to serve an assured purpose for specific situations. For example, in order to win friends in the third world countries, communist nations like the erstwhile Soviet Union as well as China had sent coaches and initiated other sporting facilities as a foreign policy tactic.[3] Furthermore, at times, when a nation does not have enough international political and economic recognition, such states deliberately attend international sporting events like the Olympics in the pursuit of international recognition.[4]

From a Chinese perspective, sports brings the whole population together without differentiating whether they are rich, poor, educated or uneducated. By analyzing political or historical process through the lens of sports, one tends to ignore the social or political divisions of a society. Apart from expressing national sentiments and simultaneously acting as an agent of international recognition, sports offer a crucial method of studying cultural, societal and people-to-people interactions. Major sporting events bring the world together and offer cross-cultural networking. By linking sports culture to globalization, new dimensions about the global culture and development in economy can be traced.[5] International sporting event is a form of semi-official diplomacy setup and is not only an important supplement to national diplomatic relations, but it can also play a buffer and transition role to resolve contradictions and disputes between countries. People of all religious beliefs and customs accept sports and therefore it is believed that sports engagement can lead to friendly international environment of cooperation.[6]

Chinese scholars consider public diplomacy as a major facet of the Chinese soft power and such scholars often look at sports diplomacy as a sub-tenet of this public diplomacy. The ultimate diplomatic strategy is of, "peaceful development" in a "harmonious world" of "mutual benefit and mutual trust". Through sports diplomacy, China aims at building the image of a 'responsible big country' pushing itself to the status of a great power nation, which is ready to undertake international missions, for example holding successful global sports events. Such events serve China's core interests and internal affairs as formerly mentioned.[7]

Therefore, Sports diplomacy does not only reflect on building inter-cultural values but it also mediates to promote people-to-people understanding and cooperation. Through the love for sports, international sporting events act as a useful diplomatic tool that improves multilateral as well as bilateral relations between nations. Not to forget, the sporting events give nations the opportunity to bridge their trust deficit.

As sports is a major tier in shaping a nation's soft power and rests on the principles of attractiveness of culture, political values and legitimacy of foreign policies of a nation, China through sports, aims at employing the soft power of cultural diplomacy and pursue its universalistic goals.

Shu Shengfang, a scholar from the Shanghai University of Sport, rather than characterizing sports diplomacy and soft power as separate entities discusses the characteristics of "Sports soft power". Sports soft power can be defined as a nation's aim of fulfilling international strategic goals through the field of sports. In an international political competition, sports soft power reflects culture, China's code of conduct, values and political system. Sports play a significant role in globalizing cultural values of a state. Sports soft power recognizes a strong relationship between sports and the economic development of a country, which there by shapes the universal value recognition of a country. In addition, sports soft power leads to overall enhancement of national strength in China and this contributes to the 'peaceful rise' and in building a 'harmonious society'. Therefore, sports soft power has far reaching practical and theoretical significance.

But what happens to this soft power and the future of sports as well as the sports diplomacy when the world is hit by a pandemic?

Looking at sport from the lens of diplomacy has unquestionably heightened with the onset of globalization. Globalization is the most significant and crucial factor that has led to an increased cross-border flow of people, money, tourism as well as sports and sporting events. Globalization made the transnational flow of people so comfortable, easy as well as crucial that itparadoxically became the reason of the present human-to-human spreading coronavirus pandemic. SARS-Cov-2 has caused serious repercussions to the globally dispersed businesses and it has created such a strong fear that the world is thinking of moving towards domestically dependent structures.[8] While the world did recover from the methodical shocks of SARS and the 9/11,[9] the speed at which COVID-19 has escalated on a global scale posits a challenge of a different degree.

History and Recent Dynamics of Sports in China

The modern sports in China has, from the beginning steered under the nationalistic banner and its victories in sports have always aimed at reflecting the supremacy of its political ideology and bolster its international image.

After founding of the People's Republic of China (PRC), China realized the importance of sports in building diplomatic relations and being internationally recognized. It created the State Physical Culture and Sports Commission (SPCSC) in 1952 in order to organize resources for elite sports in PRC. Beijing was extremely interested in building professional athletes in order to gain international pride through international sport events and for this purpose, China used to invite several experts from Socialist countries to train the Chinese athletes. However, during the earlier years, China's aim was to win friends rather than medals and Premier Zhou Enlai stressed upon the importance of friendship more than the competition.[10]

In 1963, China became an important member of the Jakarta founded, Games of the New Emerging Forces (GANEFO) and this offered Beijing with an excellent opportunity to develop friendships with the third world countries. After isolation during the Cultural Revolution, China again resumed its sports diplomacy in 1972 and this time, it chose to play the role of a benefactor where it uplifted the sports facilities for the third world countries which reflected China's soft power enhancement.

The Ping-Pong diplomacy of China is celebrated as the best form of sports diplomacy, which helped to normalize relations between China and the US. However, this was not all. China has also improvised its relations with Australia, Canada, Singapore and Malaysia through table-tennis.[11]

Following the Ping-Pong diplomacy and cultural revolution, Deng Xiaoping's reform and opening policies brought significant changes in the nation's sports. Sports became an element of embracing capitalism with Chinese characteristics and essentially served the function of promoting socialism and nationalism. The 1984 Summer Olympics gave its sports, a crucial step to advance into the world and break out of Asia.[12] China stood fourth in the medal standing[13] arousing patriotism. China observed that sports could play a great role in awakening nationalism.

China's outstanding performance in Asian Games ever since 1982 also added to its diplomatic advantages. Asian Games 1990 specifically reflected upon the close relationship between the sports and politics. As the Asian Games were hosted by China just after the 'Tiananmen Square Incident' of 1989, the Games were important for China to win back foreign investors and to gain back its self-esteem. The official slogan of 'Unity, Friendship, Progress' reflected China's political interest through the games as it wanted to win back, the trust and confidence from the Western as well as the Eastern worlds.[14]

Similarly, the Beijing Olympics 2008 added great value to China's diplomatic undertakings. More than four billion people around the globe watched the opening ceremony of Beijing Olympics[15]. Beijing Olympics coincided with China's move towards internationalization while demonstrating postulations of 'peaceful rise' and exhibiting China's cultural advancements. The three concepts of 'Green Olympics', 'People's Olympics' and 'High-tech Olympics' were highly lauded by the international organizations. In addition, it won 51 gold medals and marked an unprecedented win by grabbing the top position in the 2008 Olympics gold medal table with an overall second position[16]. Given the development challenges and conducting the games in a rapidly growing city like Beijing, UN Environment Programme's (UNEP) post-Olympic report highly lauded China's efforts to promote environment sustainability through the games.[17] From once being called the 'sick man of Asia' to China, now standing at the top position in the Asian Games and Olympics is truly commendable.

The Chinese Dream of Sports

Ever since Xi Jinping has taken over as the President of China, the central government has attached more importance to the role of sports diplomacy. Chinese scholar, Liu Naibaostates that under the new leader, China's diplomacy in the new era will characterize "honesty, sincerity, benefit and tolerance".[18] Following the 18th National Congress of the Communist party, Chinese President, Xi Jinping envisioned two centenary goals for China and called it the "Chinese Dream". The first goal focuses on building a "moderately well off society" by 2021 and second, to build a "strong, democratic, civilized, harmonious, and modern socialist country" by 2049.[19]

At the 19th National Congress of the Communist Party, Xi Jinping stated how competitive sports and Fitness-for-All programmes have been undergoing extensive development in enhancing China's cultural soft power and international influence. He appreciated the support of the people in embracing this Chinese dream by showcasing great confidence in the Chinese culture.[20] Adhering to good neighborliness and friendship, watch and help each other, talk about equality and value emotions of other countries plays an important role in the diplomacy of the nation for the great rejuvenation of the Chinese nation and the China dream. The concept of sports diplomacy must implement "sincerity, benefit and tolerance" amongst nations in order to learn from the experiences of each other and develop together.[21]

After China stood second in the medal table at the 2012 London Olympics for the second consecutive time, mass and elite sports development became a state priority. While preparing to bid for hosting the 2022 Winter Olympics in 2015, China had already outlined its ambitious plan to encourage 300 million participations in the 2022 Beijing Winter Olympics.[22]

According to the "13th Five Year plan for Sports Development", sports industry offers great opportunities for economic growth. The plan further stated that "sports, politics, economy, society and culture" will be interdependent and with information, globalization and networking, this "new diplomatic strategy will provide a broad stage for displaying the soft power of sports culture" and 2022 Beijing Olympics will aim at representing the international influence of Chinese sports strictly following the ideological path of socialism with Chinese characteristics, ultimately delivering the "iconiccause" of the "great revival" of the Chinese nation.[23]

While football is the most important sports in China, alongside it, China aims to also excel in basketball and volleyball, collectively called the 'three big ball sports'. In February 2020, the Chinese women basketball team edged Spain in the Olympic qualifiers in Belgrade and secured their berth for the upcoming Tokyo Olympics.[24] The China's women's volleyball team won Olympic gold medals in 1984, 2004 and 2016 and it is all set to ace at the Tokyo Olympics.[25]

The COVID-19 virus has certainly backfired on the Chinese dream of becoming a sports super power status. The 2020 Chinese Super League (CSL), which was scheduled to take place from February up until October 2020, has been postponed and may start by late June or early July.[26] The CSL is one of the most famous professional soccer leagues in the country and runs under the authorisation of the Chinese Football Association. The league began in 2004 with 12 clubs but it currently has 16 registered clubs that have hired famous international players as wellcoaches.[27] It is apprehended that the CSL might also have to do away with several coaches and international players, given the travel restrictions on entering China.[28]

In September 2019, China published the "Outline for the Construction of a powerful country". Deputy director of the State Sports General Administration, Li Jianming introduced three-stage strategic objectives, nine projects, five strategic tasks and six policy guidelines to pursue China into a world sports power by 2020, 2035 and 2050. The plan embodied ideas of reform and innovation emphasizing on the improvisation of policy measures which would result in enhancing the social and market forces. Development of sports industry will encourage the overall situation of social and economic development and support the Chinese dream of realizing the great rejuvenation of the Chinese nation.[29] By 2035, 45% population are expected to be involved in regular fitness exercising, up from 33.9% in 2018.[30]

China's football fortunes have been made a national priority and surpassing the earlier goal of having 20,000 academies by 2020, it now plans to have 50,000 football academies in the country by 2025 in order to achieve its ambition of becoming a soccer superpower.[31]

However, when the world is hit by a pandemic, to implement such characteristics of diplomacy becomes challenging especially for the nation from where it emerges. In 2003, during SARS, China struggled to convince the world of its preparedness as a host of the 2008 Beijing Olympics. Relations between China and majority of nations of the world turned pessimistic. China was accused of not being transparent enough about the virus. The International Ice Hockey Federation called off the Women's ice hockey, which was to be held in Beijing in April.[32] World Track Cycling Championship was moved to Europe from Shenzhen, Guangdong. China was also forced to pull out of the world volleyball championship[33] and several other sports governing bodies demanded a ban on the Asian Athletes especially Chinese in order to safely conduct international tournaments.

Sports Economy and COVID-19

China's 13th Five Year plan for Sports Development released in 2016 estimated the annual growth rate of the sports industry to be faster than the economic growth rate and it estimated the national sports industry to exceed 3 trillion yuan by the end of 2020. By the end of 2018, the total assets of sports industry legal entities was 3,149.82 billion yuan.[34] China's National Bureau of Statistics and General Administration of Sports have announced that total sports sector output grew 15.3% in 2018 and the sports industry accounted for 1.1% of the GDP of China.[35] It is the fastest growing global sports market. The official 2018 National Sports Industry Scale and Value-added data report stated,[36]

> "From the perspective of the internal structure of the sports industry, the sports service industry maintains a good development momentum, with an added value of 653 billion yuan, accounting for 64.8% of the sports industry, an increase from the previous year; of which, the sales, rental and The trade agency has the largest scale, with an added value of 232.7 billion yuan, accounting for 23.1% of the total added value of the sports industry. The added value of the manufacturing of sports goods and related products was 339.9 billion yuan, accounting for 33.7% of the added value of the entire sports industry. The added value of the construction of sports facilities is 15 billion yuan, accounting for 1.5% of the added value of the entire sports industry.

Ever since the world was hit by COVID-19, sports seem to have suddenly disappeared. An ESPN data predicted a $12 billion loss to the US sports industry and a lay off of hundreds of thousands of employees. Emsi's Analysis of data from Bureau of Labor statistics predicted that 3 million jobs and 524 occupations are dependent on sports. Most of these workers are dependent on regular paychecks.[37] A survey conducted by Statista in US stated that 71 per cent respondents are 'much less likely' to go for a sporting event to protect themselves from COVID-19.[38] Since, there are no matches being played and with every sports rescheduling its tournaments, the broadcasting commitments are not being met.

Table 8.1: 2018 年全国体育产业状况
(China's National Sports Industry Status 2018)

Category Name	*Total (100 million yuan)*		*Structure(%)*	
	Total Output	*Value Added*	*Total Output*	*Value Added*
Sports industry	26579	10078	100.0	100.0
Sports service industry	12732	6530	47.9	64.8
Sports management activities	747	390	2.8	3.9
Sports competition performance	292	103	1.1	1.0
Sports fitness leisure activities	1028	477	3.9	4.7
Stadium and facility management	2632	855	9.9	8.5
Sports brokers and agents, advertising and exhibitions, performance and design services	317	106	1.2	1.1
Physical education and training	1722	1425	6.5	14.1
Sports Media and Information Service	500	230	1.9	2.3
Sports goods and related products sales, rental and trade agency	4116	2327	15.5	23.1
Other sports services	1377	616	5.2	6.1
Manufacturing of sports goods & related products	13201	3399	49.7	33.7
Construction of sports facilities	646	150	2.4	1.5

Source: National Bureau of Statistics, People's Republic of China

The sports economy runs from the media right sales, through broadcasting, commercial advertising and sale of match day tickets. This income is then distributed amongst the participating teams or clubs. Apart from this, athletes simultaneously have their individual paid sponsorship contracts signed with the clubs that they represent as well as they have their own D2C (direct-to-consumer) broadcasting contracts. The postponement and suspension of live sports events is a major setback to the broadcasters causing losses of hundreds of millions of dollars as the advertising revenue cuts off. The National Basketball Association (NBA), which is the America's largest professional basketball association, alone, is estimated to cause $481m loss to Disney media networks and $210m to Turner broadcasting network.[39] Given the foremost rule of social distancing, the virus has very clearly and directly impacted the match day ticketing business. Pre- match as well as match day logistics have nullified given the cancellation or axing of almost every sports event in the world. This has also caused unemployment of the live audience management workforce.

The 2020 Tokyo Olympics is the most crucial sporting event to have been affected due to the outbreak of the novel coronavirus. In the history of Olympics, this is the fourth time that the Olympics have been cancelled, the other two were at the times of World War I (1916) and World war II (1940, 1944). The event has now been postponed to take place from July 23, 2021 to August 8, 2021. Japan's

National Audit Board is estimating an additional cost of $22.3 billion into the preparations for Tokyo Olympics.[40] These include re-renting of venues, re-booking of hotels, labour costs, security logistics and likewise.

NBA's which would have generated $9 billion this season is anticipated to cost $2 billion losses due to its indefinite suspension[41]. Similarly, the Chinese Baketball League (CBL) was to finish its regular season by March 2020 and there are no new scheduled dates for the same either. CBL too, just like the NBA is facing tremendous revenue loss due to a halt in media broadcasting and more importantly losing out on international sponsors due to the lack of confidence in China, given that the Sars-Cov-19 was born in Wuhan, China. After the 2016 13th Five Year Plan for sports development, CBL, just like the Chinese football league, started to transition into a commercialised sports. Therefore, the impact is incomparable to what these sports faced during the 2003 SARS crisis. Infact, many Chinese players have started to seek opportunities elsewhere, given that the future of CBL seems unclear.

The famous English Premier League which has the world's top football players assigned under 20 different clubs is set to inevitably pay $420 million to broadcasters as reimbursement of matches that could not be played due to the virus.[42] The league is not certain if it will be able to complete this year's season as there is a lack of collective will amongst the authorities and the clubs. Number of clubs of the globally renowned, Spanish football league, La Liga like FC Barcelona[43] and Atletico Madricreduced the salaries of its players and staff in order to cope with the abrupt revenue loss.

China's leading football club, Liaoning FC is on the verge of a permanent closure. The club could not pay the footballers their salary ever since 2019 and with the virus going on, the club's financial misconduct has further exacerbated.[44] Another league club, Tianjin Tianhai announced that it was looking to handover ownership free of charge after its former owner, Quanjian was enmeshed in a national scandal of being responsible for a child's cancer death[45]. The club's assets are an estimate $100 million. Due to COVID-19's impact on the economy and employment worldwide, the Chinese Football Association published, "Proposal on Properly Adjusting Salaries of Men's Football Professional Clubs and Their Players and Coaches, and Overcoming Difficulties". It outlined adjustments and negotiations for players and coaches and recommended a salary adjustment reference ratio between 30 percent and 50 percent.[46]

COVID-19 has caused fatal disruptions to the sports ecosystem. The sports industry in macroeconomic terms, faces the challenges of reorganizing its workforce operations, audience and fan management, venue strategies, investments including sponsorship contracts and broadcasting, legal and financial consequences. The world of sports faces the challenge of working around new technologies in order to channelize and maintain the interests of its fans and subsequently, require new strategies to keep the business and finances flowing.

Conclusion

Though the 'High Tech, people's, green' Beijing Olympics coincided with the China's move towards internationalization while demonstrating postulations of 'peaceful rise' and exhibiting China's cultural advancements, China's hosting of such mega events indicate its bilateral and multilateral economic growth through foreign ventures and interactions. However, amidst the virus, this effort of maintaining a positive international image and postulating economic heights through sports will be nearly impossible for China. The First reason for this is the cancellation of all major events, with further chances of postponement of the Hangzhou Asian Games 2022. Secondly, the public opinion on China has hit a new low according to the Pew Research Centre. A Pew poll of 1000 American adults conducted in March stated 66 percent of an unfavorable view of China. Seven in ten Americans (71 percent) lack confidence in President Xi Jinping.[47] In fact, the pandemic has taken a harsh toll on China's international relations with Sweden becoming the first European country to clamp down on all the Confucius Institutes in the country. Matt Schrader, a China analyst from the German Marshall Fund asserted that Confucius institutes are "propaganda tools" and promote hostility to liberal thoughts of freedom of speech, rights to information and other state-approved liberal narratives. In the name of cultural soft power, these institutes are used as a base to gather intelligence and military information of other countries.[48]

Beijing plans to be a world-class soccer competitor by 2050 and during a friendly match between youth teams of China and Germany in Berlin in July, 2017, President Xi Jinping said that Beijing wants to enhance cooperation and exchanges with Germany in order to internally rise in the sports of football. However, recently German Chancellor Angela Markel urged China to be more transparent about the birth of SARS-CoV-2. Moreover, German Tabloid, *Bild* in an article drafted a $162 billion bill to China against the damages caused by China due to COVID-19 raising new controversies and indicating strained relations between the two countries.[49] In June 2019, China and Australia entered into their third year of the China-Australia Sports Summit. This platform serves to the growth of sports industry and helps in strengthening sports and cultural ties between the two countries. However, Covid 19 has brought a bittern turn between Australia and its number one trading partner. Australia demanded an investigation on China in relation to the spread of

Figure 8.1: U.S. Views of China: Increasingly Negative Amid Coronavirus Outbreak 2020

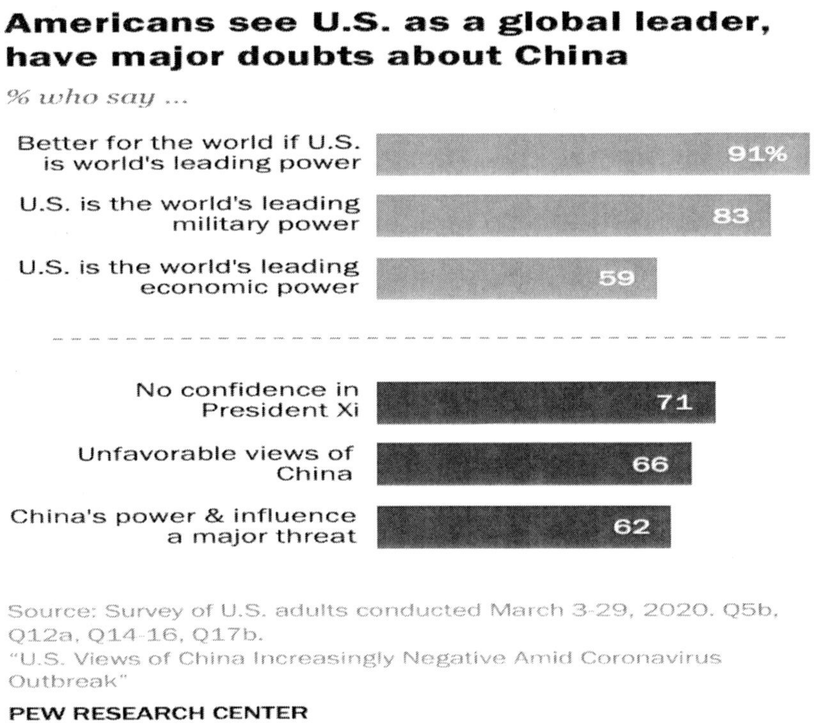

COVID-19. This led to the further escalation of trade tensions between the two countries with China threatening Australia of economic consequences.[50]

While US and China were already engaged in military, economic, technological and ideological competitions, the pandemic has worsened the already hostile Sino-US relationship and both countries are playing blame games against each other. While US President, Donald Trump raised several debates by calling COVID-19 as "Chinese Virus",[51] China has not shied away from accusing the US Military to have brought the coronavirus to China during the Military World Games, which were held in Wuhan in October, 2019.[52]

COVID-19 has worsened the gap of trust deficit between China and other nations. This is now factually applicable and suitable to the present pandemic scenario given the fact that the China broke its promise of closing the wet markets back in 2003 during the outbreak of SARS. Despite several health warnings about how wet markets could cause a global public health hazard, China reopened these markets within a year back then.

While it may take a while for the sports industry to get back to its pre-pandemic form of conducting live matches and engaging live audiences and fans, China continues to work towards its ambitions of becoming a super power in sports. Despite the outbreak of the novel coronavirus, which has brought the whole world to a halt, China continues to play its "stadium diplomacy". In the name of "friendship" stadiums, China built its first stadium called the Amaan stadium in Zanzibar, Tanzania in 1970. As of now, China has built more than 100 stadiums in the developing countries[53] and this is one of the many building structures that China exports to the under-developed countries This form of diplomacy has helped China in postulating its image of a "responsible great power". In November 2019, China "donated" a 50,000-seater "mini-football stadium" to Tunisia worth \$87,843.[54] China has now started constructing a \$1.7 billion brand new stadium in Guangzhou. The project is being carried out by Evergrande, which is owned by one of the richest men in China. The company confirmed that it intends to build two more stadiums with a capacity of 80,000 people each. It is designing world's largest football stadiums for the FIFA Club world cup to be in held in 2021 and AFC Asian Cup in 2023.[55] These newly revamped stadiums are eying at the goal of holding the World Cup in 2030. The "Bird's Nest" designed for 2008 Beijing Olympics became a significant tourist attraction and China is continuing to modernize such attractions, such as the revamp project of the Shanghai Stadium, the biggest stadium in the city of Shanghai.

COVID-19 has not just caused losses to commercial sports but it has also put the traditional fitness culture to a complete halt. Fitness has become highly digitalized with fitness companies moving the entire idea of sports and wellness to their online portals. China launched over 13 home fitness exercise guides through its official WeChat profile. Along side, Shanghai Administration of sports launched a WeChat online programme too where Chinese Olympic medalists displayed their home fitness regimes[56]. The Guangzhou Sports Bureau and the Guangzhou Sports Federation launched "Online walking Challenge" and "Online Riding Challenge" on May 1st, the May Day holiday and released 20,000 sports coupons worth 150 Yuan each.[57] Such strategies are helping China in mirroring with the interests of its citizens and simultaneously encouraging the goal of mass fitness amid the pandemic. Publicizing health and sports with the help of high profile athletes aids China in improvising its image in the eyes of its citizens and showcases that Beijing values its people. It is also helpful in keeping the nationalistic sports sentiments of the people affixed and high.

Many Chinese sports stars made significant donations to help fight COVID-19. Chinese former tennis super star, Li Na donated 3 million Yuan to her hometown, Wuhan, to fight the pandemic. 2018 Asian Footballer of the year, Wang Shuang donated 600,000 Yuan.[58] Yao Ming, the NBA basketball superstar and the president of the Chinese Basketball Association has become a setting example amongst the sports superstars worldwide. Yao raised donations within the CBA and managed to donate more that 3 million Yuan. He continued to raise donations worldwide to provide necessary medical supplies but this was not all. He was also seen donating blood as there was shortage of blood donors due to the nationwide lockdown.[59] This perfectly signified the transnational role that sports plays in bringing together countries. The current pandemic might have subdued the political phenomenon of sports by curtailing opportunities of political friendship on the sidelines of a live sports event for the leaders, but the athletes have showcased immense togetherness reaffirming the ultimate goals of sports, unity and understanding.

The World Health Organisation warned that the world would have to learn to live with COVID-19 and just like HIV, it may never completely go away.[60] This unprecedented pandemic will unleash containment strategies by mandatory provisions of maintaining social distance and developing alternative public health policies. Global unity is the need of the hour as it's a matter of life and death and sports too will have to unfold new gaming strategies. Undeniably, present relations between China and the major nations of the world stands pessimistic and therefore, the future bans and freezing of sports events as a means of retaliation could unfold the political usage of sports vis-à-vis China.

NOTES

1 Stuart Murray, "The two Halves of Sports-Diplomacy", *Diplomacy & Statecraft*, *23*(3), p.576-592, 2012

2 Penelope Kissoudi, "Sport, Politics and International Relations in the Twentieth Century", *The International Journal of the History of Sport*, *25*(13), p.1689-1689-1706, November 2008,

3 Trevor Taylor, Sport and International Relations: A Case of Mutual Neglect in *The Politics of Sport*, pp. 27-48 (Manchester: Manchester University Press ,1986)

4 Penelope Kissoudi, "Sport, Politics and International Relations in the Twentieth Century", *The International Journal of the History of Sport*, *25*(13), November 2008, p.1689-1706

5 Xu Guoqi, "*Olympic Dreams: China and Sports*" (Cambridge: Harvard University Press, 2008)

6 Li Xiang-ru, et.al, "关于新中国体育外交 的回顾与研究", [A historical review of the Sports Diplomacy since the founding of the People's Republic of China], *The Capital College of Physical Education, Beijing*, January 2003.

7 Yin Xiaoling and LIU Lianfa, 我国体育外交演进的历史逻辑与观念变革 [The Historical Logic and Conceptual Change of China's Sports Diplomacy], *Journal of Sports and Science*, p.53-58, *37* (4), July 2016

8 Mie Oba, "Coronavirus and the Future of Globalization", *The Diplomat*, March 18, 2020, at <https://thediplomat.com/2020/03/coronavirus-and-the-future-of-globalization/>

9 Dhruva Jaishankar, "A global pandemic and globalisation", *Observer Research Foundation*, April 12, 2020, at <https://www.orfonline.org/research/a-global-pandemic-and-globalisation-64468/>

10 Wang Guanhua, "Friendship First: China's Sports Diplomacy during the cold war", *The Journal of American-East Asian Relations, 12*(3), p.133-153, January 2003

11 Ibid

12 Grant Jarvie, et.al, *"Sport, Revolution and the Beijing Olympics"* (Berg, 2008)

13 "23rd Olympic Games: Los Angeles 1984", *Official Website of the Chinese Olympic Committee*, March 27, 2004, at <http://en.olympic.cn/games/summer/2004-03-27/121671.html>

14 Fan Hong & Liu Zhouxiang, "China, the Asian Games and Asian Politics (1974-2006), *The International Journal of the History of Sport*, p. 98-112, *29*(1), 2012

15 "Over 4 billion people watch Beijing Olympics ceremony ", *Xinhua*, August 17, 2008, at <https://www.chinadaily.com.cn/olympics/2008-08/17/content_6942533.htm>

16 See "2008 Beijing Summer Olympics Medals- Totals by Country", at <http://www.espn.com/olympics/summer08/medals>

17 Bhavna Singh, "*China's Discursive Nationalism: Contending in Softer Realms*", (New Delhi: Pentagon Press, 2012)

18 Liu Naibao, et.al., "新时代体育外交的理念、行为主体与战略诉求", [The Concept, Subject and Strategy of Sports Diplomacy in the New Era], *Journal of Sports and Science, 39* (3), 2018

19 "China a step closer to centenary goals", Xinhua, October 9, 2017 at <https://www.chinadaily.com.cn/china/2017-10/09/content_33029203.htm>

20 Xi Jinping, "Secure a Decisive Victory in Building a Moderately Prosperous Society in All Respects an Strive for the Great Success of Socialism with Chinese Characteristics for a New Era", speech delivered at the 19th National Congress of the Communist Party of China, *Xinhua Net,* October 18, 2017, at <http://www.xinhuanet.com/english/download/Xi_Jinping's_report_at_ 19th_CPC_National_Congress.pdf>

21 Liu Naibao, et.al., "新时代体育外交的理念、行为主体与战略诉求", [The Concept, Subject and Strategy of Sports Diplomacy in the New Era], *Journal of Sports and Science, 39* (3), 2018

22 Jinming Zheng, et.al, "Sport Policy in China (Mainland)", *International Journal of Sport Policy and Politics*, p.469-491, May 2018

23 "The 13th Five-Year Plan for Sports Development", *General Administration of Sports of China*, May 5, 2016, at <http://www.sports.cn/sire/hydt/2016/0505/278641.html>

24 "China women's basketball qualifies for Tokyo Olympics", *Xinhua Net*, February 8, 2020, at <http://www.xinhuanet.com/english/2020-02/08/c_138766640.htm>

25 "Women's volleyball: China drawn with USA, Russia at Tokyo Olympics", *CGTN*, February 1, 2020, at <https://news.cgtn.com/news/2020-02-01/Women-s-volleyball-China-drawn-with-USA-Russia-at-Tokyo-Olympics-NION233MFW/index.html>

26 "2020 Chinese Super League could start in June, says club chief", *China Daily*, April 20,2020, at <http://global.chinadaily.com.cn/a/202004/20/WS5e9cf328a3105d50a3d17474.html>

27 See official website of the Chinese Football Association Super League, at <http://csl-news.9h-sports.com/d_news_aHR0cHM6Ly9zdGF0aWMtY3NsLjloLXNwb3J0cy5jb20vaDUvbmV3cy8yMDE5MTIzMS8xNDU3MjIyOTcwMzUuaHRtbA==.html>

28 "Football: Chinese Super League could kick off without foreign stars", *Channel News Asia*, May 8, 2020, at <https://www.channelnewsasia.com/news/sport/football-chinese-super-league-could-kick-off-without-foreign-12714964>

29 "Outline for Building a Powerful Country for Sports" Creates a New Situation in Sports Development", *China Sports New*, September 3, 2019, at <http://www.sports.cn/cydt/gldt/2019/0903/289740.html>

30 "China publishes outline to build itself into leading sporting power", *Xinhua*, September 2, 2019, at <http://www.xinhuanet.com/english/2019-09/02/c_138358500.htm>

31 "China announces plans to build 50,000 soccer academies by 2025", *Sports Illustrated*, February 22, 2017, at <https://www.si.com/soccer/2017/02/22/china-50000-soccer-academies-2025-csl>

32 "Virus forces teams home", *BBC*, March 31, 2003 at <http://news.bbc.co.uk/sport2/hi/other_sports/2902227.stm>

33 "SARS Fears Force China to Exit Volleyball", *The Associated Press*, May 7, 2003 at <https://apnews.com/ff75581f28c9a34bc2a7d6c605a7ee44>

34 "China's sports industry has vigorous development prospects", *Fifteenth Report of the Fourth National Economic Census*, January 20,2020, at <http://www.stats.gov.cn/tjsj/zxfb/202001/t20200120_1724133.html>

35 Kelvin Tan, "China claims 15.3-per-cent growth in sports sector in 2018", *Sports Business,* January 21, 2020, at <https://www.sportbusiness.com/news/china-claims-15-3-per-cent-growth-in-sports-sector-in-2018/>

36 "2018 National Sports Industry scale and Value Added Announcement", *National Bureau of Statistics*, January 20, 2020, at <http://www.stats.gov.cn/tjsj/zxfb/202001/t20200120_1724122.html>

37 "Sudden vanishing of sports due to coronavirus will cost at least $12 billion, analysis says", *ESPN*, May 1, 2020, at <https://www.espn.in/espn/otl/story/_/id/29110487/sudden-vanishing-sports-due-coronavirus-cost-least-12-billion-analysis-says>

38 Christina Gough, "COVID-19: Public opinion on going to sporting events as of April 2020", *Statista* at <https://www.statista.com/statistics/1104527/sporting-event-visitors-covid/>

39 Murad Ahmed, et.al, "Global sports suffers multibillion-dollar coronavirus hit", *Financial Times*, March 14, 2020, at <https://www.ft.com/content/f5f5e870-6541-11ea-b3f3-fe4680ea68b5>

40 Michelle Bruton, "Financial ramifications of coronavirus canceling Tokyo Olympics would be 'Massive'", *Forbes*, April 28, 2020, at <https://www.forbes.com/sites/michellebruton/2020/04/28/financial-ramifications-of-coronavirus-canceling-tokyo-olympics-would-be-massive/#615ffe6a772a>

41 Matt Johnson, "NBA could lose $2 billion if season canceled due to covid-19?", *SportsNaut*, at <https://sportsnaut.com/2020/05/nba-could-lose-2-billion-if-season-canceled-due-to-covid-19/>

42 Dan Roan, et.al, "Premier League Clubs facing £340m TV refund even if season resumes", *BBC*, May 11, 2020, at <https://www.bbc.com/sport/football/52579299>

43 The world's number one football star, Lionel Messi represents FC Barcelona.

44 "Chinese Super League: once-dominant Liaoning face closure as players go unpaid", *South China Morning Post*, April 5, 2020, at <https://www.scmp.com/sport/football/article/3078487/chinese-super-league-once-dominant-liaoning-face-closure-players-go>

45 Phoebe Zhang, "Chinese health product firm Quanjian scandal widens as public anger grows", *South China Morning Post,* January 6, 2019, https://www.scmp.com/news/china/society/article/2180749/chinese-health-product-firm-quanjian-scandal-widens-public-anger

46 "Chinese Football Association's initiative to reduce wages: work together to overcome difficulties", *China Sports News*, May 9, 2020, at <http://sire.sports.cn/hydt/tycydt/2020/0509/323111.html>

47 Kat Devlin, et.al, "U.S. Views of China Increasingly Negative Amid Coronavirus Outbreak", *Pew Research,* April 21, 2020, at <https://www.pewresearch.org/global/2020/04/21/u-s-views-of-china-increasingly-negative-amid-coronavirus-outbreak/>

48 Pratik Jakhar, "Confucius Institutes: The growth of China's controversial cultural branch", *BBC News*, September 7, 2019, at <https://www.bbc.com/news/world-asia-china-49511231>

49 "German tabloid sends $162-billion bill to China as 'Covid-19 damages'", *The Hindu Business Line*, April 22, 2020, at <https://www.thehindubusinessline.com/news/world/german-tabloid-sends-162-billion-bill-to-china-as-covid-19-damages/article31403658.ece>

50 Rod Mcguirk, "China warns Australia it could face boycotts over call for an independent inquiry into coronavirus", *Time*, May 1, 2020, at <https://time.com/5830675/china-australia-coronavirus-inquiry/>

51 "Trump has no qualms about calling coronirus the 'Chinese Virus'. That's a dangerous attitude, experts say", *The Washington Post*, March 20,2020, at <https://www.washingtonpost.com/nation/2020/03/20/coronavirus-trump-chinese-virus/>

52 "US sparks word war against China on COVID-19", *Global Times*, March 14, 2020, at <http://www.globaltimes.cn/content/1182511.shtml>

53 Charlie Q.L. Xue, et.al., "Architecture of 'Stadium Diplomacy'- China-aid sport buildings in Africa", *Habitat International*, 90:101985, August, 2019

54 "China donates mini-football stadium to Tunisia", *Xinhua*, November 26, 2019, at <http://www.xinhuanet.com/english/africa/2019-11/26/c_138582898.htm>

55 "China building toward World Cup dream", *China Daily*, April 27, 2020, at <https://www.chinadaily.com.cn/a/202004/27/WS5ea63491a310a8b241151d69.html>

56 "Olympic champs become online fitness coaches amid epidemic", *Xinhua Net*, February 11, 2020, at <http://www.xinhuanet.com/english/2020-02/11/c_138774850.htm>

57 "Guangzhou launches online sports events", *China Sports* News, May 8, 2020, at <http://www.sports.cn/cydt/jsby/2020/0508/323036.html>

58 Chan Kin-Wa, "Coronavirus: retired tennis star Li Na donates 3 million yuan to support hometown fight against epidemic", February 7, 2020, South China Morning Post, at, <https://www.scmp.com/sport/china/article/3049465/coronavirus-retired-tennis-star-li-na-donates-3-million-yuan-support>

59 "Yao Ming leads world of Chinese basketball to help fight against COVID-19", *CGTN*, March 31, 2020, at <https://news.cgtn.com/news/2020-03-31/Yao-Ming-leads-world-of-Chinese-basketball-in-fight-against-COVID-19-PjxHMrwoVy/index.html>

60 "This virus may never go away, WHO says", *Al Jazeera*, May 14, 2020, at <https://www.aljazeera.com/news/2020/05/virus-200513190939371.html>

THE EXTERNAL DIMENSIONS

9

Calibrated and Effective: Taiwan's Response to COVID-19

Sana Hashmi

Introduction

Taiwan's response to the novel COVID-19 has won praises across the world. As of May 31, it had 442 positive cases of COVID-19 with seven deaths. With a population of 23.78 million and given the proximity with Mainland China, Taiwan has been able to successfully mitigate the threat from the virus. COVID-19 affected Taiwan in two waves. The first wave was when the outbreak began in Wuhan and the second wave coincided with the spread to the rest of the world. The first positive case was detected in Taiwan on January 21, 2020. From January 21 to February 29, only 39 confirmed cases were registered in Taiwan. What may be primarily characterised as imported cases, Taiwan began to see an increase in the number of cases by the end of March. In April, a small cluster emerged when Dunmu, a naval fleet, returned to Taiwan after a goodwill visit to Palau, one of its 15 diplomatic allies. 700 sailors were quarantined and as a part of contact tracing, 200,000 people were asked to self-monitor their health. However, unlike most countries, Taiwan has had no community outbreaks and 350 to 360 cases are imported. It is remarkable that despite the proximity with China, it has been able to contain the virus. More than 400,000 Taiwanese work in Mainland China. Given the timing of the outbreak in China, it was expected that several Taiwanese living in China would return to Taiwan for the Lunar New Year celebration and Taiwan will become one of the most affected countries.

Taiwan's successful management of the pandemic and the subsequent appreciation accompanied with wide reportage has irked China, which is struggling to prove that it acted responsibly and the China model is the only successful way to tackle COVID-19. For years, Chinese leadership has been attempting to shrink Taiwan's international space but the management of COVID-19 has provided sufficient exposure to Taiwan and helped it in fostering better understanding about the island nation. One important development has been that this unprecedented situation has made a distinction between China and Taiwan clearer at a wider stage.

Taiwan's Government Response

Taiwan is one of the few countries that has successfully managed to contain the virus in a timely fashion. The reason behind its success lies in the fact that the administration acted promptly. Its success has boosted the argument that democracies too could manage it well without taking harsh measures. In President Tsai Ing-wen's words, "A combination of efforts by medical professionals, government, private sector and society at large has armoured our [Taiwan's] country's defences. The painful lessons of the 2003 Severe Acute Respiratory Syndrome (SARS) outbreak, which left Taiwan scarred with the loss of dozens of lives, put our government and people on high alert early on."[1] Even when no country was even aware of the existence of COVID-19, Taiwan started taking measures. It was the first to notify the World Health Organization (WHO) about the potential health threat from a novel virus in December 2019. A series of notifications was also uploaded on the website of Taiwan's Center for Disease Control (CDC). Taiwan was probably the first country to have put in place policies and precautionary measures. The administration began to issue advisory and prepare for the potential outbreak as early as the first week of January 2020. To gather further information and prepare better for the outbreak, two medical representatives from Taiwan-Commander Chuang Yin-ching from the Communicable Disease Control Medical Network and the Medical Officer Hung Min-nan from the CDC visited Wuhan. On their return, further precautionary measures were placed. It was on January 20 that the CDC issued the travel advisory to Taiwanese citizens asking them to take necessary measures while travelling to Wuhan by raising the travel notice level for Wuhan to Level 2.[2] After two days on January 22, the level was further raised to 3 and Taiwanese nationals were asked to avoid non-essential travel to Wuhan. Subsequently, on January 25, the warning level was raised to 3 for the entire province of Hubei and 2 for the rest of Mainland China. The warning level was raised to 3 for Mainland China on January 28. Several restrictions and advisories were issued for Mainland Chinese travelers which included barring of the Chinese citizens coming from Wuhan. Sensing the threat,

Taiwan began to screen flights arriving from Wuhan as early as December 31, 2019.

One of the key features of Taiwan's response is transparency. Seemingly, information flow from the Taiwan government has been transparent. Number of positive COVID-19 cases and the number of tests conducted each day are listed on the website on Taiwan's CDC. There is a sense of accountability and trust between the government and citizens. There has been constant assurance from the government side. On January 20, the CDC announced that the "government had under its control a stockpile of 44 million surgical masks, 1.9 million N95 masks, and 1100 negative-pressure isolation rooms."[3] Another important consideration is that given that Taiwan is excluded from all the high-level inter-state and WHO-led meetings, it began to act on its own by formulating its own strategy without little or no help and information flow in Taiwan from the WHO. Taiwan Foreign Minister Joseph Wu explained, Taiwan's approach included an "early and active campaign to diagnose, track, isolate and mitigate cases."[4] According to Wu, Taiwan's government response has been eight fold: "First, quick response; second, early deployment/screening; third, transparency; fourth, export ban, ration and rapid increase of production on critical supplies; fifth, whole-of-government approach and coordination among different ministers, departments and agencies; six, rearrangement of the medical institutions to meet the emergency requirements; seventh, preventive measures of in-hospital outbreaks; and eighth, contact tracing".[5]

Taiwan was able to contain the virus without taking harsh measures because of a mix of factors. First, Taiwan has prior experience in dealing with the SARS. When the SARS outbreak hit Taiwan which resulted in more than 650 cases and 181 deaths (much more than COVID-19 causalities), Taiwan was left alone to deal with it. Chan Chang-chuan, Dean, National Taiwan University's College of Public Health remarked, "What we learned from SARS was that we need to be very skeptical with data from China. We learned very harsh lessons then and that experience is something other countries do not have."[6] To prepare better for the outbreak of the next virus, Taiwan began to form a structured and institutional response. CDC was established in 1999. In 2004, the Communicable Disease Control Act was amended and the National Health Command Center (NHCC) was established. It is under the CDC which is "to serve as a unified central command system for disaster prevention. The NHCC provides decision-makers with comprehensive information about disasters as they unfold, as well as associated resources issues. It also coordinates communications among central, regional, and local governments as part of disease prevention and control efforts. Its wide-ranging use of both hardware and software and its efficient channels of communication have established the NHCC as a holistic information platform."[7]

It already had an epidemic prevention strategy in place which came in handy. As soon as the first case was diagnosed, measures such as temperature monitoring and sanitization were put in place at public places. Temperature monitoring became a common practice before entering public transport and public/private office, educational institutes and other major places. Apart from this, quarantined protocols were put in place and it was mandatory to observe self-quarantine for Taiwan nationals and foreigners entering Taiwan from high-risk areas primarily Mainland China from February 6. Quarantine for people arriving from high-risk areas is important to ascertain the source of the infection. Social distancing has also been encouraged wherever is possible.

Second, there was a quick response with affirmative actions from the administration. Taiwan government observed the situation in China and took prompt actions. Starting February 7, visitors from Mainland China, Hong Kong and Macau were barred to enter the country if they had a prior history of visit to these places within a span of 14 days. Taiwanese nationals, however, were given an exemption. On February 10, this restriction was extended to foreigners even transiting through these places and it was mandatory for anyone who visited China to self-quarantine for two weeks. Foreigners were barred to enter Taiwan when the virus was spread to the rest of the world and the number of cases began to increase in Taiwan.

Third, the preventive measures are supported by the high-quality healthcare system. Taiwan healthcare has been ranked the best by the Global Health Care Index.[8] National Health Insurance (NHI) was introduced in 1995 and now 99 percent of the population has access to healthcare. Taiwan was one of the worst affected by SARS in 2003. Learning from its past experience, it has expanded monitoring and healthcare gradually to prepare for an inevitable pandemic. One such move was to combine the efficient healthcare with the data gathering for better preparing the medical frontliners. One such example was the development of a patient-centered system called PharmaCloud in 2013. According to the official sources:[9]

> "Using the NHI's virtual private network system, PharmaCloud allows medical institutions to view the past three months of a patient's medication history, which has helped improve the quality of hospital visits and reduced unnecessary wastage of medical resources. The government then built upon and expanded the system to create the NHIMediCloud System in 2015, introducing 12 additional categories of data into the database, including traditional Chinese medicine, detailed surgical records, and vaccination history. The government continued to optimise the management of cloud-based medical information and has now initiated a system called My Health Bank that allows citizens to

access the cloud for themselves. After registering their NHI cards, users can log on the system to check their medical history without having to use a smart card read."

Dr. Alan Hao Yang, Deputy Director at the Institute of International Relations, National Chengchi University, provided six pointers for Taiwan's success:[10]

- *Experience in [Health] Crisis Management*: The experience from dealing with the SARS helped Taiwan in tackling the COVID-19 challenge. With a sense of accountability, the government adopted whole-of-government approach accompanied by the strict protocol. Mandatory wearing of masks in public transport, an awareness drive, banning flights from the epicenter of the virus, tracing and screening of people with recent travels from China, were among the key measures.
- *Inter-agency Data Integration*: Unlike other countries, Taiwan effectively conducted contact tracing and made the information readily available to frontliners. Corroborating data from the National Health Insurance Administration (NHIA) and the National Immigration Agency proved helpful in identifying the source as also protecting the lives of the medical frontliners.
- *Public Education and Transparency:* Effective and transparent communication between the government and the people through the corresponding agencies/ministries is arguably one of the instrumental reasons for Taiwan's successful management of the virus. The Central Epidemic Command Center (CECC) and the Ministry of Health and Welfare hold daily press briefings disseminating important information regarding the virus, including relevant statistics, update on recent cases, protocols, and high-risk areas to avoid.
- *Digital Social Innovation:* Proactive civil society participation and social innovation helped in plugging gaps across sectors. Spearheaded by Audrey Tang, Taiwan's Digital Minister, greater involvement of civilians and tech volunteers was made possible. This can be seen in the various applications launched to aid data gathering and sharing, whether for up-to-date information on which pharmacies have stocks of masks or data on areas recently visited by positive cases among others. Such innovations have made it possible to better integrate government efforts with social participation, encouraging the latter to be more vigilant and determined to stay updated with relevant knowledge regarding the virus. Social media has also actively played a vital role in information dissemination. Taiwan CDC regularly sends updates through an official LINE account (疾管家).

- *Reliable Public Service*: Even before the situation was declared as a global pandemic, Taiwan started taking necessary precautions of mobilising frontline services such as research and testing centers, and CDC hotlines for inquiries and advise. The government also called on PPE manufacturers early on to halt exports of masks and to focus on production to augment local supplies.
- *Compliant and Informed Public*: It is important to give the credit to Taiwanese people as well who obeyed the rules. Government precautions mean nothing if not for a cooperative constituency. In Taiwan, the public rely on available information about the virus and heed warnings seriously. It helps that the Taiwanese population also know the extent of services available to them under the NHI, which effectively reduces the cost entailed by testing, hospitalisation, and medicine.

Apart from taking measures to contain the virus, Taiwan ramped up the production of face masks, PPE and other required medical equipment for domestic consumption and later, for importing purpose. According to Bonnie Glaser, Senior Adviser for Asia and Director, China Power Project at the Center for Strategic and International Studies:

> "Taiwan's achievement is exemplary. Importantly, Taiwan's government has won the public's confidence. 95 percent of people adhere to quarantine rules. Technology has been used very effectively to monitor individuals, and conduct contact tracing. Disinformation about the virus has been countered expeditiously. Unlike most other countries, the schools and businesses have mostly remained open. Life has not been disrupted in the way that it has in most countries."[11]

While there have been several factors behind Taiwan's impeccable response and success in mitigating the threat from the virus, the crux is that the government took prompt actions at the right time. The onus was not only on the administration but each citizen played his part in curbing this challenge. It is important to look at Taiwan's response as the Island nation managed to deal with it effectively on its own.

Taiwan Model for COVID-19

While almost half of the world had to resort to either partial or complete lockdown, Taiwan is a live example of how a democracy could handle a pandemic successfully, without any major harm to human lives and disruption to day-to-day routine. It has proven that effective governance helped it to contain the virus. Taiwan's Vice President Chen Chien-jen, who is also a renowned epidemiologist, explained that Taiwan's response to COVID-19 could be defined by "prudent action, rapid response and early deployment."[12]

Bonnie Glaser explains that "the Taiwan model phrase is being used to describe Taiwan's handling of COVID-19. More broadly, it is highlighting the success of Taiwan's democracy. Obviously, Taiwan's democracy contains many elements that are similar to other democracies, but it is the only Chinese democracy in the world. Facing a major threat from the People's Republic of China (PRC) and international isolation, Taiwan has been able to provide its people with good governance, which many democracies aspire to do but have not succeeded."[13] In terms of the pandemic, Taiwan model is characterised by reasonable social distancing, strict quarantine protocols, testing, isolation and treatment. This led to containment of the virus, prevention of community spread, and way towards complete elimination. Taiwan's response resonates with the point made by Prof. Amitav Acharya that "the present crisis underscores the reality that effective governance trumps material power rank (economic or military) in coping with global threats."[14]

Taiwan's government response has been explained aptly by Chung Kwang Tien, Taiwan Representative to India Ambassador. In an interview to an Indian Newspaper, he remarked that:[15]

> "Taiwan's strategy has been to identify the infected people, trace their contacts and isolate everyone involved, preventing the virus from spreading to the community. In addition, Taiwan has established a comprehensive national disease prevention mechanism: this includes digitised disease monitoring systems, stringent border quarantine measures, extensive community-based countermeasures, advanced medical preparedness, an abundant stock of preventive medical appliances and resources, concise guidelines and information for the reference of the general public, and annual disease prevention and control drills."

While Taiwan had prior experience in dealing with the epidemic, its response to COVID-19 may be characterised by preparedness accompanied with transparency, accountability, and promptness. Its model is different from other countries such as China which had to resort to complete lockdown with harsh measures, the United States which had to shut down the economy, and India, which also had to resort to different phases of lockdown. Taiwan model has proven successful. It did not have to resort to any kind of lockdown or shutting down the economy. Taiwan model does not only include the containment of the virus, but also extending a helping hand to countries in need. It has donated surgical masks, PPE, and other medical equipment to allies, New Southbound policy countries and other distressed countries.

Taiwan's COVID-19 Diplomacy

2019 was not a good year for Taiwan in terms of diplomatic capital. It lost its diplomatic allies and now has diplomatic ties with 15 countries only. While countries across the world have been cautious in progressing political ties with Taiwan, COVID-19 has provided Taiwan with a rare window of opportunity to reach out to countries. It is seizing the opportunity to push for greater international space. It has been utilising this situation to reach out to countries and boost its international visibility. Policy makers, scholars and journalists across the world are appreciating Taiwan's response to the virus. The calls have been made for including Taiwan in the WHO and also imitate Taiwan model to contain the spread of the virus.

Taiwan has been promptly helping its diplomatic allies. It has donated masks, PPE and other necessary medical equipment. Taiwan model and its subsequent outreach to Europe and countries under the New Southbound Policy have generated hope that China's aspiration to shrink Taiwan's international space has met with a deadlock at the moment. Taiwan has stepped up its medical diplomacy. In the times when China is selling the masks and other required equipment, Taiwan is donating millions of masks to the affected countries. Taiwan is the second largest producer of masks after China and has ramped up its production further to meet domestic needs and importing the masks. Taiwan's Economics Minister Shen Jong-chin announced that Taiwan is currently producing 15 million masks each day.[16] In March, the government relaxed the ban on masks export which was imposed on January 24. Taiwan is producing as many as 17 million masks a day now and masks and sanitisers have made a comeback in the retail market in Taiwan. Amid skepticism about the quality of masks, testing kits and other medical equipment from China, the quality of masks and other equipment from Taiwan is of superior quality. In this context, Chen Chern-chyi, Director-General of the Ministry of Economic Affairs' Bureau of Foreign Trade pointed out, "Taiwan is manufacturing certified and high-quality products to help combat the COVID-19 pandemic worldwide. Many of the products have also secured certification in other countries. The nation provides certified and effective disease-prevention products to the world. People can be reassured that products with Taiwan Excellence Awards certification are safe, reliable and high-quality."[17]

One of the beneficiaries is the United States. Taiwan Foreign Minister Joseph Wu stated Taiwan will donate 100,000 face masks per week to the United States, while the United States will provide 300,000 hazmat suits for Taiwan in future if the need arises.[18] In April, Taiwan donated 400,000 masks to the United States. The United States has been vocal about its support to Taiwan. The United States Mission in the United Nations tweeted in support of Taiwan. It said, "the UN was founded to serve all voices, welcome a diversity of views and perspectives and promote human rights. Barring Taiwan from setting foot on UN grounds is an affront not just to the proud Taiwanese people, but to the UN principle."[19] COVID-19 has further escalated tension between China and the United States. Donald Trump has been critical of China's hiding of information and mismanagement of the virus at home, calling it a deliberate attempt to spread the virus across the world. Amid the trade war and hostility in the Indo-Pacific, the relations have hit the rock bottom with the blame game on COVID-19. Minxin Pei, Professor at the California's Claremont McKenna College and a Non-Resident Senior Fellow at the German Marshall Fund opines, "Far from catalysing global cooperation, the pandemic may well lock the United States and China into a vicious cycle of escalation, leading directly to full-blown conflict."[20] The United States has withheld the funding for the WHO and also criticised it for Taiwan exclusion. A State Department Spokesperson remarked, "The United States is deeply disturbed that Taiwan's information was withheld from the global health community, as reflected in the WHO's January 14, 2020 statement that there was no indication of human-to-human transmission."[21] The United States accused "The WHO of choosing politics over public health". "On March 18, Taiwan authorities signed a deal with the American Institute in Taiwan, the US quasi-embassy in Taipei, on anti-coronavirus co-operation. China blasted the agreement as "a political plot to pursue independence with the help of the epidemic."[22]

Taiwan diplomacy is not restricted to just its diplomatic allies and the United States. It has reached out to Europe as well. It has adopted mask diplomacy, which has worked to its advantage. In April, at least seven million surgical masks were donated to the European countries and European Union (EU). EU Commissioner for Crisis Management Janez Lenarčič responded to Taiwan's donation, "*In these difficult times, international cooperation is crucial. We highly appreciate Taiwan's gesture of solidarity with its donation of medical masks to the EU. The Commission's Emergency Response Coordination Centre has facilitated the delivery of 1 million these masks to Spain and Italy, which were a direct donation to the European Union. The remaining 5.9 million masks are being provided through bilateral channels to other Member States.*"[23] Additionally, in an unprecedented move, on April 2, EU Commissioner, Ursula von der Leyen also tweeted thanking Taiwan for the donation. She remarked, "The EU thanks Taiwan for its donation of 5.6 million masks to help fight the coronavirus. We really appreciate this gesture of solidarity. This global virus outbreak requires international solidarity and cooperation."[24] Taiwan reached a cooperative agreement with Czech Republic for cooperation and collaboration on COVID-19, while it donated nine ventilators to Taiwan. It has also expanded cooperation and extended a helping hand to countries under the scope of New Southbound policy. On March 30, Taiwan announced that on the basis of reciprocity, while it will receive alcohol required for manufacturing hand sanitisers from Australia, it will export non-woven fabric for mask production to Australia.[25] Taiwan donated one million masks to India in early May.

President Tsai has also been active on social media platforms and actively pronouncing its gratitude to leaders and officials supporting Taiwan. On April 1, she stated:

> "In times of crisis, countries around the world must come together. Taiwan is indispensable to global efforts to stop the spread of COVID-19, but no country can stop this virus alone. That is why we are willing to offer medical supplies to countries most in need. We need to step up cooperation, and that means sharing experience and material, and working together to develop treatments and vaccine. Pandemics cannot be stopped by one country alone. Donate surplus masks and other supplies to allies and countries hit hardest by the virus."[26]

Alexander C. Huang from Tamkang University pointed out, "It is a rare opportunity for Taiwan as usually when Taiwan gets on international news, there is either a crisis in the Taiwan straits or a natural disaster."[27] Taiwan leadership has been using this opportunity to spread awareness about Taiwan. For instance, Taiwanese Ministers and representatives are writing opinion pieces in foreign newspapers. Taiwan medical aid and diplomacy is helping Taiwan in projecting its soft power. Its medical diplomacy has become an important part of reaching out to countries amid China's attempts to minimise Taiwan's international space. Though COVID-19 has highlighted Taiwan's ability to help countries in need, its medical diplomacy did not begin with COVID-19. Taiwan has been emphasizing on strengthening medical cooperation between Taiwan and countries under the New Southbound Policy. In 2018, Executive Yuan announced:[28]

> "The New Southbound medical cooperation and industrial chain development program was launched in 2018 to promote medical cooperation with India, Indonesia, Malaysia, the Philippines, Thailand and Vietnam. On June 1 this year, the government announced that it would establish one medical center in each of these countries, for the purposes of promoting medical personnel training, building bridges between health care industries, providing health consultation for Taiwanese expatriates, creating a culture-friendly medical environment, surveying medical regulations and market conditions, and integrating information. The program has plans to establish a disease prevention technology transfer center to enhance the region's communicable disease prevention capabilities, as well as a health information services center for people going to and coming from the New Southbound countries for work."

Taiwan's diplomacy has helped it in expanding its outreach to countries across the world. Its approach has been swift for countries and also for foreigners residing/ stuck in Taiwan. For foreigners working/studying in Taiwan, the administration made it easier to have access to the rationed masks, and extended the visas for foreigners on visitors'/tourist visas. Through its diplomacy, it presented China with a challenge that is attempting to take advantage of situation at the global stage.

Cross-Strait Complexity

The status of Taiwan is a complicated issue from the sovereignty perspective. Since 1949, Taiwan has been a core issue for the Chinese leadership. On the eve of the establishment of the PRC, Mao Zedong proclaimed that any country wanting to establish diplomatic relations with the PRC needs to relinquish ties with Taiwan. He stated:[29]

> "In order to make a clean break with the foreign policy of the old and semi-colonial China and uphold the independence and sovereignty of New China, we should "start anew" and "put the house in order before inviting guests". That is to say China renounced all the diplomatic relations the Kuomintang Government had established with foreign countries, treated heads of foreign diplomatic missions accredited to Old China as ordinary foreign nationals instead of diplomatic envoys; reviewed all the treaties and agreements Old China had concluded with foreign countries; gradually cleared up the prerogatives and influence the imperialist countries had in China; and established new diplomatic relations with other countries on the basis of mutual respect for sovereignty and territorial integrity, and equality and mutual benefit."

While the Chinese leadership has always emphasized on One-China policy and advocated for Taiwan's peaceful reunification with the Chinese motherland on the basis of 'One Country, Two Systems' principle–similar to what the CCP has applied in Hong Kong and Macau, in the past. China became more aggressive and attempted to shrink Taiwan's international space. It has registered strong protests even when countries attempt to step up cooperation with Taiwan. This has made countries such as the United States, Australia and India cautious while bolstering ties with Taiwan. This had led to marginalisation of Taiwan and left the potential of ties with Taiwan underutilised. Chinese leadership is witnessing strong opposition from the Taiwanese leadership now. Democratic Progressive Party (DPP)'s Tsai has been in power since May 2016 and came back to power after a landslide victory in January 2020. On the 40th anniversary of "Message to Compatriots in Taiwan, Xi remarked: "The historical and legal facts, that Taiwan is part of China and the two sides across Taiwan Straits belong to one and the same China, can never be altered by anyone or any force... The principles of peaceful reunification and one country, two systems are the best approach to realising national reunification... Political parties and all sectors on both sides of the Straits may recommend representatives to conduct extensive and in-depth democratic consultation on the basis of the common political foundation of upholding the 1992 Consensus and opposing 'Taiwan independence'."[30] In response to this, President Tsai stated, "I must emphasise that we have never accepted the "1992 Consensus". I want to reiterate that Taiwan absolutely will not accept one country, two systems. The vast majority of Taiwanese also resolutely oppose "One Country, Two Systems", and this opposition is also a "Taiwan consensus" ... mean that grassroots public opinion in Taiwan favors abandoning our sovereignty."[31] To manage Cross-Strait ties, Tsai illustrated four musts:[32]

> "China must face the reality of the existence of the ROC (Taiwan) and not deny the democratic system that the people of Taiwan have established together; Second, must respect the commitment of the 23 million people of Taiwan to freedom and democracy, and not foster divisions and offer inducements to interfere with the choices made by the people of Taiwan; Third, must handle Cross-strait differences peacefully, on the basis of equality, instead of using suppression and intimidation to get Taiwanese to submit; and Fourth, it must be governments or government-authorised agencies that engage in negotiations. Any political consultations that are not authorised and monitored by the people cannot be called 'democratic consultations. This is Taiwan's position, a democratic position."

Taiwan's handling of the virus and its diplomacy has made cross-strait ties further strained and tensions more explicit. The praises for Taiwan and the call for its inclusion in the WHO has created unease in China. Despite the threat looming large from the virus, China's attention on Taiwan has been intact. As the virus has spread worldwide, China has started to change the narrative and the Chinese diplomats based in foreign countries have begun the damage control exercise. While some of the Chinese diplomats are working towards projecting China as a 'friendly and helpful' country, other diplomats have taken the responsibility of targeting Taiwan. For instance, the Spokesperson of the Chinese Embassy in India, Ji Rong expressed strong discontent on Indian media reportage on Taiwan's response to COVID-19 by issuing a statement: "The WHO is a specialised agency of the United Nations restricted to only sovereign states. Any questions about Taiwan's participation in international organisations must be arranged under the One-China principle."[33] Even China's Ministry of Foreign Affairs Spokeswoman Hua Chungying on Taiwan's donating the masks to the United States warned, "In the current extraordinary period, mutual assistance and support are all welcomed. But I still want to remind the US and Taiwan that if someone tries to take advantage of the epidemic to impair China's core interests, they must be cautious." China even accused Taiwan of 'venomously' attacking the WHO and taking advantage of the crisis for seeking independence.[34]

According to Bonnie Glaser:

> "Even before the outbreak of COVID-19, China was stepping up military, diplomatic and economic pressure on Taiwan. This is likely to continue and perhaps be ratcheted up further. Beijing is worried that Taipei will use the pandemic to increase its international support. It has warned Taiwan not to exploit the opportunity to push for independence. China is closely watching the potential for a referendum in 2021 on revising the ROC constitution. It is also worried about the trend of strengthening US-Taiwan ties. Over the next four years of DPP rule in Taiwan, China will take a range of steps to prevent Taiwan from challenging its sovereignty claims. It is unlikely, however, that China will use military force in the near term. It has a very large tool box of other measures it can use to influence and punish Taiwan."

The virus has added another dimension to the already complex cross-strait ties. China even refused to allow repatriation of Taiwanese nationals stuck in Mainland China. While some of the major countries are struggling to deal with the pandemic at home, China is using this opportunity to ramp up its military presence in the Taiwan Strait. In an article, Bonnie Glaser and Matthew P. Funaiole mention, "The People's Liberation Army Air Force (PLAAF) and Navy (PLAN) have conducted as many as 10 transits and military exercises near Taiwan since mid-January, including multiple deliberate incursions into Taiwan's airspace."[35] This is also to showcase its capabilities and willingness to use force if the need arises.

WHO and Taiwan

It is not common to see a tussle between an international body/agency and a state. Tensions have flared up between Taiwan and the WHO over the former's exclusion and non-sharing of information. As mentioned, on December 31, Taiwan alerted the WHO about the possible human-to-human transmission of a SARS-like virus in Wuhan through an email to International Health Regulations (IHR). Taiwan informed the WHO that through internet sources, it has learnt that in Wuhan, people were getting infected with atypical pneumonia who were being treated in isolation and that there is a likelihood of human-to-human transmission.[36] Asking for establishing information sharing platform and get sufficient information from the WHO, Ministry of Health remarked that, "Given the lack of clarity at the time, as well as the many rumors that were circulating, Taiwan's aim was to ensure that all relevant parties remained alert, especially since the outbreak occurred just before the Lunar New Year holiday, which typically sees tremendous amounts of travel."[37]

Taiwan's exclusion from the WHO is directly linked to China's opposition to its membership and attempts to shrink its global exposure. In 2009, Taiwan was given the status of an observer in the World Health Assembly (WHA), committee governing the WHO. Former President of Taiwan Ma Ying-jeou, who later went on to have met Xi in Singapore in 2015, negotiated with Beijing for entry in the WHA. Beijing agreed on a condition that Taiwan was listed as a province of China in WHA proceedings and publications. WHO confidential memo consisting the details of the deal was leaked in 2010 and led to outrage in Taiwan. It was mentioned in the memo that the only terminology to be used within the WHO would be Chinese Taipei and Taiwan to be regarded as a province of China. Taking into account the representation of China in the WHO, health agencies should refrain "from actions which could constitute or be interpreted as recognition of a separate status of Taiwanese authorities and institutions from China."[38] The memo further mentioned:

> "There has been no change in the status of Taiwan Province of China within the WHO. Information related to the Taiwan Province of China must be listed or shown as falling under China and not separately as if they referred to a state."[39] The memo also mentioned that Taiwan was to be excluded from the IHR, which allows information sharing among members in an event of epidemic outbreak. Tsai, then DPP's chairperson called it called it a "serious" and "regrettable" incident and if this becomes Taiwan's method of participating in international organisations, it will have a deep impact on our country's global position and international space."[40]

When Tsai came to power, she refused to accept One-China principle. As a result, WHA observer status was taken away from Taiwan in 2016 and since then any attempts for acquiring the observer status has gone in vain.[41] WHO has attracted criticism for kowtowing to China. Countries such as Canada, Japan and the United States have showed support for Taiwan's participation in the WHO. Japanese Prime Minister Shinzo Abe stated, "It is necessary for Taiwan to join the WHO. Under the premise of epidemic prevention and public health policies, 'political stances' should be overruled. Otherwise, maintaining the health of the entire region and further preventing the spread of infection will become a difficult problem."[42] Canadian Prime Minister Justin Trudeau also voiced Canada's support for Taiwan's WHO membership, "As we did during the time of the SARS virus, we support Taiwan's meaningful participation in international multilateral forums especially when its presence provides important contributions to the global public good. We believe that Taiwan's role as an observer in World Health Assembly meetings is in the best interests of the international health community and is also an important partner in the fight...we welcome participation from the entire international community to promote global health. That is why we have long taken this position."[43]

United States Department of State voiced its support for Taiwan's participation in the WHO. It stated, "Recently, the United States and Taiwan announced enhanced cooperation on preventing the spread of COVID-19. Working with Taiwan and like-minded countries to expand Taiwan's international participation is an important part of that effort. Countries around the world can benefit from better understanding the Taiwan Model, as well as the generous contributions and impressive expertise Taiwan – a vibrant democracy and force for good – brings to the global community."[44] U.S.-China Economic and Security Review Commission published an issue brief on how China is using COVID-19 to bully Taiwan and called out WHO for Taiwan's exclusion. It was highlighted, "WHO officials consistently ignored Taiwan's attempts to exchange information about the virus and share best practices for containing it. Meanwhile, Beijing ramped up military pressure on Taiwan through a series of coercive exercises."[45]

In its defence amid rising criticism, the WHO stated, "The question of Taiwanese membership in WHO is up to WHO Member States, not WHO staff. However, WHO is working closely with all health authorities who are facing the current coronavirus pandemic, including Taiwanese health experts."[46] China has also come in defence of the WHO. Media Spokesperson in the Chinese Embassy in India, Ji Rong stated, "The DPP, since taking power (in Taiwan) in 2016, has been stubbornly adhering to Taiwan's independence separatist stance, constantly challenging the One-China principle, thus undermining the political foundation for the region's participation in the WHO."[47] China's Ministry of Foreign Affairs Spokesperson Hua Chunying has said:[48]

> "The United States government and the Taiwan region are fully aware that WHO members must be sovereign countries. According to arrangement between China and WHO, medical and health experts in the Taiwan region can, on the precondition of the one-China principle, participate in WHO's technical activities in their own capacity. With International Health Regulations (IHR) contact point in the Taiwan region, it has no problem at all in accessing WHO information on global public health emergencies, including notifications and cooperation on epidemics. I hope certain people will refrain from politicising the pandemic."

Clearly, instead of debating the merits and demerits of Taiwan's participation, China has tried to twist the narrative to the sovereignty issue and make it look like a challenge to its One-China policy.

Taiwan's Political Debate

With Taiwan's response, the approval rating of Tsai has gone up. She had already taken some landmark decisions in her first term such as legalising same sex marriage and formal apology to indigenous people. At the external front, Taiwan increased its outreach by initiating the New Southbound Policy and has been assertive with China. Though losing allies has been a setback for Taiwan but the New Southbound Policy has yielded results. One important development was the change of the name of representative office in Japan to include Taiwan in it. The United States enacted Taipei Act which would facilitate greater cooperation between the United States and Taiwan.

Exclusion from the WHO and China's aggression have sparked domestic debates in Taiwan. Tsai's assertive posture towards China is one of the reasons for her high public approval rating. However, Taiwan leadership had to deal with some criticism as well. One view was that Taiwan was not testing enough as there might be affected people who are asymptomatic. Since there was no community outbreak, the leadership relied on quarantine and contact tracing instead of mass testing. According to Minister of Health and Welfare Chen Shih-chung, "50 regional hospitals and medical centres and 167 community hospitals and clinics to create a tiered system for testing."[49] According to the official stand, the infection rate is low and the absence of community outbreak does not make the case for mass testing. On April 28, Chen further added that "Of the 60,956 people tested, only 429 were confirmed to be infected with COVID-19, and that the authorities could not identify the source of infection in only 10 cases.... With an infection rate of around 0.7 percent among those tested and 0.009 percent among those who reported COVID-like symptoms, there is no need to move toward mass testing, as public health experts have been advocating."[50]

Second, in January, despite just a handful of positive cases, countries such as Italy and the Philippines had banned flights to and from Taiwan. Also, Taiwanese abroad were misconstrued as Chinese and were mistreated at some places. This created discomfort at the domestic level. Lack of awareness and confusion about the official name of Taiwan (Republic of China) and the PRC led to the demand of changing the official name of the ROC to Taiwan or Republic of Chunghwa. Taiwan's New Power Party (NPP) conducted a poll in March and according to the poll results, 51.2 percent strongly supported the suggestion that China should be dropped from the official name, 23.1 percent were supportive, 10.8 percent disagreed, and 6.4 percent strongly disagreed, while 8.5 percent expressed no clear opinion."[51] There have been calls to change the name of the State airlines as well, from China Airlines to Taiwan Airlines. Though the leadership expressed solidarity towards these calls for the name change, they have been cautious in touching such a sensitive topic and emphasised that at the moment, the focus should be on fighting the pandemic. In this context Joanne Wu, Ministry of Foreign Affairs Spokesperson stated, "According to the constitution, the official name is the ROC and that the word Taiwan was already added to passport covers in 2003. In the future, if there is consensus between the ruling and opposition parties on this new name, the Foreign Ministry shall cooperate in handling it."[52] Taiwan's successful response and diplomacy has led to a number of tweets from countries across the world with the hashtag Taiwan is helping! Taiwan can help!

Conclusion

Taiwan's handling and successful management of COVID-19 has improved its image worldwide and put it back on the global map. There is a silver lining for Taiwan in this grim situation. It has shaped countries' perception about Taiwan. While China hid the information at the crucial time and mismanaged the situation, Taiwan showed the world how to contain the virus successfully and responsibly. It has not only managed the situation well at home, but also helped the international community by donating the essential medical supplies. This has presented the world with an alternate and a more responsible 'China'.

Taiwan has used this opportunity to its advantage. Its response to COVID-19 domestically and medical outreach to countries worldwide have helped it in expanding its international space. It has certainly strengthened Taiwan's aspiration to boost its international cooperation. Post-pandemic world might see escalation in cross-ctrait ties and a more assertive and aggressive China but what is certain is that this has created greater space for Taiwan at a wider global stage.

NOTES

1 Tsai Ing-wen (2020), "President of Taiwan: How My Country Prevented a Major Outbreak of COVID-19", 16 April 2020, https://time.com/collection/finding-hope-coronavirus-pandemic/5820596/taiwan-coronavirus-lessons/, accessed online 16 April 2020.

2 Taiwan Center for Disease Control (2020), "Two experts from Taiwan visit Wuhan to understand and obtain information on severe special infectious pneumonia outbreak; Taiwan CDC raises travel notice level for Wuhan to Level 2", 20 January 2020, https://www.cdc.gov.tw/En/Bulletin/Detail/jFGUVrlLkIuHmzZeyAihHQ?typeid=158, accessed online 28 March 2020.

3 C Jason Wang Chun Y Ng, and Robert H Brook (2020), "Response to COVID-19 in Taiwan: Big Data Analytics, New Technology, and Proactive Testing", 3 March 2020, https://jamanetwork.com/journals/jama/fullarticle/2762689, accessed online 20 March 2020.

4 Joseph Wu (2020), "Transcript: Taiwan's Strong COVID-19 Response: Remarks by Foreign Minister Joseph Wu", 10 April 2020, https://www.hudson.org/research/15919-transcript-taiwan-s-strong-COVID-19-response-remarks-by-foreign-minister-joseph-wu, accessed online April 12, 2020.

5 Ibid.

6 Michelle Yun (2020), "How Taiwan is Containing Coronavirus – Despite Diplomatic Isolation by China", 13 March 2020, https://www.theguardian.com/world/2020/mar/13/how-taiwan-is-containing-coronavirus-despite-diplomatic-isolation-by-china, accessed online 20 March 2020.

7 Taiwan's Center for Communicable Disease (2018), "NHCC", 31 January 2018, https://www.cdc.gov.tw/En/Category/MPage/gL7-bARtHyNdrDq882pJ9Q, accessed online 29 March 2020.

8 Chang-Chin Tu (2020), "Lessons from Taiwan's experience with COVID-19", https://www.atlanticcouncil.org/blogs/new-atlanticist/lessons-from-taiwans-experience-with-COVID-19/, accessed online 7 April 2020.

9 Ministry of Foreign Affairs of the Republic of China (2020), "Taiwan's Comprehensive National Health Insurance System and Our Experience of Fighting the SARS Epidemic", April 2020, https://www.mofa.gov.tw/Upload/RelFile/2890/172272/1-1Taiwan%27s%20comprehensive%20national%20health% 20insurance%20system%20and%20our%20experience%20of%20 fighting%20the%20SARS%20epidemic.pdf, accessed online 02 May 2020.

10 In an email interview with author, 12 May 2020.

11 In an email interview with author, 13 May 2020.

12 Smith Nicola (2020), "Taiwan's Vice-President Chen Chien-jen on His Country's Fight with COVID-19", 18 April 2020, https://www.telegraph.co.uk/global-health/science-and-disease/taiwans-vice-president-chen-chien-jen-countrys-fight-COVID-19/, accessed online 19 April 2020.

13 In an email interview with author, 13 May 2020.

14 Acharya, Amitav (2020), "How Coronavirus May Reshape the World Order", 18 April 2020, https://nationalinterest.org/feature/how-coronavirus-may-reshape-world-order-145972, accessed online 19 April 2020.

15 Tuteja, Ashok (2020), "Saturday Interview-Taiwan will Help India with COVID-19", 18 April 2020, https://www.thestatesman.com/exclusive-interviews/saturday-interview-taiwan-will-help-india-COVID-19-1502878704.html, accessed online 20 April 2020.

16 Ching-Tse Cheng (2020), "Taiwan's Daily Production of Face Masks Soon to Reach 15 Million", 6 April 2020, https://www.taiwannews.com.tw/en/news/3911053, accessed online 8 April 2020.

17 Shelly Chan (2020), "Virus Outbreak: Taiwan Produces High-Quality Medical Gear to Help World Fight Virus: Ministry", 5 May 2020, https://www.taipeitimes.com/News/taiwan/archives/2020/05/05/2003735849, accessed online 10 May 2020.

18 Everington Keoni (2020) "Taiwan to Donate 100,000 Masks Per Week to US", 18 March 2020, https://www.taiwannews.com.tw/en/news/3899531, accessed online March 20, 2020.

19 Lederer Edith M. (2020), "US Tweets Support for Taiwan, Sparking Opposition from China", 2 May 2020. https://abcnews.go.com/US/wireStory/us-tweets-support-taiwan-sparking-opposition-china-70468629, accessed online 5 May 2020.

20 Minxin Pei (2020), "COVID-19 is Finishing off the Sino-American Relationship", 29 April 2020, https://www.project-syndicate.org/commentary/china-america-relations-after-covid19-pandemic-by-minxin-pei-2020-04, accessed online 30 April 2020.

21 The Straits Times (2020), "Coronavirus: US Criticises WHO for Ignoring Taiwan Warnings", 10 April 2020, https://www.straitstimes.com/world/united-states/coronavirus-us-criticises-who-for-ignoring-taiwan-warnings, accessed online 10 April 2020.

22 Peel Michael and Katherin Hille (2020), "Taiwan to donate 10m masks to Europe and US", 01 April 2020. https://www.ft.com/content/e47a8cf4-786d-4367-a589-054a6a198840, accessed online 01 April 2020.

23 European Commission (2020), "Coronavirus: Taiwan's Aid to the EU Delivered to Spain and Italy", 09 April 2020, https://ec.europa.eu/commission/presscorner/detail/en/ip_20_643, accessed online 05 May 2020.

24 EU Commissioner, Ursula von der Leyen's tweet available on xhttps://twitter.com/vonderleyen/status/1245399247232684034?lang=en, accessed online 02 April 2020.

25 Peel Michael and KatherinHille, "Taiwan to Donate 10m Masks to Europe and US", 01 April 2020, https://www.ft.com/content/e47a8cf4-786d-4367-a589-054a6a198840, accessed online 01 April 2020.

26 Office of the President of the Republic of China (2020), "President Tsai's Address on COVID-19 Cooperation", 01 April 2020, https://english.president.gov.tw/News/5989, accessed online 01 April 2020.

27 Ruwitch John (2020), "Taiwan's Coronavirus Monment: And Delicate Balancing Act", 30 April 2020, https://www.npr.org/2020/04/29/847308433/taiwans-coronavirus-moment-and-delicate-balancing-act, accessed online 30 April 2020.

28 Executive Yuan (2020), "Taiwan Promotes Medical Cooperation with New Southbound Countries", 14 June 2020, https://english.ey.gov.tw/Page/61BF20C3E89B856/1b6c017c-49f0-4536-803b-bc7f0b94b4b9, accessed online 04 April 2020.

29 Ministry of Foreign Affairs of the People's Republic of China, "Formulation of Foreign Policy of New China on the Eve of its Birth", https://www.fmprc.gov.cn/mfa_eng/ziliao_665539/3602_665543/3604_665547/t18057.shtml, accessed online 17 March 2020.

30 The State Council Information Office of the People's Republic of China (2019), "Highlights of Xi's Speech at Taiwan Message Anniversary Event", 02 January 2019, http://english.scio.gov.cn/topnews/2019-01/02/content_74334053.htm, accessed online 03 March 2020.

31 Office of the President of the Republic of China (Taiwan) (2019), "President Tsai Issues Statement on China's President Xi's Message to Compatriots in Taiwan", 02 January 2019, https://english.president.gov.tw/News/5621, accessed online 07 April 2020.

32 Ibid.

33 The Indian Express (2020), "Reports advocating Taiwan's participation in WHO violated 'one-China' principle: Chinese embassy", 01 April 2020, https://indianexpress.com/article/world/taiwan-who-china-6339762/, accessed online 01 April 2020.

34 Al Jazeera (2020), "China Calls Taiwan's Attacks on WHO 'Venomous'", 10 April 2020, https://www.aljazeera.com/news/2020/04/china-calls-taiwan-attacks-venomous-200410075151269.html accessed online 12 April 2020.

35 Glaser Bonnie and Matthew P. Funaiole (2020), "China's Provocations around Taiwan aren't a Crisis", 15 May 2020, https://foreignpolicy.com/2020/05/15/chinas-provocations-around-taiwan-arent-a-crisis/, accessed online 17 May 2020.

36 Op. cit, no. 3.

37 Ministry of Health and Welfare of the Republic of China (2020), "The Facts Regarding Taiwan's Email to Alert WHO to Possible Danger of COVID-19", 11 April 2020, https://www.mohw.gov.tw/cp-115-52687-2.html. accessed online 12 April 2020.

38 Vincent Y. Chao, Shih Hsiu-chuan and Shelley Huang (2011), "WHO Memo Sparks Outrage in Taiwan", 10 May 2011, https://www.taipeitimes.com/News/front/archives/2011/05/10/2003502850, accessed online 12 March 2020.

39 Ibid.

40 Ibid.

41 Wilfred Chen (2020), "The WHO Ignores Taiwan. The World Pays the Price", 03 April 2020, https://www.thenation.com/article/world/taiwan-who-coronavirus-china/, accessed online 05 April 2020.

42 Everington Keoni (2020), "Taiwan Thanks Japan, Canada for Backing WHO Bid", 01 January 2020, https://www.taiwannews.com.tw/en/news/3867837, accessed online 19 March 2020.

43 Toronto Sun (2020), "CHEN: China Needs to Stop Blocking Taiwan from the WHO", 01 February 2020, https://torontosun.com/opinion/columnists/chen-china-needs-to-stop-blocking-taiwan-from-the-who, accessed online 19 March 2020.

44 US Department of State (2020), "Virtual Forum on Expanding Taiwan's Participation on the Global Stage", 02 April 2020, https://www.state.gov/virtual-forum-on-expanding-taiwans-participation-on-the-global-stage/, accessed online 02 April 2020.

45 Lloyd-Damnjanovic Anastasya (2020) "Beijing's Deadly Game: Consequences of Excluding Taiwan from the World Health Organization during the COVID-19 Pandemic", 12 May 2020, https://www.uscc.gov/research/beijings-deadly-game-consequences-excluding-taiwan-world-health-organization-during-covid, accessed online 12 May 2020.

46 WHO (2020), "Information Sharing on COVID-19", 29 March 2020, who.int/news-room/detail/29-03-2020-information-sharing-on-COVID-19, accessed online 04 April 2020.

47 Dikshit Sandeep (2020), "Indian Media's Reporting on Taiwan has China Fuming", 01 April 2020, https://www.tribuneindia.com/news/nation/indian-medias-reporting-on-taiwan-has-china-fuming-63745, accessed online 01 April 2020.

48 Ministry of Foreign Affairs of the People's Republic of China (2020), "Foreign Ministry Spokesperson Hua Chunying's Regular Press Conference on April 3, 2020", 03 April 2020, https://www.fmprc.gov.cn/mfa_eng/xwfw_665399/s2510_665401/2511_665403/t1765751.shtml, accessed online 15 April 2020.

49 Chen Shih-chung (2020), "Taiwan's Coronavirus Protocol Shows How it is Done", 02 May 2020, https://www.thehindu.com/opinion/op-ed/taiwans-coronavirus-protocol-shows-how-it-is-done/article31484681.ece, accessed online 02 May 2020.

50 Focus Taiwan (2020), "Taiwan's COVID-19 Infection Rate Does Not Justify Mass Testing: CECC", 28 April 2020, https://focustaiwan.tw/society/202004280019, accessed online 30 April 2020.

51 Everington Keoni (2020), "Over 70 percent Favor Removing China from Taiwan Passport", 30 March 2020, https://www.taiwannews.com.tw/en/news/3907124, accessed online 02 April 2020.

52 Blanchard Ben (2020), "In Taiwan, Anger at China over Virus Drives Identity Debate", 01 April 2020, https://www.reuters.com/article/us-health-coronavirus-taiwan-china/in-taiwan-anger-at-china-over-virus-drives-identity-debate-idUSKBN21J4JK, accessed online 05 April 2020.

10

Fraying but Far from Broken: China-US Relations and COVID-19

Rukmani Gupta

The COVID-19 pandemic has brought to the fore underlying antagonisms in the relationship between China and the United States (US), exposing the deep-seated mistrust between the two nations. The already delicate relationship had just begun to stabilize after the vicissitudes of protracted trade negotiations in early January 2020 when an acrimonious blame-game over COVID-19 came to be played from diplomatic rostra. Given the personalities involved and the growth of nationalism in both countries, it is unlikely that the bilateral relationship will recover to the semblance of constructive cooperation achieved under the Obama administration. The reasons for this are varied and complex, not only related to the immediate problem of the global pandemic, but the increasingly divergent world views of the two countries.

The changing rhetoric on COVID-19

The US' Centre for Disease Control and Prevention issued its first travel advisory for China, related to the spread of respiratory illness in Wuhan, on 6 January 2020 and passenger screening was announced for those arriving in the US from Wuhan on 16 January 2020. Even as the first case of the illness in the US was confirmed on January 21st, President Trump praised Chinese efforts to tackle the disease in a tweet on 24 January.[1] This was when 830 of the total 896 positive cases of the disease globally were in China.[2] By 2 February, the US had banned entry to travelers from China and those with recent travel history to the country.

Until the end of February, President Trump repeatedly expressed his confidence in Chinese President Xi Jinping's ability to handle the fallout of the coronavirus and contain it.[3] By this time, on 11 February 2020, the International Committee on Taxonomy of Viruses (ICTV) had announced "severe acute respiratory syndrome coronavirus 2 (SARS-CoV-2)" as the name of the new virus responsible for respiratory illness identified in Wuhan and the disease itself was named "COVID-19" by the World Health Organization (WHO). A month later, on 11 March 2020, WHO classified COVID-19 as a pandemic. By this date, the US had reported 696 positive cases of the disease[4] even as Chinese infections had soared to over 80,000. As infection rates in the US rose exponentially, so did the US administration's view of Chinese culpability in the spread of the disease.

In February 2020, despite efforts by Republican senator Tom Cotton to link the coronavirus to the Wuhan Institute of Virology[5], a press statement by the US Secretary of State, Michael Pompeo, referred to the contagion as "Novel Coronavirus"[6]. However, by March the US Secretary of State began referring to the contagion as the "Wuhan Virus",[7] shunning the taxonomy adopted by the ICTV. President Trump too repeatedly referred to the contagion as a "Chinese Virus".[8] The attempt to identify SARS-CoV-2 as a distinctly "Chinese" phenomenon by US government officials[9] unsurprisingly led to a swift response from the Chinese government. Chinese Ministry of Foreign Affairs (MFA) spokesperson Geng Shuang condemned Pompeo's use of the term "Wuhan Virus"[10] as "despicable" and later urged the US to stop making "unwarranted accusations against China". The Chinese diplomatic corps seems to up the ante with a tweet by the deputy director of the Chinese MFA Information Department, Zhao Lijian, speculating that perhaps it was the US Army that spread the disease when it participated in October 2019 World Military Games in Wuhan.[11] It has been speculated that President Trump desisted from using the "Chinese Virus" terminology as a consequence of Chinese Ambassador Cui Tiankui's remarks dismissing allegations that the coronavirus was manufactured in a lab.[12]

In spite of reduced references to the "Chinese virus" and earlier statements regarding data sharing,[13] by late March 2020 US government officials repeatedly criticized the Communist Party of China for its handling of the coronavirus outbreak and suggested a lack of transparency in Chinese efforts and communication with the world on the nature of disease[14] citing the silencing of Wuhan doctor Li Wenliang as an example. The implication was that this botched attempt at silencing doctors led to a rampant spread of COVID-19.[15] By this time, the US had over 42,000 positive cases of COVID-19 – about half the number of positive cases reported in China.[16] Although US news media has been critical of US government's messaging on the COVID-19 pandemic, highlighting the utility of attacks on China in an election year,[17] this has not deterred the Trump administration. A report carried by Bloomberg on 1 April 2020 quoted unnamed sources as alleging that the US intelligence community had concluded that China had concealed the extent of the spread of the disease.[18] Hua Chunying, MFA spokesperson dismissed US reports of a cover-up by China and highlighted instead the inability of the US to take the situation seriously and a bungled government response.[19] White House officials seemed to once again suggest the involvement of the Wuhan Institute of Virology in the spread of COVID-19[20] and indicated that investigations of Beijing's handling of the outbreak were ongoing.[21] These allegations were denied by MFA spokespersons who in turn accused the US of spreading disinformation.[22] On 30 April 2020, the US Office of the Director of National Intelligence issued a press statement concurring with the scientific opinion that the COVID-19 virus was not manmade although it did not rule out accidental leak from the laboratory in Wuhan.[23] These exchanges indicate that assigning culpability for the pandemic has become the focal point of global and domestic messaging for the US. By 1 May 2020, while the number of Chinese confirmed cases remained constant at around 84,000, the number of COVID-19 cases in the US had risen exponentially to over 1 million with over 50,000 deaths[24] – the largest of any country in the world.

On 30 April 2020, New China TV – the official YouTube channel of Chinese state news agency Xinhua – released a short satirical video titled "Once upon a virus..." mocking US allegations against China on the handling of the coronavirus outbreak.[25] The Chinese position on US allegations is essentially that the US did not take the threat seriously enough early on and did little to prepare for it. Therefore, according to Chinese commentary, US officials are using China as a scapegoat before the domestic audience in order to deflect responsibility for government inaction in order to win the 2020 Presidential election.[26] US-led construction of a negative public opinion on China is viewed as highlighting US discomfort with China's status as a strategic competitor and "the price China has to pay for growing stronger".[27] These explanations notwithstanding, China continues to deflect US questions back at it. A commentary carried by Xinhua listed five questions that Washington "needs" to answer. These included the role of a US Army biological research facility in Maryland; the precise date of local transmission in the US; whether the US was slow in its response to the pandemic leading to an aggravation of worldwide spread and; the reasons the US seeks to blame China for the disease.[28] Drawing primarily from reports in US news media, the commentary demonstrates that China is willing and able to use the US playbook in attempting to shape public opinion by appealing to fringe elements. To provide a rebuttal against US allegations of Chinese culpability for the pandemic, Xinhua published a report responding to 24 such allegations related to COVID-19.[29] Some of the most important are tabulated below.

Table 10.1: 24 Allegations of the US and China's Response

	US Allegation	*Chinese Response*
1.	COVID-19 is a "Chinese Virus"	WHO say naming of a disease should not be associated with any particular country or place
2.	Wuhan is the origin of the virus	Origin of the virus is unknown, Wuhan was the first to "report" the virus
3.	Virus is manmade, likely at the Wuhan Institute of Virology	Available scientific evidence indicates the virus is natural in origin
4.	The virus leaked accidentally from the Wuhan Institute of Virology	There is no evidence of this. The institute in question does not have the capability to design and synthesise new coronavirus
5.	China is responsible for the spread of the virus	China took the most stringent measures for containment
6.	Chinese contracted the virus because they eat bats	Bats are not a part of regular Chinese diet
7.	China is opening wildlife "wet" markets	There are no so-called "wildlife wet markets" in China. China has passed legislation banning all illegal hunting and trade of wild animals
8.	A cover-up by the Chinese government led to the spread of the virus	China took the best measures it could when facing an unknown contagion. It has provided timely and transparent information
9.	China arrested Dr. Li Wenliang a whistle-blower	Dr Li Wenliang was not a whistle-blower, he was not arrested
10.	Chinese disclosure of information on human-to-human transmission of the virus was late	China gave timely information to the WHO and the US knew of the dangers associated with the virus all along

There is clearly little appetite for self-reflection on the part of China in the face of US allegations. This is evident in the responses regarding its actions in the wake of a new coronavirus disease. That wildlife trade within China has been on-going despite existing legislation is well documented.[30] Even in the wake of COVID-19, wildlife trade will likely continue in some shape and form.[31] Also, while Dr Li Wenliang's actions was not defined as that of a "whistle-blower" by China, he was asked to reconsider his assessment of a new coronavirus disease and was penalized for raising the alarm – which was rescinded only after an enquiry.[32] The shortcomings in Chinese assessments notwithstanding, the US position on China's responsibility is far from disinterested and often in direct conflict with scientific opinion.

It's the economy!

The Trump administration's disenchantment with China predates the COVID-19 pandemic. While campaigning for the 2016 Presidential election, China was very much a central talking point[33] for Trump. As the Republican frontrunner and the then Republican candidate, Trump promised to declare China a currency manipulator[34] and raise tariffs on Chinese goods.[35] Galled at the growing trade deficit with China, he asserted that the US was being used as a "piggy bank" to rebuild China.[36] Renegotiating a trade deal with China has been a key foreign policy goal for the Trump administration.

With the view to address perceived unfair advantages enjoyed by China in its economic relations with the US and by compelling China to negotiate a new trade deal, the Trump administration had imposed multipletranches of tariffs on Chinese goods throughout 2018 and 2019. The first of these was announced by the Office of the US Trade Representative (USTR) in June 2018, imposing 25 percent additional tariff on imports of Chinese goods valued at USD 34 billion. According to the USTR, the additional tariffs were in response to findings that "China's acts, policies and practices related to technology transfer, intellectual property, and innovation are unreasonable and discriminatory, and burden U.S. commerce".[37] China's Ministry of Commerce (MOFCOM) retaliated to this within hours with additional tariffs on US goods worth USD 34 billion.[38] The USTR announced a second tranche of 25 percent additional tariff on Chinese goods worth USD 16 billion in August 2018 as part of the US response to "China's unfair trade practices related to the forced transfer of American technology and intellectual property".[39] MOFCOM announced similar additional tariff on US imports to China valued at USD 16 billion.[40] The third tranche of tariffs was announced in September 2018 by the USTR. This imposed an additional tariff of 10 percent on Chinese imports to the US valued at USD 200 billion, with the provision to increase additional tariff to 25 percent by January 2019.[41] China's response was to impose 10 percent additional tariff on imports from the US valued at USD 60 billion.[42] In May 2019, a fourth tranche announced by the USTR increased tariff levels from 10 percent to 25 percent on Chinese goods worth USD 200 billion.[43] Huawei, one of China's foremost technology companies, was added to the US Department of Commerce's entities list restricting its economic activity in the US.[44] MOFCOM responded with additional tariffs of up to 25 percent on US imports to China worth USD 60 billion.[45] In June 2019, the State Council of China released a White Paper on trade titled "China's position on the US-China Economic and Trade Consultations.[46] This document lays out the Chinese perception of the so-called "trade-war" that characterises US actions as unilateral and coercive, taking no account of the progress made by China on safeguarding intellectual property rights and ultimately harming not only for Chinese trade but also ordinary US consumers.[47] In early August 2019, the Trump administration threatened additional 10 percent tariff on further Chinese goods worth USD 300 billion and soon after the Chinese Renminbi fell to its lowest level against the US dollar in over a decade. This devaluation prompted the US Department of Treasury to designate China as a currency manipulator[48] for the first time since 1994. USTR announced 10 percent additional tariff on Chinese goods worth USD 300 billion on 13 August 2019.[49] China imposed additional tariffs upto 10 percent on US goods valued at USD 75 billion[50] in response to what the MOFCOM termed as "unilateral escalation of the trade friction".[51]

In January 2020, the two countries signed a "phase one" trade agreement. Under this agreement, the US rolled back tariffs from 15 percent to 7.5 percent on USD 120 billion worth of Chinese goods although tariffs remained in place on Chinese goods valued at USD 250 billion. China for its part committed to increase purchases from the US by USD 200 billion over two years. This would be above the baseline imports of USD 185 billion US goods. Additionally, China also committed to reducing additional tariffs imposed on US goods.[52] Two days before the agreement was signed, the US dropped its designation of China as a currency manipulator.[53]

The protracted nature of this 18-month long trade war underlines the importance accorded by the Trump administration to achieving a favourable balance of trade with China. Given the long-standing resentment that China had successfully "cheated" the international economic system[54] it is unsurprising that COVID-19 is being viewed by many as an opportunity to punish China economically. Even as he continues to make China a central theme of his re-election campaign[55], President Trump has warned China against seeking a revision of its obligations under the trade deal, suggesting that he would scrap the entire deal if China could not keep up its commitments to increase US imports by USD 200 billion.[56] Given that the International Monetary Fund has projected global growth to fall to -3 percent in 2020,[57] it is unlikely that China will be able to meet its commitments under the trade deal in face of declining demand at home and abroad.

Media reports also indicate that the White House prioritised concerns about China's role in the pandemic over the trade deal.[58] Various options are reportedly under consideration to punish China financially including lifting its sovereign immunity enabling American lawsuits seeking compensation for losses as a result of COVID-19; new sanctions and non-tariff trade restrictions.[59] Lawsuits have already been filed by American officials and organizations against China's complicity in the pandemic[60] and been dismissed by MFA spokespersons as ridiculous and frivolous.[61] The White House has also indicated incentivising the return of production lines back to the US.[62] This sentiment seems to have emerged from the struggle to maintain supply chains through the Chinese lockdown in the wake of COVID-19 and suggest attempts to decouple from the Chinese economy. While it remains to be seen what success the US achieves with such proposals, it is clear that Sino-US economic relations are at a precarious turning point. Chinese commentators had already expressed their reservations to the trade agreement as a ceasefire rather than a long-term truce in the economic competition between the US and China. While stabilizing Chinese exports in the short term, the trade agreement has been viewed as unfavourable to China in the medium and long term.[63] In an interview with People's Daily and Central Radio and Television in December 2019, the Chinese Foreign Minister had remarked that US unilateral actions had damaged the mutual trust between the two countries, effectively undoing the progress made over 40 years of bilateral relations.[64] Chinese intellectuals identify a dual purpose in the Trump administration's economic policies towards China – an expansion of US commercial interest in China while constraining the growth of Chinese power by delaying its technological progress.[65] In light of these perceptions, it is clear that further economic pressure will only deepen the divide between the world's two largest economies and disrupt global economic stability.

Figure 10.1: US Trade in Goods with China (in USD Million)

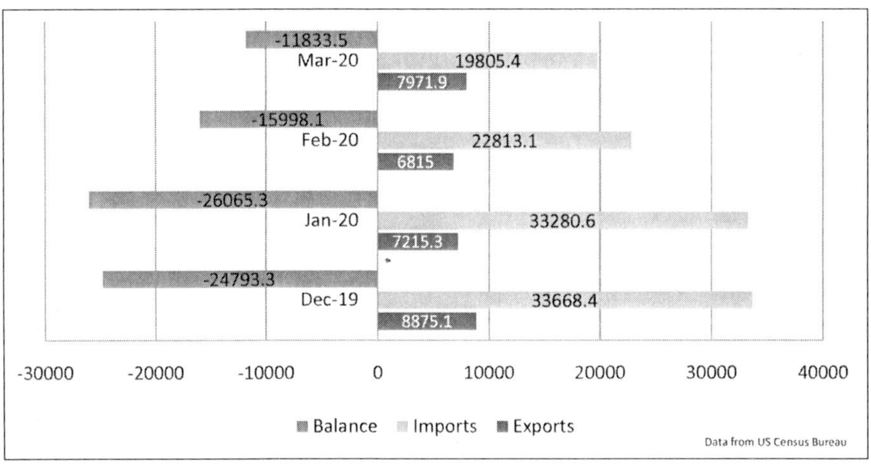

Military competition

The US has also been critical of Chinese military activities in the Indo-Pacific and the South China Sea in particular, condemning what it has termed as Beijing's "bullying" tactics[66]. Even while battling COVID-19, China did not suspend military activity in contested waters of the South China Sea. At a time when other states in its immediate neighbourhood prioritized containing the spread of the disease, China continued to reinforce its claims through military exercises and drills. The frequency of PLA activity around Taiwan and the disputed regions of the South China Sea may be interpreted as a demonstration of PLA's resolve and capabilities being unaffected by the pandemic.

The US Navy's Ticonderoga-class guided-missile cruiser *USS Shiloh* transited the Taiwan Strait on 16 January 2020.[67] Coming soon after the reelection of Taiwan's President Tsai Ing Wen, who opposes closer relations with China, MOFA spokesperson Geng Shuang's remarks that China had closely monitored the US vessel and that Taiwan was the most important and sensitive issue in US-China relations.[68] On 23 January, PLA's Su-30 and Y-8 aircraft flew to the Western Pacific through the Bashi Channel south of Taiwan. Two days later, multiple PLA aircraft including KJ-500 early warning aircraft and H-6 bombers flew the same route. February too witnessed increased military activity around Taiwan including joint naval and air drills south of the island, and flights to the Western Pacific during which PLA aircraft briefly crossed the median line in the Taiwan Strait.[69] The US Air Force flew a MC-130J special missions aircraft flew north to south along Taiwan's airspace along the Taiwan Strait and two B-52 bombers flew along Taiwan's east coast[70]. Another USN Ticonderoga-class guided-missile cruiser transited the Taiwan Strait two days after the US Air Force's flyover. In March 2020, the PLA conducted an unusual nighttime aerial exercise near Taiwan that included J-11 fighters and KJ-500 early warning aircraft.[71] Remarks on these drills by PLA Eastern Command spokesperson, Senior Colonel Zhang Chunhui, referred to "Taiwan secessionist forces"[72] thereby indicating that the rare drills were intended to deter any moves towards Taiwan's independence. Subsequently, a USN Arleigh Burke-class guided-missile destroyer transited through the Taiwan Strait in what was termed "a routine Taiwan Strait transit" according to a spokesperson for US 7th Fleet.[73] PLA spokesperson, Ren Guoqiang characterized the transit as provocative and damaging to China's security interests. In April, PLA's aircraft carrier, *Liaoning*, undertook a training mission sailing through waters near Japan and Taiwan and into the South China Sea near Vietnam[74]. USN vessels undertook two more transits through the Taiwan Strait in April 2020[75]. Both China and the US have increased the frequency of military activity in the area around Taiwan. Given that reunification with Taiwan is a core interest for China, the special relationship with the US enjoyed by the island is a constant source of irritation for Beijing. In March 2020, President Trump signed the Taipei Act which, in the most simple terms, calls for deeper economic and trade relations with Taiwan; strengthening Taiwan's diplomatic and international engagement by altering US relations and; assist Taiwan to gain entry to international organizations. In the wake of the COVID-19 pandemic, the US has called for Taiwan to join the WHO.[76]

The US conducts "Freedom of Navigation Operations" (FONOPs) close to Chinese claimed features in the South China Sea to challenge what are perceived as China's unilateral expansionist claims. The first FONOP of 2020 was conducted in late January with a USN Independence-class littoral combat ship passing close to Fiery Cross Reef[77] - which is home to one of three new airstrips constructed by China in the Spratly islands. In March, a USN destroyer sailed closed to the Paracel islands inviting a warning from the spokesperson of the PLA's Southern Theatre Command.[78] Subsequently, The Theodore Roosevelt Carrier Strike Group, America Expeditionary Strike Group and 31st Marine Expeditionary Unit conducted expeditionary strike force operations in the South China Sea.[79] In response, China organised live-fire drills involving sub-surface, surface and air platforms from the Southern Theatre Command[80] and also conducted anti-submarine warfare drills.[81] On 18 April, China's State Council approved the creation of two district administrations to cover the Paracel and Spratly islands.[82] A day later, China released names and coordinates for islands, reefs and undersea entities in the South China Sea[83] to bolster its sovereign claims over these features. These moves by China were heavily criticised by the parties to the territorial and maritime disputes in the region. The attempt to "regularise" Chinese names and administrative control of disputed areas indicates that China does not seek dialogue in the South China Sea and is keen to establish de facto control over the region. April witnessed increased presence of the US military in the South China Sea. Two more FONOPs were conducted by USN vessels– one in the Paracel islands and the other in Spratly islands.[84] Three US Navy vessels also conducted naval exercises with an Australian Navy frigate in the SCS.[85] Two US Air Force bombers also conducted a 32-hour round-trip sortie over the South China Sea.[86] China has opposed the increased presence of what it terms "foreign militaries" in the South China Sea.[87]

As with Taiwan, China is wary of US diplomatic and military engagement with ASEAN members. Even with a focus on tackling the global pandemic, US engagement with ASEAN has involved a critique of Chinese activities in the South China Sea. This is evident in the US Secretary of State, Michael Pompeo's press statement from 23 April 2020 which characterizes Beijing's actions in the South China Sea as part of "long-term threats to…shared security" and calls attention to China's exploitation of the COVID-19 crisis by continuing its provocative behavior.[88] Chinese media highlighted the PLA's readiness to tackle US military provocations in a post-pandemic worldwhile reporting on China's naval exercises in early May 2020.[89]

A global contest for power

Underlying the diplomatic, economic and military wrangling between the US and China is the strategic competition for power in the international order. The National Security Strategy released by the Trump administration in 2017 states, "China and Russia challenge American power, influence, and interests, attempting to erode American security and prosperity."[90] The document further asserts that, "competitors such as China steal U.S. intellectual property valued at hundreds of billions of dollars. Stealing proprietary technology and early-stage ideas allows competitors to unfairly tap into the innovation of free societies." It is thus clear that China's growth is viewed through a zero-sum prism by the Trump administration. Long accustomed to its preeminence in the international order, the US is unwilling to accommodate any change in the status quoin spite of the "America First" strategy of the current US administration. Since coming into office, President Trump has withdrawn from multilateral agreements and international forums that have been viewed as unfavourable to US interests. The most important of these have been the Paris Agreement on Climate Change and the Joint Comprehensive Plan of Action (JCPOA). Both these withdrawals have brought the US in conflict with China which exemplifies the differences in the world views of the two states.

The Trump administration rationale for withdrawal from the Paris agreement was that it places undue burden on the US economy.[91] President Trump himself has often stated that he does not believe in climate change.[92] For China, US withdrawal from the Paris Agreement entailed reaffirming its own status as a responsible country that meets its international obligations in contrast to the US.[93] Furthermore, Chinese official commentary emphasized the need for collective action to tackle what was a global problem and China's willingness to work with the international community to maintain a hard-won consensus.[94] Similarly, President Trump's unilateral withdrawal from JCPOA was predicated on objections about the negotiations by the Obama administration and assertions that it enabled Iran to build nuclear weapons.[95] It has been speculated that the Trump administration's support for Israel played an important role in decisions regarding the JCPOA.[96] After its exit from the JCPOA, the US introduction economic sanctions to prevent Iranian oil exports. In defiance of US sanctions, which targeted Chinese individuals as well as COSCO subsidiaries,[97] China remains one of the largest importers of Iranian oil, even as the volume of its imports has reportedly fallen significantly.[98] In early January 2020, Chinese and American officials were reportedly still in talks to further curb Chinese imports of Iranian oil.[99] In the wake of the COVID-19 pandemic, China has reiterated its commitment to aid Iran in fighting the pandemic and urged the lifting of economic sanctions that hinder Iran's ability to fight the disease.[100] US Secretary of State,

Michael Pompeo, has accused China, Russia and Iran of carrying out disinformation campaigns related to the pandemic aimed at disparaging US efforts.[101]

The Trump administration has repeatedly threatened to withdraw from international organisations that it determines as being unfair to the US. The Trump administration has been critical of the World Trade Organization (WTO) for its inability to tackle the challenge presented by China's "non-market practices"[102] and officials have called China's accession to the WTO in 2001 a mistake.[103] Amid trade negotiations with China and other countries in 2018, President Trump had indicated the possibility of pulling out from the WTO[104] if it continued to treat its largest investor poorly.[105] In April 2020, the Trump administration suspended US funding to the WHO pending a review into the institution's response to the pandemic and its assessment of China's response to the outbreak.[106] This announcement came in the wake of increasing US criticism of China's role in the pandemic. The WHO has consistently praised China's handling of the pandemic and its swift response to the outbreak.[107] China expressed its "grave concerns" over the US suspension of funding for the WHO and urged the country to fulfill its international obligations.[108] In May 2020, President Trump announced US withdrawal from the WHO.[109] The Trump administration has invariably expressed US role in international institutions through a comparison of funding support relative to that provided by China. This has enabled Chinese rhetoric to portray US actions as self-serving while emphasizing China's commitment to the international community as a responsible major power.[110]

Prospects for the future of bilateral relations

The relationship with China was described as "frustrating and disappointing" by White House Press Secretary, Kayleigh McEnany, in early May 2020.[111] This in a way sums up the perspective of the Trump administration. The 2017 National Security Strategy makes clear that support for China's rise and hoping for its liberalization through integration into the international order was a mistake. Therefore, it was always unlikely that the Trump administration would work towards greater accommodation with China. What was unexpected was the extent to which it would seek to punish China for not falling in with the White House's wishes. The trade war with China is just one example. Although numerous studies and opinion polls warned against implementing significantly higher tariffs on Chinese goods imported to the US, the Trump administration seemed to push through with them on near-ideological grounds. A Congressional Budget Office's report released in January 2020[112] suggests that tariffs are expected to reduce average real household income in the US by 1,277 USD in 2020. The gross domestic product for the US was also expected to be reduced by 0.5% in view of rising prices and unsteady business outlook.

US action and rhetoric have rung alarm bells in China. This has led to a reassessment of not only American attitude toward China and the international community but also a rethinking into China's actions and postures. According to some Chinese thinkers, American leadership was predicated upon balance between the pursuit of the US national interest and maintaining order within the international system. Since, in comparison to emerging countries the US receives diminished benefits from the international system, it is now unwilling to continue to invest in it. This unwillingness to invest in or lead the international order is not assessed as impacting American hegemony through the exercise of hard power.[113] The US is therefore expected to become more unilateral in its actions within the international system. China on its part is viewed successfully utilizing soft power, making it more adaptable than the US and promoting greater stability in the international system.[114] For other scholars, the actions of the US fall have been a wake-up call for China to take cognizance of the hitherto unthinkable. The first of these is the sheer the extent of American disaffection with China and the effort expended to paint China in a poor light. The second is the ruthlessness with which the US has dealt with China. The imposition of wide-ranging tariff barriers was unprecedented indicating that the US was willing to sacrifice trade relations which have always been the focal point of the relationship. The third unexpected issue that China must come to terms with is that fact that despite building positive relations with much of the world, no country was willing to voice support for China even in the face of unreasonable American trade policies. Finally, despite the deep divide between democrats and republicans in domestic US politics, there seems to be united front on China related issues.[115] In light of these unexpected realisations, China must reevaluate its understanding of the US to recognize the centrality of domestic politics, trade and self-interest in American interaction with other countries.[116] The central framework of the bilateral relationship comprising of strategic security, ideology, economic and trade issues and Taiwan is assessed to have remained constant, but US mentality that has changed in light of China's development.[117] Chinese commentators suggest that in order to deal with the US, China will have to avoid any direct challenge to the US authority since it is unlikely to be successful, given American strategic influence in the international system.[118] Others emphasise the centrality of external relations in China's developmental aims which require the avoidance of direct confrontation and utilizing a mix of tension and cooperation to achieve its goals.[119] While differences exist between Chinese commentators on China's ability to match US power[120], it is noteworthy that the US is expected to attempt a containment of China.[121] In that sense, conflict is deemed unavoidable. In view of these assessments it is likely that Chinese diplomatic response to US rhetoric critical of China will remain robust even as Chinese leadership seeks to arrive at an accommodation with the Trump administration. The use of "wolf warrior" diplomats[122] in strenuously negating and deflecting criticism of China will become entrenched. This is evident in the four-fold increase in social media activity by Chinese diplomats from April 2019 to April 2020.[123] Although Chinese statements and commentaries indicate that it currently seeks to avoid direct confrontation, China can be expected to continue pursing military and diplomatic policies that exacerbate tensions with the US. Rather than a change in Chinese policies towards the US, the author anticipates a deepening of Chinese engagement with other countries to bolster international support. This will however require a degree of transparency regarding motives as well as acceptance of criticism that China may not be amenable to.

NOTES

1 Trump Donald J. (2020), Twitter post, 25 January 2020, https://twitter.com/realDonaldTrump/status/1220818115354923009?s=20, accessed online 3 April 2020.

2 World Health Organisation (2020), "Novel Coronavirus (2019-nCoV) Situation Report – 4", 24 January 2020, https://www.who.int/docs/default-source/coronaviruse/situation-reports/20200124-sitrep-4-2019-ncov.pdf?sfvrsn=9272d086_8, accessed online 3 April 2020.

3 White House, Office of the Press Secretary (2020), "Remarks by President Trump, Vice President Pence, and Members of the Coronavirus Task Force in Press Conference", 27 February 2020 https://www.whitehouse.gov/briefings-statements/remarks-president-trump-vice-president-pence-members-coronavirus-task-force-press-conference/, accessed online 3 April 2020; White House, Office of the Press Secretary (2020), "Remarks by President Trump, Vice President Pence, and Members of the Coronavirus Task Force in Press Conference", 29 February 2020, https://www.whitehouse.gov/briefings-statements/remarks-president-trump-vice-president-pence-members-coronavirus-task-force-press-conference-2/, accessed online 3 April 2020.

4 World Health Organisation (2020), "Coronavirus Disease 2019 (COVID-19) Situation Report – 51", 11 March 2020, https://www.who.int/docs/default-source/coronaviruse/situation-reports/20200311-sitrep-51-COVID-19.pdf?sfvrsn=1ba62e57_10, accessed online 3 April 2020.

5 Firozi Paulina (2020), "Tom Cotton keeps repeating a coronavirus conspiracy theory that was already debunked", 17 February 2020, https://www.washingtonpost.com/politics/2020/02/16/tom-cotton-coronavirus-conspiracy/, accessed online 3 April 2020.

6 Pompeo Michael R. (2020), "The United States Announces Assistance To Combat the Novel Coronavirus", U.S. Department of State, 07 February 2020, https://www.state.gov/the-united-states-announces-assistance-to-combat-the-novel-coronavirus/, accessed online 3 April 2020.

7 Pompeo Michael R. (2020), "Secretary Pompeo's Remarks to the Press", U.S. Department of State, 05 March 2020, https://www.state.gov/secretary-pompeos-remarks-to-the-press/,accessed online 3 April 2020; Pompeo Michael R. (2020), "Secretary Michael R. Pompeo's Remarks to the Press", 17 March 2020, https://www.state.gov/secretary-michael-r-pompeo-remarks-to-the-press-6/, accessed online 3 April 2020.

8 Trump Donald J., Twitter post, 17 March 2020, https://twitter.com/realdonaldtrump/status/1239685852093169664?lang=en, accessed online 3 April 2020.

9 The attempt to identify the contagion as distinctly Chinese or Asian led to an upsurge of racist attacks on US citizens and visitors of Asian heritage. The Asian Pacific Policy and Planning Council began documenting racist incidents in the wake of COVID-19 on 18 March 2020. For further

information, please see Russell Jeung, "Incidents of Coronavirus Discrimination March 19-25, 2020 - A report for A3PCON and CAA", http://www.asianpacificpolicyandplanningcouncil.org/wp-content/uploads/A3PCON_Public_Weekly_Report_3.pdf,accessed online 3 April 2020 ; and "In One Month, STOP AAPI HATE Receives almost 1500 Incident Reports of Verbal Harassment, Shunning and Physical Assaults" http://www.asianpacificpolicyandplanningcouncil.org/wp-content/uploads/Press_Release_4_23_20.pdf, accessed online 3 April 2020.

10 Ministry of Foreign Affairs of the P.R.C., "Foreign Ministry Spokesperson Geng Shuang's Regular Press Conference on March 9, 2020", 9 March 2020, https://www.fmprc.gov.cn/mfa_eng/xwfw_665399/s2510_665401/2511_665403/t1753656.shtml, accessed online 3 April 2020.

11 Li Jianzhao, Twitter Post, March 12, 2020, https://twitter.com/zlj517/status/1238111898828066823?lang=en, accessed online 3 April 2020.

12 Swan Jonathan and Bethany Allen-Ebrahimian (2020), "Top Chinese official disowns U.S. military lab coronavirus conspiracy", 22 March 2020, https://www.axios.com/china-coronavirus-ambassador-cui-tiankai-1b0404e8-026d-4b7d-8290-98076f95df14.html, accessed online 3 April 2020.

13 White House, Office of the Press Secretary (2020), "Remarks by President Trump, Vice President Pence, and Members of the Coronavirus Task Force in Press Conference", March 12, 2020 at https://www.whitehouse.gov/briefings-statements/remarks-president-trump-vice-president-pence-members-coronavirus-task-force-press-conference-3/, accessed online 3 April 2020.

14 Sugeno Mikio and Tsuyoshi Nagasawa (2020), "Pompeo blasts China over coronavirus 'disinformation'" 31 March 2020, https://asia.nikkei.com/Editor-s-Picks/Interview/Pompeo-blasts-China-over-coronavirus-disinformation, accessed online 3 April 2020.

15 U.S. Department of State (2020), "Secretary Michael R. Pompeo With Tony Perkins of Washington Watch", 24 March 2020, https://www.state.gov/secretary-michael-r-pompeo-with-tony-perkins-of-washington-watch-2/, accessed online 3 April 2020.

16 World Health Organisation (2020), "Coronavirus Disease 2019 (COVID-19) Situation Report – 64", 24 March 2020, https://www.who.int/docs/default-source/coronaviruse/situation-reports/20200324-sitrep-64-COVID-19.pdf?sfvrsn=723b221e_2, accessed online 3 April 2020.

17 For example see Klein Betsy (2020), "Campaign follows Trump's lead, hitting China and Biden amid coronavirus crisis", 20 March 2020, https://edition.cnn.com/2020/03/19/politics/trump-campaign-china-email/index.html, accessed online 3 April 2020.

18 Wadhams Nick and Jennifer Jacobs (2020), "China Concealed Extent of Virus Outbreak, U.S. Intelligence Says", 02 April 2020, https://www.bloomberg.com/news/articles/2020-04-01/china-concealed-extent-of-virus-outbreak-u-s-intelligence-says, accessed online 3 April 2020.

19 Ministry of Foreign Affairs of the P.R.C. (2020), "Foreign Ministry Spokesperson Hua Chunying's Regular Press Conference on April 2, 2020", 02 April 2020, https://www.fmprc.gov.cn/mfa_eng/xwfw_665399/s2510_665401/2511_665403/t1765251.shtml, accessed online 3 April 2020.

20 Ibid.

21 White House, Office of the Press Secretary (2020), "Remarks by President Trump, Vice President Pence, and Members of the Coronavirus Task Force in Press Briefing", 27 April 2020, https://www.whitehouse.gov/briefings-statements/remarks-president-trump-vice-president-pence-members-coronavirus-task-force-press-briefing-33/, accessed online 3 April 2020.

22 Hua Chunying (2020), Twitter post, 27 April 2020, https://twitter.com/SpokespersonCHN/status/1254783225559306245?, accessed online 3 April 2020.

23 Office of the Director of National Intelligence (2020), "Intelligence Community Statement on Origins of COVID-19", 30 April 2020, https://www.dni.gov/index.php/newsroom/press-releases/item/2112-intelligence-community-statement-on-origins-of-COVID-19, accessed online 3 April 2020.

24 World Health Organisation (2020), "Coronavirus Disease 2019 (COVID-19) Situation Report-102", 01 May 2020, https://www.who.int/docs/default-source/coronaviruse/situation-reports/20200501-COVID-19-sitrep.pdf?sfvrsn=742f4a18_4, accessed online 3 May 2020.

25 New China TV (2020), "Once upon a virus…", 29 April 2020, https://www.youtube.com/watch?v=Q5BZ09iNdvo, accessed online 3 April 2020.

26 China.com (2020), "蓬佩奥再口出狂言，中国岂能任你摆布?" [Pompeo once again spoke wildly, will China be controlled by you?], 04 May 2020, https://military.china.com/topic/37527485.html, accessed online 3 May 2020.

27 Global Times (2020), "Political motives behind China smears: Global Times editorial", 27 April 2020, https://www.globaltimes.cn/content/1186941.shtml, accessed online 3 May 2020.

28 Xinhuanet (2020), "Spotlight: Five questions Washington needs to answer on coronavirus pandemic", 04 May 2020, http://www.xinhuanet.com/english/2020-05/04/c_139029131.htm, accessed online 3 May 2020.

29 "Reality Check of US Allegations Against China on COVID-19", 10 May 2020, http://www.xinhuanet.com/english/2020-05/10/c_139044103.htm, accessed online 3 May 2020.

30 Wilson Centre (2020), "Wild Laws: China and Its Role in Illicit Wildlife Trade", 02 June 2016, https://www.wilsoncenter.org/event/wild-laws-china-and-its-role-illicit-wildlife-trade, accessed online 3 May 2020..

31 Stanway David (2020), "China legislators take on wildlife trade, but traditional medicine likely to be exempt", 21 May 2020, https://in.reuters.com/article/health-coronavirus-china-wildlife/china-legislators-take-on-wildlife-trade-but-traditional-medicine-likely-to-be-exempt-idINKBN22X077, accessed online 3 May 2020..

32 Chun Han Wong (2020), "China Rescinds Penalty for Late Doctor Who Warned About Coronavirus", Wall Street Journal, 19 March 2020, https://www.wsj.com/articles/china-rescinds-penalty-for-late-doctor-who-warned-about-coronavirus-11584637545, accessed online 3 May 2020.

33 BBC (2020), "Trump accuses China of 'raping' US with unfair trade policy", 02 May 2016, https://www.bbc.com/news/election-us-2016-36185012, accessed online 3 May 2020.

34 Trump Donald J. (2016), "Donald Trump's Contract with the American Voter", 22 October 2016, https://assets.donaldjtrump.com/_landings/contract/O-TRU-102316-Contractv02.pdf, accessed online 3 May 2020.

35 Reuters (2020), "Trump targets China trade, says plans serious measures", 26 August 2016, https://www.reuters.com/article/us-usa-election-trump-china-idUSKCN10Z2JN, accessed online 3 May 2020.

36 Teague Beckwith Ryan (2020), "Read a Transcript of the First Presidential Debate Between Hillary Clinton and Donald Trump", 27 September 2016, https://time.com/4508768/presidential-debate-trump-clinton-transcript/, accessed online 3 May 2020.

37 Office of the U.S. Trade Representative (2020), "USTR Issues Tariffs on Chinese Products in Response to Unfair Trade Practices", 15 June 2018, https://ustr.gov/about-us/policy-offices/press-office/press-releases/2018/june/ustr-issues-tariffs-chinese-products, accessed online 3 May 2020.

38 Ministry of Commerce P.R.C. (2018), "China imposes counter tariffs on US products", 06 July 2018, http://english.mofcom.gov.cn/article/counselorsreport/europereport/201807/20180702764612.shtml, accessed online 3 May 2020.

39 Office of the U.S. Trade Representative (2018), "USTR Finalizes Second Tranche of Tariffs on Chinese Products in Response to China's Unfair Trade Practices", 07 August 2018, https://ustr.gov/about-us/policy-offices/press-office/press-releases/2018/august/ustr-finalizes-second-tranche, accessed online 3 May 2020.

40 Ministry of Commerce P.R.C. (2018), "China's additional tariffs on $16 billion of U.S. goods", 15 August 2018,http://english.mofcom.gov.cn/article/counselorsreport/americaandoceanreport/201808/20180802775808.shtml, accessed online 3 May 2020.

41 Office of the U.S. Trade Representative (2018), "USTR Finalizes Tariffs on $200 Billion of Chinese Imports in Response to China's Unfair Trade Practices", 18 September 2018, https://ustr.gov/about-us/policy-offices/press-office/press-releases/2018/september/ustr-finalizes-tariffs-200, accessed online 3 May 2020.

42 Ministry of Commerce P.R.C. (2018), "Announcement on Levying Tariffs on Goods and Commodity Imports from the US", 19 September 2018, http://english.mofcom.gov.cn/article/newsrelease/significantnews/201809/20180902790073.shtml,accessed online 3 May 2020; See also Ministry of Commerce P.R.C. (2018), "中华人民共和国商务部公告2018年第63号" [Announcement No. 63 of 2018 by the Ministry of Commerce of the People's Republic of China], 13 September 2018, http://www.mofcom.gov.cn/article/b/g/201809/20180902786225.shtml, accessed online 3 May 2020; and P.R.C. State Council Customs Tariff Commission (2018), "国务院关税税则委员会公告2018年第6号" [Announcement No. 6 of 2018 of the Customs Tariff Commission of the State Council], 09 September 2018, http://www.mofcom.gov.cn/article/b/g/201809/20180902788950.shtml,accessed online 3 May 2020.

43 Office of the U.S. Trade Representative (2019), "Statement By U.S. Trade Representative Robert Lighthizer on Section 301 Action", 05 October 2019, https://ustr.gov/about-us/policy-offices/press-office/press-releases/2019/may/statement-us-trade-representative, accessed online 3 May 2020.

44 U.S. Department of Commerce Bureau of Industry and Security (2020), "Huawei Entity List and Temporary General License Frequently Asked Questions (FAQs)", 18 May 2020, https://www.bis.doc.gov/index.php/documents/pdfs/2447-huawei-entity-listing-faqs/file, accessed online 3 May 2020.

45 Ministry of Commerce of the P.R.C. (2019), "China to increase tariffs on imported U.S. products", 14 May 2019, http://english.mofcom.gov.cn/article/counselorsreport/americaandoceanreport/201905/20190502862572.shtml, accessed online 3 May 2020.

46 State Council of the P.R.C. (2019), "China's Position on the China-US Economic and Trade Consultations", 02 June 2019, http://english.www.gov.cn/archive/white_paper/2019/06/02/content_281476694892692.htm, accessed online 3 May 2020.

47 For a succinct summary of key points see Xinhuanet (2020), "China releases white paper on its position on economic and trade consultations with US", 02 June 2019, http://www.xinhuanet.com/english/2019-06/02/c_138110173.htm, accessed online 3 May 2020.

48 U.S. Department of the Treasury (2020), "Treasury Designates China as a Currency Manipulator", 05 August 2019, https://home.treasury.gov/news/press-releases/sm751, accessed online 3 May 2020.

49 Office of the U.S. Trade Representative (2020), "USTR Announces Next Steps on Proposed 10 Percent Tariff on Imports from China", 13 August 2019, https://ustr.gov/about-us/policy-offices/press-office/press-releases/2019/august/ustr-announces-next-steps-proposed, accessed online 3 May 2020.

50 Xinhuanet (2020), "China to impose additional tariffs on U.S. imports worth 75 bln USD", 24 August 2019, <http://www.xinhuanet.com/english/2019-08/24/c_138332912.htm, accessed online 3 May 2020.

51 Ministry of Commerce P.R.C. (2019), "Regular Press Conference of the Ministry of Commerce (August 22, 2019)", 23 August 2019, http://english.mofcom.gov.cn/article/newsrelease/press/201909/20190902895452.shtml, accessed online 3 May 2020.

52 Reuters (2020), "What's in the U.S.-China Phase 1 trade deal", 15 January 2020, https://

www.reuters.com/article/us-usa-trade-china-details-factbox/whats-in-the-us-china-phase-1-trade-deal-idUSKBN1ZE2IF, accessed online 3 May 2020.

53 Shalal Andrea and Alexandra Alper (2020), "U.S. Treasury drops China currency manipulator label ahead of trade deal signing", 14 January 2020, https://www.reuters.com/article/us-usa-trade-china/u-s-treasury-drops-china-currency-manipulator-label-ahead-of-trade-deal-signing-idUSKBN1ZC2FV,accessed online 3 May 2020.

54 White House, Office of the Press Secretary (2019), "Remarks by President Trump at the Economic Club of New York", 12 November 2019, https://www.whitehouse.gov/briefings-statements/remarks-president-trump-economic-club-new-york-new-york-ny/, accessed online 3 May 2020.

55 Economic Times (2020), "Trump warns China of consequences if found 'knowingly responsible' for COVID-19", 19 April 2020, https://economictimes.indiatimes.com/news/international/world-news/trump-warns-china-of-consequences-if-found-knowingly-responsible-for-COVID-19/articleshow/75230647.cms?from=mdr, accessed online 3 May 2020.

56 Economic Times (2020), "Trump threatens to terminate trade deal if China does not honour it citing coronavirus crisis", 22 April 2020, https://economictimes.indiatimes.com/news/international/business/trump-threatens-to-terminate-trade-deal-if-china-does-not-honour-it-citing-coronavirus-crisis/articleshow/75285941.cms, accessed online 3 May 2020.

57 Gopinath Gita (2020), "The Great Lockdown: Worst Economic Downturn Since the Great Depression", 14 April 2020, https://blogs.imf.org/2020/04/14/the-great-lockdown-worst-economic-downturn-since-the-great-depression/, accessed online 3 May 2020.

58 Mason Jeff, Matt Spetalnick and Humeyra Pamuk (2020), "Trump threatens new tariffs on China in retaliation for coronavirus", 01 May 2020, https://in.reuters.com/article/health-coronavirus-usa-china/trump-threatens-new-tariffs-on-china-in-retaliation-for-coronavirus-idINKBN22D47E, accessed online 3 May 2020.

59 Stein Jeff, Carol D. Leonnig, Josh Dawsey and Gerry Smith, "U.S. Officials crafting retaliatory actions against China over coronavirus as President Trump fumes", 30 April 2020, https://www.washingtonpost.com/business/2020/04/30/trump-china-coronavirus-retaliation/, accessed online 3 May 2020.

60 Madhukalya Anwesha (2020), "$20 trillion lawsuit against China! US group says coronavirus is bioweapon", 02 April 2020, https://www.businesstoday.in/current/world/usd-20-trillion-lawsuit-against-china-us-group-says-coronavirus-bioweapon/story/399071.html, accessed online 3 May 2020; also Economic Times (2020), "US State files lawsuit against China on COVID-19 handling", 23 April 2020 https://economictimes.indiatimes.com/news/international/world-news/us-state-files-lawsuit-against-china-on-coronavirus-handling/articleshow/75286051.cms?from=mdr, accessed online 3 May 2020.

61 Ministry of Foreign Affairs of the P.R.C. (2020), "Foreign Ministry Spokesperson Geng Shuang's Regular Press Conference on April 22, 2020", 22 April 2020, https://www.fmprc.gov.cn/mfa_eng/xwfw_665399/s2510_665401/2511_665403/t1772428.shtml, accessed online 3 May 2020.

62 The White House (2020), Twitter post, May 4, 2020, https://twitter.com/WhiteHouse/status/1257294185314607107, accessed online 5 May 2020.

63 ANTAI (2020), "2020-中美关系能否掀开新篇章?" [Will 2020 China-US relations open a new chapter?], Nantong Antai Machinery Co. Ltd., 01 May 2020, http://www.ntatjx.com/20200105113740494.html, accessed online 5 May 2020.

64 Sina (2019), "王毅：共同把中美关系扳回健康发展的轨道" [Wang Yi: Jointly bring Sino-US relations back to the track of healthy development], 23 December 2019, https://finance.sina.com.cn/china/gncj/2019-12-23/doc-iihnzahi9497003.shtml, accessed online 5 May 2020.

65 Wu Xinbo (2020), "特朗普政府重构中美关系的抱负与局限" [Trump Administration's Aspirations and Limitations in Reconstructing Sino-US Relations], 27 March 2020, http://www.iis.fudan.edu.cn/6a/7d/c6852a223869/page.htm, accessed online 5 May 2020.

66 Congressional Research Service (2020), "U.S.-China Strategic Competition in South and East China Seas: Background and Issues for Congress", 28 May 2020, https://crsreports.congress.gov/product/pdf/R/R42784, accessed online 5 May 2020.

67 Werner Ben (2020), "USS Shiloh Transits Taiwan Strait a Week After Presidential Election", 17 January 2020, https://news.usni.org/2020/01/17/uss-shiloh-transits-taiwan-strait-a-week-after-presidential-election, accessed online 5 May 2020.

68 Ministry of Foreign Affairs of the P.R.C. (2020), "Foreign Ministry Spokesperson Geng Shuang's Regular Press Conference on January 17, 2020", 17 January 2020, https://www.fmprc.gov.cn/mfa_eng/xwfw_665399/s2510_665401/2511_665403/t1733473.shtml, accessed online 5 May 2020.

69 For a review of these exercises, see: Dotson John (2020), "Military Activity and Political Signaling in the Taiwan Strait in Early 2020", 01 April 2020, https://jamestown.org/program/military-activity-and-political-signaling-in-the-taiwan-strait-in-early-2020/, accessed online 5 May 2020.

70 Focus Taiwan (2020), "Three American military planes fly past Taiwan: MND", 12 February 2020, https://focustaiwan.tw/politics/202002120015, accessed online 5 May 2020.

71 Lu Li-shih (2020), "PLA exercises cause for concern", 03 April 2020, https://www.taipeitimes.com/News/editorials/archives/2020/04/03/2003733893, accessed online 5 May 2020.

72 Liu Xuanzun (2020), "PLA warplanes conduct rare nighttime exercises near Taiwan: reports", 17 March 2020, https://www.globaltimes.cn/content/1182876.shtml, accessed online 5 May 2020.

73 Werner Ben (2020), "China Calls USS McCampbell Taiwan Strait Transit 'Provocative'", 27 March 2020, https://news.usni.org/2020/03/27/china-calls-uss-mccampbell-taiwan-strait-transit-provocative, accessed online 5 May 2020.

74 Focus Taiwan (2020), "Chinese aircraft carrier maneuver aimed at achieving multiple results", 26 April 2020, https://focustaiwan.tw/cross-strait/202004260009, accessed online 5 May 2020.

75 Reuters (2020), "U.S. Navy destroyer transits Taiwan Strait on same day as Chinese drills", 11 April 2020, https://in.reuters.com/article/taiwan-security-usa/u-s-navy-destroyer-transits-taiwan-strait-on-same-day-as-chinese-drills-idINKCN21T034, accessed online 5 May 2020; and Lagrone Sam (2020), "Two U.S. Warships Pass Through Taiwan Strait in 7th Transit Since 2018", 29 April 2020, https://news.usni.org/2019/04/29/two-u-s-warships-pass-through-taiwan-strait-in-7th-transit-since-2018, accessed online 5 May 2020.

76 Lynch Colum (2020), "WHO Becomes Battleground as Trump Chooses Pandemic Confrontation Over Cooperation", 29 April 2020, https://foreignpolicy.com/2020/04/29/world-health-organization-who-battleground-trump-taiwan-china/, accessed online 5 May 2020.

77 Ziezulewicz Geoff and Shawn Snow, "Navy conducts year's first FONOP in South China Sea", 28 January 2020, https://www.navytimes.com/news/your-navy/2020/01/28/navy-conducts-years-first-fonop-in-south-china-sea/, accessed online 5 May 2020.

78 CGTN (2020), "China slams U.S. warship's trespassing in South China Sea", 11 March 2020, https://news.cgtn.com/news/2020-03-11/China-slams-U-S-warship-s-trespassing-in-South-China-Sea-OLSr9ThNE4/index.html, accessed online 5 May 2020.

79 Huynh Nicholas (2020), "Theodore Roosevelt, America strike groups conduct expeditionary strike force training", 17 March 2020, https://www.cpf.navy.mil/news.aspx/130567, accessed online 5 May 2020.

80 Liu Xuanzun (2020), "Chinese Navy holds drills amid US violation", 02 April 2020, https://www.globaltimes.cn/content/1184586.shtml, accessed online 5 May 2020.

81 Ng Teddy (2020), "Chinese naval planes conduct anti-submarine drills in South China Sea", 21 March 2020, https://www.scmp.com/news/china/military/article/3076273/chinese-naval-planes-conduct-anti-submarine-drills-south-china, accessed online 5 May 2020.

82 State Council of the P.R.C. (2020), "State Council approves establishing of two districts in Sansha city", 18 April 2020, http://english.www.gov.cn/statecouncil/ministries/202004/18/content_WS5e9ae179c6d0b3f0e9495d49.html, accessed online 5 May 2020.

83 Shumei Leng (2020), "Names of islands, reefs in South China Sea released", 19 April 2020, https://www.globaltimes.cn/content/1186084.shtml, accessed online 5 May 2020.

84 Lendon Brad (2020), "US Navy stages back-to-back challenges to Beijing's South China Sea claims", 30 April 2020, https://edition.cnn.com/2020/04/30/asia/south-china-sea-us-navy-freedom-of-navigation-intl-hnk/index.html, accessed online 5 May 2020.

85 Greene Andrew (2020), "South China Sea tensions rise as Australian frigate exercises with US warships", 22 April 2020,https://www.abc.net.au/news/2020-04-22/tensions-rise-in-south-china-sea-after-us-australia-exercises/12171806,accessed online 5 May 2020.

86 Air Force Technology (2020), "US Air Force bombers conduct sorties over South China Sea", 01 May 2020, https://www.airforce-technology.com/news/us-air-force-bombers-sorties-south-china-sea/, accessed online 5 May 2020.

87 Zhang Zhihao (2020), "PLA slams naval drills in South China Sea", 01 May 2020, https://www.chinadaily.com.cn/a/202005/01/WS5eab62dca310a8b2411530ee.html, accessed online 5 May 2020.

88 Pompeo Michael R. (2020), "The United States and ASEAN Are Partnering To Defeat COVID-19, Build Long-Term Resilience, and Support Economic Recovery", 22 April 2020, https://www.state.gov/the-united-states-and-asean-are-partnering-to-defeat-COVID-19-build-long-term-resilience-and-support-economic-recovery/, accessed online 5 May 2020.

89 Liu Xuanzun (2020), "China conducts naval drills in S. China Sea, prepares for post-pandemic US military provocations", 05 May 2020, https://www.globaltimes.cn/content/1187466.shtml, accessed online 5 May 2020.

90 White House (2017), "National Security Strategy of the United States of America December 2017", https://www.whitehouse.gov/wp-content/uploads/2017/12/NSS-Final-12-18-2017-0905.pdf, accessed online 5 May 2020.

91 Pompeo Michael R. (2019), "On the U.S. Withdrawal from the Paris Agreement", U.S. Department of State, 04 November 2019, https://www.state.gov/on-the-u-s-withdrawal-from-the-paris-agreement/, accessed online 5 May 2020.

92 BBC (2018), "Trump on climate change report: 'I don't believe it'", 26 November 2018, https://www.bbc.com/news/world-us-canada-46351940, accessed online 5 May 2020.

93 Li Haidong (2019), "US withdrawal from Paris Agreement shows it is an untrustworthy partner", 11 November 2019, https://www.globaltimes.cn/content/1169687.shtml, accessed online 5 May 2020.

94 Ministry of Foreign Affairs of the P.R.C. (2017), "Foreign Ministry Spokesperson Hua Chunying's Regular Press Conference on June 2, 2017" 02 June 2017, https://www.fmprc.gov.cn/mfa_eng/xwfw_665399/s2510_665401/t1467465.shtml, accessed online 5 May 2020.

95 Office of the Press Secretary of the USA (2018), "Remarks by President Trump on the Joint Comprehensive Plan of Action", 08 May 2018, https://www.whitehouse.gov/briefings-statements/remarks-president-trump-joint-comprehensive-plan-action/, accessed online 5 May 2020.

96 Zurcher Anthony (2018), "Three reasons behind Trump ditching Iran deal", 08 May 2018, https://www.bbc.com/news/world-us-canada-43902372, accessed online 5 May 2020.

97 Al Jazeera (2019), "US 'concerned' over untrackable China ships carrying Iran oil", 16 October 2019, https://www.aljazeera.com/news/2019/10/concerned-untrackable-china-ships-carrying-iran-oil-191016081016944.html, accessed online 5 May 2020.

98 Reuters (2019), "China's Iran oil imports plunge as U.S. sanctions bite", 27 July 2019, https://www.reuters.com/article/us-china-economy-trade-crude/chinas-iran-oil-imports-plunge-as-us-sanctions-bite-idUSKCN1UM0CB, accessed online 5 May 2020.

99 Scheid Brian (2020), "US, Chinese officials in talks on halting imports of Iranian crude", 13 January 2020, https://www.spglobal.com/platts/en/market-insights/latest-news/oil/011320-us-chinese-officials-in-talks-on-halting-imports-of-iranian-crude, accessed online 5 May 2020; The US has accused Chinese firm Huawei of supporting Iranian government's surveillance of protestors in the country in violation of US economic sanctions. See Radio Free Europe Radio Liberty (2020), "U.S. Accuses China's Huawei Of Helping Iran Track Protesters", 14 February 2020, https://www.rferl.org/a/us-accuses-huawei-aiding-iran-track-protesters/30433636.html, accessed online 5 May 2020.

100 Ministry of Foreign Affairs of the P.R.C. (2020), "Foreign Ministry Spokesperson Zhao Lijian's Regular Press Conference on March 5, 2020", 05 March 2020, https://www.fmprc.gov.cn/mfa_eng/xwfw_665399/s2510_665401/2511_665403/t1752564.shtml, accessed online 5 May 2020.

101 Beavers Olivia (2020), "Pompeo says China, Russia, Iran are spreading disinformation about coronavirus", 20 March 2020, https://thehill.com/policy/national-security/488659-pompeo-says-china-russia-iran-are-spreading-disinformation-about, accessed online 5 May 2020.

102 Office of the U.S. Trade Representative (2018), "2017 Report to Congress On China's WTO Compliance", January 2018, https://ustr.gov/sites/default/files/files/Press/Reports/China%202017%20WTO%20Report.pdf, accessed online 5 May 2020.

103 Wroughton Lesley (2018), "Trump administration says U.S. mistakenly backed China WTO accession in 2001", 20 January 2018, https://www.reuters.com/article/us-usa-trade-china/trump-administration-says-u-s-mistakenly-backed-china-wto-accession-in-2001-idUSKBN1F82U1, accessed online 5 May 2020.

104 Wang Christine (2018), "Trump threatens to withdraw from World Trade Organization", 30 August 2018, https://www.cnbc.com/2018/08/30/trump-threatens-to-withdraw-from-world-trade-organization.html, accessed online 5 May 2020.

105 Kucik Jeffrey (2018), "Why Trump's wrong about WTO treating US unfairly", 04 September 2018, https://theconversation.com/why-trumps-wrong-about-wto-treating-us-unfairly-102562, accessed online 5 May 2020.

106 Klein Betsy and Jennifer Hansler (2020), "Trump halts World Health Organization funding over handling of coronavirus outbreak", 15 April 2020, https://edition.cnn.com/2020/04/14/politics/donald-trump-world-health-organization-funding-coronavirus/index.html, accessed online 5 May 2020.

107 India Today (2020), "Amid attack from Trump, WHO praises China for handling coronavirus pandemic", 02 May 2020, https://www.indiatoday.in/world/story/amid-attack-from-trump-who-praises-china-for-handling-coronavirus-pandemic-1673609-2020-05-02, accessed online 5 May 2020.

108 Ministry of Foreign Affairs of the P.R.C. (2020), "Foreign Ministry Spokesperson Zhao Lijian's Regular Press Conference on April 15, 2020", 15 April 2020, https://www.fmprc.gov.cn/mfa_eng/xwfw_665399/s2510_665401/2511_665403/t1770103.shtml, accessed online 5 May 2020.

109 Ehley Brianna and Alice Miranda Ollstein (2020), "Trump announces U.S. withdrawal from the World Health Organization", 29 May 2020, https://www.politico.com/news/2020/05/29/us-withdrawing-from-who-289799, accessed online 5 May 2020.

110 Xi Jinping (2020), "Unity and Cooperation Are the International Community's Most Potent Weapon to Overcome the Pandemic", *Qiushi Journal*, 12 (2), 43, 2020, http://english.qstheory.cn/2020-04/22/c_1125885463.htm, accessed online 5 May 2020.

111 Office of the Press Secretary of the USA (2020), "Press Briefing by Press Secretary Kayleigh McEnany", 06 May 2020, https://www.whitehouse.gov/briefings-statements/press-briefing-press-secretary-kayleigh-mcenany-050620/, accessed online 5 May 2020.

112 Congressional Budget Office of the USA (2020), "The Budget and Economic Outlook: 2020 to 2030", January 2020, https://www.cbo.gov/publication/56073, accessed online 5 May 2020.

113 Jin Canrongand Wang Heyi (2020), "当前国际秩序的"美国困境" [The current international order's "American dilemma"], 30 March 2020, http://bjrb.bjd.com.cn/html/2020-03/30/content_12453838.htm, accessed online 5 May 2020.

114 Ibid.

115 Dai Xu (2020), "2020 年的中美关系中国人有4个没想到必须重新认识美国 [China-US relations in 2020 gave Chinese people four realisations to understand the US anew]", 24 March 2020, https://military.china.com/retie/37506750.html, accessed online 5 May 2020.

116 Ibid.

117 Zhang Hongzhi (2020), "新形势下中美关系的再认识 [Understanding China-US relations again under new circumstances]", 31 March 2020, https://www.dswxyjy.org.cn/n1/2020/0331/c427152-31656012.html, accessed online 5 May 2020.

118 Dai Xu (2020), "2020 年的中美关系中国人有4个没想到必须重新认识美国 [China-US relations in 2020 gave Chinese people four realisations to understand the US anew]", 24 March 2020, https://military.china.com/retie/37506750.html, accessed online 5 May 2020.

119 Zhang Hongzhi (2020), "新形势下中美关系的再认识 [Understanding China-US relations again under new circumstances]", 31 March 2020, https://www.dswxyjy.org.cn/n1/2020/0331/c427152-31656012.html, accessed online 5 May 2020.

120 Jin Canrong, "中国完全破解美国军事威胁 [China has already resolved the threat from the US]", Sina, at https://k.sina.cn/article_1558148043_m5cdf73cb03300qzhq.html?from=mil; See also, "张召忠解读中美军力差距有多大：中国20年也追不上 [Zhang Zhaozhong assesses how big the gap between Chinese and American military is: China cannot catch up in even 20 years]", https://mil.sina.cn/sd/2017-03-29/detail-ifycstww1779357.d.html; "美国和中国军力差不多？张召忠：千万不要有这种想法太危险" [The US and China have similar military strength? Zhang Zhaozhong: This kind of thinking is too dangerous], QQ, May 25, 2017, https://v.qq.com/x/page/m05079s729k.html, accessed online 5 May 2020.

121 Zhang Hongzhi (2020), "新形势下中美关系的再认识 [Understanding China-US relations again under new circumstances]", 31 March 2020, https://www.dswxyjy.org.cn/n1/2020/0331/c427152-31656012.html, accessed online 5 May 2020.

122 For an exposition on China's "Wolf warrior" diplomacy during the pandemic see Kuwahara Kyoko (2020), "China's 'Wolf Warrior Diplomacy': The Limitations and Challenges Exposed by the Corona Crisis", 16 May 2020, https://www.jiia.or.jp/en/strategic_comment/2020/05/jiia-strategic-comments-2020-11.html, accessed online 5 May 2020.

123 Scott Mark (2020), "Chinese diplomacy ramps up social media offensive in COVID-19 info war", 29 April 2020, https://www.politico.com/news/2020/04/29/chinese-diplomacy-ramps-up-social-media-offensive-in-COVID-19-info-war-220738, accessed online 5 May 2020.

11

China-Russia and COVID-19

Sakshi Anand

Introduction

Since the establishment of the diplomatic ties between People's Republic of China and Soviet Union in 1949, the relationship between both the countries has seen many ups and downs. The ties which came to a standstill during the Cold War era have seen a gradual improvement after the establishment of the Russian Federation in 1991. The partnership has evolved from being defined as a "Strategic Partnership" in 2001 to that of a "Comprehensive Strategic Partnership" in 2010 and upgraded to a "Comprehensive Strategic Partnership of Coordination for a New Era" in 2019. The relationship has witnessed unprecedented growth after the West had imposed sanctions on Russia during Ukraine crisis in 2014, and Russia thus began looking towards the East. Hence, since 2013 President Xi and President Putin have met more than 30 times indicating greater confidence and trust at the political level. But corona virus is now a new elephant in the room conflicting enormous losses to both China and Russia with potential to redefine global power equations and make China Russia "Frenemies".

Historically, the relationship between China and Russia has undergone dynamic changes. This leaves an imprint on the current relationship as well. At a time when the entire world has fallen into a deep crisis driven by the Corona virus pandemic and has started questioning China's role, it becomes interesting to see how China's closest major power ally in the present scenario, Russia responds to the crisis. The aim of the paper is to analyse the China-Russia relationship during the COVID-19 epidemic and its impact on both countries.

Before we discuss the COVID-19 issue, a brief review of the views of scholars on bilateral relations between China and Russia is due. Despite closer political ties, mutual suspicion and mistrust persists in the China-Russia relationship due to their historical memories and fear of Chinese aggression in Russian Far East. Dr. Sayana Namsaraeva argues that this mistrust operates not only at the individual level, but also at the level of the state at the China-Russia border.[1] Fu Ying echoes the idea by pointing out that as the power gap between the two countries will grow, so will their mutual suspicion against each other's foreign policies.[2] Pointing out the bleak picture of the economic relationship between China's Northeast and Russia's Far East, Feng Shaolei and Cui Heng have highlighted that between 2009-2018, the two sides achieved a project completion rate of only 28 percent. Also, the number of registered Chinese companies in the Russian Far East declined from 162 in 2015 to 125 in 2017.[3] Bobo Lo terms the relationship as 'Axis of Convenience' saying that it is pragmatic and tactical with strategic calculus in mind.[4] Li Mingjiang and Angela Poh opines that common desire of both countries to challenge US hegemony has brought them together despite lingering problem of mistrust and asymmetry. They put forward that the relationship has move beyond axis of convenience to a fully-fledged strategic partnership.[5] Moving a step further, Alexander Gabuev has stated that the pressure from the West post Ukraine crisis has pushed Russia closer to China and has forced Russia to become China's junior partner and the asymmetry continues to increase.[6] Alexander Lukin underlines that the rapprochement between China and Russia have occurred because they share similar view on geopolitical situation of the world. But closeness in China-Russia ties cannot be termed as an alliance. Both China and Russia will continue to maintain their relationship with other countries based on their interests.[7]

From the above arguments it is clear that closer political ties between China and Russia is driven by external powers which has not yet brought closer people-to-people ties as desired. Unleashing of COVID-19 pandemic where China is largely seen as a culprit by most of the West and where Russia has become one of the worst hit countries, has put their relationship in test. Whether Russia will stand by China or remain neutral or side with the Western world is of paramount importance to China's stand and authority on the global platform.

Russia's response at the onset of the virus outbreak in China

Looking at the internal measures taken by Russia to stop the spread of coronavirus from China, it was interestingly amongst countries which took the most stringent measures. Russia was one of the first countries to close its border with China on January 30 after the news of few confirmed cases and one death came out from

Heilongjiang region in late January.[8] 16 out of 25 border points were closed swiftly.[9] It also stopped issuing electronic visas to Chinese visitors and students except for diplomatic and official visitors. Rail and air traffic between the two sides were stopped except the charter flights and flights of Aeroflot between Moscow and Beijing, Shanghai and Guangzhou.[10]

For Chinese students studying in Russian universities, students arriving after 15 February 2020 were instructed to be self-isolated for two weeks and vacations were extended for those who remained in China. Students also faced discrimination while travelling in metro where people tried to move away from Chinese nationals and also through taxis which refused to take Chinese passengers.[11] Chinese citizens were monitored and were told to fill a form in public transport.[12] In February, police in Moscow were ordered to raid various places in search of Chinese people to curb the spread of virus.[13,14] Violation of quarantine procedures also led to deportation of some Chinese students staying in Russia.[15] Russian police reportedly took action against Chinese citizens for evading quarantine measures.[16] At some places, there were protests by locals near the quarantine centres having Chinese citizens. Moreover, some Taiwanese mistaken as Chinese were put into quarantine.[17]

At other level, in the beginning, Russian Prime Minister, Mikhail Mishustin said on February 3 that foreigners testing positive would be sent back, however, there was no such mention afterwards.[18] As a show of support to China at the international stage, the Russian side was quick to denounce attack on China over coronavirus.[19] Later on February 5, President Putin appreciated measures taken by China to counter the spread of infection.[20] He also praised China's handling of the COVID-19 situation during a phone call with President Xi Jinping on 19 March 2020.[21] Russia sent 23 tonnes of medical assistance to China on February 9.[22] Russia also offered help to China on developing vaccine for the virus.[23] Moreover, Russia was the first country to send a delegation of five epidemic prevention experts team to help China in fighting the epidemic and for technical exchanges on epidemic prevention on February 5.[24] At the same time, Russia also evacuated its citizens from the epicentre of the virus, Wuhan.[25]

To note public perception in Russia on China's role, English media in Russia largely remained silent on the origin of coronavirus in China.[26] However, few Russian language media and blogs like Nezavisimaya Gazeta (dated March 4) criticised China on not standing with Russia in the oil price war between Russia, Saudi Arabia and the US.[27] Konstantin Eggert, an independent journalist questioned Russia's silence on China.[28] An article in Kommersant by Sergei Strokan mentioned that China has gone offensive by shifting the blame on the US.[29] Despite China-Russia propaganda blaming the US for the origin of the virus, general public do believe that the virus has its origins from a Chinese lab.[30] According to reports, social media also responded negatively for China.[31] There has also been news of crowds moving away from Chinese people.[32]

Chair of Asia-Pacific Program at Carnegie Moscow Center, Alexander Gabuev noted that despite Russia officially offering support and admiration for China's effort in controlling the virus, privately senior officials have expressed concerns that arise due to lack of transparency by China. He also emphasised that the situation has raised anti-China sentiments among the citizens and the government wants to answer people's concern.[33] Other noted scholar, Dmitri Trenin argued that the outbreak had put relations between the two countries under strain, but the two countries have passed the test.[34] In yet another instance, while many Russian media have largely blamed US for the origin of the virus, a researcher at Engelhardt Institute of Molecular Biology in Moscow, Petr Chumakov highlighted that China did something which gave the virus the ability to infect human cells.[35]

The Spread of the Virus in Russia

Due to these proactive and strict measures, Russia was largely able to evade the virus from Feb to the mid-March, however Russian and foreign travellers coming from other countries like Italy may have spread the infection in Russia afterwards.[36] The COVID-19 virus ultimately dwarfed all the strict actions of Russia to ultimately turn it into a country with second highest rate of spread of virus.[37] Inspired by China, Russia rushed to build a hospital specially for coronavirus patients by late March.[38] The Russian Army is currently building 16 coronavirus special hospitals. An analysis by Moscow based private lab said in May that one out of seven healthy Russians may have been infected with coronavirus.[39] According to the World Health Organisation (WHO), over 4693 deaths were reported in Russia till May 31.[40]

The situation later became so devastating that even Russian Prime Minister, Mikhail Mishustin could not escape from the virus infection.[41] Figure 11.1 mentions the rising trend of the number of corona cases in Russia till May 2020.

As far as Central Asia is concerned which are also neighbouring countries of Russia and China, number of reported cases and deaths as per WHO data are less as compared to Russia. Kazakhstan reported the highest number with 10,858 COVID-19 cases, while Turkmenistan did not report any cases till May 31. However, countries like Tajikistan and Turkmenistan are said to have under reported cases.[42] Tajikistan also reported second highest number of cases (3,807) and highest number of deaths (47) in Central Asia due to coronavirus. The total number of coronavirus cases and deaths in Central Asia can be seen in Fig. 11.2.

Figure 11.1: Total Number of Corona Cases in Russia from February to May 2020

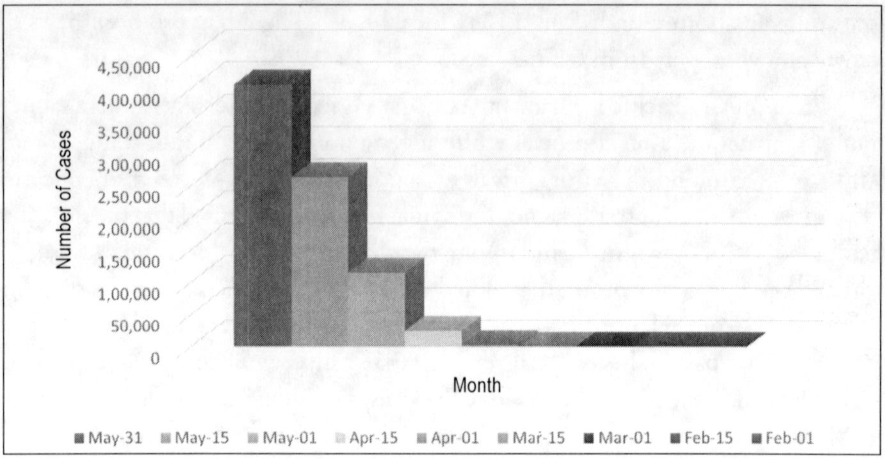

Source: World Health Organisation.

Figure 11.2: Total Number of Corona Cases in Central Asia till May 2020

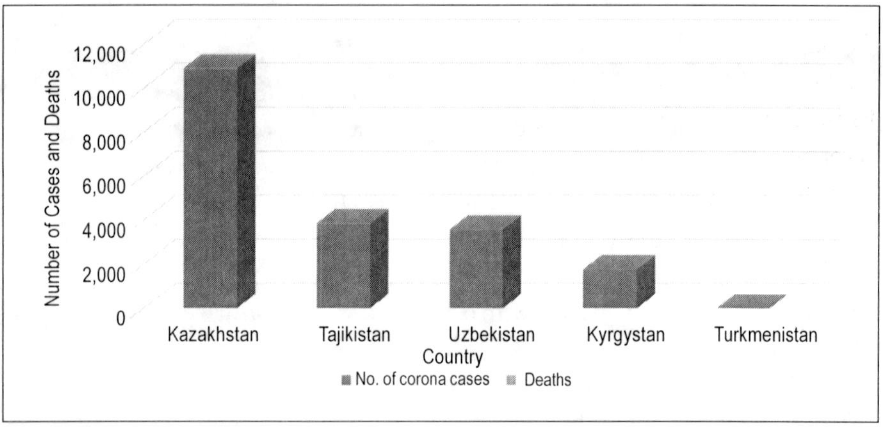

Source: World Health Organisation.

Chinese response against Russian Actions

At the diplomatic level, China's Foreign Minister, Wang Yi thanked Russia for its assistance and support in fighting the virus.[43] However, China has also expressed its dissatisfaction over Russia's treatment of its citizens in Russia. With regard to the report of Russian authorities checking passport of Chinese citizens in public places and other measures, the Chinese embassy letter dated Feb 24 stated that Russian authorities should be moderate and non-discriminative against Chinese as only Chinese citizens were inspected.[44] The letter highlighted that the special monitoring of Chinese nationals did not even existed in countries like US and other Western countries.[45]

With respect to Chinese media, *Global Times* (dated February 19) was quite critical of Russia's handling of the situation openly stating that the two countries have some divergences regarding the coronavirus situation, though underlining that it is understandable.[46] In another article, (dated March 3) it was critical of Russia's handling of the situation and the problems that Chinese students had to face because of measures taken by the authorities.[47] Media sources like 'The Paper' have also highlighted the difficulties that the Chinese students had to undergo in Russia.[48] The Chinese social media users were also critical of Russia's discrimination against the Chinese citizens.[49] Shi Yinhong, an International Relations expert at Renmin University argued that the pandemic had cast a shadow over relations between China and Russia due to Moscow's decision to close the border in late January despite Chinese opposition.[50] On the contrary, there were also reports that praised treatment of Chinese patients in Russia.[51] Li Lifan, a scholar at Chinese Academy of Social Sciences holds a view that Moscow's treatment of Chinese citizens triggered a backlash on social media, but these could hardly derail bilateral relationships.[52]

Reverse Flow of the Epidemic

China with all its might, strict quarantine measures and aggressive testing of virus was largely able to contain the virus by March while the rest of the world including Russia started reeling under the devastation of the corona virus. As the number of coronavirus cases in Russia increased, the number of people coming back to China from Russia also increased. Large numbers of Chinese nationals travelling from Russia turned the bordering town of Suifenhe in Heilongjiang Province into a hotspot.[53] The imported cases overwhelmed the local health resources which led to closure of border on 7 April 2020. Around mid-April, Suifenhe had more than 300 infected cases. While another city of Heilongjiang, Mudanjiang bordering Russia became second Chinese city after Wuhan to order mass testing for its 2.8 million people.[54] Other cities close to Russia like Shulan in Jilin Province and Manzhouli in Inner Mongolia were also closed due to increased influx of cases from Russia.[55] Reportedly, Heilongjiang province was also offering cash rewards upto 5000 Yuan for reports about illegal crossing of border from Russia to China.[56] Around 2,850 guards were deployed on the China-Russia border to prevent illegal crossings.[57] Additionally, operation of some flights also added to the spread of virus from Russia to even deep inlands of China. 60 Chinese citizens coming from a flight from Russia to Shanghai on April 10 were tested positive for the novel coronavirus.[58]

Reportedly, this led to speculations and anger in the Chinese social media that Russian authorities were hiding the extent of the spread of the disease in Russia.[59] The closure of the Suifenhe Port also led to disagreements between the two sides as

Russia wanted to send back Chinese nationals, however the Chinese side was not ready.[60] Wu Dahui, a professor at Tsinghua University describes this as the inability of the Russian side to take care of stranded Chinese.[61] Another expert, Shi Yinhong from Renmin University blamed Russia for mishandling of the outbreak and the risk that it brought to China.[62] *Global Times* also criticised Russia over its failure to control coronavirus cases and blamed Russia for being the largest source of imported cases.[63] On the contrary, Dmitry Peskov, Kremlin spokesman disagreed with the Chinese media criticism on the rising number of cases of infection in China due to returnees from Russia.[64] He stated that:

> "We hear that there is now an exchange of criticism over coronavirus between different countries, which is played like ping pong. We Consider this to be a thankless exercise."

Likewise, the Governor of Primorsky Oleg Kozhemyako retorted that the Chinese citizens who travelled from Moscow to the border to go to China led to the spread of the disease in the Russian Far-East regions.[65] Authorities of Primorsky Krai announced that they planned to return around 330 stranded Chinese nationals back to China, but later they removed the announcement from their website.[66]

Chinese Assistance

China which had largely contained the virus in its own territory by the time of worsening of crisis in Russia was quick to support and provide assistance to Russia. As soon as the number of cases began increasing in Russia, China sent 25.5 tons of medical supplies to the country on 2 April 2020. A 10-member medical team was sent by China to Russia on 11 April 2020 to assist Russia on the prevention, control, diagnosis and treatment of COVID-19. This team had experts specializing in laboratory testing, epidemiologists with specialization in prevention and control of infectious diseases, pulmonologists, intensive care and traditional Chinese medicine experts from the Chinese Centre for Disease Control and Prevention, the Heilongjiang Provincial Centre for Disease Control and Prevention and four hospitals in the province. The team also brought medical supplies including surgical masks, N95 masks and PPE kits.[67] Russia also received millions of masks and testing kits via Chinese assistance through entrepreneur Jack Ma's Ali Baba.[68] Other Chinese companies such as the Greenwood International Trade Center in Moscow and Russian branch of Industrial and Commercial Bank of China have also donated medical supplies to Russia.[69]

Chinese President in a telephone conversation with Russian President Putin on 16 April 2020 assured Russia in the procurement of medical supplies. In March, China Sinopharm International Corporation and Russia reached an agreement to supply millions of face masks and protective suits to Russia. Subsequently, China sent 20 million face masks in April[70] Chinese assistance to Russia in this critical time received praise from Russian netizens.[71] In addition, Russian Prime Minister issued an order on April 16 to use the Chinese drug Hydroxychloroquine which is still not registered in Russia.[72]

Russia-China Political Coordination over the Pandemic

Russia was on the forefront to defend China when western countries were targeting China for the severe spread of virus all over the world. The Russian government displayed show of solidarity with the Chinese and pledged to counter the politicisation of the coronavirus pandemic. President Putin said that the country will work closely with China under United Nations (UN) to fight the pandemic. He also stated that the aim to discredit China was not acceptable.[73] Russia's Foreign Minister, Sergei Lavrov criticised western countries demanding China for reparations.[74] China with the help of Russia vetoed against a discussion in the UN Security Council over the coronavirus pandemic.[75] Russia also introduced a resolution in UN as a show of solidarity with China. The text contains provisions about "*unacceptability of stigmisations of states, peoples and individuals with regard to pandemic, and the need to circulate only reliable and science-based information about it*". Russia also took the opportunity to include "rejection of unilateral sanctions" in the text.[76]

Russia rejected US call on investigating the source of coronavirus saying it is not proper to blame any nation for the origin of the virus without evidence.[77] Moreover, according to reports, China and Russia can also initiate an investigation of bio-labs around the world, including P3 and P4 labs run by the US, at the United Nations. Russia joined hands with China in defending the role of WHO with Russian Foreign Minister, Sergei Lavrov saying criticism about the role of WHO in the pandemic as unfair.[78] The two countries have endorsed each other's narrative on the issue. For instance, various Russian media sources and Russian linked social media accounts alleged US hand behind the outbreak, perpetuating Chinese claims.[79] China's Foreign Ministry Spokesperson, Geng Shuang on 29 April 2020 also supported Moscow's concern over the presence of US labs in former Soviet Union countries for creating bioweapons.[80] China and Russia have taken the opportunity to improve their global image by providing humanitarian assistance in many countries. Russia also helped China in delivering medical supplies to Moldova by providing its military aircraft.[81]

Notwithstanding, China-Russia coordination amidst the pandemic, Russia's coordination with the US cannot be ignored. Russia delivered protective gears and ventilators to the US. In return, the US also delivered ventilators to Russia.[82] Furthermore,

Trump also mediated between Russia and Saudi Arabia to end the spat resulting due to drop in oil prices following the pandemic. Consequently, the two leaders also issued a statement on 25 April 2020 commemorating the 75th anniversary of the first meeting between American and Soviet troops on the banks of the Elbe River in 1945.[83]

Impact on Russia

Notwithstanding the outbreak, the trade volume between the two countries rose by 3.4 percent in the first quarter of 2020. China's import from Russia increased by 17.3 percent from last year to USD 16.2 billion, while exports declined by 14.6 percent to reach USD 9.15 billion.[84] Lower oil price has given China an opportunity to fill its reserves. In April 2020, China increased its import of oil by 18 percent to 7.2 million tons overtaking Saudi Arabia to become largest partner of Russia. However, given the deteriorating condition of virus in Russia and worldwide, overall impact of COVID-19 is going to be devastating. According to Li Xin, director of the Institute for Eurasian Studies under the National Institute for SCO, trade between China and Russia may drop 50 percent in 2020.[85] The annual bilateral trade trend over the years between the two countries is mentioned in the Fig. 11.3. Decline in demand for hydrocarbons and lower oil price will also impact the Russian economy as it heavily depends on revenues from oil and gas. The spread of virus and lockdown has already led to reduction in gas demand from Europe.[86] No matter, China's purchase of oil from Russia increased in the first quarter of 2020 but lower oil prices will only increase Russia's dependence on China.[87] The turmoil has also impacted Russian stock markets and the value of Ruble.

Figure 11.3: China-Russia Bilateral Trade

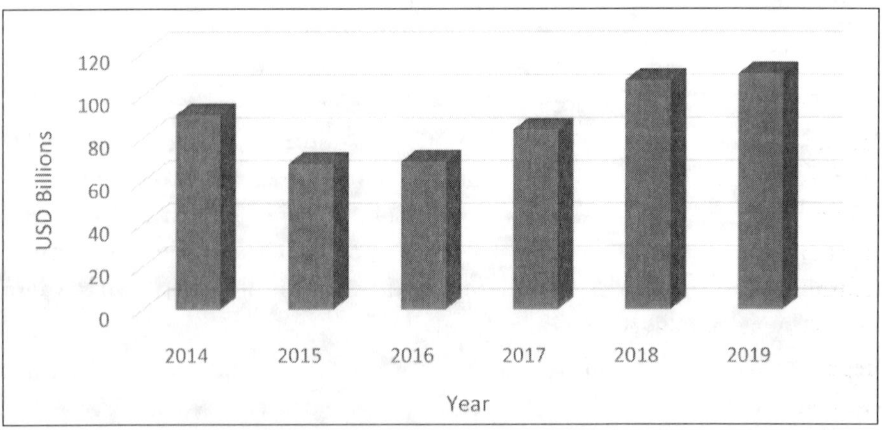

Source: National Bureau of Statistics.[88]

The coronavirus has deeply impacted the Russian tourism industry. Bilateral tourism will also be impacted as large number of Chinese tourists visit Russia every year. According to Association of Russian Tour Operators, the tourism industry will lose around USD 400 million if ban is not lifted before 2020 summer.[89] The Russian Far East which heavily depends on China's trade and tourism is also impacted due to the outbreak. For instance, Russian farmers suffered due to limitations in the supply of Russian fish to China which accounts for 70 percent of the total exports.[90] Cessation of delivery from China led to spike in vegetable prices in places like Blagoveshchensk.[91] Hotels and Restaurants which depended on Chinese, Japanese and Korean tourists in the Far East have no visitors. Owners of apartments rented out to foreign tourists will suffer losses. Russian dependence on Chinese labourers will also impact the economy of the Russian border region.[92] Additionally, according to Deputy Transport Minister, Alexander Yurchik, suspension of flights to China and the lost incurred had cost USD 25.2 million to Russian aviation industry. Further, according to the estimates of the head of the Federal Air Transport Agency, Alexander Neradko losses of Russian Airlines could be more than USD 1.35 billion.[93]

Igor Nikolayev of Grant Thorntan estimates that the unemployment could hit 15 percent by 2020 in Russia.[94] According to Russian Audit Chamber Chief, Alexei Kudrin, the Russian economy is expected to fall between 3 to 5 percent even if it is moderately hit from the virus outbreak; while other Russian economists expect the economy to fall by 9 percent.[95] According to the Chief Economist of VEB.RF (a national economic development institution of Russia), Andrey Klepach, the recovery of the Russian economy will begin in Q3 of 2020 by best possible estimates.[96] There also rests risks of opportunistic takeovers by China to which already many countries have taken actions to restrict.[97] However, since the pandemic is still beginning to peak in Russia with number of cases increasing in thousands per day uncertainty lies ahead.[98]

The impact of coronavirus on demography will be noteworthy as around 29 percent of the Russian population is above 55 by July 2018 estimate.[99] The Russian population is already shrinking as the country's natural population declined at an 11 year low in 2019.[100] In addition to it, the pressure on Russian healthcare system cannot be ignored as Medical professionals are reportedly committing suicide out of stress and pressure.[101] 101 Russian medics have died from coronavirus till May.[102]

The sudden leap in number of cases has revealed Russia's unpreparedness. Few reports suggest that Russian federal regions are implementing their own decision without any coordination with Moscow. This highlights the disagreements between centre and federal regions.[103] Also there were reports of protest in North Ossetia in

April.[104] Besides, virtual online protests also took place throughout Russia on April 2020 against inadequate actions taken by the authorities to contain the spread of virus.[105]

Impact on China

Notwithstanding, robust growth of the bilateral trade between China and Russia in the first quarter, the trade ties has been impacted. Fall in demand from the Russian side such as of industrial machinery have impacted Chinese exports. Suppliers of heavy industrial machinery in Wuhan have experienced fall in new orders by over 50 percent in January and February.[107]

As condition in Russia worsens, Chinese business and cross-border trade on the border areas like Suifenhe have been impacted. Heilongjiang Province which accounts for about one-fifth of China's total trade with Russia is facing weak demand. Timber industries of bordering areas are also receiving very few orders and Chinese owners of farms in Russia are also facing uncertainty.[108] Chinese companies in Russia involved in tourism, hospitality, trade and construction are facing a business slump. The halt in tourism in Russia has led to return of many of the Chinese tour guides and Chinese chefs in the restaurants to their homeland.[109] The deteriorating situation led the local government of Suifenhe to announce measures to support local companies by issuing USD 63 million loans to 83 local business, 5 percent discount on electricity charge and subsidies.[110] Cross-border e-commerce has also gone down due to cancellation of orders and decline in demand.[111] Nevertheless, impact on Chinese side will be less serious as compared to the Russian side.

Assessment

So far China and Russia have followed a very pragmatic policy and have refrained from engaging in a blame-game at a higher level. Russia has provided political and moral support to China. Moving a step further, President Putin and President Xi are also planning to visit each other later this year.[112] However, the anti-China sentiments and the 'Yellow Peril fear' among the Russian public is hard to change easily which is well reflected by their behaviour during the pandemic. Similarly, the historical enmity and the perception that Russia has occupied a large area of Chinese land still persist among the Chinese citizens. These sentiments rebounds during sensitive times, no matter how peaceful the bilateral political ties are. According to a January 2020 survey by Levada Analytical Center, a Russian non-governmental research organisation, the very positive attitude towards China has declined from 16 percent in November 2019 to 12 percent in January 2020, whereas, very negative attitude for China has increased from 6 percent in November 2019 to 8 percent in

January 2020.[113] This gap in bilateral ties may also give opportunity for countries like US to reset ties with Russia to counter China. However, the possibility is rare since it will come with number of compromises.

Russia needs Chinese money to sort out its economic woes, while China finds a strong partner in Russia to support it in countering western criticism. The duo has a common interest in opposing the west, due to the pressure created by sanctions against Russia and US-China trade friction. Therefore, differences at the domestic level do not get reflected in the international platform. Unlike China's aggressive behaviour in other countries, its behaviour with Russia has been very complaisant. Russia's support to China and coordination with China in the international platform signals that they both need each other to counter the west. Therefore, China has got a phenomenal support from Russia at the international level. In return, Russia got appreciation and stronger Chinese support to fight the virus.

The impact that the virus had at bilateral level may be solved by top leadership, but the overall impact on Russia's internal situation is alarming. China may not be impacted much by the slowdown in trade relations because China's export to Russia is not much in comparison to other countries like US, Japan and South Korea. But if we look at the impact of the pandemic on internal situation of Russia, Russia has been hard hit by the crisis as seen from fall in Ruble due to weak oil demand. The long-term impact on economy will further increase Russia's woes which is already grappling with economic crisis. Russia's economic crisis will worsen after the pandemic is over which may tilt Russia even closer to China and increase its dependency on China. Threat to economic stability of the country could also pose a threat to the position of the ruling elite of Russia. It has also opened the door to strengthen China's 'Health Silk Road' and introduce and market China's traditional medicine in Russia. China is already working to increase medical tourism from Russia, Central Asia and other neighbouring countries. It has built a hospital for Russian patients in Heihe region of Heilongjiang province.[114]

As the number of cases are rapidly growing inside Russia, it also has an ever-growing internal dissent of its population to satisfy as well as answer their queries. Notwithstanding, China's medical support and assistance, the anti-China sentiments among the common citizens will rise at least for some time. In all likelihood it will have to take dual stands, one to appease its own population in which it will remain silent about China's role and the impact of COVID-19 on Russian economy, and the other to defend beleaguered China on international stage. China may have to turn a blind eye to the indifferences meted to its citizens on Russian soil and students in Russia in lieu of Russia's support on international platform. It will require a very high degree of shrewd diplomacy to contain and complement contradictory stances on part of both countries.

NOTES

1 Namsaraeva Sayana, "Deja vu of Distrust in the Sino-Russian Borderlands", in Caroline Humphrey, Ed. *Trust and Mistrust in the Economies of China-Russia borderlands*, Amsterdam, Amsterdam University Press, 2018.

2 Fu Ying (2016), "Are China and Russia Partnering to Create an Axis", 20 October 2016, https://eng.globalaffairs.ru/articles/are-china-and-russia-partnering-to-create-an-axis/, accessed online 21 March 2020.

3 Feng Shaolei and Cui Heng (2019), "Developing the Far East and Chinese-Russian Relations: New Perceptions and New Practices", 30 September 2019, https://eng.globalaffairs.ru/articles/developingthe-far-east-and-chinese-russian-relations-new-perceptions-and-new-practices/, accessed online 23 March 2020.

4 Lo Bobo, *Axis of Convenience*, London, Brookings Institution Press, 2008.

5 Li Mingjiang and Poh Angela, "The Indispensable Partner: Russia in China's Grand Strategy", in Jo Inke Bekkevold and Bobo Lo, Ed. *Sino-Russian Relations in the 21st Century*, Switzerland, Palgrave Macmillan, 2019.

6 Gabuev Alexander, "Unwanted but Inevitable: Russia's Deepening Partnership with China Post Ukraine", in Jo InkeBekkevold and Bobo Lo, Ed. *Sino-Russian Relations in the 21st Century*, Cham, Palgrave Macmillan, 2019.

7 Lukin Alexander, *China and Russia: The New Rapprochement*, Cambridge, Polity Press, 2018.

8 Urankyzy Aruuke (2020), "The Coronavirus in Russia: What is the State of Preparedness", 07 April 2020, https://researchcentre.trtworld.com/publications/info-packs/the-coronavirus-in-russia-whatis-the-state-of-preparedness, accessed online 21 April 2020.

9 The Moscow Times (2020), "Russia Closes Far East Border Over Coronavirus", 30 Jan 2020, https://www.themoscowtimes.com/2020/01/30/russia-closes-far-east-border-over-coronavirus-a69100, accessed online 5 Feb 2020.

10 Zuenko Ivan (2020), "The Coronavirus Pandemic and the Russo-Chinese Border", 09 May 2020, http://www.theasanforum.org/the-coronavirus-pandemic-and-the-russo-chinese-border/#a8, accessed online 21 May 2020.

11 Qi Shuyang (2020), "全球战疫·连线丨一位在俄中国留学生的亲历、观察和呼吁", 29 Feb 2020, https://www.thepaper.cn/newsDetail_forward_6236097, accessed online 01 March 2020 ; Chirikov Sergey (2020), "People leer at me like I am a leper", 25 Feb 2020, https://meduza.io/en/feature/ 2020/02/24/people-leer-at-me-like-i-m-a-leper, accessed online 05 March 2020; Guancha (2020), "莫斯科在防止新型冠状病毒肺炎 COVID-19 疫情上的措施遭到中国使馆批评", 28 Feb 2020, https://user.guancha.cn/main/content?id=251618&s=fwzxfbbt, Accessed 01 March 2020.

12 Chirikov Sergey (2020), "People leer at me like I am a leper", 25 Feb 2020, https://meduza.io/en/feature/2020/02/24/people-leer-at-me-like-i-m-a-leper, accessed online 05 March 2020.

13 Daily Mail Online (2020), "Russian police raid homes and businesses in search of Chinese people to stop the spread of corona virus", 23 Feb 2020, https://www.dailymail.co.uk/news/article-8034317/Moscow-targets-Chinese-raids-amid-virus-fears.html, accessed online 24 Feb 2020.

14 Meduza (2020), "We decided to defend our home", 11 Feb 2020, https://meduza.io/en/feature/2020/02/11/we-decided-to-defend-our-home, accessed online 11 Feb 2020.

15 Embassy of the PRC in Russia (2020), "中国驻俄罗斯使馆高度关注中国公民被遣返事", 05 March 2020, http://ru.chineseembassy.org/chn/ggl/t1752594.htm, accessed online, 10 March 2020; Litvinova Daria (2020), "Russia deports Chinese for violating self-quarantine rules, 20 March 2020, https://abcnews.go.com/International/wireStory/russia-deports-chinese-violating-quarantine-rules69706271, accessed online 24 March 2020.

16 Li Zhen (2020), "China complains of unfair treatment of Chinese in Russia amid coronavirus fears", 29 Feb 2020, https://sg.news.yahoo.com/china-complains-unfair-treatment-chinese 120354148.html, assessed online 29 Feb 2020.

17 Tetrault- Farber Gabriella (2020), "China to Russia: End discriminatory coronavirus measures against Chinese", 26 Feb 2020, https://www.themoscowtimes.com/2020/02/26/china-to-russia-enddiscriminatory-coronavirus-measures-against-chinese-a69416, accessed online 29 Feb 2020.

18 Ellayatt Holly (2020), "Russia may deport any foreigners found with coronavirus, prime minister says", 03 Feb 2020, https://www.cnbc.com/2020/02/03/russia-could-deport-any-foreigners-foundwith-coronavirus-mishustin.html, accessed online 04 Feb 2020.

19 TASS (2020), "Russian envoy says attacks on China over coronavirus 'unjustified, unfounded'", 14 Feb 2020, https://tass.com/politics/1120253, accessed 16 Feb 2020.

20 TASS (2020), "Putin notes 'decisive, vigorous' measures taken by China to fight coronavirus", 05 Feb 2020, https://tass.com/politics/1116753, accessed online 07 Feb 2020.

21 CGTN (2020), "Xi Jinping, Vladimir Putin discuss strengthening cooperation on fighting COVID19 by phone", 20 March 2020, https://newsaf.cgtn.com/news/2020-03-20/Xi-Jinping-holds-phonetalk-with-Vladimir-Putin-OZQc5Mm5Ow/index.html, accessed online 25 March 2020 .

22 TASS (2020), "China thanks Russia for its assistance in fighting coronavirus", 09 Feb 2020, https://tass.com/society/1118097, accessed online 01 March 2020.

23 TASS (2020), "Russia ready to help China develop vaccine against novel coronavirus", 31 Jan 2020, https://tass.com/society/1115171, accessed online 01 March 2020.

24 The Paper (2020), "全球战疫·连线丨一位在俄中国留学生的亲历、观察和呼吁", 29 Feb 2020, https://www.thepaper.cn/newsDetail_forward_6236097, accessed online 01 March 2020; Global Times (2020), "Russian netizens praise China's medical aid", 12 April 2020, https://www.globaltimes.cn/content/1185400.shtml, accessed online 22 April 2020; Ministry of Foreign Affairs of the PRC (2020), "Foreign Ministry Spokesperson Geng Shuang's Daily Briefing", 10 Feb 2020, https://www.fmprc.gov.cn/mfa_eng/xwfw_665399/s2510_665401/2511_665403/t1743009.shtml, accessed online 10 March 2020.

25 Embassy of the PRC in Russia (2020), "俄驻华大使表示不会撤离所有在华侨民", 05 February 2020, http://ru.chineseembassy.org/chn/ggl/t1740700.htm, accessed online 10 April 2020.

26 TASS (2020), "Scientists debunk rumors of unnatural coronavirus origin", 20 February 2020, https://tass.com/science/1122269, accessed online 01 March 2020.

27 The Asan Forum (2020), "Country Report: Russia", 30 March 2020, http://www.theasanforum.org/country-report-russia-march-2020/, accessed online 01 April 2020.

28 Ibid.

29 Ibid.

30 Youtube (2020), "What Russians Think About Coronavirus?", 15 March 2020, https://www.youtube.com/watch?v=-JClprScd2s, accessed online 14 April 2020.

31 CGTN (2020), "Xi Jinping, Vladimir Putin discuss strengthening cooperation on fighting COVID19 by phone", 20 March 2020, https://newsaf.cgtn.com/news/2020-03-20/Xi-Jinping-holds-phonetalk-with-Vladimir-Putin-OZQc5Mm5Ow/index.html, accessed online 15 March 2020.

32 Couch Emily (2020), "Russia's Chinese Dream in the Era of COVID-19", 27 March 2020, https://www.wilsoncenter.org/blog-post/russias-chinese-dream-era-COVID-19, accessed online 30 March 2020.

33 The Moscow Times (2020), "Russia Gets Tough on Coronavirus. And What Does Surkov's Departure Say About Modern Russia", 20 Feb 2020, https://www.themoscowtimes.com/2020/02/20/russiagets-tough-on-coronavirus-and-what-does-surkovs-departure-say-about-modern-russia-2-a69369, accessed online 20 Feb 2020.

34 Huang Kristin and Zhou Laura (2020), "Coronavirus poses test for Russia and China's friendship", 17 May 2020, https://www.scmp.com/news/china/diplomacy/article/3084704/coronavirus-posestest-russia-and-chinas-friendship, accessed online 17 May 2020.

35 The Moscow Times (2020), "Russian TV Runs Conspiracy Theory Blaming Trump for Coronavirus", 06 February 2020, https://www.themoscowtimes.com/2020/02/06/russian-tv-runs-conspiracytheory-blaming-trump-for-coronavirus-a69189, accessed online 10 March 2020; Geopolitica (2020), "Former Putin's Aide: Coronavirus is the US biological weapon", 13 March 2020, https:// www.geopolitica.ru/en/news/former-putins-aide-coronavirus-us-biological-weapon, accessed online 01 May 2020; Stewart Will (2020), "CORONA BLAME Wuhan lab 'did absolutely crazy things' to manipulate coronavirus into infecting humans, Russian microbiologist claims", 23 April 2020, https://www.thesun.co.uk/news/11462934/coronavirus-wuhan-lab-russia-microbiologist-claims/, accessed online 01 May 2020.

36 Reuters (2020), "Russian citizen who returned from Italy diagnosed with coronavirus: RIA cites ministry", 02 March 2 2020, https://www.reuters.com/article/us-health-coronavirus-russia/russiancitizen-who-returned-from-italy-diagnosed-with-coronavirus-ria-cites-ministry-idUSKBN20P1JH, accessed online 5 May 2020; Uscinski Joseph E. and Enders Adam M, "The Coronavirus Conspiracy Theory", 30 April 2020, https://www.theatlantic.com/health/archive/2020/04/what-cancoronavirus-tell-us-about-conspiracy-theories/610894/, accessed online 7 May 2020.

37 Graham Emma, Roth Harrison Andrew and Farrer Martin (2020), "Russia now has second-highest rate of COVID-19 spread as other countries ease restrictions", 02 May 2020, https://www.theguardian.com/world/2020/may/02/new-york-nursing-home-reports-98-coronavirusdeaths-in-horrifying-outbreak, accessed online 2 May 2020.

38 The Moscow Times (2020), "Moscow Workers Race to Finish 'Chinese-Inspired' Virus Hospital", 21 March 2020, https://www.themoscowtimes.com/2020/03/21/moscow-workers-race-to-finishchinese-inspired-virus-hospital-a69706, accessed online 25 April 2020.

39 The Moscow Times (2020), "Coronavirus in Russia", 04 June 2020, https://www.themoscowtimes.com/2020/06/04/coronavirus-in-russia-the-latest-news-june-4-a69117, accessed online 4 June 2020.

40 WHO, "Russian Federation", https://covid19.who.int/region/euro/country/ru, accessed online 01 June 2020.

41 BBC News (2020), "Coronavirus: Russian PM Mishustin tests positive for virus", 30 April 2020, https://www.bbc.com/news/world-europe-52491205, accessed online 15 May 2020.

42 Otorbaev Doozmart (2020), "Coronavirus Crisis and Central Asia's Diverse Responses", 30 May 2020, https://www.financialexpress.com/opinion/coronavirus-crisis-and-central-asias-diverse-covidresponses/1975532/, accessed online 4 June 2020 ; Eurasianet (2020), "Tajikistan Strains Credibility with Apparent COVID-19 Turnaround", 22 May 2020, https://eurasianet.org/tajikistan-strainscredibility-with-apparent-COVID-19-turnaround, accessed online 04 June 4, 2020.

43 Ministry of Foreign Affairs of the PRC (2020), "Wang Yi: Facing the Common Threat, China and Russia Will Continue to Firmly Support Each Other", 16 Feb 2020, https://www.fmprc.gov.cn/mfa_eng/zxxx_662805/t1746146.shtml, accessed 18 April 2020.

44 Embassy of PRC in Russia (2020), "中国驻俄罗斯使馆同莫斯科市政府就俄方采取的涉我公民防疫措施进行沟通" 17 March 2020, http://ru.chineseembassy.org/chn/ggl/t1750245.htm, accessed online 23 March 2020; Liu Zhen (2020), "China complains of unfair treatment of Chinese in Russia amid coronavirus fears", 29 February 2020, https://sg.news.yahoo.com/china-complainsunfair-treatment-chinese-120354148.html, accessed online 19 March 2020 .

45 Farber Gabrielle-Tétrault (2020), "China to Russia: End discriminatory coronavirus measures against Chinese", 26 Feb 2020, https://www.reuters.com/article/us-china-health-moscow-letter/china-

torussia-end-discriminatory-coronavirus-measures-against-chinese-idUSKCN20K1HU, accessed online 20 march 2020.

46 Global Times (2020), "Russian ban on Chinese visitors regrettable but understandable: experts", 09 Feb 2020, https://www.globaltimes.cn/content/1180092.shtml, accessed online 27 March 2020.

47 Global Times (2020), "Dozens of Chinese citizens forcibly quarantined and deported in Russia amid coronavirus", 03 March 2020, https://www.globaltimes.cn/content/1181467.shtml, accessed online 05 March 2020.

48 The Paper (2020), "全球战疫·连线丨一位在俄中国留学生的亲历、观察和呼吁", 29 February 2020, https://www.thepaper.cn/newsDetail_forward_6236097, accessed online 7 March 2020.

49 KXAN36 (2020), "Chinese experts evaluated the effects of coronavirus on relations with Russia", 07 May 2020, http://www.kxan36news.com/chinese-experts-evaluated-the-effects-of-coronavirusonrelations-with-russia, accessed online 10 May 2020.

50 Huang Kristin and Zhou Laura (2020), "Coronavirus poses test for Russia and China's friendship", 17 May 2020, https://www.scmp.com/news/china/diplomacy/article/3084704/coronavirusposestest-russia-and-chinas-friendship, accessed online 17 May 2020.

51 "在俄罗斯的中国新冠病人：就当是一场重感冒", Sina Feb 5, 2020, Accessed 13 May 2020, http://news.sina.com.cn/s/2020-02-05/doc-iimxxste8909630.shtml

52 Huang Kristin and Zhou Laura (2020), "Coronavirus poses test for Russia and China's friendship", 17 May 2020, https://www.scmp.com/news/china/diplomacy/article/3084704/coronavirusposestest-russia-and-chinas-friendship, accessed online 17 May 2020.

53 India Today (2020), "China toughens restrictions on border with Russia as imported coronavirus cases hit record", 13 April 2020, https://www.indiatoday.in/world/story/china-toughensrestrictionson-border-with-russia-as-imported-coronavirus-cases-hit-record-1666298-2020-04-13, accessed online 13 April 2020.

54 The Hindu Business Line (2020), "Second Chinese city orders mass testing for COVID-19 after Wuhan", 04 June 2020, https://www.thehindubusinessline.com/news/world/second-chinesecityorders-mass-testing-for-COVID-19-after-wuhan/article31745017.ece#, accessed online 4 June 2020.

55 Financial Express (2020), "Is Covid 19 Virus Changing? New Coronavirus Cases in China takes Longer time to test Negative", 21 May 2020, https://www.financialexpress.com/lifestyle/health/isCOVID-19-virus-changing-new-coronavirus-patients-in-china-take-longer-time-to-test-negative/1965887/, accessed online 31 May 2020.

56 Ministry of Foreign Affairs of the PRC (2020), "Foreign Ministry Spokesperson Zhao Lijian's Regular Press Conference", 14 April 2020, https://www.fmprc.gov.cn/mfa_eng/xwfw_665399/s2510_665401/2511_665403/t1769716.shtml, accessed online 9 May 2020.

57 Wang Qi (2020), "3,000 guards on China-Russia border block illegal entries", 06 May 2020, https://www.globaltimes.cn/content/1187570.shtml, accessed online 10 May 2020.

58 Ministry of Foreign Affairs of the PRC (2020), "Foreign Ministry Spokesperson Zhao Lijian's Regular Press Conference", 13 April 2020, https://www.fmprc.gov.cn/mfa_eng/xwfw_665399/s2510_665401/2511_665403/t1769241.shtml, accessed online 28 April 2020.

59 Xu Xiaofei (2020), "Infodemic infects Chinese-Russian relations", 12 April 2020, https://eurasianet.org/infodemic-infects-chinese-russian-relations, accessed online 16 April 2020.

60 Wang Qi and Yang Sheng (2020), "China, Russia appear to be in discord over whether to re-open land port amid pandemic", 09 April 2020, https://www.globaltimes.cn/content/1185193.shtml, accessed online 11 April 2020.

61 Ibid.

62 Huang Kristin and Zhou Laura (2020), “Coronavirus poses test for Russia and China's friendship”, 17 May 2020, https://www.scmp.com/news/china/diplomacy/article/3084704/coronavirus-posestest-russia-and-chinas-friendship, accessed online 17 May 2020.

63 Global Times (2020), “Russian alarm on imported infection risk”, 13 April 2020, https://www.globaltimes.cn/content/1185509.shtml, accessed online 22 April 2020.

64 TASS (2020), “Kremlin says countries should drop accusations and join efforts to fight COVID19”, 15 April 2020, https://tass.com/politics/1145107, accessed online 17 April 2020.

65 Brendan Cole (2020), “Russian Governor Fears Chinese Citizens Have Spread Coronavirus in His Region After Beijing Closes Border”, 09 April 2020, https://www.newsweek.com/russian-governorfears-chinese-citizens-have-spread-coronavirus-his-region-after-beijing-closes-1497106, accessed online 15 May 2020.

66 Yang Tommy (2020), “Unease at the border: Russia and China seek to downplay COVID-19 outbreak in Suifenhe”, 18 April 2020, https://www.theguardian.com/world/2020/apr/18/unease-at-theborder-russia-and-china-seek-to-downplay-COVID-19-outbreak-in-suifenhe, accessed online 19 April 2020.

67 National Health Commission of the PRC (2020), “Chinese medical team arrives in Moscow “, 13 April 2020, http://en.nhc.gov.cn/2020-04/13/c_79117.htm, accessed online 30 April 2020.

68 Al Jazerra (2020), “Russia latest country to receive coronavirus kits from Jack Ma”, 27 March 2020, https://www.aljazeera.com/news/2020/03/russia-latest-country-receive-coronavirus-kits-jack-ma200326215605441.html, accessed online 19 May 2020.

69 Ma Jingjing and Zhao Juecheng (2020), “Virus hits Chinese firms in Russia”, 16 April 2020, https://www.globaltimes.cn/content/1185821.shtml, accessed online 26 April 2020.

70 TASS (2020), “China to deliver 80 mln face masks to Russia in April-early May”, 04 April 2020, https://tass.com/society/1140305, accessed online 10 April 2020 ; Belt and Road Portal (2020), “Freight train loaded with 20 mln masks departs China for Russia”, 21 April 2020, https://eng.yidaiyilu.gov.cn/qwyw/rdxw/123486.htm, accessed online 7 May 2020.

71 Wan Lin, Qu Pei and Xu Keyue (2020), “Russian netizens praise China's medical aid”, 12 April 2020, https://www.globaltimes.cn/content/1185400.shtml, accessed online 13 April 2020.

72 Embassy of the PRC in Russia (2020), “俄罗斯总理签署政府令允许使用未在俄注册的中国产羟氯喹治疗新冠肺炎患者或疑似患者”, 17 April 2020, http://ru.chineseembassy.org/chn/ggl/t1770990.htm, accessed online 29 April 2020 .

73 Zhou Laura (2020), “Don't make pandemic political': Xi and Putin show united front as China criticised over coronavirus handling”, 17 April 2020, https://www.scmp.com/news/china/diplomacy/article/3080386/dont-make-pandemic-political-xi-and-putins-show-united-front, accessed online 19 April 2020.

74 TASS (2020), “Lavrov castigates attempts to make China pay reparations for COVID-19 damages”, 14 April 2020, https://tass.com/politics/1144557, accessed online 20 May 2020.

75 The Statesman (2020), “China obstructs discussion on Coronavirus in UNSC, blocks draft seeking ‘full transparency’”, 27 March 2020, https://www.thestatesman.com/world/china-obstructs discussion-coronavirus-unsc-blocks-draft-seeking-full-transparency-1502870418.html, accessed online 21 May 2020.

76 Permanent Mission of the Russian Federation to the United Nations (2020), “Press release on consideration by the UN General Assembly of a Declaration on Solidarity in Countering COVID19 Pandemic”, 02 April 2020, https://russiaun.ru/en/news/pressrelease_020420, accessed online 18 April 2020.

77 Ellyatt Holly (2020), “Russia tries to stay neutral as US-China tensions rise over coronavirus' origin”, 24 April 2020, https://www.cnbc.com/2020/04/24/russia-says-coronavirus-origin-is-unknown-asus-china-tensions-rise.html, accessed online 19 May 2020.

78 InfoRos (2020), "Lavrov slams criticism of WHO's activities amid pandemic as unfair", 27 April 2020, http://inforos.ru/en/?module=news&action=view&id=108173, accessed online 12 May 2020.

79 The Moscow Times (2020), "Russian TV Runs Conspiracy Theory Blaming Trump for Coronavirus", 07 February 2020, https://www.themoscowtimes.com/2020/02/06/russian-tv-runs-conspiracytheory-blaming-trump-for-coronavirus-a69189, accessed online 30 March 2020 ; South China Morning Post (2020), "Coronavirus: Russia pushing fake news about US using outbreak to 'wage economic war' on China, officials say", 23 February 2020, https://www.scmp.com/news/world/ russia-central-asia/article/3051939/coronavirus-russia-pushing-fake-news-about-us-using, accessed online 28 February 2020.

80 Bhadrakumar M.K (2020), "Russia-China Entente Deepens in the Shadow of the Pandemic", 04 May 2020, https://www.newsclick.in/Russia-China-Entente-Deepens-Shadow-Pandemic-USA, accessed online 10 May 2020.

81 Ministry of Foreign Affairs of the PRC (2020), "Foreign Ministry Spokesperson Geng Shuang's Regular Press Conference", 22 April 2020, https://www.fmprc.gov.cn/mfa_eng/xwfw_665399/s2510_665401/2511_665403/t1772428.shtml, accessed online 27 April 2020.

82 NPR (2020), "U.S. Sends Ventilators To Russia In $5.6 Million Coronavirus Aid Package", 21 May 2020, https://www.npr.org/sections/coronavirus-live-updates/2020/05/21/860143691/u-s-sendsventilators-to-russia-in-5-6-million-coronavirus-aid-package, accessed 28 May 2020.

83 Raghvan P.S. (2020), "COVID-19 Gathers Force", 06 May 2020, https://anantacentre.in/russiareview/russia-review-april-2020, accessed online 11 May 2020 .

84 Xinhua (2020), "China-Russia Trade up 3.4 pct in Q1", 23 April 2020, http://www.xinhuanet.com/english/2020-04/23/c_139002268.htm, accessed online 23 April 2020.

85 Xie Jun and Yin Yeping (2020), "Pandemic curbing China-Russia trade", 07 May 2020, https://www.globaltimes.cn/content/1187700.shtml, accessed online 10 May 2020.

86 Kapitonov Sergei (2020), "European Lockdown Hits Russia's Gas Market", 17 April 2020, https://carnegie.ru/commentary/81580, accessed online 24 May 2020.

87 The Moscow Times (2020), "Coronavirus Hits Russian Markets", 01 May 2020, https://www.themoscowtimes.com/2020/05/01/russia-coronavirus-ruble-stock-market-reaction-live-updatesa69640, accessed online 7 May 2020.

88 National Bureau of Statistics of China, "Annual", http://data.stats.gov.cn/english/easyquery.htm?cn=C01, accessed online 14 May 2020.

89 Wong Kai Ho (2020), "How Will the Coronavirus Outbreak Affect Russia-China Relations?", 14 March 2020, https://thediplomat.com/2020/03/how-will-the-coronavirus-outbreak-affect-russiachina-relations/, accessed online 30 March 2020.

90 Saveliev Alexander (2020), "Coronavirus closes Chinese corridor to Far Eastern Farmers", 13 February 2020, https://en.eastrussia.ru/material/koronavirus-udaril-po-rybodobytchikam-dfo/, accessed online 25 May 2020.

91 Higgins Andrew (2020), "Businesses 'Getting Killed' on Russian Border as Coronavirus Fears Rise", 24 February 2020, https://www.nytimes.com/2020/02/24/world/europe/coronavirus-russia-chinacommerce.html, accessed online 24 March 2020.

92 Zuenko Ivan (2020), "The Coronavirus Pandemic and the Russo-Chinese Border", 09 May 2020, http://www.theasanforum.org/the-coronavirus-pandemic-and-the-russo-chinese-border/#a8, accessed online 12 May 2020.

93 UrankyzyAruuke (2020), "The Coronavirus in Russia: What is the State of Preparedness", 07 April 2020, https://researchcentre.trtworld.com/publications/info-packs/the-coronavirus-in-russia-whatis-the-state-of-preparedness, accessed online 21 April 2020.

94 Cordell Jake and Zakharin, Stanislav (2020), "Analysts Fear the Economic Impact of Russia's April Coronavirus Shutdown Will Be Catastrophic", 03 April 2020, https://www.themoscowtimes.com/2020/04/02/russia-economy-coronavirus-analysts-fear-economic-impact-russias-april-coronavirusshutdown-catastrophic-a69851, accessed online 5 April 2020.

95 Avdaliani Emil (2020), "Coronavirus Is Hitting Russia on More than the Economy", 17 April 2020, https://besacenter.org/perspectives-papers/coronavirus-russia-economy/, accessed online 18 April 2020.

96 InfoRos (2020), "Russia's economic recovery will begin in Q3 of 2020", 13 April 2020, http://inforos.ru/en/?module=news&action=view&id=107508, accessed online 15 April 2020.

97 India Today (2020), "As global economies dwindle, world wakes up to China's hostile takeovers amid pandemic", 21 April 2020, https://www.indiatoday.in/business/story/world-wakes-up-to-chinahostile-takeovers-of-companies-amid-COVID-19-pandemic-1669240-2020-04-21, accessed online 29 April 2020.

98 The Asan Forum (2020), "Country Report: Russia", 30 March 2020, www.theasanforum.org/country-report-russia-march-2020/, accessed online 16 May 2020.

99 Index Mundi (2020), "Russia Demographic Profile 2019", https://www.indexmundi.com/russia/demographics_profile.html, accessed online 15 May 2020.

100 Ibid.

101 Radio Free Europe (2020), "Third Russian Doctor Mysteriously Falls From Hospital Window Amid Coronavirus Outbreak", 04 May 2020, https://www.rferl.org/a/third-russian-doctor-mysteriouslyfalls-from-hospital-window-amid-coronavirus-outbreak/30591638.html, accessed online 9 May 2020 .

102 The Moscow Times (2020), "Coronavirus in Russia", 04 June 2020, https:// www.themoscow times.com/2020/06/04/coronavirus-in-russia-the-latest-news-june-4-a69117, accessed online 4 June 2020.

103 Avdaliani, Emil (2020), "Coronavirus Is Hitting Russia on More than the Economy", 17 April 2020, https://besacenter.org/perspectives-papers/coronavirus-russia-economy/, accessed online 18 April 2020.

104 Sokolov, Denis (2020), "COVID-19 is a Threat to Putin", 14 April 2020, https://www.4freerussia.org/COVID-19-is-a-threat-to-putin/, accessed online 18 April 2020.

105 Free Russia (2020), "Virtual Protests in Russia "Dispersed" by Government-Controlled Yandex", 27 April 2020, https://www.4freerussia.org/blog/, accessed online 30 April 2020.

106 Levada Centre (2020), "The Russian Political System", 13 April 2020, https://www.levada.ru/en/2020/04/13/the-russian-political-system, accessed online 30 April 2020.

107 Yang Kunyi (2020), "China-Russia trade grows despite coronavirus pressure but braces for shrinking Russian demand", 25 March 2020, https://www.globaltimes.cn/content/1183697.shtml, accessed online 30 March 2020.

108 Global Times (2020), "Spreading Pandemic in Russia Deals Blow to Chinese Investors", 13 May 2020, https://www.globaltimes.cn/content/1188289.shtml, accessed online 15 May 2020; Wu, Huizhong (2020), "Remote Chinese city hit by coronavirus after weeks of feeling safe", 16 April 2020, https://www.reuters.com/article/us-health-coronavirus-china-border/remote-chinese-city-hitby-coronavirus-after-weeks-of-feeling-safe-idUSKCN21Y0J2, accessed online 27 May 2020.

109 Ma Jingjing and Zhao, Juecheng (2020), "Virus Hits Chinese Firms in Russia", 16 April 2020, https://www.globaltimes.cn/content/1185821.shtml, accessed online 18 May 2020.

110 Xie Jun and Yin Yeping (2020), "Pandemic Curbing China-Russia Trade", 07 May 2020, https://www.globaltimes.cn/content/1187700.shtml, accessed online 10 May 2020.

111 Zhang Hongpei (2020), "Cross-border e-commerce feels the pinch due to coronavirus outbreak", 22 March 2020, https://www.globaltimes.cn/content/1183349.shtml, accessed online 29 April 2020; Global Times (2020), "Spreading Pandemic in Russia Deals Blow to Chinese Investors", 13 May 2020, https://www.globaltimes.cn/content/1188289.shtml, accessed online 15 May 2020

112 Zhou Laura (2020), "Russia summits are on the cards for Xi Jinping in July", 20 May 2020, https://www.scmp.com/news/china/diplomacy/article/3085344/russia-summits-cards-chinese-presidentxi-jinping-july, accessed online 31 May 2020

113 Levada Centre (2020), "Russia and the West", 28 February 2020, https://www.levada.ru/en/2020/02/28/russia-and-the-west/, accessed online 31 May 2020.

114 National health Commission of the PRC (2017), "New hospital in Heihe to serve Russian patients", 31 August 2017, http://en.nhc.gov.cn/2017-08/31/c_72411.htm, accessed online 30 May 2020.

12

China-EU Relations and COVID-19

Tenzin Lhadon

Xi Jinping is seen by many as the most powerful leader after Mao Zedong through quickly consolidating his position and becoming the core leader of the Chinese Communist Party (CCP) through an anticorruption campaign. Xi Jinping is also considered a 'game changer' since, under his governance, there were many significant changes in Chinese domestic politics and foreign policy.[1] China's re-emergence as a global power in the form of bold regional initiatives such as the Asian Infrastructure Investment Bank (AIIB) and the One Belt One Road (OBOR), later renamed as Belt and Road Initiatives (BRI), and China's assertive role in East and South China Sea has been interpreted by several Chinese scholars (Yan 2014, Wang and Zeng 2016, Zhou 2019) as a shift in China's grand strategy from Deng Xiaoping's 'keeping a low profile' to displaying its global ambitions by asserting its core interests. Thus, it was observed that "With China's re-emergence as a global power, its current President Xi Jinping has attracted enormous public and academic attention both domestically and internationally".[2]

Xi Jinping in his work report of the 19th National Congress stated that national rejuvenation has been the greatest dream of the Chinese people since modern times and the dream of the Chinese people is closely connected to the dreams of people of other countries.[3] Beijing views the achievement of 'national rejuvenation' as essential in advancing socialism in the country. However, Elizabeth Economy believes that the rejuvenation of the Chinese nation is not only a powerful vision, but also a patriotic call to arms, drawing inspiration from past history and the ideals of present socialism to promote unity inside China and a strong influence abroad.[4]

However, the central question of this paper is focused on the outbreak of COVID-19 pandemic, what are the implications for Xi Jinping's regime and the projected vision of his desired world order while Chinese influence and leverage continue to grow in Europe. Beijing's adamant pursuit over creating a Sino-centric world order has been noticed during the pandemic outbreak, which has placed much spotlight on China's actions which have been deemed as bullying, threatening and provocative in nature.[5] Therefore, another question with regard to the China–EU equation is: has China's Sino–centric strategy intensified and has there been a specific modulation of strategy in key areas of Europe due to the outbreak of the pandemic in early 2020. Furthermore, how would this then affect China's relationship with the EU?

China's Foreign Policy: Revisiting the Middle Kingdom Framework

China under Xi Jinping has undergone major changes in some of its established norms, namely the rejection of the collective leadership system introduced during and after Deng Xiaoping for Xi's centralized rule over China, making him the paramount leader of the country.[6] Xi Jinping's centralization of power through several institutional reforms has brought the party-state's military, security, foreign affairs, and economic and domestic issues directly under his control.[7] Xi led an anti-corruption campaign to strike against many powerful figures to regain Communist Party's credibility among the public. But apprehension exists among many that Xi Jinping is creating a cult of personality who removed the term limits of his presidency by revising the Chinese constitution. His accession to power in 2012 redirected Chinese foreign policy, where he combined new ideas (China Dream), new policies (comprehensive diplomacy and security), new institutions (AIIB) and new projects (BRI) to build a 'community of shared destiny'.[8] China has always criticized the current international system and international order as being Eurocentric or that is in favor of developed countries (US and European countries) therefore, it often asserts opposition to hegemonism. However, there is a larger question about whether China is seeking a Sino-centric network of economic, political and cultural relations or whether it's current policies have an internationally recognized legal and ethical legitimacy in their introduction of new ideas, norms and rules. Elizabeth Economy believes that Xi Jinping's "vision contains an implicit fear that an open door to Western political and economic ideas will undermine the power of the Chinese state".[9] The foundation of China's foreign relations, especially with Western countries, has always been on the basis of the 'five principles of peaceful coexistence, from Mao Zedong to Xi Jinping. Along with the five principles of peaceful coexistence, Xi Jinping also pursued forging a new form of international relations that featured mutual respect, fairness, justice, and win-win cooperation, as highlighted in the

2018 policy paper on EU.[10] The new generation of Chinese leaders, known as the 'fifth generation', that is headed by Xi Jinping, the President of the PRC and Chairman of the Central Military Commission (CMC), has put forth a series of important ideas and concepts for China's diplomacy in the new era such as the new type of big power relations. The concept was proposed in 2012 when Xi Jinping became the new leader, while emphasizing other ideas such as the two centenary goals which included building a community of common destiny, Chinese dream, national rejuvenation and Xi's pet project, the BRI.

> "Under the guidance of Xi Jinping Thought on Socialism with Chinese Characteristics for a New Era, China will stay committed to pursuing peaceful development, comprehensively deepening reform and breaking new grounds in opening-up on all fronts, and building a new type of international relations and a community with a shared future for mankind in order to create new opportunities for and make fresh contributions to world peace and development".[11]

The 'Thought on Socialism with Chinese Characteristics for a New Era' builds on and further 'enriches' Marxism-Leninism, Mao Zedong Thought, Deng Xiaoping Theory, the Theory of Three Represents, and the Scientific Outlook on Development and strives to achieve national rejuvenation.[12] In Xi's understanding, it is essential to have a peaceful environment for China to achieve national rejuvenation, where there is friendship and peaceful coexistence and mutual respect for each other in an international environment. China professes to pursue an independent foreign policy, free of foreign aggression and interference under any pretext and seeks common development. The BRI is one project that China claims will help develop countries and pursue common prosperity. Xi Jinping's BRI is an ambitious foreign and economic policy which aims to strengthen Beijing's economic leadership through deepening the integration of policy, infrastructure, trade, financial and people-to-people connectivity throughout Asia, Europe, Africa and other interested partnering countries, as enumerated in Xi's speech at the opening of the Belt and Road Forum in 2017. "Many foreign policy analysts view this initiative largely through a geopolitical lens, seeing it as Beijing's attempt to gain political leverage".[13] Peter Caiwho believes that Xi's BRI is crucial to the task of upgrading China's industry and exporting China's technological and engineering standards.[14] The BRI announced at the end of 2013 in Kazakhstan and Indonesia under the proposed project called the Silk Road Economic Belt and the 21st Century Maritime Silk Road, both of which falls under the Belt and Road Initiative.[15] The BRI is not just about increasing connectivity in infrastructure or for economic development but also includes deepening policy connectivity. The BRI aims to complement the development strategies of countries and promote complementarity between China's development plan and other countries that are part of the initiative.[16] A number of cooperation agreements on policy connectivity and action plans were signed between China and a number of countries.[17] This will not only lead to greater integration but will let China have more access into the policy implementation of major projects of other nations. The financial connectivity of the BRI involved multiple forms of financial cooperation between China and other countries part of the BRI, the AIIB, the Silk Road Fund and the 17+1 financial holding company between China and Central and Eastern European countries. Such cooperation has constructed these new financial mechanisms that complement existing financial institutions such as the World Bank.[18] Although China maintains that ambitious projects like the BRI is complementary in nature with the existing international institutions, at the same time China also questions the existing international order and sees the need to change it. The BRI as a whole is akin to another form of foreign policy because it incorporates the three pillars (political – social – economic) of China's relation with foreign countries: deepening policy connectivity, increase trade connectivity and strengthen people-to-people connectivity. Xi's effort in strengthening people-to-people connectivity through establishing the educational Silk Road and the health Silk Road, along with cooperation in science, education, culture, health and exchanges can be analyzed as how China sees its rejuvenation in terms of soft power, thereby maintaining close contact between people as the key to sound state-to-state relations.[19] Xi Jinping considers the BRI as a road to prosperity because he believes that development holds the master key to solving all problems.[20] It is interesting to note that William Callahan stressed that through the BRI, Beijing seeks to deepen connectivity in the regional countries by developing shared beliefs and norms that will build the 'community of shared destiny' which is a Sino-centric regional order.[21] This Sino-centric regional order takes inspiration from Chinese traditional idea of peripheral diplomacy that assumes Beijing at the center of the new regional order, while neighboring countries are at the margins.[22] This is part of Xi Jinping's strategy to rework the norms, rules, and institutions of global governance that is presently seen as the Western-led liberal order to a Chinese-style globalization.[23] A question that arises then is that with Xi defying the existing rule-based international order, one that is supported by and upheld by the European Union (EU), how will this in turn alter the power balance between China and the EU. The current international order that has kept the balance between various nations for decades has to now deal with Beijing's economic power backing up its aspired alternative world order, one that will presumably hinder European security, norms, beliefs and the foundations of its institutions. However, the EU's response, pertaining to safeguarding its economic interest and in making credible policies among the 27 European countries has been weak. Moreover, China's increasing leverage in some EU member states has moved the latter to block EU criticism of China's human rights record.[24] With China's increasing assertiveness in its geopolitics, the relations between China and the EU has turned sore. Evidently, EU not only labelled Beijing as an "economic competitor" but as a "systemic rival promoting alternative models of governance".[25] However, according to Ian Bond, "EU made no proposals for how it could resist the systemic challenge or promote its own values in response. Yet it must."[26]

The 'Unhealthy' New Silk Road

The year 2020 will be remembered as one of the most challenging times in human history. The COVID-19 pandemic has devastated lives, crippled economies, and brought the world to a standstill. While the virus was detected in December 2019 in Wuhan, where the virus originated, debates regarding how China handled the pandemic in its early stage and whether it should be held responsible for all the damages the pandemic caused around the world is an ongoing issue. Furthermore, questions arise whether the pandemic has changed the nature of China's relation with its foreign counterpart. In particular, China's relation with the EU has been facing various issues along with the pandemic. Although President of the European Council, Charles Michel spoke of the necessity and opportunity that he sees in engaging and cooperating with China, he recognizes that the EU does not share the same values, political systems, or approach to multilateralism.[27] Amid these issues, the EU is faced with increasing number of cases of people infected with the COVID-19 virus. Some of the worst hit pandemic countries in the world include many European countries as the virus continued to sweep across Europe. The number of cumulative cases of COVID-19 and cumulative death in Europe is shown in Figures 12.1 and 12.2. As the Figures indicates, there is a steep increase in both cumulative cases and cumulative deaths from March till June.

Figure 12.1: Number of Cumulative Cases of COVID-19 in the EU member States' Nations

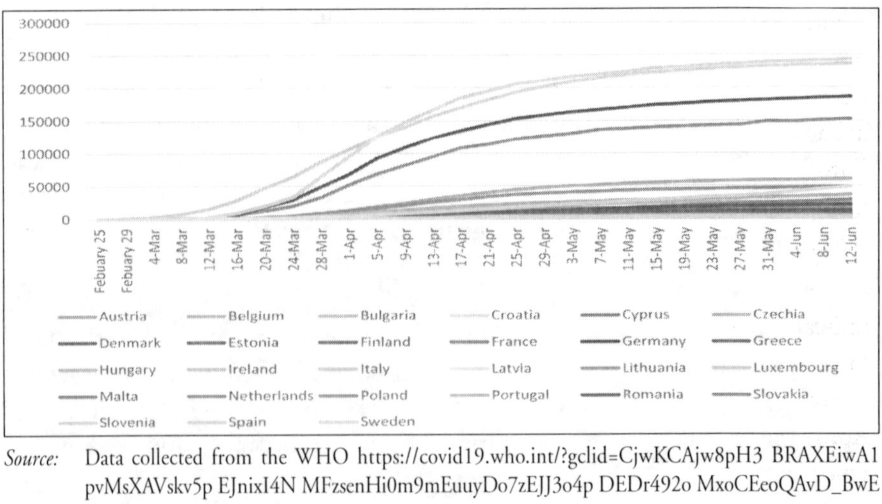

Source: Data collected from the WHO https://covid19.who.int/?gclid=CjwKCAjw8pH3 BRAXEiwA1 pvMsXAVskv5p EJnixI4N MFzsenHi0m9mEuuyDo7zEJJ3o4p DEDr492o MxoCEeoQAvD_BwE

Figure 12.2: Number of Cumulative Deaths Caused by COVID-19 in the EU Member States' Nations

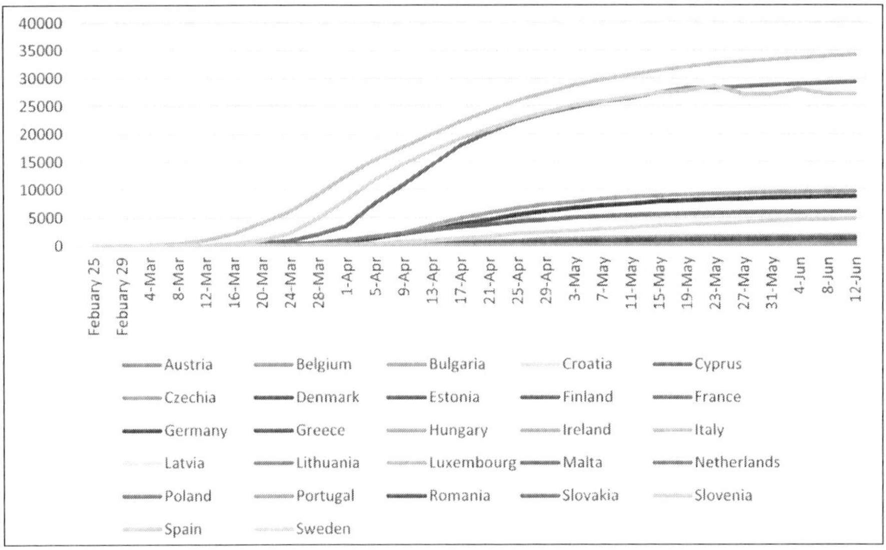

Source: Data collected from the WHO https://covid19.who.int/?gclid=CjwKCAjw8pH 3BRAX Eiw A1pv MsXAVskv5pEJnixI4NMFzsenHi0m9mEuuyDo7zEJJ3o4p DEDr 492oMxo CEeoQAvD_BwE

As the pandemic continued to sweep across Europe, the number of cases continued to rise. It has not only become a significant challenge for the EU to collaborate, but the EU has also shown weaknesses in responding immediately to the needs of the situation under the pandemic. The pandemic not only caused substantial damages in all the European countries but more so, the pandemic has caused far-reaching damages to some of the most populated and major economic centers. For instance, the four hardest-hit European countries are, Spain, Italy, Germany and France which are the same four countries that detected the virus in late January, as shown in Table 12.1. Although there is no definite explanation of the origin of the virus in Europe, there are measures undertaken to curb the spread of virus. At present, these four European countries have overtaken China in the number of COVID-19 cases, indicating the severity of the situation.

Figures 12.3, 12.4, 12.5, and 12.6 shows the four hardest-hit European countries indicating that in all these countries, the cases of COVID-19 in February was lower with a sudden rise in late March. The highest increase in the number of cumulative cases and deaths due to the pandemic in these four countries was in April, May and June as shown in Figure 12.3, 12.4, 12.5, and 12.6 below. As reported, Europe in early April remained the epicenter of the coronavirus pandemic

Table 12.1: Detection of COVID-19 cases in the European Countries

Name of EU member states	*First COVID-19 entry date*	*Latest COVID-19 Cumulative Case on June 14, 2020*	*Latest COVID-19 Cumulative Death on June 14, 2020*
France	24/01/2020	152460	29335
Germany	28/01/2020	186269	8787
Finland	29/01/2020	7087	325
Italy	29/01/2020	236651	34301
Spain	31/01/2020	243605	27136
Sweden	31/01/2020	50931	4874
Belgium	04/02/2020	59918	9650
Austria	25/02/2020	17014	677
Croatia	25/02/2020	2251	107
Greece	26/02/2020	3112	183
Romania	26/02/2020	21679	1391
Denmark	27/02/2020	12139	597
Estonia	27/02/2020	1973	69
Netherlands	27/02/2020	48640	6057
Lithuania	28/02/2020	1763	75
Czechia	01/03/2020	9991	329
Ireland	01/03/2020	25295	1705
Luxembourg	01/03/2020	4063	110
Latvia	02/03/2020	1097	28
Portugal	02/03/2020	36463	1512
Hungary	04/03/2020	4064	559
Slovenia	04/03/2020	1492	109
Poland	05/03/2020	29017	1237
Slovakia	06/03/2020	1545	28
Malta	07/03/2020	646	9
Bulgaria	08/03/2020	3266	172
Cyprus	09/03/2020	980	18

Source: Data collected from the WHO https://covid19.who.int/?gclid=CjwKCAjw8pH3 BRAXEiw A1pvMs XAVskv5pEJnixI4 NMFzsenHi0m9mEuuyDo7zEJJ3o4p DEDr492o MxoCEeo QAvD_BwE

with nearly 50,000 dead and more than 600,000 infected.[28] In Spain, the total number of Coronavirus cases has reached 293,352 with no recovery cases[29] while Italy has reached 238,499 cases, Germany has reached 192,119 and France with 160,750 cases. These four European countries are also one of the largest economies in the EU with substantial influence outside Europe. As the situation in this region became worse, the respective governments introduced new measures to curb the virus from spreading, such as calling for national lockdowns, freezing international travels and brought new regulations to stay under quarantine.

Figure 12.3: Spain with the highest number of cumulative cases and deaths of COVID-19

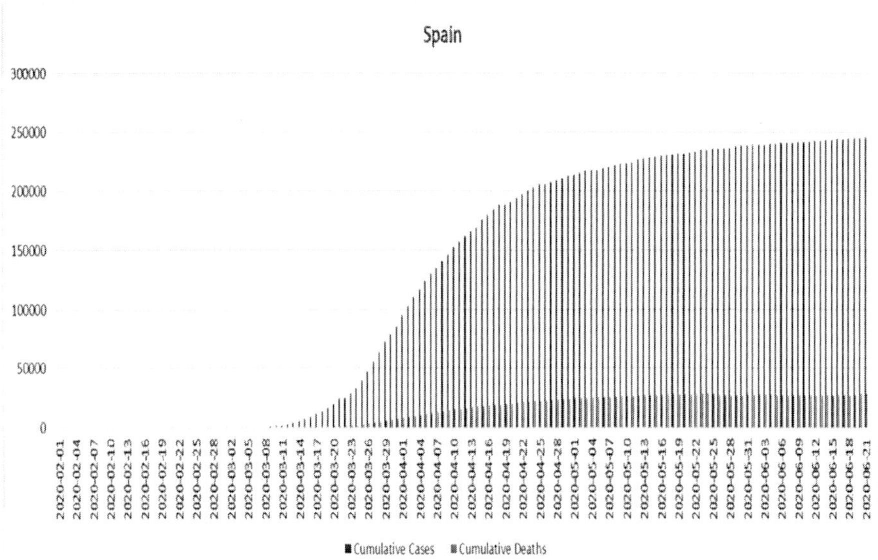

Source: Data collected from the WHO https://covid19.who.int/?gclid=CjwKCAjw8pH3 BRAXEiwA1pv MsXAVskv5pEJnixI4NMFzsenHi0m9mEuuyDo7zEJJ3o4p DEDr492o MxoCEeoQAvD_BwE

Figure 12.4: Italy with second highest number of cumulative cases and deaths of COVID-19

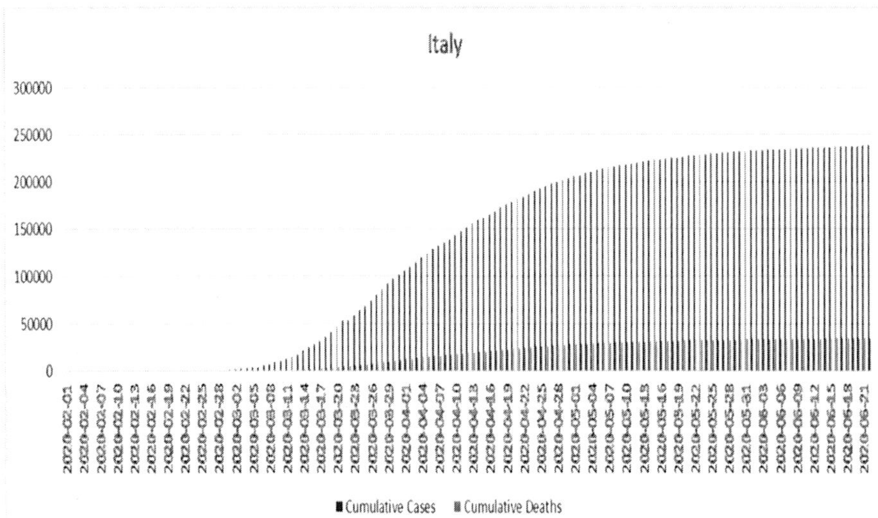

Source: Data collected from the WHO https://covid19.who.int/?gclid=CjwKCAjw8pH3 BRAXEiwA1 pvMsXAVskv5pEJnixI4NMFzsenHi0m9mEuuyDo7zEJJ3o4pDEDr492o MxoCEeoQAvD_BwE

Figure 12.5: Germany with third highest number of cumulative cases and deaths of COVID-19

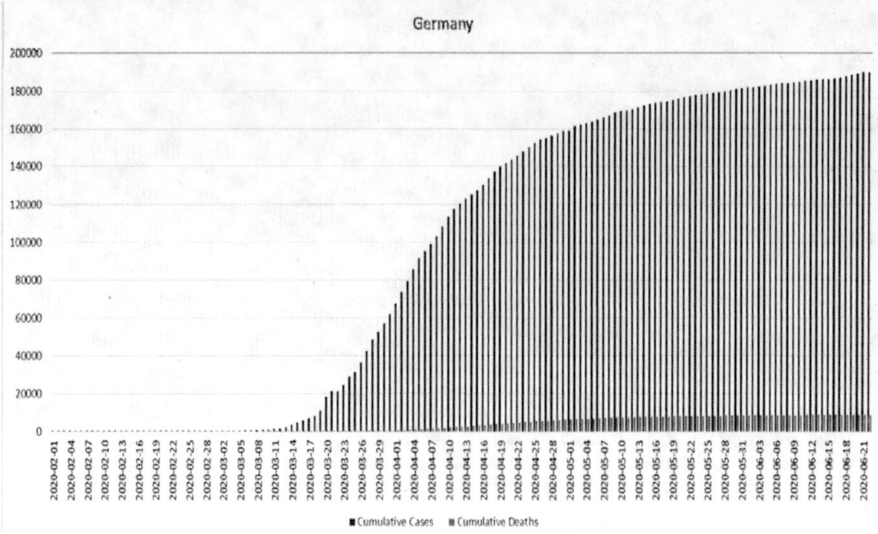

Source: Data collected from the WHO https://covid19.who.int/?gclid=CjwKCAjw8pH3 BRAXEiw A1 pvMsXAVskv5pEJnixI4NMFzsenHi0m9mEuuyDo7zEJJ3o4pDEDr492o MxoCEeoQAvD_BwE

Figure 12.6: France with fourth highest number of cumulative cases and deaths of COVID-19

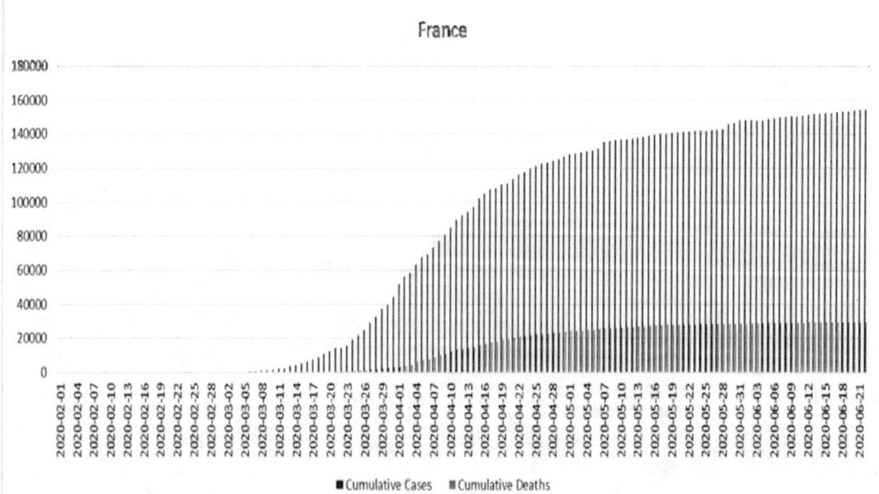

Source: Data collected from the WHO https://covid19.who.int/?gclid=CjwKCAjw8pH3 BRAXEiwA1pv MsXAVskv5pEJnixI4NMFzsenHi0m9mEuuyDo7zEJJ3o4pDEDr492o MxoCEeoQAvD_BwE

As the pandemic continued to sweep across Europe, the respective domestic governments of each European country have imposed national lockdowns to curtail the widespread propagation of the virus. Due to the rapidly spreading nature of the COVID-19 cases in Europe, it was expected of the EU to provide the necessary emergency assistance to the pandemic hit European nations. However, when the EU failed in its capacity to make a collective decision to immediately provide medical assistance, or curtail the widespread pandemic by closing borders or imposing lockdowns to minimize the damage, it was the European nations and its leaders who took care of the situation individually. The chaos that the pandemic brought has not only wrecked the EU's stability, but has also seen European governments misleading Brussels about their preparedness, then hoarded essential equipment and haphazardly shut their borders, disrupting commerce and stranding citizens.[30] The EU's initial response towards stabilizing the situation inside Europe has been weak, leaving the task to individual nations and leaders. This, according to Abhimanini Sawhney, indicates a significant deviation from the EU's usual policy of transnational cooperation and regional collaboration which resulted in excessive strain on the medical and healthcare resources of nations like Italy and Spain.[31] While the outbreak of the COVID-19 pandemic in EU nations was detected in late January and in early February (see Table 12.1), EU's collective response to the pandemic only began in March through setting up of a Coronavirus response team–led by five commissioners. The Union also instituted a "Coronavirus Response Investment Initiative," to mobilise funds for national healthcare systems, set up SURE (Support mitigating Unemployment Risks in Emergency) to protect unemployment, launched program like the Pandemic Emergency Purchase Programme (PEPP) worth €750 billion to counter the monetary risks and introduced various other initiatives and programmes to reduce the spread of virus and ensure stability within the EU.[32]

However, with the absence of EU's immediate response to the outbreak of the pandemic in Europe, especially in countries like Italy and Spain where the number of infected cases of pandemic kept increasing, the situation opened the door for other nations to step in. China in particular took the opportunity in providing medical assistance to Italy and Spain. China's first team arrived on March 12 in Rome with essential medical supplies and equipment and later helped the hard-hit Spain with the same resources.[33] However, Chinese increasing influence via its 'medical assistance' that is termed 'medical diplomacy' was received with suspicion and resentment. It was reported that politicians in Berlin, Paris, London and Brussels were expressing concern over Beijing's narrative on COVID-19, which hints at a deeper resentment against Beijing.[34] The growing Chinese presence in Europe via its medical supplies has given China a greater foothold in Europe and has furthered its BRI agenda, which may potentially compromise the EU's broader strategic interests. The Chinese State Councilor and Foreign Minister Wang Yi pointed out that China's assistance towards countries including Spain demonstrated "the international humanitarian spirit and the concept of a community with a shared future for mankind, with no extra political conditions or geopolitical private interests".[35] This is clearly a strong indication of China's response to the growing insecurity of the EU leaders to Beijing's overtures.

Furthermore, Beijing's engagement with the world community through its own initiatives like the BRI has been seen focusing on advancing China's international prestige and its national interest. In recent years, one of the highpoints of China's EU strategy has been Beijing's active engagement with its 17+1 group during the pandemic, a move that has attracted speculation from various quarters.[36] The EU is on alert due to the increasing Chinese presence through its growing investment and financial groupings like the 17+1 between China and Central and Eastern European countries. The 17+1 grouping include 12 EU member states – Estonia, Latvia, Lithuania, Poland, the Czech Republic, Slovakia, Hungary, Romania, Bulgaria, Croatia, Slovenia and Greece – and five aspiring members – Serbia, Bosnia and Herzegovina, Montenegro, Albania and North Macedonia. In a sign of according greater significance to this development, President Xi Jinping replaced Li Keqiang as the host for the 2020 'Cooperation between China and Central and Eastern European Countries' meeting. The cooperation initiative, that was previously called 16+1 initiative between China and 16 Central and Eastern European Countries (CEEC), had Greece joining in April 12, 2019.[37] Observers remarked that Xi's presiding over the 2020 CEEC meeting is evidence of Beijing deepening its relations with the European countries amid rising tensions between China and the US. There always seems to be a spillover effect of China's rivalry with the US over Europe. Although China claims that the initiative is not intended to weaken the EU, Wang Yiwei, a professor of international relations at the Renmin University of China in Beijing, states that the European countries are part of the initiative not only because of economic reasons but also because of the leverage that China has over the EU.[38] Noting China's growing presence in the EU, the 2019 Joint Communication specified that "in cooperating with China, all Member States, individually and within sub-regional cooperation frameworks, such as the 16+1 format, have a responsibility to ensure consistency with EU law, rules and policies".[39] The indication of the EU's frustration against Beijing's 17+1 group is evident while China continues to be engaged in the delivery of medical supplies to targeted regions in Europe amid the pandemic. Although Zhang Ming, head of the Chinese Mission to the EU, said the fight against the virus had nothing to do with the social system or geopolitics,[40] there are rising apprehensions against Chinese activities in some parts of Europe during the pandemic and it is seen as an extension to the BRI, which is also termed "the Health Silk Road".

Although Chinese investment in the European region has been critically viewed, some European countries including Hungary, Poland, Greece, Portugal, Luxembourg, and Italy have already joined the BRI. In fact, Italy is now the first G7 nation and one of the founding members of the EU to sign up to the trade initiative. However, other European leaders have expressed their dissatisfaction and concern over Chinese investment in regions that are strategically and commercially important links within European states. The EU has been reviewing its China policy and making members aware of the national security risk posed by foreign investment in critical assets, technologies and infrastructure. German Chancellor Angela Merkel, French President Emmanuel Macron and European Commission President Jean-Claude Juncker all signaled that China should further open its markets before they consider joining the BRI. Shannon Tiezzi observed that the BRI is more symbolic than substance and that there is no guarantee of increase in Chinese investments as seen in the case of Poland (the first European country to support the BRI) after its backing failed to yield expected rise in Chinese funds.[41]

Despite the EU's growing concern, Xi Jinping expects that more European countries will join in the project. It was argued that the primary purpose behind the win-win economic opportunities the BRI provides for various countries is to use China's economic leverage to build a network of new institutions, new ideas, new projects to build a Sino-centric 'community of shared destiny', which will in turn make China a normative power that sets rules for a new global governance.[42] China reiterates that it is against using force or coercive methods in international relations yet issues that it deems are against its core interests have received aggressive reactions from Beijing in the past, ranging from threats of economic sanctions to international indictment. More importantly, Xi's consolidation of power has seen harsh crackdowns on various individuals and groups that raised issues regarding human rights and on various occasions European leaders have taken strong stands on these issues. For instance, President of France, Macron continues to raise concerns on the question of respecting fundamental rights in China particularly regarding China's oppression of the Uyghur ethnic group that has potentially irked Xi Jinping.[43] Taking EU as one of the most important partner in China's foreign relations, one of the key theme of Xi Jinping's foreign policy was comprehensiveness and coordination which is reflected in China-EU relations. While the BRI is portrayed as an inclusive project, several major countries such as the US, Western European countries (excluding Italy), Japan and India are absent from this plan.

However, the *Global Times* claims that China's achievement in the struggle against the COVID-19 pandemic has placed questions on Western democratic decision-making mechanisms and their belief in human rights without explaining how they purport to do so.[44] The question still remains, does Beijing intend to make its advancement at the expense of creating differences and division among the EU member countries. If Beijing's efforts to divide and rule in the EU is, in all sense, real and applied, the EU leadership might need to reconsider its partnership with Beijing and assess the 'Chinese threat' in order to safeguard EU's unity and stability. Interestingly, China has attempted to divert the EU's integration issues and its declining strength and international influence towards the handling of the pandemic. It is clear from both sides that competition will increase in the post-pandemic era but the question remains whether competition will exceed cooperation and how it will change the dynamics of China-EU relations.

China-EU rift amid COVID-19 pandemic

The China-EU relations before and after the pandemic present two different pictures. The positivity in China-EU relations in 2019 led toward the upcoming major summits that were on the 2020 agenda, namely, the China-Central and Eastern European Countries Summit, the 22nd EU-China Summit, and a special Leipzig EU-China Summit. The Chinese Academy of Social Sciences in late 2019 reported that the EU-China relations showed a steady trend of improvement, emphasizing that EU-China cooperation has a solid foundation, and their cooperation mechanisms are becoming increasingly mature.[45] However, right before the spread of the COVID-19 pandemic, the nature of China-EU relations took a shift after the EU labeled Beijing as "economic competitor and a systemic rival promoting alternative models of governance".[46] It was the EU's most critical response to Beijing issued in early 2019. The Joint Communication by the European Commission set out a 10-point action plan to establish a more balanced relationship with China. As reflected in the Communication, Beijing's growing presence, political influence and its global ambition to lead, has caused a rift between China and the EU. Interestingly, Yang Fengmin, Director of the European Institute at East China University of Science and Technology, writes that the EU does not have the intention to become a global hegemon and that it is not a cause for any serious political obstacles between the EU and China.[47] Does that mean China truly sees itself moving towards its global ambition to lead and, since the EU does not pose a challenge, it would lead to a stable relationship? In Beijing's quest for its global ambition to lead, the US poses a more forceful competitor to China than Europe. For instance, Wang Yiming, researcher at Renmin University notes that the 2019 EU's Strategic Communication on China is the offshoot of the US pressuring the EU to adjust its perception of China and to be more assertive.[48] The negative perception of China is prevalent in the EU as well as among European policy makers and European members. This negative perception, seen in the form of Europe adopting more of an assertive approach, is a sign of the EU's wariness of China's increasing presence in the economically weaker Central and Eastern European countries, thereby undermining the EU solidarity.[49]

As a reaction against China's growing influence, an alliance was formed by senior lawmakers from eight democracies including the US to counter China. The Inter-Parliamentary Alliance on China (IPAC) was launched on June 5, 2020 to foster deeper collaboration between like-minded legislators to work towards reforms on how democratic countries should approach China. One of the purpose of the inter-parliamentary alliance was to work towards making sure China upheld the standards of the international order, including upholding human rights values.[50] While announcing the formation of the alliance, the US senator from Florida, Marco Rubio noted that, "China, under the rule of the Chinese Communist Party represents a global challenge".[51] The global resentment against China's Sino-centric regional order under Xi Jinping has been in the spotlight during the COVID-19 pandemic. China's handling of the coronavirus to constantly being involved in bullying as well as threatening countries economically and politically has put it under global scrutiny. As mentioned earlier, there is also an increasing concern from Europe (especially from the Western European countries) on the growing geopolitical power and assertiveness from China. Incidentally, a historic meeting between Xi Jinping and EU leaders that was supposed to be held in September has been postponed indefinitely.[52] Josep Borrell, EU's foreign affairs chief, shared the view that "COVID-19 pandemic could be seen as a turning point in the power shift from West to East" and has also pointed out that the "current relations between Brussels and Beijing weren't always based on trust, transparency and reciprocity".[53] Despite the trust deficiency in China-EU relations, the significance of the relationship was maintained, if not increased, due to various reasons including China's trade war with the US, the bilateral investment agreement between China and the EU, the meeting between Xi Jinping and the European heads of state in Leipzig, Germany and in the China-EU Summit. Moreover, it has been argued in a report by the Chinese Academy of Social Sciences in May 2020 that it is in the interest of both sides to maintain a good and stable Sino-European relation.[54]

The significance of China-EU partnership entails cooperation at various levels, namely, the political, economic and cultural or people-to-people exchange which was enumerated in China's EU policy paper of 2003 and in every consecutive policy paper thereafter. President Xi Jinping notes that the EU has been China's largest trading partner for 14 years in a row and China has been the EU's second largest trading partner. Developing a sound relationship with the EU has long been a foreign policy priority for China, which was recently highlighted by Zhang Ming, head of the Chinese Mission to the EU. Celebrating the 45th anniversary of the establishment of China-EU diplomatic ties on May 6, Zhang expressed the damage the COVID-19 pandemic had caused for the international community.[55] However, he left out how the pandemic posed an unprecedented challenge for its political systems. In one revealing case, as reported by Matt Apuzzo of The New York Times, the Chinese government threatened the EU officials for documenting its push on spreading disinformation about the COVID-19 pandemic.[56] Beijing's threat not only proved effective as, it was successful in quickly blocking the release of the document. However, Zhang Ming quickly denied engaging in such acts of disinformation and outright dismissed the speculation. Furthermore, China's Ministry of Commerce spokesperson, Gao Feng said, "China opposes distortion of facts, evading responsibilities and politicizing the COVID-19 battle."[57] He further remarked that the concerned countries and politicians should stop having a confrontation mentality against China amid the COVID-19 situation.[58]

The relationship continues to suffer after the outbreak of the COVID-19 and has exposed some fundamental differences between the two. Recently, in a revealing case, Yang Peng, a researcher from Beijing Center for Diseases Prevention and Control (Beijing CDC) claimed that the genome sequencing showed that the coronavirus came from Europe.[59] Additionally, Chinese experts argue that the pandemic was caused by imported seafood that was contaminated by the coronavirus in Europe before being delivered to China.[60] Earlier, a Chinese diplomat accused the American army for exporting the virus to China.[61] While an independent investigation into the origin of the virus has been called by many Western governments, an idea supported by the European Union as well, the diplomatic tensions over the origin of pandemic will nevertheless add to the rift between China and the EU.

While the diplomatic relationship between China and the EU deteriorated during and due to the COVID-19, there are various issues raised from "wolf warrior diplomacy" adopted by several Chinese officials to popular perception that China is responsible for the COVID-19 pandemic to issues surrounding "medical diplomacy". These all pointed towards what John Seaman, of the French Institute, called as China's public diplomacy gone into overdrive however well it appears coordinated, with varying degrees of dogmatism, divisiveness and moderation.[62]

China is a rising power, and it is increasingly a nation under construction in terms of building its image on a global stage. The fact that China hid the first cases of Coronavirus outbreak reveals that Beijing places its national interest before its citizens. Therefore, human rights do not always appear in their agenda. For China, defending its national interest and its image has been the ultimate state priority. It is highly conscious of how it presents itself to the world, due to fear of losing face, Beijing went to extreme measure in blacklisting whistleblowers (most of whom are renowned doctors) who first spread the news about coronavirus despite the government crackdown. The Chinese diplomats have responded aggressively to global criticism for its handling of the pandemic.

The pursuits behind Beijing flexing its diplomatic muscles in trying to divert global scrutiny over the origin of the virus, or how it has been handled poorly at the beginning, or defy any accusations towards the Chinese government, is tied to its larger foreign policy objectives. China's concern and its great challenge is seemingly in guarding its international image or convey a moral upright and ethical China to a global community using both covert and overt tactics. China used the pandemic to display its normative power while the government has been suspected of engaging in systematic propaganda and disinformation campaign.[63] In fact, the EU foreign policy chief accused China of trying to create differences among the EU members. The European chief explicitly shared the view that publicity and politicization of COVID-19 pandemic campaign should be avoided.

The Perennial Issues of Human rights, Tibet and Taiwan between China and EU

During the COVID 19 pandemic, the issues of Tibet and Taiwan resurfaced between China and the EU. Despite the changing relationship between the two entities, the decades' long discussion and disagreement between them on these problematic matters continues to be a strain on their relationship. China's Jiang Duan, Minister Counselor at the Permanent Mission of the PRC, was appointed to the Human Rights Council's Consultative Group in April 2020 for a year long term. Jiang Duan will play a key role in selecting human rights investigators in various United Nations bodies.[64] Human rights activists around the world criticized the appointment, in particular its relation to the United Nations and the founding principles of the Organization. Given the recent occurrences of human right violations in China amid its crackdown on whistleblowers on the coronavirus pandemic, accusations have been leveled at the UN on its decision to appoint a representative from Beijing to oversee the UN's work on human rights.

Moreover, in the latest published report by Freedom House, which rated 210 countries and territories, Tibet was placed second on the list of the least free countries in the world after Syria for the fifth consecutive year.[65] The report by the Freedom

House revealed an intensification of State led pressure on civil liberties over the past few years, when censorship and surveillance reached new extremes.[66] On a more revealing note, the Human Rights Watch on March 5, published a report on China's bilingual education policy in Tibet, highlighting that the policy has accelerated the demise of Tibetan-medium instruction in primary schools in Tibetan areas.[67] The report not only reveal the threats faced by the Tibetan language under the guise of improving access to education, but it also exposed the underneath state propaganda unleashed in the name of "strengthening the unity of nationalities".[68] Sophie Richardson, who heads the China section, concludes that China's bilingual education policy is motivated by political imperatives rather than educational ones. She accused the Chinese government for violating its international legal obligations to provide Tibetan-language instruction to Tibetans. The Tibetan language activist Tashi Wangchuk was also arrested in 2016 and charged with inciting separatism. The demolition of monasteries in Tibet continues, while the rising number of self-immolations against the repressive policies endures. All these reports on human rights violations was released during the outspread of coronavirus around the world.

An important development between China and Czech Republic unfolded during the time when China's economic and political strength was hit by the COVID-19 pandemic. Calling China an "unreliable partner", the mayor of Prague urged other European members to be cautious as well. On January 12, 2020 Zdenek wrote that he could not sign an agreement that forced Prague to "speak out against the independence of Tibet and Taiwan".[69] However, Prague's termination of its relations with Beijing is not only unanticipated but rather a bold move played by the local city government. Apparently, Beijing's sister-city partnership with Prague ended when the city refused to commit to the "One China" policy. The One China policy is an obligation that Beijing adamantly makes on all the countries while establishing relations with them. The policy is a basis of legitimacy asserted by the PRC to denote that both Taiwan and Tibet belong to a single entity, the PRC. The Chinese government, in fact, condemned Prague for violating the One China policy and China's core interest. While Prague Mayor Zdenek Hrib approached Taiwan on the ground that both nations share democratic values and respect fundamental human rights and cultural freedom, he also criticized Chinese policies in Tibet. Prague's stand on these issues, despite the probability of losing much vaunted Chinese business is an oddity in International Relations where many other countries have agreed to Beijing's demands when establishing economic relations with it.

Both Tibet and Taiwan issues have been major factors, playing an important role in European countries relations with China, and in this case Czech's relation with China. With China's economic expansion as well as political commitment, a greater number of countries are increasingly bandwagoning with Beijing, evidently seen with the recent visit of Xi Jinping to Nepal and Myanmar.

China is aggressively moving towards realizing Xi's vision of a "rejuvenated China", and it's "China Dream" of reclaiming its supposed seat at the head of the table of nation states. Its economic and political policies is reflected in its ambitious BRI, the ADB, the SCO, the RECP deal and its increasing influence in the south east Asian CPTPP agreement. As the country attempts to secure its paramount position as well as securitize its internal differences with regard to Tibet, Xinjiang and Taiwan by receiving the acquiescence of other countries to its claims, Prague's stand on rejecting Beijing's political and economic clout by standing in solidarity with global norms of democracy and freedom is perhaps a testament to a new approach to international relations, one where normative questions of human rights and freedom seem to take precedence over the material issues of economics.

Conclusion

Following the outbreak of the COVID-19 pandemic, Beijing quickly moved towards securing its image, both internationally and domestically. China responded by sending its medical teams to Iran, Iraq, Italy, Serbia and Cambodia, claiming that the government has provided 83 countries and international organizations with emergency assistance to tackle the pandemic.[70] Through such goodwill, Beijing not only hopes to garner positive responses to its global image, but strategically influence the emotions of the people of these countries. Italy in particular has been severely hit by the pandemic and Beijing was quick to seize the opportunity to downplay the role of the EU and European countries. In fact, Chinese media platforms quickly made and circulated a video of Italians praising Chinese generosity.[71] There is a perception, in that China has gained much ground in creating a global image, one defined by generosity, benevolence and sympathy during the COVID-19 pandemic coupled with strong diplomatic influence at the international level.

On the other hand, the outbreak of the COVID-19 pandemic, nonetheless, has increased global attention and scrutiny over China's policies. Using both overt and covert tactics, Beijing was able to pressure foreign officials whose opinions went against its policies. Beijing seems adamant to use the pandemic as a platform to exhibit its diplomatic muscle, particularly its soft power diplomacy. These incidents might have increased China's leverage, but they do not necessarily translate into favorable perceptions because there are limitations to China's soft power due to rising skepticism from world leaders and communities on China's handling of the COVID–19 pandemic.

In a fund-raising effort spearheaded by the EU that brought many countries around the world to pledge their contributions in an effort to develop a vaccine to stop the virus, China has made no financial pledge despite the fact that the pandemic that spread from Wuhan has brought immense disaster around the world.[72] China's lack of transparency, suspicious death toll rate, refusing to allow international experts, blocking Chinese scientists from probing the origin of the disease, threatening officials for documenting the Chinese government's push in spreading disinformation about the COVID–19 pandemic and its approach towards cutting Taiwan off from the World Health Assembly as an observer has added to the global suspicion.[73] Several countries now want an inquiry into the roles of both WHO and China, with China being increasingly belligerent in its response to such demands. China's proactive public diplomacy amid COVID-19 pandemic indicates that Beijing is using all its might and force to protect its national interest, continues to expand its reach and promote the success story of China's fight against COVID-19 and countering narratives critical of China, thereby solidifying its position inside and outside China.

The geopolitical leverage via the BRI is an attempt to not only export China's ideals, ideology and belief but it is also an attempt to gain more political and economic leverage, with Europe being seen as an important partner in this equation. When Italy was severely hit by the pandemic and China came forth with its assistance, the Italian Prime Minister was quoted saying, "China has come to us in our hour of need", thereafter the camaraderie extended to Italy becoming the first G-7 member country to sign with China a memorandum of understanding to jointly advance the construction of the China-proposed BRI.[74] While China's "medical diplomacy" might have succeeded in promoting its soft power in few targeted regions, others interpret the new confrontational approach as the "wolf-warrior diplomacy."[75] It is a new approach adopted by the Chinese officials that is more assertive and proactive, and a transition of Chinese diplomacy from conservative, passive and low-key.

In a nutshell, 2019 saw China being put under pressure and questioned for its internal policies towards its ethnic minority communities in Tibet and Xinjiang while the large-scale protests in Hong Kong revealed the insecurity of Beijing with regard to its "One country, Two System" arrangement. Similarly, China's BRI initiative as well as border issues with India, Japan and the rest of South East Asia saw it being flanked on multiple sides. The COVID–19 pandemic brought an immediate blanket cover on all these issues and the global world shifted its entire focus on dealing with the situation, so much so that China received positive adulation from WHO and even President Trump for its role during the initial spread of the disease[76]. The present situation, five months after China closed down the Wuhan region, is very different. The US is increasingly turning antagonistic towards Beijing while a large section of the global community has started to view Xi's policies with great apprehension. Furthermore, the Hong Kong protests has picked up steam again due to China's new proposed legislation that threatens to strip away at the already failing Hong Kong autonomy, while its coercive stance towards Taiwan has brought the Cross-Strait relations under rising pressure. 2020 may have started off well for China's foreign policy and as a shield for its internal maneuvers but it seems that the magic has worn off, revealing the foundational ruptures between Beijing's propagandist claims and the reality that it attempts to hide from the rest of the world.

NOTES

1 Wang Zhengxu and Zeng Jinghan, "Xi Jinping: the game changer of Chinese elite politics?" *Contemporary Politics*, 22(4), (April 28, 2016) pp. 469-486 at https://www.tandfonline.com/doi/abs/10.1080/13569775.2016.1175098?journalCode=ccpo20

2 Ibid

3 Xi Jinping, "Secure a Decisive Victory in Building a Moderately Prosperous Society in All Respects and Strive for the Great Success of Socialism with Chinese Characteristics for a New Era", *Xinhuanet,* May 12, 2020 at http://www.xinhuanet.com/english/download/Xi_Jinping's_report_at_19th_CPC_National_Congress.pdf

4 Elizabeth C. Economy, "China's Imperial President, Xi Jinping tightens his grip", *Foreign Affairs,* 93(6), 80-86 at https://www.jstor.org/stable/24483923?seq=1

5 Mark J. Valencia, "As the world focuses on COVID-19, is China exploiting the distraction in the South China Sea? Only if you believe US propaganda", *South China Morning Post,* June 12, 2020 at https://www.scmp.com/comment/opinion/article/3081472/world-focuses-COVID-19-china-exploiting-distraction-south-china-sea

6 Ibid

7 Wang Zhengxu and Zeng Jinghan

8 William A Callahan, "China's "Asia Dream": The Belt Road Initiative and the new regional order", *Asian Journal of Comparative Politics*, 1(3): 226-243 at https://journals.sagepub.com/doi/abs/10.1177/2057891116647806

9 Elizabeth C. Economy, "China's Imperial President, Xi Jinping tightens his grip", *Foreign Affairs,* 93(6), 80-86 at https://www.jstor.org/stable/24483923?seq=1

10 Xi Jinping, "Secure a Decisive Victory in Building a Moderately Prosperous Society in All Respects and Strive for the Great Success of Socialism with Chinese Characteristics for a New Era", *Xinhuanet,* May 12, 2020 at http://www.xinhuanet.com/english/download/Xi_Jinping's_report_at_19th_CPC_National_Congress.pdf

11 China's Policy Paper on the European Union, "Mission of the People's Republic of China to the European Union", *Mission of the PRC to the EU,* April 10, 2020 at http://www.chinamission.be/eng/zywj/zywd/t1227623.htm

12 Xi Jinping, "Secure a Decisive Victory in Building a Moderately Prosperous Society in All Respects and Strive for the Great Success of Socialism with Chinese Characteristics for a New Era", *Xinhuanet,* May 12, 2020 at http://www.xinhuanet.com/english/download/Xi_Jinping's_report_at_19th_CPC_National_Congress.pdf

13 Peter Cai, "Understanding China's Belt and Road Initiative", *Lowy Institute for International Policy,*

March 22, 2017 at https://www.lowyinstitute.org/publications/understanding-belt-and-road-initiative

14 Ibid

15 "Full text of President Xi's speech at opening of Belt and Road forum", *Xinhuanet*, May 30, 2020 at http://www.xinhuanet.com/english/2017-05/14/c_136282982.htm

16 Ibid

17 Ibid

18 Ibid

19 Ibid

20 Ibid

21 William A Callahan, "China's "Asia Dream": The Belt Road Initiative and the new regional order", *Asian Journal of Comparative Politics*, 1(3) (May 16, 2016) : 226-243 at https://journals.sagepub.com/doi/abs/10.1177/2057891116647806

22 Ibid

23 Ibid

24 Helena Smith, "Greece blocks EU's criticism at UN of China's human rights record", *The Guardian,* March 14, 2020 at https://www.theguardian.com/world/2017/jun/18/greece-eu-criticism-un-china-human-rights-record

25 European Commission, "EU-China – A strategic outlook", *European Commission,* March 20, 2020 at https://ec.europa.eu/commission/sites/beta-political/files/communication-eu-china-a-strategic-outlook.pdf

26 Ian Bond, "Europe Must Stand Up to China Before It's Too Late", *Foreign Policy,* June 19, 2020 at https://foreignpolicy.com/2020/06/16/europe-must-stand-up-to-china-before-its-too-late/

27 European Council, "EU-China Summit: Defending EU interests and values in a complex and vital partnership - Press release by President Michel and President von der Leyen", *Council of European Union*, June 20, 2020 at https://www.consilium.europa.eu/en/press/press-releases/2020/06/22/eu-china-summit-defending-eu-interests-and-values-in-a-complex-and-vital-partnership/

28 David M. Herszenhorn and Sarah Wheaton, "How Europe failed the Coronavirus Test", *Politico,* June 20, 2020 at https://www.politico.eu/article/coronavirus-europe-failed-the-test/

29 Ibid

30 Ibid

31 Abhimanini Sawhney, "The potential fallouts of EU's collective response to COVID19", *ORF*, June 20, 2020 at https://www.orfonline.org/expert-speak/the-potential-fallouts-of-eus-collective-response-to-covid19-65619/

32 Ibid

33 Cui Mu, "COVID-19: China steps in to help Italy battle the virus", *DW*, June 20, 2020 at https://www.dw.com/en/COVID-19-china-steps-in-to-help-italy-battle-the-virus/a-52901560

34 Japan Times, "China's coronavirus diplomacy has finally pushed Europe too far", *The Japan Times*, June 20, 2020 at https://www.japantimes.co.jp/news/2020/04/22/asia-pacific/politics-diplomacy-asia-pacific/china-coronavirus-diplomacy-europe/#.XvCFeWgzbIU

35 "China to continue helping Spain fight COVID-19 epidemic: FM", *Xinhuanet*, June 20, 2020 at http://www.xinhuanet.com/english/2020-05/13/c_139051653.htm

36 Emilian Kavalski, "China's 16+1 is Dead? Long Live the "17+1", *The Diplomat*, June 20, 2020 https://thediplomat.com/2019/03/chinas-161-is-dead-long-live-the-171/

37 David Lee, "17+1 breaks myth of China wedge in Europe", *CGTN*, June 3, 2020 at https://news.cgtn.com/news/3d3d774e3345444d34457a6333566d54/index.html

38 Laura Zhou, "Chinese President Xi Jinping to take over as host of '17+1' summit with European leaders", *South China Morning Post*, June 2, 2020 at https://www.scmp.com/news/china/diplomacy/article/3044359/chinese-president-xi-jinping-take-over-host-171-summit

39 European Commission, "EU-China – A strategic outlook", *European Commission*, March 20, 2020 at https://ec.europa.eu/commission/sites/beta-political/files/communication-eu-china-a-strategic-outlook.pdf

40 EURACTIV Network, "Capitals Special Edition – How effective is China's 'mask diplomacy' in Europe?", *EURACTIV.com*, June 12, 2020 at https://www.euractiv.com/section/politics/news/capitals-special-edition-how-effective-is-chinas-mask-diplomacy-in-europe/

41 Shannon Tiezzi, "Xi Jinping in Europe: A tale of 2 countries", *The Diplomat*, June 30, 2019 at https://thediplomat.com/2019/03/xi-jinping-in-europe-a-tale-of-2-countries/

42 William A Callahan, 2016

43 Shannon Tiezzi, 2019

44 "2020 a critical year for China-EU relations after pandemic", *Global Times*, June 3, 2020 at https://www.globaltimes.cn/content/1187765.shtml>

45 Viviana Zhu, "EU-China: A Fairly Smooth Road Ahead" in "EU-China, Towards a Chinese Win", in Institut Montaigne's *China Trends*, June 11, 2020 at https://www.institutmontaigne.org/documents/china-trends/china-trends-5-EN-web.pdf

46 European Commission, March 20, 2020

47 Viviana Zhu, June 11, 2020

48 Ibid

49 Aryaman Bhatnagar, "Reset in EU-China relations tougher in a post Covid19 world", *Observer Research Foundation*, June 10, 2020 at https://www.orfonline.org/expert-speak/reset-in-eu-china-relations-tougher-in-a-post-covid19-world-65012/

50 IPAC, Inter-Parliamentary Alliance on China, May 30, 2020 at https://www.ipac.global/

51 SidharthShekhar, "To counter 'authoritarian' China, senior lawmakers from eight democracies unite to form new coalition", *Timesnownews.com*, July 5, 2020 at https://www.timesnownews.com/international/article/to-counter-authoritarian-china-senior-lawmakers-from-eight-democracies-unite-to-form-new-coalition/602799

52 Stuart Lau, "China trying to divide and rule in Europe, EU foreign policy chief Josep Borrell says", *South China Morning Post*, June 8, 2020 at https://www.scmp.com/news/china/diplomacy/article/3084684/china-trying-divide-and-rule-europe-eu-foreign-policy-chief

53 Associated Press, "EU's top diplomat calls for 'more robust' stance on China as US power starts to wane", *South China Morning Post*, May 30, 2020 at https://www.scmp.com/news/china/diplomacy/article/3085967/eus-top-diplomat-calls-more-robust-stance-china-us-power

54 Viviana Zhu, June 11, 2020

55 Xinhua, "More important than ever to keep China-EU relations in good shape: Chinese envoy", *Xinhua*, May 7, 2020 at http://www.xinhuanet.com/english/europe/2020-05/07/c_139036131.htm

56 Matt Apuzzo, "Pressured by China, E.U. Softens Report on COVID-19 Disinformation", *The New York Times*, May 30, 2020 at https://www.nytimes.com/2020/04/24/world/europe/disinformation-china-eu-coronavirus.html

57 CGTN, "China exports medical supplies to fight COVID-19", *CGTN*, June 11, 2020 at https://news.cgtn.com/news/2020-04-09/China-is-willing-to-provide-medical-supplies-to-other-countries-PycamD9Fny/index.html

58 Ibid

59 Liu Caiyu and Zhang Hui, "Source of Beijing cases renews speculation over COVID-19 origin", *Global Times*, June 20, 2020 at https://www.globaltimes.cn/content/1191679.shtml

60 Ibid
61 Maha Siddiqui, "China Faces International Pressure as India Joins 61 Nations to Seek 'On-site' Probe into COVID-19 Origin", *News18*, June 20, 2020 at https://www.news18.com/news/india/trouble-for-china-as-india-61-nations-to-seek-probe-into-coronavirus-crisis-2624579.html
62 Jamie Dettmer, "China's 'Wolf Warrior' Diplomacy Prompts International Backlash", *VOA*, June 20, 2020 at https://www.voanews.com/COVID-19-pandemic/chinas-wolf-warrior-diplomacy-prompts-international-backlash
63 Stuart Lau, "China trying to divide and rule in Europe, EU foreign policy chief JosepBorrell says", *South China Morning Post*, June 8, 2020 at https://www.scmp.com/news/china/diplomacy/article/3084684/china-trying-divide-and-rule-europe-eu-foreign-policy-chief
64 Marco Respinti, "U.N. Human Rights Council: More than 100 Organizations Protest China's Selection as a Member of the Consultative Group", *Bitter Winter*, June 7, 2020 at https://bitterwinter.org/china-and-un-human-rights-council/>
65 Freedom House, "Freedom House rates 210 countries and territories in Freedom in the World, and 65 countries in Freedom on the Net", *Freedom House*, April 6, 2020 at https://freedomhouse.org/countries/freedom-world/scores
66 Ibid
67 Human Rights Watch, "China's "Bilingual Education" Policy in Tibet", *Human Rights Watch*, April 6, 2020 at https://www.hrw.org/report/2020/03/04/chinas-bilingual-education-policy-tibet/tibetan-medium-schooling-under-threat
68 Ibid
69 Agence France-Presse, "Prague mayor hits out at 'unreliable' China, as Czech capital switches from Beijing to Taipei in twinning deal", *South China Morning Post*, February 14, 2020 at https://www.scmp.com/news/china/diplomacy/article/3045739/prague-mayors-hits-out-unreliable-china-czech-capital-swaps
70 CGTN, "COVID-19: China has provided emergency assistance to over 80 countries and organizations", *CGTN*, May 26, 2020 at https://news.cgtn.com/news/2020-03-26/COVID-19-China-provides-assistance-to-83-countries-organizations—Pauc1WnMPu/index.html
71 Theresa Fallon, "China, Italy, and Coronavirus: Geopolitics and propaganda", *The Diplomat*, May 26, 2020 at https://thediplomat.com/2020/03/china-italy-and-coronavirus-geopolitics-and-propaganda/
72 Matina Stevis-Gridneff and Lara Jakes, "World Leaders Join to Pledge $8 Billion for Vaccine as U.S. Goes It Alone", *The New York Times*, May 16, 2020 at https://www.nytimes.com/2020/05/04/world/europe/eu-coronavirus-vaccine.html
73 Lily Kuo, "Coronavirus outbreak: senior US official accuses China of lack of transparency", *The Guardian*, May 26, 2020 at https://www.theguardian.com/world/2020/feb/14/coronavirus-china-not-being-honest-says-us-as-wartime-measures-widened
74 Xinhua, "Spotlight: Italy, China stand together in joint fight against COVID-19", *Xinhua*, June 8, 2020 at http://www.xinhuanet.com/english/2020-05/27/c_139092441.htm
75 Zhu Zhiqun, "Interpreting China's 'Wolf Warrior Diplomacy'", *The Diplomat*, June 1, 2020 at https://thediplomat.com/2020/05/interpreting-chinas-wolf-warrior-diplomacy/
76 Xinhua, "China deserves appreciation for efforts, sacrifices in fighting epidemic: WHO chief", *Xinhua*, May 18, 2020 at http://www.xinhuanet.com/english/2020-02/16/c_138789289.htm

13

China-Japan Relations under COVID-19: Immunity of the Ties Tested Against the Virus

Amrita Jash

Introduction

Citing the coronavirus outbreak in Wuhan in China, on 17 January 2020, a confectionary shop in Hakone, in Japan's Kanagawa prefecture displayed at the storefront a sign board saying: "Chinese are banned from entering" and "I'd hate to have the virus scattered about (here)".[1] In justifying the 'ban', the owner of the shop stated: "I want to take measure to defend my shop against the Wuhan virus, so I don't want Chinese nationals to enter".[2] This reaction came in response to Japan's report of its first COVID-19 case in Kanagawa on 15 January. Such anti-Chinese sentiment if sparked further will be critical to China-Japan relations.

Given the logic of Japan's geographical proximity, intense people-to-people and economic exchanges with China – the virus spread in Japan should have been explosive. As noted in other affected countries such as Italy and the United States, the aging population has been most sensitive to the virus exposure. This very aspect of 'high elderly demographic' which constitutes over a quarter of Japanese population (as noted in Figure 13.1) in all likelihood, makes Japan more vulnerable to the COVID-19 outbreak than any of China's neighbours. However, surprisingly; in Japan, this scenario has been ruled out despite its aged population.

As of 30 April, total number of confirmed cases reported were 14,088 with total death toll of 415; and out of the 47 prefectures in Japan, 46 prefectures had reported cases of COVID-19. Wherein, Tokyo prefecture had the highest number with 4152 cases, followed by Osaka prefecture with 1625 cases. What adds to this trend, as noted by Japanese government is that 61 per cent of infections are those with unknown routes of transmission[4] – calling for an increasing rate of the daily risk of infection.

Figure 13.1: Population ages 65 and above (% of total population), 1960-2018

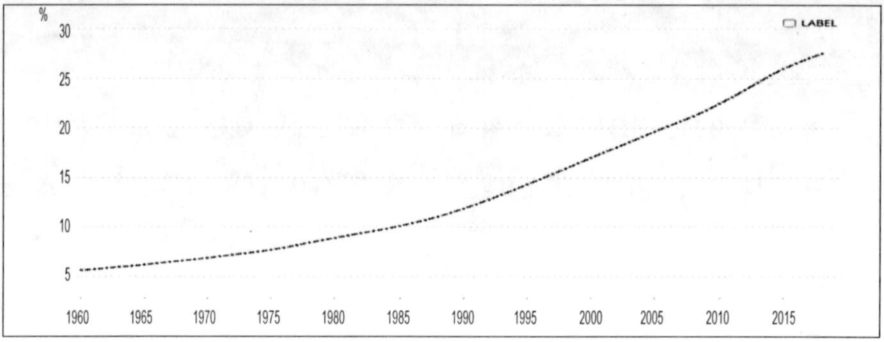

Source: The World Bank.[3]

With the rapid spread of the virus and the damages incurred, it becomes imperative to understand the consequences of the COVID-19 on China's ties with Japan. In view of this, the Chapter analyses the 'impact of COVID-19 on Japan' as the key indicator and determinant to provide a detailed assessment of the likely implications that will be witnessed in China-Japan ties under the COVID-19 effect. The nodal point of enquiry is to test: Whether Beijing-Tokyo ties will experience a de-coupling as witnessed in case of Beijing's ties with Washington. The centrality of the Chapter lies in examining two perspectives: First, has COVID-19 imposed a roadblock to the brimming Beijing-Tokyo bonhomie. Second, is there a possibility for the relations to witness a diplomatic upswing against the odds of the virus outbreak.

The Virus makes its way from Wuhan to Tokyo: Implications for Japan

In global transmission, Japan was the first country after China to be affected by COVID-19, but despite its highest percentage of aged population who are vulnerable to the virus, it failed to emerge as an epicentre as that of Italy or the United States. On 15 January, Japan's Ministry of Health, Labour and Welfare (MHLW) reported an imported case of laboratory-confirmed 2019-nCoV from Wuhan[5] – becoming the second country to report a confirmed case outside of China. In addition, at the initial stages of the global spread of the virus, Japan also reported the third-highest number of coronavirus cases after China and South Korea.

In Japan, the initial majority of the cases were reported in the port of Yokohama in the Diamond Princess cruise ship. Wherein, out of 3,711 passengers and crew, 712 (19.2 per cent) tested positive of the virus[6]-making it the largest cluster of cases outside China. Given the surge of infections, the ship was put under quarantine since 5 February in the event of a former passenger testing positive after disembarking in Hong Kong. The trajectory of the spread of COVID-19 are shown in Figures 13.2, 13.3 and 13.4.

Figure 13.2: Trend of daily coronavirus cases reported in Japan (until 18 May 2020)

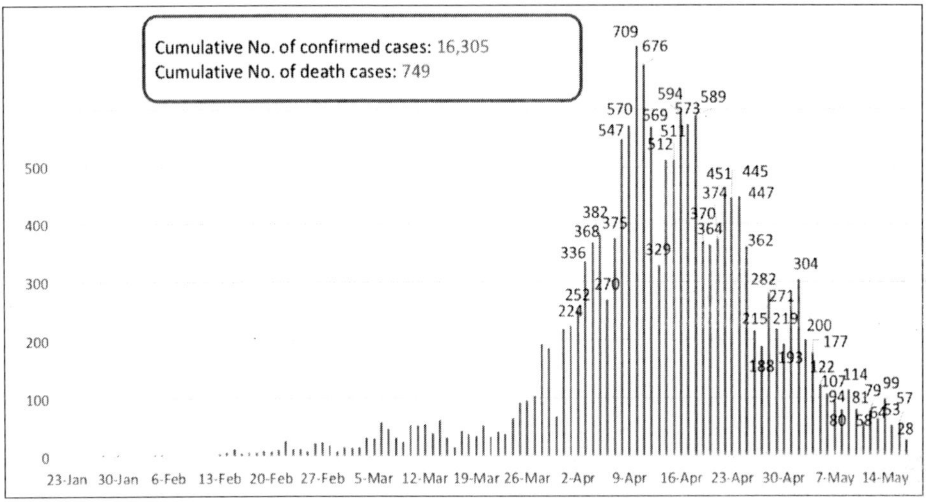

Source: MHLW, Japan.[7]

Figure 13.3: Trend of COVID-19 Outbreak in Japan (until 25 April 2020)

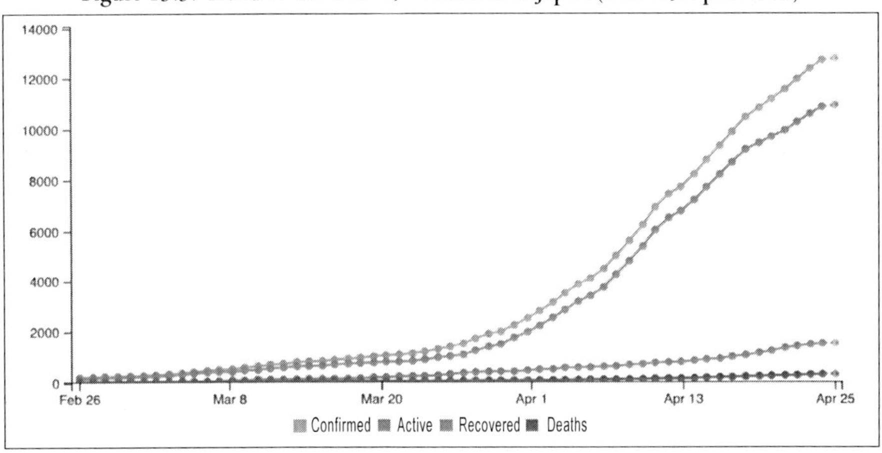

Source: Japan COVID-19 Coronavirus Tracker.[8]

Figure 13.4: Trajectory of COVID-19 Outbreak by Prefecture (> 100 Cases)

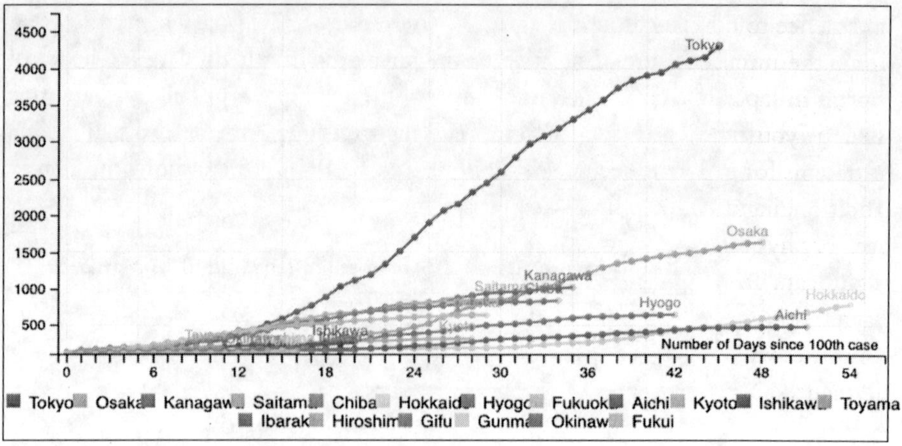

Source: Japan COVID-19 Coronavirus Tracker.[9]

What is noteworthy is that although Japan is not immune from the viral infection; but it still appears to be an exceptional case in the global mapping, despite its crowded cities and mainly, aged population.

Table 13.1: Record of COVID-19 in Japan (until 15 July 2020)

Parameters	*Numbers*
Infected in Japan	22081
Returnees from China on government Charter Flights	15
Cases Confirmed in Airport Testing	412
Total Infections	22508
Total Deaths	984
Total Recoveries	18545

Source: Adapted from Nippon.com (based on data collected from Japan's MHLW).[10]

From the above data combined with the global trajectory of the virus outbreak, it can be rightly stated that Japan appears to be an exception as compared to the other countries. This can be explained in a three-fold perspective: First, despite its geographical proximity to China, Japan has failed to exhibit a spike as witnessed in the viral outbreaks in China, South Korea, Italy and the United States. Second, although Japan was the second country to declare the virus infection, the trajectory of the viral outbreak remains to be comparatively low, mainly in terms of the extent of spread.[11] And third, the number of infections have increased but the mortality rate remains to be significantly low (as noted in Figure 13.2), when compared to China, United States, Italy, Iran, Spain, France, United Kingdom and South Korea. These exceptions have positioned Japan in a better place than most countries in 'flattening the curve'.

In Japanese view, social and cultural norms that impose self-discipline and obedience to official guidance are one of the reasons Japan has so far managed to limit the number of infections. As Kazuto Suzuki suggests that prevalent social norms in Japanese society such as: "you should not cause trouble to other people" and "if you don't take care of yourself and become ill, that is taken as causing problems for other people" – have led people to comply with strict controls.[12] In addition, ingrained Japanese habits such as handwashing and wearing of masks, the lack of physical contact habits such as handshakes and hugs are argued to have been significant in stemming the virus spread in Japan. In view of this, to correlate Japan's lower rate of infection to its lower rate of testing as compared to other countries will be faulty.[13] The details of Japan's testing of virus infections is noted in Figure 13.5.

Figure 13.5: Trend of the Capacity and the number of COVID-19 cases tested per day (until 16 May 2020)

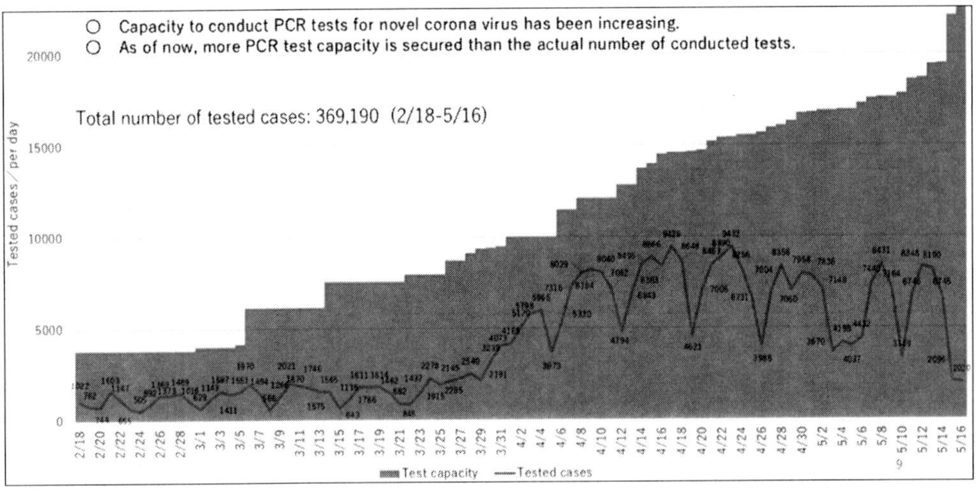

Source: MHLW, Japan.[14]

As noted, unlike other countries, Japan exhibits lower rate of mortality as well as lack of overwhelming of hospitals- further clarifying Japan's exceptionalism to COVID-19. However, although Japan has not faced a devastation as that of China, Italy and the United States, but this does not make COVID-19 less of a concern for the Japanese government. To note, in the past, Japan was one of the few Asian countries to be spared from the SARS epidemic in 2003; but under COVID-19, the situation in Japan is not the same.

While the number of overall cases is still relatively low; but unless the pace of increase is slowed, Japan could face the same situation as most affected countries. If not in numbers as compared to others, but for Japan the concern remains over the rise of cases at an alarming rate (as new cases are reported every day), with Tokyo showcasing a surge in cases. For instance, on 22 April, Costa Atlantica, an Italian cruise ship docked for repairs in Nagasaki carrying 623 crew members (with no passengers) reported 34 COVID-19 cases-making it the second such incident after the Diamond Princess.[15]

Like most affected countries other than China; in Japan too, the surge in infections is mainly argued to be the importation of cases from abroad. However, what has raised alarms is that in a growing number of cases the transmission route could not be traced. Acting on the situation, on 7 April, Japanese Prime Minister Shinzo Abe declared a "state of emergency" in accordance with article 32 of the Act on Special Measures, with effect in seven prefectures of Tokyo, Kanagawa, Saitama, Chiba, Osaka, Hyogo and Fukuoka.[16] However, taking stock of the severity with 200 new cases reported on one day (the highest figure to date), on 17 April Abe declared a nationwide state of emergency until 6 May.[17] Given this contingency, if not by striking numbers, COVID-19 has affected Japan's global aspirations, both significantly and symbolically. This is caused by the postponement of the Tokyo 2020 Olympics and Paralympics (set to run 24 July to 9 August and the Paralympics 25 August to 6 September) rescheduled for 23 July to 8 August 2021. Agreeing to the postponement over cancellation, Prime Minister Abe stated that Japan will fulfill its responsibility as the host nation "to prove that humanity has beaten the novel coronavirus".[18] This decision calls for both economic and political aftershocks for Japan given the outbreak caused at a critical time when Japan was planning an economic recovery.

With this, Japan's economy gets the hardest hit-faced with the "biggest crisis in post-war era", as stated by Abe.[19] For the Games were an opportunity to upswing Japan's staggering economy, the cancellation of which is argued to lead Japan into a full-blown recession- as the economic output in the last quarter of 2019 was down 7.1 percent. As Goldman Sachs estimates that Japan's economy will now contract at a 4.5 per cent rate in the first quarter and drop an additional 7.2 per cent in the second quarter.[20] With $12.6 billion as the final cost of hosting the Olympics,[21] the suspension cost is estimated to be $6 billion – almost a third of the entire cost.[22] Furthermore, what also adds to the monetary loss of Japan is the symbolic cost that is weighed by- the loss of opportunity in showcasing to the world a revitalised Japan after years of economic slowdown, and the loss of geopolitical primacy caused by being outranked as world second largest economy by China in 2010. It remains undisputable that for Japan to watch China's economic rise was far more uneasy than any other major country.

In addition, the economic burden on Japan is also affected by the hard hit tourism sector due to the viral outbreak. More specifically, Tokyo's over reliance on Chinese tourism further puts the economy at risk – mainly hurting consumption resulted from decline in Chinese tourists. To avert the economic crisis caused by the pandemic, Japanese government on 7 April (partly revised on 20 April) adopted its biggest-ever emergency economic package of $990 billion (108 trillion yen) equivalent to about 20 per cent of its gross domestic product (GDP).[23] But will Abe's stimulus policy help stabilise the economy remains questioned. As Takahide Kiuchi, executive economist at the Nomura Research Institute pointedly notes that – "[o]nly after the coronavirus issue is put to rest, most of the items pushing up GDP will be spent and exert an economic boost effect," [...] So the package will fail to offset the immediate negative impact stemming from the declaration of the state of emergency".[24]

But despite the economic downturn; Abe, unlike his ally Trump, has maintained restraint in criticising Beijing over its handling of the virus. On the contrary, unlike the United States, Australia, Singapore and other countries that imposed blanket ban on visitors from China, Japan restricted entry from only two provinces- Hubei and Zhejiang. In addition, Japan also was one of the first countries to fly aid packages especially personal protective equipment (PPE) to Wuhan. Tokyo's such an attitude has been helpful for Beijing but has created "doubts" over Abe's administration amongst Japanese- raising speculations over whether it is "appropriate for the nation".[25] This brings into perspective the impact of COVID-19 on Japan's political leadership, mainly the government's competency in dealing with the pandemic. With elections in 2021, Abe's voter support are showing signs of decline, as a poll published by Sankei newspaper showed support falling 8 percentage points to 36 per cent,[26] while conservative Yomiuri newspaper noted that 52 per cent of respondents were dissatisfied with Abe's handling of the virus spread.[27] These falling numbers are critically damaging to guarantee Abe's premiership in the upcoming elections. The query is: Will the sliding support push Abe to re-think Japan's China policy?

It appears that Japan's relations with China under COVID-19 seems to be largely immuned; however, the implications of the virus outbreak is creating a divide within Japan. To argue so, the increasing cases of infections have resulted into a political and economic instability in Japan, calling for the query: How long will Japan maintain its considerate behaviour towards China? As Noriyuki Kawamura have stated: "China's initial response to the virus was insufficient. [But] [t]he question is what Japan will do when those problems are exposed. Will it criticise China or close its eyes?".[28] However, so far, choosing reciprocity over animosity has been the choice between Tokyo and Beijing.

Beijing-Tokyo Ties: The Hits and Misses under COVID-19

China-Japan relationship is primarily characterised as 'hot economics, cold politics'. Wherein, the recent signs of thaw between the two countries reflect the adage that in international politics there are no permanent enemies or friends, just permanent interests. However, the thaw has been met with the COVID-19 crisis. But what is noteworthy is that the crisis hits the relationship at a time when the ties are both politically and economically much deeper than ever.

A. Diplomatic High-Tone

The most significant impact of the virus outbreak has been the postponement of Xi Jinping's state visit to Japan scheduled early April and no new date has yet been set. Xi's visit was proposed by Abe on the sidelines of the 2019 G20 Summit in Osaka, which also marked Xi's first visit to Japan. However, Xi's 2020 visit would have marked a major diplomatic event in Sino-Japanese ties as the first state visit by a Chinese leader to Japan since May 2008. Also reciprocal to Abe's visit 2018 visit to China that marked the first formal visit to Beijing by a Japanese leader in seven years.

Table 13.2: Chinese Leaders State Visit to Japan (1972 onwards)

Year	*Chinese Leaders Visiting Japan*
1980	Premier Hua Guofeng
1998	President Jiang Zemin
2008	President Hu Jintao

Source: Prepared by the Author.

Xi's visit would have marked the fourth state visit by a Chinese leader since 1972. The most important aspect of the visit was the Xi-Abe consensus on drafting a plan to stabilise the ties. The logic of 'stability' is well-noted in the intentions, as at the G20 Summit in Osaka, Xi claimed the ties to be at a "new historical starting line";[29] while simultaneously, Japan's 2019 *Diplomatic Bluebook* emphasised that stabile ties not just "essential" for the two countries but also, for dealing with regional and international issues.[30] The public opinion in both countries highlight the same sentiment as that of the political leadership. As the 2019 Genron NPO Report notes that 60 per cent of the Chinese and 50 per cent of the Japanese believe that a "new, stronger cooperating relationship" is necessary for peace in East Asia and for the stable development of the global economy.[31]

In fulfilment of this common objective, a political document by Xi was on the cards in his Tokyo visit[32] – which would have marked the fifth of its kind since the 1972 normalisation of ties. At present, the four documents that lay the political foundation of China-Japan relations are: (a) the China-Japan Joint Statement of 1972, (b) the China-Japan Treaty of Peace and Friendship of 1978, (c) the China-Japan Joint Declaration of 1998 and (d) a joint statement on advancing relations in 2008. Wherein, the spirit of the four documents in Chinese view includes learning from history, peaceful coexistence, mutual respect, friendship for generations, mutually beneficial cooperation and common development.[33] The fifth document by Xi would have further strengthened the political foundation.

Unlike the past diplomatic overtures, the postponement of Xi's visit does not call for a diplomatic fallout, as public health concerns rather than anything political have acted as the cause. As noted, despite the crisis, both sides expressed reluctance in calling off the event. This is evident from China's top diplomat, Yang Jiechi's[34] visit to Tokyo amidst the COVID-19 crisis in late February – a precursor to the preparations of Xi's Tokyo visit. Yang's visit not only exemplified the interest to go with the existing plan but also highlighted the importance China attaches to its Japan ties and vice-versa. Other than Xi's visit, Yang's agenda also entailed co-chairing the 8th China-Japan High-level Political Dialogue with Head of Japan's National Security Council Shigeru Kitamura on 28 February.

Against the COVID-19 crisis, Yang pointedly expressed that the "[Chinese] believe after the test of the epidemic, the lasting friendship between China and Japan will increasingly become the aspiration and action of the two peoples".[35] Yang's such an outlook can be argued to be bolstered by the Chinese interest to maintain stable ties with Japan given the virus issue has greatly severed China's major diplomatic ties with the United States and Europe. To which, Japanese side expressed the interest to "strengthen information sharing, experience sharing and technical cooperation with the Chinese side in the field of public health security to jointly safeguard international public health security".[36] However, the political exchanges did not make any mention of any form of cooperation in dealing with non-traditional security issues, despite the COVID-19 crisis. As also noted in Yang's meeting with Prime Minister Abe, both sides pledged to step up public health cooperation to contain the outbreak of coronavirus[37] – no political agreement has been signed, making it more of a rhetoric between the two countries than a reality.

Apart from the high-level visits, the warmth was also highlighted in the diplomatic exchanges between China and Japan. Most notably, China's expression of gratitude towards Japan set a new precedent given in the past, China expressed discontent over Japan's wartime atrocities. Chinese Foreign Ministry Spokesperson, Hua Chunying praised Japan by saying: "Since the outbreak of the epidemic, the Japanese government and people have expressed sympathy, understanding and support to us. [...] We will keep these in our heart. What the virus has done is cruel and will not last.

What the people has done is touching and will be remembered forever".[38] Beijing's such an emotional overtone towards Tokyo came as a response to Japan's kind gesture given the boxes of masks donated to China came with a written verse in Chinese "Although we are in different places, we are under the same sky".[39] In addition, Japanese government and businesses were amongst the first to have donated China masks, goggles, protective suits and other supplies for epidemic prevention and control, as enlisted in Table 13.3. Most notably, Japan's ruling Liberal Democratic Party (LDP) Diet members donated a portion of their March salaries (5000 yen) to China's fight against COVID-19 – a sum totalling 2 million yen (18,170 dollars).[40] To note, Japan's helping attitude towards China is not new. As during the 2003 SARS outbreak, Japan sent medical teams, medicine and medical equipment to China to help stem the spread of the virus.

Table 13.3: Japan's 'Means and Ways' to Help China

Sl. No.	*Japan's Donation to China*
1	Japan's Oita Prefecture, a sister prefecture of Wuhan, sent 30,000 masks, 600 sets of protective clothing, and 400 goggles to Wuhan.
2	Japanese city of Mito donated 50,000 masks to its Chinese sister city Chongqing.
3	Japanese city of Okayama donated 22,000 face masks to its sister city Luoyang.
4	Japanese students of Zhangbin Erhu College in Nagoya donated 50,000 medical masks, 8,000 protective masks, and 200 sets of protective clothing to the Chinese city of Nanjing.
5	Japanese company Ito-Yokado donated a million masks to China. While.
6	Japanese corporations like Maeda Construction, Air Water, and MUJI provided protective supplies.
7	Japan's Youth Development Association donated masks and thermometers to China.

Source: Prepared by the Author with reference to various Chinese and Japanese sources.

In response, China too sent testing kits to Japan as the Diamond Princess got quarantined, while Chinese billionaire Jack Ma donated a million masks to Japan.[41] In addition, Huawei donated masks to a university hospital in Nagoya that treated Chinese passengers on the Diamond Princess.[42] Additionally, China has also recommended Avigan, an anti-viral drug produced by Japan's Fujifilm Holdings Corp., to be an effective treatment for the coronavirus.[43] These actions demonstrate a 'new thinking' in China-Japan relations- exemplifying a departure from the old trend of diplomatic spats. These instances reflect that unlike China's other diplomatic ties, its equation with Tokyo under the virus outbreak have witnessed a new high, if not low. Japan's helping hand to China does go with the proverb – A friend in need is a friend in deed.

However, despite such visible cordiality, signs of criticism are getting surfaced in Tokyo's diplomatic tone. As noted, hinting at China's mismanagement of COVID-19, on 2 April, Japan's Deputy Prime Minister Taro Aso in his parliament address vehemently stated: "It shouldn't be called the WHO. It should be renamed the CHO [China Health Organization]".[44] This official remark by Japan is reflective of the fact that all is not well in the ties, as seen on the surface. With the social and economic disparity on the rise due to COVID-19, it is unlikely that Japan's criticism of China will fade away, rather more likely to get severe.

B. The Sink in the Economic Ship

The economic relationship between Beijing and Tokyo is one of the largest in the world and has significantly grown in terms of both trade and investment. The bilateral trade relationship ranks as the third- largest in the world, with China being Japan's largest trading partner, accounting for one-fifth of its trade, and Japan ranks third amongst China's major trading partner. In the first two months of the outbreak, the total value of the China-Japan trade was RMB 274.95 billion- down by 15.3 per cent and accounting for 6.7 per cent of China's total foreign trade.[45] This highlights the imminent impact of COVID-19 on the trade partnership raising serious long term concerns.

As noted, Chinese imports to Japan witnessed a drastic fall in February,[46] with imports plummeting by 47.1 per cent year on year.[47] The shutting down of Chinese production units led to Japanese manufacturers starve of parts. For instance, For instance, in March, Nissan Motor Corp. has been forced to close down production in several domestic assembly factories, including Tochigi and Fukuoka, due to a shortage of Chinese parts.[48] The fall was mainly in imports of clothing and apparel (65.7 per cent), smartphones and other communication devices (45.3 per cent), and PCs and other computers (37.2 per cent).[49]

Invariably, Japan's exports to China fell by only 0.4 per cent due to fall in the shipment of automobiles, semiconductors and other electronic components.[50] To note, Japan exports a far larger share of parts and partially finished goods to China than other major industrial nations. Thereby, the skewed export-import balance resulted into Japan's first trade surplus with China since March 2018 and the largest surplus to date. In addition, Japanese businesses in China faced a severe setback, such as: half of global clothing giant UNIQLO's 750 stores in China remain suspended; retail chain Muji suspended operations at its 17 stores in Wuhan and automobile giants such as Toyota, Honda and Mazda faced delays in reopening of factories in various Chinese cities.[51] Within Japan, the businesses that are significantly affected are: Toyota Motor Corp., Honda Motor Co., Mazda Motor Corp., Nissan Motor Corp., Asahi Group Holdings Ltd., Hanwa Co., Ltd., Kirin Holdings Co. Ltd.,

Ajinomoto Co. Inc., Yamazaki Baking Co., Ltd., Coca-Cola Co., Ltd., and others.[52] Of which, automobiles are most affected given China is one of Japan's largest foreign automobile markets.

These contingencies indicate the likely impact of the viral outbreak in disrupting the supply chain between the two major trading partners- affecting both trade as well as investments between the two countries. For China is Japan's largest export market with the bilateral trade exceeding US$300 billion; while Japan's total investment in China amounts to US$120 billion dollars with 10-billion-dollar worth of commodities, which are manufactured in China by Japanese companies and exported to the United States each year.[53] However, this economic interdependency will face a significant downturn as a result of Japan's withdrawal of its business from China. Against the economic halt caused by COVID-19, Japan has already expressed intention to reduce its reliance on Chinese manufacturing base.[54] In doing so, Tokyo plans to shift the manufacturing of high-added-value products back to Japan, and for production of other goods to be spread across Southeast Asia.[55] This Japanese intention is well-witnessed in Abe's stimulus package. Wherein, of the ¥243.5 billion of the support package, ¥220 billion is for companies shifting production back to Japan and ¥23.5 billion for companies moving production to other countries.[56] This move by Japan runs in contrast to its warmth towards China in the initial phase of COVID-19.

To this Japanese move, Beijing in its response, as stated by Zhao Lijian – "China has achieved remarkable results in fighting the virus and resuming normal socioeconomic development. We hope other countries [Japan] can also take measures to avoid further impacts on the world economy and global supply chains. We need to make concerted efforts to safeguard the stability of global supply chains and bring the world economy back onto the normal track".[57]

Against this Chinese intention, it is important to highlight that the initial disruption to businesses was caused by the Wuhan epidemic followed by the spread of the pandemic in Italy and other parts – thus, affecting the infrastructure and global networks of supply chains. Moreover, as China functions as the "World's Factory", a halt in China causes a halt everywhere in the globe, as evident from the Wuhan epidemic.

What further adds to Japan's economic woes in relation to China is the disruption in tourism. Japan's services trade has been driven by a significant boom in inbound tourists; wherein, Chinese tourists have been the key to the boom. In 2019, 9.6 million Chinese visited Japan- marking a new record high by equating to one-third of total visitors.[58] As noted, since 2007, the number of Chinese tourists to Japan has increased ten-fold from being 940,000, with a significant rise since 2014, as noted in Figure 13.6.[59] Specifically, in 2003, that marked the SARS epidemic, there were about 449,000 visitors to Japan from mainland China.[60]

Figure 13.6: Chinese Visitor Numbers to Japan (since SARS in 2003)

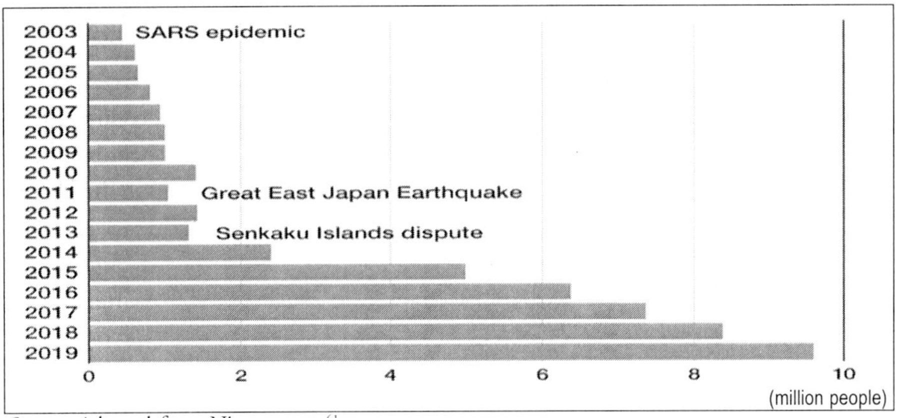

Source: Adapted from Nippon.com.[61]

As noted, of the total ¥4.81 trillion of the overseas spending in Japan in 2019, China accounted for ¥1.8 trillion-equivalent to 36.8 per cent of total visitor spending in Japan.[62] China's annual spending in Japan has significantly increased as noted in Figure 13.7.

Figure 13.7: Annual Spending by Chinese Visitors in Japan

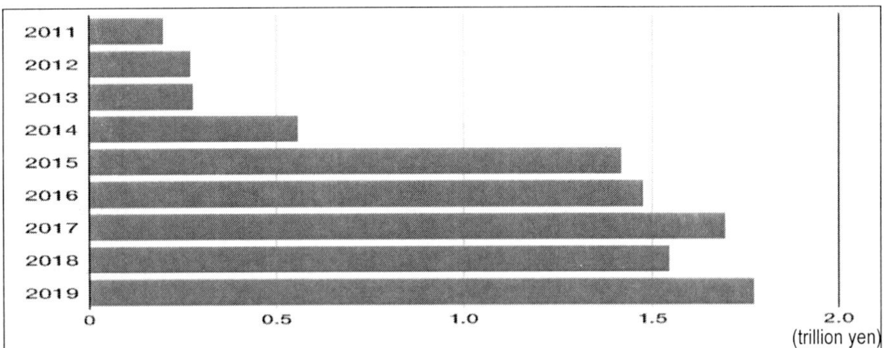

Source: Adapted from Nippon.com.[63]

With Chinese tourists acting as a significant source of revenue, COVID-19's initial hit to Japanese economy came with Beijing's decision to block outbound tour groups during the Lunar New Year holidays to stem the spread. This would have otherwise witnessed an influx of tourists in Japan. With the spread of the pandemic resulting into international travel bans, COVID-19 has severely affected Japan's tourism industry in particular.

Figure 13.8: Monthly Trend of Chinese Visitors to Japan

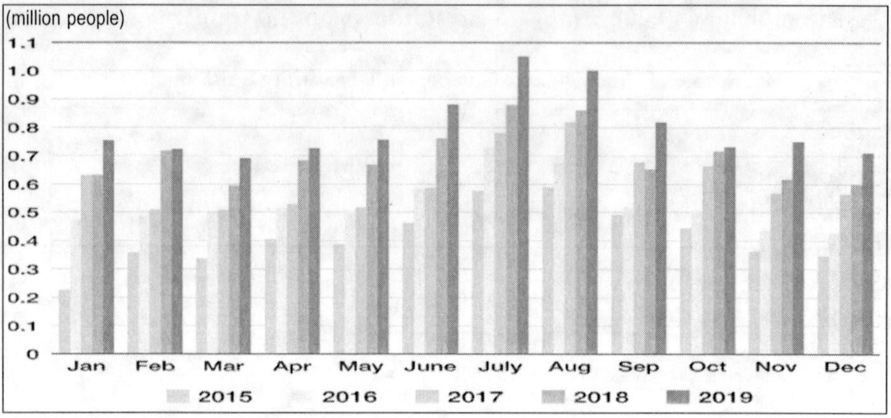

Source: Adapted from Nippon.com.[64]

As noted above, the period between June-August is the peak of Chinese visitors to Japan. In view of this, in 2020, this trend will witness a sharp decline due to COVID-19. In Japanese view, if the Chinese tourist numbers tumble at the same rate as experienced during the three-months SARS outbreak, Japanese growth could be cut by 0.2 percentage point; and if the virus outbreak stays over a year, then that would result into a cut by 0.45 percentage point.[65] These projections signify the severe damage caused to the Japanese economy by the virus. Furthermore, it is also to suggest that if there was no COVID-19, Japan would have witnessed a further spike in Chinese tourists due to the 2020 Tokyo Olympics- providing a significant boost to Japanese economy. However, even if the outbreak comes under control by this period, Chinese tourism in Japan undoubtedly will still experience a significant low.

These economic contingencies thereby act as key roadblocks that would affect the stability in China-Japan ties. Thereby, Japan's economic recovery will then act as a decisive factor in shaping the economic ties between the two trading partners – both in scale as well as scope.

Amidst COVID-19, Old Troubles Still Play Out: Tensions in the East China Sea

On 30 March, a Chinese fishing boat collided with Japan's Maritime Self-Defense Force's (JMSDF's) Hatakaze-class guided missile destroyer JS Shimakaze in the East China Sea. The collision occurred in east of Zhoushan in China's Zhejiang province. Asserting its claims, Chinese Foreign Ministry remarked that: "The collision took place in China's coastal waters and the activities of Japan's MSDF vessel there endangered the safety of Chinese boats".[66] Expressing its concern, Beijing also posited that "China is in close communication with Japan and hopes to find out the cause soon to avoid the recurrence of such incidents".[67] The Japanese Ministry of Defence cited that the vessel was on patrol after departing from Sasebo in Nagasaki Prefecture and that it will cooperate with the coast guard's investigation along with launching a probe panel within the MSDF as well.[68]

Beijing's such a response appears to be passive as compared to its past reactions towards Tokyo as noted in two key incidents: First, in September 2010, a Chinese fishing boat collided with two Japanese Coast Guard vessels in waters off the Diaoyu/Senkaku Islands. Second, in September 2012, the Japanese Government's nationalized the Diaoyu/Senkaku Islands. Both these incidents sparked severe criticism from Beijing resulting into diplomatic fallout as well as increased anti-Japanese sentiment in China. Asserting its claims, in November 2013, China unilaterally established an Air Defence Identification Zone (ADIZ) in the East China Sea. These three incidents in the East China Sea plummeted the bilateral ties to their worst level since the two governments normalised diplomatic relations in 1972. Given these episodes, the issue of sovereignty and maritime rights in the East China Sea has surfaced overtime between China and Japan.

In recent times, the trend in the East China Sea is exemplified by an uptick in China's military activism towards Japan to assert its claims. This is mainly noted in two areas: First, Chinese incursions into Japan's airspace, wherein Japan's Air Self Defense Force (JASDF) intercepted China's military aircrafts (both PLAAF and PLAN),[69] 523 times between 1 April and 31 December 2019- marking a 9.9 percent increase compared to 2018 and the second highest total for the period.[70] Second, China's increasing naval activities into the 24-nautical-mile (nm) contiguous zone and 12nm territorial sea around the Diaoyu/Senkaku Islands, as noted in Figure 13.9.

Figure 13.9: Number of Chinese Government Vessels in Diaoyu/Senkaku's Contiguous Zone/Territorial Sea (2009-Present)

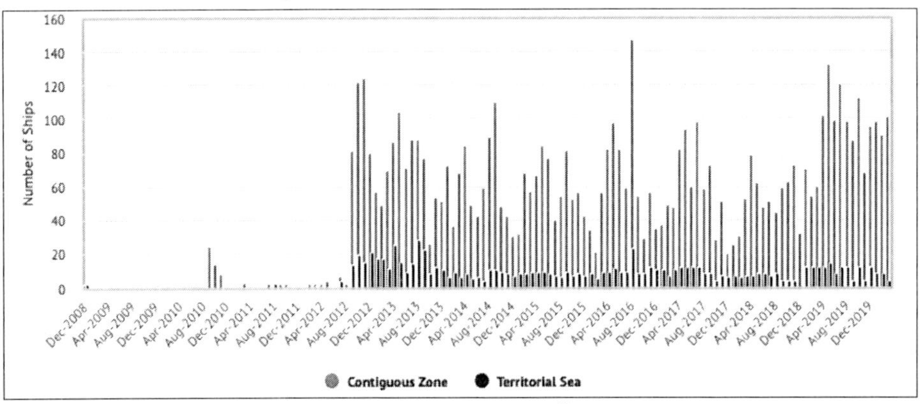

Source: Adapted from Asia Maritime Transparency Initiative.[71]

Therefore, China's not so aggressive reaction to Japan in the recent collision appears to be an intentional oversight. China's such an approach can be attributed to its reciprocity towards Tokyo's non-critical attitude of Beijing over COVID-19. However, amidst the virus crisis, Chinese government ships continue to patrol around the Japanese-administered islands; such as in April, Japan reported of the presence of four Chinese ships in what it claims to be its territorial waters.[72] China's such activities of intrusion in Japanese claimed waters is well-witnessed in Figure 13.10.

Figure 13.10: Records of Intrusions of Chinese Government and Other Vessels into Japan's Territorial Sea (Japanese view)

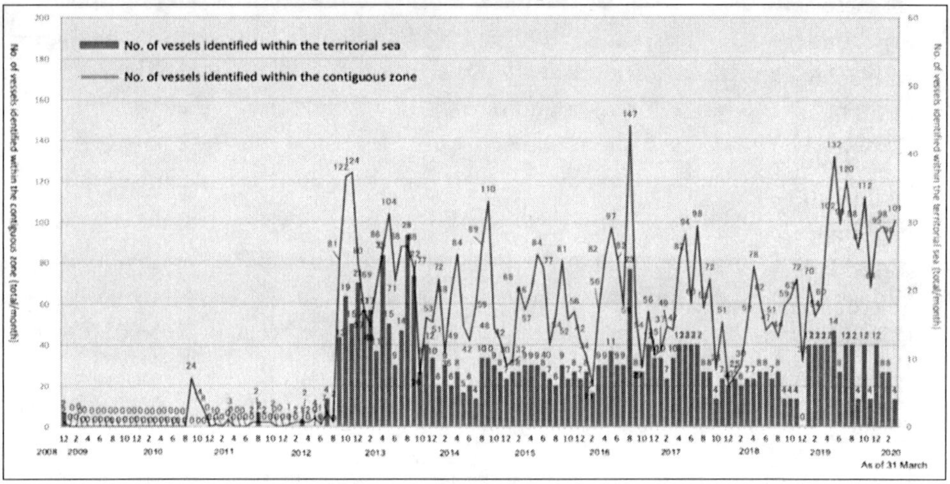

Source: Adapted from Ministry of Foreign Affairs of Japan.[73]

Thereby, with high stakes involved and no resolution reached, the East China Sea remains far from being settled between China and Japan. To which, the COVID-19 crisis does not make much difference in averting the risks of contingencies. Rather if the ties take a downturn under the virus outbreak as that of China and the United States, the East China Sea will become the flashpoint of power projections between Beijing and Tokyo.

Will China Taste its Own Medicine from Japan: Possibilities over COVID-19

In addition to the East China Sea dispute, troubles between China and Japan can also be witnessed in other areas. For instance, against the heavy health and economic costs incurred by COVID-19, countries such as the United States and Germany have called for China to compensate for the pandemic-related losses. This very aspect of 'making China pay' can be linked to China's own tendency towards Japan in seeking reparation over the losses induced by Japan in 1930s. Till date, Chinese plaintiffs file petitions to seek compensation from Japan over the wartime past.

If not reparation from Japan, but a similar corollary can be drawn from Japan's Official Development Assistance (ODA) to China since 1979, wherein 75 per cent of the aid has been given as yen loans. However, in 2008 Japan stopped its ODA yen loan programme to China. Owing to this transaction, Japanese view that ODA acted as an important instrument of atonement, which most Chinese view to be a series of mutually beneficial arrangements, not as gifts; and some forms of ODA are loans that are to be repaid. However, some ODA arrangements are seen by the Japanese as an important part of their penance for World War II. Applying this logic, under the irreparable damages caused to Japanese economy by COVID-19, will Japan apply a similar rule on China- seeking monetary compensation similar to ODA.

In addition to the issue of monetary compensation, the global debate on China taking full responsibility of the COVID-19 crisis is also gaining dominance. This 'repentance logic' also predominates the Sino-Japanese ties as China has continuously seeked Japan's apology over the wartime past. It is noteworthy that till date, despite Tokyo's numerous official apologies as noted in Table 13.4, resulting into Japan's 'apology fatigue', China has still held Japan accountable of not expressing a 'proper apology'. In arguing so, the key accusation of Chinese against the Japanese government is: there have been sincere apologies but "never an all inclusive apology that is not only deeply sincere, using the right language, but also inclusive of all the areas of perceived injury".[74] That is, the apology should encompass all issues such as- Japan's militarism, invasion, colonialism, comfort women, POWs, Nanjing massacre and others.

Table 13.4: Official Statements of Apologies by Japanese Leaders since 1972

Year	*Emperor/Prime Minister*	*Apologies for World War II*
1972	Tanaka Kakuei	"It is regrettable that for several decades in the past, the relations between Japan and China had unfortunate experiences. During that time our country gave great troubles to the Chinese people, for which I once again make profound self-examination" – *Speech in Beijing, September 25, 1972.*" The Japanese side is keenly aware of Japan's responsibility by causing enormous damages in the past to the Chinese people through war and deeply reproaches itself" – *Joint Communique*, September 29, 1972.
1992	Emperor Akihito	"In the long history of relationships between our two countries, there was an unfortunate period in which my country inflicted

Year	Emperor/Prime Minister	Apologies for World War II
		great suffering on the people of China. About this I feel deep sadness" – *at a banquet in the Great Hall of the People, Beijing, October 23, 1992.*
1995	Murayama Tomiichi	In the hope that no such mistake be made in the future, I regard, in a spirit of humility, these irrefutable facts of history, and express here once again my feelings of deep remorse and state my heartfelt apology" – *Statement marking the 50th anniversary of Japan's surrender, August 15, 1995.*
2003	Koizumi Junichiro	"During the war, Japan caused tremendous damage and suffering to the people of many countries, particularly to those of Asian nations. On behalf of the people of Japan, I hereby renew my feelings of profound remorse as I express my sincere mourning to the victims" – *Statement at the 58th anniversary of Japan's surrender, August 15, 2003.*
2005	Koizumi Junichiro	"Our country has caused tremendous damage and pain to the peoples of many countries, especially Asian countries, through colonial rule and invasion. Humbly acknowledging such facts of history, I once again reflect most deeply and offer apologies from my heart" – *Statement marking the 60th anniversary of Japan's surrender, August 15, 2005.*

Source: Prepared by the Author.

Taking a cue from China's own attitude towards Japan, will Tokyo apply the same tactic against Beijing on holding it accountable for the COVID-19 crisis-seeking a formal Chinese apology for the damages caused to Japan. If Japan adopts such a political tool, it will only even the score with China. However, the big question is: Will Japan act like China under the pressure of the pandemic or continue with its pacifist policy?

Conclusion

China's COVID-19 crisis is not just a health emergency but is increasingly becoming a diplomatic challenge for Beijing. Mounting criticism over China's negligence over handling of the virus outbreak has resulted into a global boycott of China. With Donald Trump leading the war of criticism towards China, other major and smaller countries are also showing signs of discontent. In view of this, Japan somewhat appears to have largely maintained restraint and adopted cordiality towards China. This is evident from China's ties with Japan that exhibited maximum cordiality in times of the COVID-19 crisis–highlighting reciprocity over animosity. However, this is not to suggest that the Sino-Japanese ties have not been affected by the COVID-19. With Japanese economy being badly hit, the trade equation between the two countries have witnessed a significant decline resulting into Japan's plans to withdraw investments from China. In addition, Chinese tourists to Japan have witnessed a sharp fall and the trend is likely to continue till the virus outbreak prevails. These spiralling economic contingencies will contribute to political divides between the two countries. As to note, unlike China's authoritarian one-party rule, Japan has a democratic polity which is already expressing signs of resentment towards China. As the COVID-19 crisis gets severe and Japan's domestic situation faces a graver emergency, Abe's interest to stabilise ties with Xi's China will face a severe scrutiny. That is to argue, Xi-Abe's top agenda of putting the relations on a stable track has been significantly challenged by the coronavirus crisis; wherein, the cordiality is likely to face a setback. In the long run, the fragility of the ties becomes the point of concern; as so far China's ties with Japan did pass the COVID-19 test. Wherein, if not economically, but the diplomatic equation between Beijing and Tokyo has so far remained significantly immuned from COVID-19. However, only time will tell, how long will this peace sustain.

NOTES

1 "Shop fearing Wuhan virus bans Chinese visitors in Hakone", *Japan Today*, 23 January 2020, https://japantoday.com/category/national/candy-shop-fearing-wuhan-virus-bans-chinese-visitors-inpopular-tourist-destination-hakone.

2 Ibid.

3 See, The World Bank, https://data.worldbank.org/indicator/SP.POP.65UP.TO.ZS?contextual=default&end=2018&locations=JP&start=1960&view=chart.

4 Ministry of Health, Labour and Welfare (2020), "Basic Policies for Novel Coronavirus Disease Control by the Government of Japan (Summary)", 28 March 2020 (Revised on 16 April 2020), https://www.mhlw.go.jp/content/10900000/000624436.pdf.

5 World Health Organization (2020), "Novel Coronavirus – Japan (ex-China)", 17 January 2020, https://www.who.int/csr/don/17-january-2020-novel-coronavirus-japan-ex-china/en/, 2020.

6 US Department of Health and Human Services/Centers for Disease Control and Prevention (2020), "Public Health Responses to COVID-19 Outbreaks on Cruise Ships-Worldwide, February-March 2020", Morbidity and Mortality Weekly Report, 27 March 2020, Vol. 69, no. 12, p. 348, https://www.cdc.gov/mmwr/volumes/69/wr/mm6912e3.htm#F1_down.

7 Ministry of Health, Labour and Welfare (2020), "Updates on COVID-19 in Japan", 18 May 2020, p. 5, https://www.mhlw.go.jp/content/10900000/000631469.pdf.

8 See, Japan COVID-19 Coronavirus Tracker, https://covid19japan.com.

9 Ibid.

10 "Coronavirus Cases in Japan by Prefecture", *Nippon.com*, 24 April 2020, https://www.nippon.com/en/japan-data/h00657/coronavirus-cases-in-japan-by-prefecture.html.

11 On April 18, Japan's COVID-19 cases rose above 10000. From the first infection case recorded on 15 January, it took around two months to reach 1,000 cases. However, the pace of infection has shown a clear increase from late March, and over the last 10 days there have been around 1,000 new cases every two days. For details see, *Nippon.com*, https://www.nippon.com/en/japan-data/h00657/coronavirus-cases-in-japan-by-prefecture.html.

12 Quoted in Kathrin Hille and Edward White (2020), "Containing Coronavirus: Lessons from Asia",

Financial Times, 16 March 2020, https://www.ft.com/content/e015e096-6532-11ea-a6cddf28cc3c6a68.

13 As noted, Japan has conducted 0.6 tests per thousand people as compared to South Korea where over 10 tests per thousand have been carried out.

14 Ministry of Health, Labour and Welfare (2020), "Updates on COVID-19 in Japan", n. 7, p. 9.

15 "Nagasaki reports 14 more coronavirus cases on Italian cruise ship", *The Japan Times*, 23 April 2020, https://www.japantimes.co.jp/news/2020/04/23/national/japan-more-coronavirus-cases-onitalian-cruise-ship-nagasaki/#.XqL7Py2B2gQ.

16 Prime Minister of Japan and his Cabinet (2020), "[COVID-19] Press Conference by the Prime Minister Regarding the Declaration of a State of Emergency", 07 April 2020, https://japan.kantei.go.jp/98_abe/statement/202004/_00001.html.

17 Prime Minister of Japan and his Cabinet (2020), "[COVID-19] Press Conference by the Prime Minister regarding the Novel Coronavirus", 17 April 2020, https://japan.kantei.go.jp/98_abe/statement/202004/_00002.html.

18 Ahiza García-Hodges, Yuliya Talmazan and Arata Yamamoto (2020), "Tokyo 2020 Olympics postponed over coronavirus concerns", *NBC News*, 24 March 2020, https://www.nbcnews.com/news/world/tokyo-2020-olympics-postponed-over-coronavirus-concerns-n1165046.

19 "BREAKING NEWS: Japan economy faces biggest crisis in postwar era: Abe", *Kyodo News*, 07 April 2020, https://english.kyodonews.net/news/2020/04/7428aca759fe-breaking-news-japaneconomy-faces-biggest-crisis-in-postwar-era-abe.html.

20 William Sposato (2020), "Japan Hopes for a Post-Coronavirus Olympics", *Foreign Policy*, 27 March 2020, https://foreignpolicy.com/2020/03/27/cancellation-abe-japan-holds-out-post-coronavirus olympic-hopes/.

21 "Tokyo 2020 Olympics unveil final budget of $12.6 billion", *France 24*, 20 December 2019, https://www.france24.com/en/20191220-tokyo-2020-olympics-unveil-final-budget-of-12-6-billion.

22 David Hutt (2020), "Japan Olympics postponed – what does that mean for the economy?", *Asia Fund Managers*, 31 March 2020, https://www.asiafundmanagers.com/GBR/japan-olympicspostponed/.

23 The package aims at five objectives, including to:
   (i) develop preventive measures against the spread of infection and strengthen treatment capacity (expenditure of 0.5 per cent of GDP),
   (ii) protect employment and businesses (16.0 per cent of GDP),
   (iii) regain economic activities after containment (1.6 per cent of GDP), (iv) rebuild a resilient economic structure (3 per cent of GDP), and
   (v) enhance readiness for the future (0.3 per cent of GDP). The key measures comprise cash handouts to every individual and affected firms, deferral of tax payments and social security contributions, and concessional loans from public and private financial institutions.

   See, International Monetary Fund, "Policy Responses to COVID-19", https://www.imf.org/en/Topics/imf-and-covid19/Policy-Responses-to-COVID-19#J.

24 Quoted in Keita Nakamura (2020), "FOCUS: Japan's biggest-ever stimulus package likely to entail more steps", *Kyodo News*, 08 April 2020, https://english.kyodonews.net/news/2020/04/63e35b6a1696-focus-japans-biggest-ever-stimulus-package-likely-to-entail-more-steps.html.

25 Isabel Reynolds (2020), "Burden of viral outbreak threatens Abe's government and his legacy", *The Japan Times*, 02 March 2020, https://www.japantimes.co.jp/news/2020/03/02/national/politicsdiplomacy/coronavirus-shinzo-abe-government/#.XqKNaS2B1QJ.

26 Ibid.

27 Isabel Reynolds and Dandan Li (2020), "Spread of COVID-19 in Japan could hurt Abe's bid to rebuild China ties", *The Japan Times*, 21 February 2020, https://www.japantimes.co.jp/news/2020/02/21/national/politics-diplomacy/abe-china-coronavirus/#.XqL-Ki2B2gQ, accessed online 22 April 2020.

28 Ibid.

29 Kristin Huang et al. (2019), "China and Japan seek to take relationship to 'next level' as Xi Jinping state visit confirmed for spring", *South China Morning Post*, 27 June 2019, https://www.scmp.com/news/china/diplomacy/article/3016415/china-and-japan-seek-take-relationship-next-level-xi-jinping.

30 Ministry of Foreign Affairs of Japan (2019), Diplomatic Bluebook 2019, 17 October 2019, p. 51, https://www.mofa.go.jp/fp/pp/page22e_000929.html.

31 The Genron NPO (2019), "The 15th Joint Public Opinion Poll: Japan-China Public Opinion Survey 2019", October 2019, p. 11, http://www.genron-npo.net/en/archives/191024.pdf.

32 "Japan-China political document to be unveiled during Xi's state visit", *The Japan Times*, 10 January 2020, https://www.japantimes.co.jp/news/2020/01/10/national/politics-diplomacy/japan-chinacraft-new-political-document-xi-jinpings-state-visit/#.Xqx39S2B1QI.

33 "Diplomat urges improvement of China-Japan ties", *China Daily*, 26 October 2013, http://usa.chinadaily.com.cn/china/2013-10/26/content_17060914.htm.

34 Yang Jiechi is member of the Political Bureau of the Central Committee of the Communist Party of China (CPC) and Director of the Office of the Foreign Affairs Commission of the CPC Central Committee.

35 Ministry of Foreign Affairs of the People's Republic of China (2020), "The 8th China-Japan Highlevel Political Dialogue Held in Tokyo", 28 February 2020, https://www.fmprc.gov.cn/mfa_eng/zxxx_662805/t1751472.shtml

36 Ibid.

37 "China, Japan pledge cooperation in fighting COVID-19 epidemic", *Xinhuanet*, 29 February 2020, http://www.xinhuanet.com/english/2020-02/29/c_138828544.htm.

38 Ministry of Foreign Affairs of the People's Republic of China (2020), "Foreign Ministry Spokesperson Hua Chunying's Daily Briefing Online on February 4, 2020", 04 February 2020, https://www.fmprc.gov.cn/mfa_eng/xwfw_665399/s2510_665401/t1740278.shtml.

39 "Feature: Japan offers warm support to China in battle against virus outbreak", *Xinhuanet*, 13 February 2020, http://www.xinhuanet.com/english/2020-02/13/c_138779612.htm.

40 Ibid.

41 Elliot Silverberg (2020), "Better ties with China: Japan's coronavirus silver lining?", *The Japan Times*, 01 April 2020, https://www.japantimes.co.jp/opinion/2020/04/01/commentary/japan-commentary/better-ties-china-japans-coronavirus-silver-lining/#.XqCaSi2B1QI.

42 Ibid.

43 "Japan sets aside ¥243.5 billion to help firms shift production out of China", *The Japan Times*, 09 April 2020, https://www.japantimes.co.jp/news/2020/04/09/business/japan-sets-aside-¥243-5billion-help-firms-shift-production-china/#.XqQ6Ri2B1QI.

44 Quoted in Emma Colton (2020), "Japanese deputy prime minister says WHO should be renamed China Health Organization", Washington Examiner, 02 April 2020, https://www.washington examiner.com/news/japanese-deputy-prime-minister-says-who-should-be-renamed-china-healthorganization.

45 "The growing concerns behind the overall decline in China's trade", *FXStreet*, 16 April 2020, https://www.fxstreet.com/analysis/the-growing-concerns-behind-the-overall-decline-in-chinas-trade202004160931.

46 This has been the biggest drop in Chinese imports to Japan since August 1986.

47 "COVID-19 Calamity Halves Imports from China in February", *Nippon.com*, 01 April 2020, https://www.nippon.com/en/japan-data/h00678/covid-19-calamity-halves-imports-from-china-infebruary.html.

48 "Impact of COVID-19 on Japan Economy, Deviation & Trends Analysis Report, Segmentation (Automobile, Food & Beverage, Chemical, Energy, Electronic and Electrical, Aviation, Retail, Travel & Tourism and Others) and Forecast 2019-2025", *OMR Global*, March 2020, https://www.omrglobal.com/industry-reports/impact-of-covid-19-on-japan-economy.

49 Ibid.

50 "Japan's exports fall, imports from China slump as virus impact widens", *The Japan Times*, 18 March 2020, https://www.japantimes.co.jp/news/2020/03/18/business/economy-business/japans-exportsfall-imports-china-slump-coronavirus-impactwidens/#.XqRBPC2B1QI.

51 Thisanka Siripala (2020), "Will Japan's Economy Buckle Under the Coronavirus Outbreak?", *The Diplomat*, 13 February 2020, https://thediplomat.com/2020/02/will-japans-economy-buckle-underthe-coronavirus-outbreak/.

52 "Impact of COVID-19 on Japan Economy, Deviation & Trends Analysis Report, Segmentation", *OMR Global*, n. 48.

53 "Interview: China, Japan should work together as anchor, propeller for free trade system: Chinese ambassador to Japan", *Xinhuanet*, 27 June 2019, http://www.xinhuanet.com/english/2019-06/27/c_138176284.htm.

54 A February survey by Tokyo Shoko Research found 37 per cent of more than 2,600 Japanese companies that responded were diversifying procurement to places other than China due to the coronavirus crisis. Cited in, Isabel Reynolds and Emi Urabe (2020), Japan to Fund Firms to Shift Production Out of China", *Bloomberg*, 08 April 2020, https://www.bloombergquint.com/globaleconomics/japan-to-fund-firms-to-shift-production-out-of-china.

55 "Japan sets aside ¥243.5 billion to help firms shift production out of China", *The Japan Times*, n. 43.

56 Ibid.

57 Ministry of Foreign Affairs of the People's Republic of China (2020), "Foreign Ministry Spokesperson Zhao Lijian's Regular Press Conference on April 8, 2020", 08 April 2020, https://www.fmprc.gov.cn/mfa_eng/xwfw_665399/s2510_665401/t1767488.shtml.

58 Ibid.

59 Ibid.

60 Eric Johnston (2020), "How lessons learned from SARS could apply to the coronavirus outbreak", *The Japan Times*, 24 January 2020, https://www.japantimes.co.jp/news/2020/01/24/national/sciencehealth/examining-coronavirus-outbreak-lessons-learned-sars-can-apply-growing-crisis/#.XqwMii2B1QI.

61 "Chinese Visitors Spend ¥1.8 Trillion in Japan in 2019", *Nippon.com*, 12 February 2020, https://www.nippon.com/en/japan-data/h00646/chinese-visitors-spend-¥1-8-trillion-in-japan-in2019.html.

62 The overseas spending include: Taiwan- ¥550.6 bn; South Korea- ¥1420.9 bn; Hong Kong- ¥1352.4 bn and; United States- ¥1324.7 bn.

63 "Chinese Visitors Spend ¥1.8 Trillion in Japan in 2019", *Nippon.com*, n. 61.

64 Ibid.

65 Yuko Takeo (2020), "Coronavirus Could Hit Japan's Economy Harder Than SARS, Say Economists", *Bloomberg*, 27 January 2020, https://www.bloomberg.com/news/articles/2020-01-27/coronavirusseen-hitting-japan-s-economy-harder-than-sars.

66 "Japanese warship, Chinese fishing boat in collision", *The China Daily*, 01 April 2020, https://www.chinadaily.com.cn/a/202004/01/WS5e83f59ba3101282172838a0.html.

67 Ibid.

68 "SDF destroyer, fishing boat collide in East China Sea", *Kyodo News*, 31 March 2020, https://english.kyodonews.net/news/2020/03/41b8d310126e-breaking-news-sdf-warship-fishing-boatcollide-in-east-china-sea.html.

69 PLAAF–People's Liberation Army Air Force; PLAN–People's Liberation Army Navy.

70 Franz-Stefan Gady (2020), "Japan Intercepts Chinese Military Aircraft 523 Times in 9 Months", *The Diplomat*, 04 February 2020, https://thediplomat.com/2020/02/japan-intercepts-chinesemilitary-aircraft-523-times-in-9-months/.

71 Zack Cooper (2018), "Flashpoint East China Sea: Potential Shocks", Asia Maritime Transparency Initiative, 27 April 2018, https://amti.csis.org/flashpoint-east-china-sea-potential-shocks/.

72 "Japan sets aside ¥243.5 billion to help firms shift production out of China", *The Japan Times*, n. 43.

73 See, Ministry of Foreign Affairs of Japan (2020), "Trends in Chinese Government and Other Vessels in the Waters Surrounding the Senkaku Islands, and Japan's Response", 06 April 2020, https://www.mofa.go.jp/region/page23e_000021.html.

74 Darryl Lupton (2012), "Can the 'apology standoff' between China and Japan be resolved?", *Culture Mandala: The Bulletin of the Centre for East-West Cultural and Economic Studies*, Vol. 11, No. 2, pp. 20-21.

14

China's Relations with South Asian in a COVID-19 World Order

Sriparna Pathak

Introduction

The COVID-19 has changed the course of international relations, as the system sees the most powerful states of the international system ranging from the U.S. to European countries grappling with a pandemic in the absolute absence of an antidote or a vaccine. The unprecedented impacts on the system range from calls for greater medical cooperation, to possibilities of China emerging as the leader of the system to calls for the inclusion of Taiwan as a member in the World Health Organization (WHO). While all of these are issues that have existed in parts or in whole in the international system of the 21st century, the COVID-19 pandemic has also opened space for new forms of diplomacy ranging from narrative diplomacy to facemask diplomacy to medical diplomacy.

China's emergence at the international stage in the 21st century owes largely to its economic prowess, as it emerged as the manufacturing platform of the world. China's prowess in manufacturing led it to be a pole of international trade in goods, as the world became increasingly reliant on cheaply manufactured Chinese products. While China's most important trading partners remain in the West, in the countries of the U.S. and the European Union (EU), fact remains that South Asia is an important market for China as well.

However, as the world remains quarantined in the hopes that increased social distancing enforced by lockdowns will lead the virus to die its natural death, production has taken a hit and the global economy is on the verge of a recession. Steps taken to protect countries from the virus spread range from complete lockdowns to sealing of borders with neighbouring countries to cancellation of flights to and from other countries, putting arriving citizens of respective countries from other countries into compulsory quarantine among others.

South Asia has also been badly impacted by the COVID-19. In this context, it is essential to point out that China has offered medical aid and supplies to several countries of South Asia. However, what remains to be better analysed is how effective is the aid, what has been the impact of COVID-19 on China's relations with countries of South Asia, and whether China can emerge as the most important player in South Asia in the COVID-19 order. This chapter looks at the impact of the COVID-19 on individual South Asian countries, their response, particularly with respect to those arenas which might impact foreign relations with China positively or negatively. The chapter relies on primary as well as secondary sources.

COVID-19 in South Asia

While the impact of the COVID-19 is relatively less than what has been in Western countries, as the South Asian Association for Regional Cooperation (SAARC) region as a whole sees a slower increase in COVID-19 infections, especially in the numbers of critical cases. Lockdowns and stringent social distancing measures currently exist in India, Afghanistan, Bangladesh, Bhutan, Nepal, Pakistan, Sri Lanka and the Maldives. According to data published by the South Asia Economic Focus published by the World Bank in April, the eight SAARC countries account for about 1.1 per cent of the total coronavirus cases in the world, and in terms of fatalities, the SAARC total is 0.49 percentage of the total people who have died of the infection.[1] However, in another report published by the World Bank titled 'South Asia Economic Focus', it is mentioned that there will be a sharp economic slump in each of the eight countries, caused by halted economic activity, collapsing trade and greater stresses in the financial and banking sectors of the countries. The report also adds that the significant gains that South Asia has made in terms of poverty alleviation will be wiped out in all likelihood.[2]

The report goes on to predict that regional growth will fall to somewhere between 1.8 to 2.8 per cent in 2020, down from 6.3 per cent as projected six months ago. This will be the SAARC's worst performance in the last 40 years, with temporary contractions in all of the eight countries.[3] Out of the eight countries, Afghanistan has been the most vulnerable given its geographic proximity to Iran, which as of April 22 had 85,996 cases of coronavirus.[4]

While China's trade with South Asia does not represent a significant portion of China's total trade, fact remains that South Asia is an important market for China, while for the South Asian countries, China remains an important source for imports. The following graph shows China's total trade with South Asia.

Graph 14.1: China's Total Trade with South Asian countries in 2017

Unit: USD 10,000

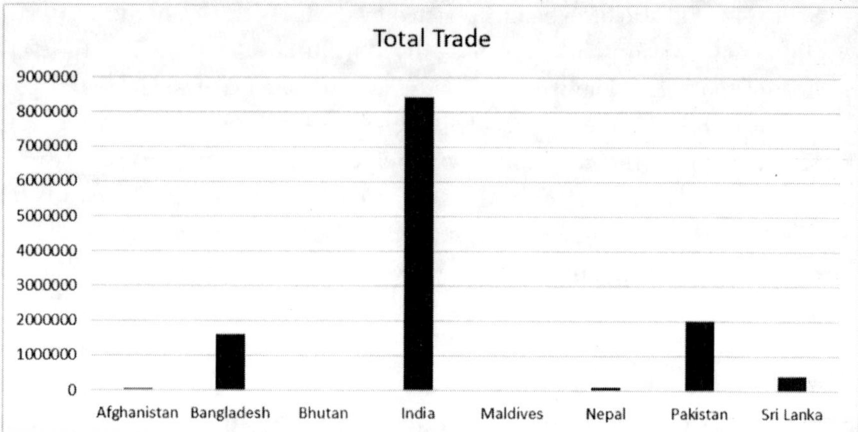

Source: China Statistical Yearbook, 2018, National Bureau of Statistics, People's Republic of China

As seen in graph 14.1, India remains the strongest trade partner for China within South Asia. In 2018, the total trade between the two countries stood at USD 95.7 billion. While India's exports stood at USD 18.83 billion, China's exports to India stood at USD 76.87 billion.[5]

In the COVID-19 situation, as stated by Chinese official date, the trade between the two countries in January and February 2020 was down 12.4 per cent. Chinese exports to India in this period stood at 67.1 billion Yuan which represented a reduction of 12.6 per cent year-on-year, while imports from India dropped by 11.6 per cent to USD 18 billion Yuan.[6] Trade remains an important facet of China's stature in international relations, and China needs continuous trade for its own economic development, like all other countries in the world. However, this is drastically set to change in the current COVID-19 world order. Before economic assessments can be made, and a post COVID-19 world order can be envisaged, it first becomes pertinent to understand the medical costs that South Asia is currently paying to control the spread of the pandemic, in order to further understand how this might affect China's relations with South Asian countries in the near future.

The following timeline shows the emergence of the first cases in the first eight countries.

Table 14.1: TimeLine of the emergence of COVID-19 in South Asia

Country	*Details of first reported case*
Nepal	On January 13, 2020, a 32-year-old Nepalese student of Wuhan University of Technology, Wuhan, PRC, returned to Nepal. He visited the Hospital in Kathmandu on 13 January. He was discharged within four days of isolation.
Pakistan	On January 29, 2020 four Pakistani students tested positive for COVID-19 in China. All four recovered by February 12, 2020. On February 26, two cases were reported from within the territory of Pakistan, both patients had returned from Iran.
India	January 30, 2020 saw the first case in India in Kerala's Thrissur District. The affected was a student, who returned from a University in Wuhan, People's Republic of China (PRC)
Afghanistan	February 24, 2020 saw the first case in Afghanistan. The affected was a 35-year-old man; a resident of Herat who had returned from Iran.
Bhutan	On March 6, a US national in Bhutan tested positive for COVID-19.
Maldives	On March 7, two confirmed cases were reported in Maldives. The two affected worked in a resort and had come in contact with an Italian tourist who tested positive after returning to Italy.
Bangladesh	On March 8, three people tested positive for the COVID-19 in Bangladesh. Two of these three people returned from Italy.
Sri Lanka	On March 11, 2020, the first positive case was reported in Sri Lanka. The infected 52-year-old tour guide had come in contact with Italian tourists

Source: News Reports, Various.

As of March 24, SAARC had reported just 1536 cases in total, and 22 deaths due to the virus. Fact remains that diagnostic testing facilities are extremely poor in each of the eight countries, and South Asia as a region is not well prepared to deal with the COVID-19. However, the SAARC nations with the exception of Pakistan have decided to collaborate with each other to deal with the COVID-19 pandemic. The Indian Army is in the process of deploying separate teams to Sri Lanka, Bangladesh, Bhutan and Afghanistan to help those countries to boost capabilities to deal with increasing counts of the COVID-19. In March, a 14 member Indian Army team was sent to Maldives to help in setting up of coronavirus testing laboratories and to train local medical professionals to fight the pandemic.[7] Nevertheless, fact remains that a closer look at unfolding COVID-19 scenarios in each of the eight SAARC countries is needed. The following sections elaborate on the prevailing situations in each of the eight countries and how relations with China and shaping up in the current COVID-19 world order.

Afghanistan

As of April 24, 2020, Afghanistan reported 1279 cases of coronavirus infections with 42 deaths.[8] In April it was reported that in Afghan President Ashraf Ghani's official residence about 20 staff have tested positive for the new coronavirus.[9] Ongoing fighting, widespread poverty and weak public health systems have not been helpful in the fight against COVID-19 in Afghanistan. In February this year, Afghanistan's public health ministry designated the Afghanistan-Japan hospital in Kabul as the capital's primary coronavirus treatment facility. However, there is a startling shortage of coronavirus tests and ventilators. In order to mitigate the spread, Afghanistan in March even released 10,000 prisoners to curb spread of coronavirus.[10] A lockdown was announced in Kabul in March itself, and in April, it has been extended for two more weeks. Operating with the paucity of funds, Afghanistan faces further shortage of funds in dealing with the pandemic as the US has cut USD 1 billion in aid to Afghanistan this year. However, the U.S. has also given aid in the form COVID-19 assistance gone to Afghanistan, which totals to roughly USD 18 million.[11] The spread of the virus in Afghanistan can be attributed to migration flows between Iran and Afghanistan. As per the International Organisation for Migration (IOM), about 2.4 million Afghans are in Iran at any given time.[12] The border between the two countries has been a well-worn path for unskilled labourers for decades. The IOM states that as many as 15,000 people crossed on some days in March between Iran and Afghanistan. Nick Bishop, who heads the IOM's coronavirus response in Afghanistan stated that "it is the only place in the world with such massive cross border returns during the COVID-19."[13]

After increasing concerns regarding the spread of the COVID-19 in Afghanistan, the Chinese Embassy in Kabul said in March that China is ready to share its experiences with Afghanistan in addition to providing health aid.[14] On April 2, 2020, China handed over the first batch of China-aided medical supplies to Afghanistan.[15] On April 13, India sent a ship through Iran's Chabahar port carrying a major consignment of wheat and hydroxychloroquine, which is being used in the fight against the coronavirus pandemic. 251 containers carrying the first Indian consignment of 5022 MT of wheat out of a total of 75000 MT from India to Afghanistan, has already been sent while the remaining consignments will follow in the next few weeks. India is gifting 5,00,000 tablets of Hydroxychloroqine to Afghanistan as well.[16]

While efforts to mitigate the pandemic's effect on health and mortality continue in Afghanistan, the economy is another arena which is bearing severe impacts of the pandemic. As per data from World Integrated Trade Solution of the World Bank, Afghanistan's top markets for exports were in Pakistan, India and China.[17] On March 16, Pakistan closed its borders with Afghanistan in its bid to control the spread of the Coronavirus.[18] Even though borders between Afghanistan and India have not been sealed, India brought back 56 of its staff and Indo-Tibetan Border Police (ITBP) personnel from Afghanistan winding down its operations at its consulates in Herat and Jalalabad in view of the increasing fears of coronavirus spread and security threats.[19] As far as China is concerned, Afghanistan sealed its borders and restricted travel to and from the People's Republic of China in February itself. Authorities in northern Badakhshan province bordering China and Tajikistan said borders with both the countries have been closed in a bid to prevent from an outbreak of coronavirus epidemic to Afghanistan.[20] As per news reports imports from China stopped over the Coronavirus outbreak. Air corridors are the most direct route for Afghan investors to send their export to China.

According to the Chamber of Commerce and Investment of Afghanistan, more than 20 tons of Afghan dry fruits and saffron are sent to China every week by Turkish airlines flights but these flights have stopped since the coronavirus outbreak.[21] Local investors also say that imports of fruits and vegetables from China have stopped. Figures from the National Statistics and Information Authority show that Afghanistan's imports from China were worth USD 1.2 billion last year. China is the second biggest exporter of goods to Afghanistan after Iran.[22]

A closer look at Afghanistan's foreign trade statistics reveals that even though it suffers from massive negative balances of trade, imports have been essential for the country. Last year, customs revenue contributed around 40 per cent of Afghanistan's annual revenue. Comparing monthly customs revenues, the February revenue was 17 percent lower than the same month last year.[23] Agriculture contributes to about 30 per cent of the gross domestic product (GDP), and contributes to about 70 per cent of employment of the population. Unemployment leading to a decline in consumption will adversely impact local demands for fresh and dry fruits, and declining returns on agricultural produce would also dampen other economic indicators through a domino effect.[24] Therefore, both medically and economically, Afghanistan is in the throes of a severe crisis.

Bangladesh

Bangladesh recorded a total of 4689 cases of coronavirus infected along with 131 deaths as of April 24, 2020.[25] Bangladesh is among the most densely populated countries in the world wit 165 million people occupying a little over 147,000 sq. km. of territory. Thus the fears that the country could be ripe for the spread of coronavirus are rampant. Prime Minister Sheikh Hasina's government while stepping up measures to tackle the pandemic chose to declare a nation-wide holiday starting on March 26 as opposed to a lockdown. The holiday has been extended several times and remains in place as of April 24, 2020. Despite the fear of community spread high in Bangladesh, fact remains that the number of tests conducted are low. In fact, the percentage of tests being carried out is among the lowest- at about 143 per one million people. According to the country's health directorate, in March this year, Bangladesh screened more than 650,000 passengers at its international airports, ports and land borders by measuring their body temperatures. However, only 28,500 people were put in quarantine and only 65 in isolation.[26] Additionally, as per news reports, hospitals refuse people with fever and cough.

An additional problem that has emerged is that among the impacted are Bangladesh's frontline healthcare workers. At least 251 doctors tested positive for coronavirus on April 23 according to the Bangladesh Doctors Foundation (BDF). The group stated that a lack of personal protective equipment (PPE) and infections from patients were responsible for the outbreak among doctors.[27] Health workers have also complained about the quality of PPE being provided to them. As demands for PPE have increased, some ready-made garment (RMG) factories started producing it. Notably, Bangladesh is the second-largest RMG exporter after China. A further reduction in the number of frontline health workers only means further reduced care for the infected patients. Bangladesh in any case has 0.5 doctors per 1000 people.[28]

In addition to the medical threat, economic threat looms large upon Bangladesh. According to the World Bank, only 15 per cent of Bangladesh's population earns more than USD 5.90 a day.[29] Most villagers rely on remittances from cities of from abroad. However, in the face of this global pandemic, people are out of work everywhere and income has shrunk even in Bangladesh.

Garment exports account for a significant percentage of Bangladesh's foreign trade. In 2019, exports of garments accounted for USD 34.12 billion or 84 per cent of Bangladesh's total exports of USD 40.53 billion.[30] It is, however, set to lose about USD 6 billion in export revenue this year amidst widespread cancellations from the world's largest retailers and brands.[31] The largest trading partners of Bangladesh are China, U.S. and India. In February itself Bangladesh suspended visa on arrival for Chinese, U.S. and Indian nationals. The land border between India and Bangladesh is however still open.[32]

In February itself, the Bangladesh Trade and Tariff Commission sounded the warning bell on the impact of the Coronavirus on Bangladesh-China trade. It said, "due to the virus outbreak, both domestic and export trade of China as come to a standstill. Its impact has already started impacting Bangladesh's trade". In its report, the Commission stated that nearly 60 per cent fabrics of woven sub-sector were imported from China, and that the negative impacts of the COVID-19 had started becoming apparent. It added that about 15-20 per cent raw materials and about 80-85 per cent of dyeing chemicals and accessories of the knitwear sector came from China; the supply chain had been clearly disrupted.[33]

The following table shows the various sub-segments of Bangladesh's industries dependent on China for foreign trade which will get affected in the economic fallouts caused by the COVID-19.

Table 14.2: Impact of Coronavirus on Bangladesh's foreign trade with China: Segment-wise outline

Industrial segment	*Dependence percentage/ degree on China*	*Projected losses to the industry*	*Reason*
Finished leather and leather goods	60-65%	USD 353 million	Curtailment of exports to China
Garment accessories' raw materials	40%	USD 176.5 million	Curtailment of imports from China
Cosmetics and toiletries	200 containers per month	USD 8.8 million	Imports suspension from China
Machinery and spare parts	80-85%	–	Imports suspension from China
Jute spun export goods	–	USD 5.32 billion	Imports suspension from China
Printing raw materials	USD 1.8 billion worth imported from China	USD 3.6 billion	Shipment suspension from China

Source: Tariff Commission of Bangladesh.[34]

Bangladesh imports roughly USD 13.85 billion worth of goods from Bangladesh while exporting USD 831 million worth of goods. In addition to the segments mentioned in Table 14.2, Bangladesh also annually imports 25 containers of medical equipment and hospital equipment from China; imports about 95 per cent of raw materials of eyewear from China along with computer accessories. All of these remain suspended currently.

In March, China provided Bangladesh with medical supplies.[35] The Chinese embassy in Dhaka said the supply included 10,000 test kits, 10,000 PPE, and 1000 infrared thermometers. In its first batch of supplies provided to Bangladesh, China had sent 500 medical kits to detect the coronavirus infection. Earlier, the Bangladesh government sent some medical equipment, including masks, to China during the coronavirus outbreak in Wuhan. In April, Bangladesh sought China's medical assistance to handle its worsening COVID-19 situation as the country's death tolls continue rising. The Foreign Ministry of Bangladesh urged China to send an expert team comprising nurses, doctors and technicians to train Dhaka's health professionals. China has agreed to provide further help, share experience and data on the virus.[36]

Bhutan

Bhutan has had seven cases of Coronavirus so far with zero death, as on April 24, 2020.[37] Despite several infrastructural challenges, Bhutan has been able to manage the COVID-19 crisis well. To begin with Bhutan does not suffer from a population of overpopulation, and hence overcrowding- one of the main transmission modes of the virus. Additionally, since the first case of the COVID-19 was reported, the people of Bhutan undertook several effective, low cost measures to ensure hygiene across the country as they set about creating quarantine zones across the country with the help of the government.[38] In addition to this, Bhutan closed its borders with India in March itself over coronavirus fears.

As far as China is concerned, the Kingdom of Bhutan and the PRC do not maintain official diplomatic relations. The PRC shares a contiguous border of 470 kms with Bhutan. In terms of trade, in 2005, total trade between China and Bhutan stood at US$ 0.47 million. According to Bhutan's trade statistics, China ranks third after India and Japan among more than 38 countries from where Bhutan imports goods and commodities. However, Chinese goods have flushed the Bhutanese market.[39] Local cross-border merchants of western district of Haa and Paro import Chinese goods on horseback from Tibetan region. The goods arrive in shops of Thimphu after five to six days of walk over rugged mountains and hills. Such an import, however, is risky for local merchants for it is illegal. Other groups of business people in Thimphu sell Chinese products imported from Indian border towns, Bangladesh and Nepal.[40] With the sealing of borders, and increased focus on cross border movement, this is going to be impacted. However, fact remains that Bhutan has maintained the supply of essential goods well. According to Foreign Ministry spokesperson Geng Shuang, Chinese officials have shared their COVID-19 experiences with South Asian countries via a video conference and countries including Bhutan, Sri Lanka, India, Nepal, Pakistan, Bangladesh and Maldives have participated in it.[41] IN February itself, India agreed to provide technical assistance to Bhutan in managing the pandemic and to screen passengers.

India

India has a reported total of 24,530 cases of coronavirus cases, with 780 deaths as of April 25, 2020.[42] While the spread has been relatively low as compared to Western countries, the spread is the highest in South Asia. India like most other countries has been plunged into a crisis by the pandemic and is struggling to step up its testing for the coronavirus. On March 24, 2020, Prime Minister Narendra Modi announced a three-week long lockdown. In April, while announcing the extension of the nationwide lockdown, the government granted approvals to a slew of domestic kit makers. India received its much-delayed order of 650,000 tests from China on April 16, 2020. In the meantime, the Indian Council for Medical Research also gave approvals to domestic companies like Ambala based Alpine Biomedicals, Pune based Immunoscience and Delhi based Nulife Care.[43] One of the biggest fallouts of the lockdown has been on migrant labour. Millions of migrant labourers are stuck in different parts of India without jobs, livelihoods, adequate shelter and essentials. Out of work and with no means of ensuring essential supplies of food, when the initial lockdown was supposed to end on March 24, thousands thronged railway stations in the hopes of being able to get back home. Some even tried walking back thousands of kilometres to their homes. Most state that their homes in villages can at least guarantee them food.[44] Uttar Pradesh for example, has among the largest number of migrant labourers who work in agriculture, factories, services and logistics in states such as Maharashtra, Gujarat, Delhi and Karnataka. A very large number, close to one million, are on their way back home.[45]

In addition to the impact on the lives and health of the people of India, the coronavirus pandemic has also led to an economic crisis. India's already slowing growth rates have further slowed after the onset of the pandemic. In terms of foreign trade, China is India's second largest trading partner after the U.S., and India imports some of the most critical inputs in segments ranging from organic chemicals to electrical machinery from China. There could be a shortage of critical inputs from China amidst the COVID-19. As per estimates published by the United Nations Conference on Trade and Development (UNCTAD) in March this year, India is among the top 15 economies which will be most affected by the slowdown induced by the COVID-19. The trade impact of the coronavirus epidemic for India is estimated to be about 348 million dollars.[46]

In March, India temporarily suspended almost all travel visas as part of its efforts to contain the pandemic. In February itself India suspended all visas issued to Chinese passport holders from the PRC, except for those from Hong Kong, Macao and Taiwan travelling from any part of the world, including from within the PRC.[47]

In March, India provided China with 15 tons of medical supplies including masks, gloves and other emergency medical equipment at a cost of about Rs. 2.11 crores.[48] In March, India received its second batch of critical medical supplies including protective gears, masks and ventilators from China.[49] In April it was reported that India did receive some PPE that failed quality tests in India. At least 50,000 of the

1.7 lakh PPE kits from China failed checks.[50] However, despite the reports of the testing kits failing quality standards in India, the Ministry of External Affairs in India said that at least 20 more flights are expected from China bringing in supplies.

In addition to the medical and economic hardships faced by India in the COVID-19 world order, China has also unleashed aggression at the borders, and on May 5, 2020, Indian and Chinese troops engaged in non-lethal face offs and skirmished along the India-China border. Skirmishes took place near the Pangong Lake in Ladakh, Nathu La pass in Sikkim, and there are several ongoing face offs at multiple locations in eastern Ladakh, along the Line of Actual Control. A significant point of focus in this context is the Galwan River valley, where China claims that India is violating Chinese sovereignty. China's officials and media claim that India is "violating" their "sovereignty and territorial integrity" and "trespassing" in the western sector currently, as if the two countries have agreed-upon maps delineating their respective borders in these areas. None exist between India and China. China is now claiming the Galwan area, which was traditionally part of the Kashmir princely state and at no point in China's history did it have control over it.[51] This attempt of China offering medical diplomacy on the one hand and upping aggression at India's borders is a usage of the carrot and stick policy, in order to ensure that India does not indulge in any activity or international coalition which China disapproves of. For the purpose, it is extending the carrot of medical diplomacy stressing on bonhomie, while using the stick of aggression at borders to remind India that it is in a subordinate position, and can be put in its place by China at any time if it takes a stance not agreeable to China.

Maldives

Maldives has reported 141 cases of Coronavirus with zero dates as of April 26, 2020.[52] The pandemic spread to Maldives in March through an Italian tourist who spent holidays in Kuredu Resort and Spa in Maldives.[53] After this, the hotel was locked down with several tourists stranded on the island. In March, the islands of Kuredu, Vilamendhoo, Batalaa and Kuramathi were placed under quarantine and schools were closed.[54] The government has turned the resort island of Villivaru into a quarantine facility, described as the "world's first coronavirus resort" where patients would enjoy free luxurious stay along with free medical care.[55] Despite the fact that the Maldivian economy is dependent on tourism, the government took the hard decision of stopping all visas on arrivals from March itself. Working with the World Health Organization, the Maldives government has taken important steps to establish isolation and quarantine facilities and prepare hospitals for testing and treatment. If COVID-19 hits local population, 60-80 percent will get infected in Maldives. With government interventions, it is hoped to be reduced by 30-40 per cent. However, like most South Asian countries, Maldives also lacks medical facilities for the ones seriously affected. In addition to the problem faced by the local population from the COVID-19, another pertinent problem exists in Maldives- that of migrant labourers primarily from Bangladesh. Two cases of COVID have been reported from amongst migrant labourers. There are roughly 100,000 migrant workers in Maldives, most of them from Bangladesh, making up about 25 per cent of the island country's population.[56] The migrant population is especially vulnerable given the fact that they live in congested shared quarters and engage in work that ensures practising social distancing is not possible.

The economic fallout of the pandemic is going to be immense for the island country, as stated by foreign affairs minister Abdulla Shahid in March during an interview with CNN. As stated by Shahid, tourist arrivals in Maldives were down by 22 per cent in March itself, and an overall drop of 35 per cent is expected this year. Shahid quoted an ADB study on the impact of COVID-19 on tourism and stated that Maldives was projected to be the second worst hit country with a reduction in 8.7 per cent of the GDP. Tourism receipts are the lifeline for the country's foreign exchange, which stands at about USD 450 million. Because of the pandemic, the government revenue is set to decline between USD 140 million to USD 440 million this year alone.[57]

Maldives has received a 14-member medical team from India along with essential medications from India. India donated three months of medicines required by Maldives. In terms of assistance provided so far to Maldives, Bangladesh has also provided significant assistance to Maldives, after India. Japan and the United States have also sent help. Chinese government has not given any assistance so far, even though the Yunnan provincial government has sent some relief assistance to Maldives.[58]

Nepal

Nepal has a total of 51 cases and zero deaths due to the COVID-19 as of April 26, 2020.[59] While the first case was detected in early January, it was only in March that Nepal went into complete lockdown, owing to the fact that the total number of infected was still in single digits till April 2. However, according to health experts, the numbers are low because of low testing. Fewer than 100 tests had been done up to April 2.[60] After the first few cases, Nepal established health desks at its international airport as well as on border checkpoints with India, beginning in the middle of January itself. Land borders with both India and China were soon sealed off, and schools and colleges closed. Quarantine centres and temporary hospitals were set up across Nepal and laboratory facilities are in the process of being upgraded and expanded.

However, the Nepal government was slow in shutting down flights despite a Supreme Court order dated 2nd March 2020 directing them to do so immediately.[61] Even as late as 18th March flights from virus infected countries continued to fly in before a ban was put into place. Surprisingly the government did not stop flights from China even then.[62] The only working thermal scanner at Tribhuvan International Airport stopped working from 8th Feb. Unchecked flow of people continued past the open border points. While the border check posts with China were closed, those with India continued to remain open until lockdown came into effect on 24th March. Hence influx of people into Nepal remained unchecked at best.[63]

A severe shortage of facemasks and protective gear as well as price hikes were reported following bans on export in India and China respectively. Some hospitals took upon the task of sewing plain clothes masks as precautions. Shortages of sanitisers were also reported.[64] Nepal has also halted all flight operations till May 15, 2020. This year was to be the Visit Nepal Year 2020, which the government has now cancelled. The economy of the country rests on foreign employment, tourism, manufacturing, trade and construction- all of which are impacted due to the COVID-19 pandemic.

On March 10, 71 Chinese workers who were employed in the construction of the Pokhara Airport, who had returned from China after undergoing a 14-day long quarantine were put into quarantine for another 14 days. Before these 36 Chinese workers who had been working on the same project had also gone through a similar quarantine process upon their return to work.[65] Between March 12-15, labour permits for all countries were suspended indefinitely. Nepal closed its land borders with India and China on March 23, 2020. Earlier, India and Nepal had decided to keep four checkpoints at the border to be operational. However, Nepal's authorities expressed concerns about the unrestricted movement of the two countries' citizens through crossings along the 1800 km border. Nepal's import-dependent economy is also vulnerable to depreciation of Indian currency to which its currency is permanently pegged, as India's economy itself slides into economic chaos caused by the pandemic.

Nepal's tourism sector has been suffering immensely due to the absence of Chinese tourists. In the first six months of 2019, at least 85,318 Chinese tourists visited Nepal which was a 19.53 percent year-on rise over the same period of 2018.[66] The Visit Nepal plan scheduled for 2020 aimed at attracting 350,000 Chinese tourists. However, in January, China instructed all travel companies to temporarily stop selling international tour packages, presenting a significant setback to Visit

Nepal 2020.[67] Number of international flights to and from Nepal had decreased by more than 50 per cent by 13 March.[68]

Nepal's manufacturing sector is also experiencing a shortage of raw materials, most of which comes from China. The construction sector for example, which imports most of its building materials from China, has also been negatively impacted. In addition to this, remittances, which contribute to more than half of Nepal's GDP have also been hit. Work permits all across the globe have been impacted.

The wholesale and retail sector has also been affected due to fall of imports from China. Foreign direct investment (FDI) has also been severely impacted. Before the emergence of the pandemic, in the first six months of the fiscal year 2019-20, FDI pledges in Nepal had increased by 315.3 per cent to Rs. 190.36 billion, as per the Department of Industry in Nepal. Most of the foreign investment commitments were from China. However, this will also be severely negatively impacted.[69]

The Chinese Embassy in Nepal, Sichuan Province and Alibaba Foundation, Jack Ma Foundation, China CAMC Engineering Company Ltd., and Sichuan Huashi Group Company Ltd. jointly donated the medical aid including kits, portable ventilators, thermometers, personal protective equipment, and surgical masks to the Nepal government.[70] As far as India is concerned, while India has already gifted 23 T of medicine to Nepal, help and support in other areas is also being extended. In order to minimize the impact of lockdowns on mutual trade between the countries, the Indian Customs has granted waivers on certain import conditions. The Certificate of Origin CoO is an important document to ascertain that provisions of the Preferential Trade Treaty are not violated. The CoO produced by local chambers of commerce in India certify items of export to be of Indian Origin, thus allowing preferential duty/NIL duty to be levied on such items. The Indian Customs has waived the requirement to produce CoO against an undertaking. This should prevent holdup at the border thus ensuring steady supply of essentials from India.[71] While this may be of some economic benefit, fact remains that Nepal, like other South Asian countries is in for a long haul in terms of medical and economic costs of the COVID-19 pandemic.

Pakistan

Pakistan has reported a total of 14,079 cases with 301 deaths as of April 28, 2020. Till March, Pakistan led South Asia with the highest number of coronavirus cases, as stated by government data. Half of these were traced to a quarantine camp on its border with Iran. Like most other countries, Pakistan has also implemented quarantines in localised areas, closed borders with neighbouring countries, levied restrictions on travel, closed schools and universities in addition to promoting social distancing and banning public events. In March itself, Pakistan sealed its borders with Afghanistan, China and Iran. Pakistan also suspended airlinks with China and Iran in March itself. On April 25, Prime Minister Imran Khan announced a 'smart lockdown', under which areas where outbreaks have taken place will be closed, while certain economic activities continue to take place. Pakistan has allowed religious congregations during Ramzan, except for in the province of Singh, where health officials have warned that the virus spread could be rapid, which is why mosques remain shut in the region. Despite having more than 10,000 cases on April 25th, Khan said that the number of cases in Pakistan are low.[72] When the COVID-19 pandemic first broke out in Wuhan, Pakistan refused to evacuate Pakistani nationals from China in a show of solidarity. Pakistan's Ambassador to China also added that Pakistani students will not be evacuated from Wuhan, since China has better medical facilities.[73]

On March 31, Pakistan even said that the transmission of the COVID-19 was not due to China; in this bid Pakistan also tried to defend its decision to not airlift Pakistani students from Wuhan during the initial days of the outbreak.[74]

Pakistan's testing rates are extremely low, as it has been testing (as of April 20, 2020) 0.4 people per 1000 people.[75] Pakistan in any case has a fragile healthcare system. As stated by the World Health Organization, Pakistan's health expenditure is just 2.9 per cent of its GDP, significantly lower than half the world's average.[76] Pakistan like several other South Asian countries suffers from a shortage of diagnostics. The emergency of the situation is revealed by what transpired at the Aga Khan University Hospital, when it closed its doors to new COVID-19 patients in late March after massive crowds of people overwhelmed the clinic, exposing the staff to infection, who suffer from a lack of protective gear in any case.[77]

The case of the quarantine center in Taftan, in Pakistan's Balochistan province is also telling of the severe medical challenges the country faces in the COVID-19 situation. The camp in Taftan was to function as a sanitary quarantine location, preventing the spread of the virus from Iran. However, there was nothing in the camp, and patients were simply made to sleep in some dilapidated tents. Basic precautionary measures to prevent the spread of the virus were also missing, and as per doctors at the camp, even people who showed symptoms were not tested or even isolated. There was a shortage of doctors in any case in addition to medical facilities. Finally protests broke out among those quarantined.[78] In addition to these cases, the province of Sindh, which has the highest number of confirmed Coronavirus cases in Pakistan, has 484 ventilators, of which 353 are working, 52 are out of order and 43 yet to be installed.[79]

Economically, Pakistan is already in an extremely difficult spot as it has to repay USD 27.8 billion worth of public debt to international creditors, which include China, the Asian Development Bank, the World Bank and the International Monetary Fund among others.[80] It also has to repay the balance of payments support it has obtained from Saudi Arabia, China. UAE and Qatar, which amounts to an additional USD 8.5 billion.[81] Pakistan has to repay China irrespective of the fact that the two describe their relations as all-weather strategic cooperative partnership and frequently vow to support each other on issues concerning each other's core interests.

Industrial production has taken a hit due to the pandemic. The Central Government has diverted most of its funds to fight the pandemic and has announced an economic package worth USD 7 billion.[82] In addition to this, the Asian Development Bank, the International Monetary Fund have also pledged or approved further loans to Pakistan.

On March 27, Pakistan opened its borders with China for a day to accept Chinese medical supplies to fight the growing coronavirus outbreak.[83] Pakistan's President Arif Alvi had visited China on March 17, and within days of the visit, China sent medical supplies to Karachi. Sindh province's Chief Minister Syed Murad Ali Shah approved the purchase of 290 ventilators, 3.2 million personal protective equipment (PPE), 100 rapid kit antigen test machines (RKATM), 100,000 testing kits, 50 RT lamp testing machines and 10,000 RT lamp kits and 29 portable X-ray machines so that testing capacity in the province could be enhanced.[84] China has also sent a medical team to Pakistan to help in training. Huang Qingzhen, a member of the expert group and the chief physician of the Center for Disease Control and Prevention of the Chinese People's Liberation Army, told reporters that after arriving in Pakistan on April 24, the expert group visited 7 medical institutions and designated hospitals in Islamabad and surrounding areas non-stop and listened to the report on the epidemic prevention measures taken by Pakistan. China's People's Liberation Army veterans are trying to help the Pakistani Army in the management of COVID-19.[85]

Despite China's generous sales of medical equipment to Pakistan, at least 5000 more ventilators are required in Pakistan![86] Islamabad had sent a large number of supplies to China when Beijing was in the throes of the virus in January. The Hunza region in Gilgit-Baltistan, Pakistan donated 7,000 surgical masks to China through the Chinese embassy in Pakistan in Islamabad on Wednesday.[87] The province donated the masks as opposed to selling them.

In addition to the disruption in international trade which Pakistan is expected to face, another blow comes in the form of that to the China Pakistan Economic

Corridor (CPEC). The much-touted economic corridor was hoped to bring infrastructural and employment benefits to Pakistan. However, in a detailed report tabled before the high-powered National Coordination Committee in Pakistan, it was suggested that Chinese companies working on CPEC projects will suffer delays and higher costs along with supply-chain and worker related disruptions will be witnessed. The report also adds that Pakistan's plan to expeditiously build Special Economic Zones (SEZs) will be thwarted or at least face delays as Chinese companies will find it hard to manage required human and capital supplies on an urgent basis.[88]

Sri Lanka

In Sri Lanka, there have been 596 cases so far with seven deaths as of April 28, 2020.[89] As compared to most other countries in the neighbourhood, Sri Lanka's cases are still relatively low. Sri Lanka's edge in healthcare is already a bright spot in South Asia. Since March, the country has been focussing on detecting infections, referring identified patients for treatment to dedicated COVID-19 centres, while isolating cases during treatment to prevent further exposure from the detected cases. Sri Lanka's primary strategy to deal with the pandemic includes contact tracing, quarantining exposed persons, active searches among close contacts through testing at the appropriate time after exposure, follow-ups and breaking links from the index cases.[90] In January this year, as one of the countries frequently visited by Chinese tourists and citizens, the Ministry of Health of Sri Lanka has received a notice from the WHO requesting that it be vigilant against the new coronavirus in Wuhan.[91] Sri Lanka also imposed a nation-wide curfew staring on March 20, 2020. There has been intermittent lifting of the curfew in selected areas which were not seen as dangerous for the spread of the deadly virus. However, the curfew has meant that several sections, with daily wage earners in particular are left with no means of livelihood. Additionally, while there are no official figures for the number of tests conducted so far, several experts have pointed out to the need to test more as the pandemic grows. Sri Lanka also needs masks, ventilators and personal protection equipment (PPE), which are in short supply.[92] The Government Medical Officers Association (GMOA), a professional body comprising of Sri Lanka's doctors, insist that the country has over 42,000 people who have had contacts with those who have tested positive for COVID-19 and that at least 1,500 tests need to be carried out daily.[93]

Between late March and early April, the Chinese government and companies that are involved in major projects in Sri Lanka have donated a large amount of masks, PPE, and test kits. Among these companies are China Merchants Port Group (CMPort), the parent company of Colombo International Container Terminals

(CICT) and Hambantota International Port Group (HIPG); CHEC Port City Colombo, the company behind the project building a financial centre on 269 hectares of land reclaimed from the sea; Metallurgical Corporation of China (MCC), which has won the contracts to build a number of infrastructure projects, including an airport highway; China National Aero-Technology International Engineering Corporation (AVIC-ENG), which built infrastructure projects from highways to water supply projects and Huawei; and a telecommunications giant with an office in Colombo.[94] Sri Lanka also received a donation of 20,000 testing kits from Alibaba Group's founder Jack Ma. Jack Ma is currently donating 1.8 million masks, 210,000 test kits, 36,000 protective suits, plus ventilators and thermometers to Afghanistan, Bangladesh, Cambodia, Laos, Maldives, Mongolia, Myanmar, Nepal, Pakistan, and Sri Lanka.[95]

The World Bank has stated that it expects a recession in Sri Lanka in the coming months with forecast growth between –3 percent to –0.5 percent for 2020.[96] Manufacturing Purchasing Managers Index (PMI) in February marginally slowed by 0.4 basis points due to a contraction in new orders and employment in the manufacturing sector. Meanwhile, Services PMI recorded a 6.8 basis point drop owing to reduction in new businesses, business activity and expectations.[97] The tourism sector which contributes significantly to the economy will also see losses. According to the Asian Development Bank's estimates on 06 March 2020, the decline in tourism revenues for Sri Lanka could range from USD 107 mn – USD 319 million. China dropped out from Sri Lanka's top 10 tourist source markets for the first time since 2012.[98] Several infrastructures and building projects have also slowdown due to the delay in procurement of materials from China and the complete stoppage of work due to the curfew.

China's COVID-19 Diplomacy in South Asia

The COVID-19 presents China with immense possibilities to emerge as a heavyweight in international relations, as the current hegemon – the U.S. finds itself like the rest of the countries across the world – a pandemic with origins in China! China has actively tried to shape narratives, and tried to deflect taking any responsibility for the initial cover up of the virus. On November 17, 2019 itself Dr. Li Wenliang – an ophthalmologist at Wuhan Central Hospital, had warned about the possible outbreak of an illness that resembled the severe acute respiratory syndrome (SARS), which is now known as COVID-19. After he shared his warnings publicly, the Wuhan police summoned him and rebuked him for spreading falsehood on the internet. The Chinese Government instead of promptly informing the World Health Organization and the rest of the world about the onset of the deadly Coronavirus, for reasons best known to it, kept the matter under wraps. The country placed it in the public domain only on 31 December 2019, which is after a delay of six weeks of occurrence.

Li eventually got infected with the coronavirus and died of it. However, even before his death he had turned into a hero for many Chinese people.[99] The suppression of Li's warnings has not been the only instance of China's suppression of information on the outbreak of the COVID-19 epidemic. In an interview with the Chinese magazine *Renwu*, which is being rapidly censored and reposted on the Chinese web, Ai Fen, director of emergency at Wuhan Central Hospital, said that superiors had reprimanded her for reporting a SARS-like virus.[100]

Li Wenliang's death caused furore among the Chinese public, and only in response to it, the central government dispatched investigators to look into the circumstances surrounding his reprimand and death. Beijing's investigators concluded that Wuhan authorities acted "inadequately" when they reprimanded the late doctor and failed to follow "proper law enforcement procedure."[101] The point to note is that the investigators did not mention what the response to Li's warnings should have been. This was a clear attempt at narrative shaping not just for domestic consumption but for international consumption as well. The attempt was to portray China as having a responsible system of governance that takes gross miscarriages of justice into cognisance.

The myriad sale of medical equipment that China is currently undertaking to the world is an extension of its aid diplomacy. China touts its aid as being that of no-strings attached. However, how "no strings" have played out for Sri Lanka when China took over its Hambantota port when Sri Lanka could not repay China's loans is a known fact. In addition to creating dependence on China for medical aid in the current situation, what China's medical diplomacy is also doing is revenue creation for China through sales of medical equipment. In the absolute dearth of vaccines, antidotes, medical gear, ventilators and even face masks, the world is scrambling for supplies.

China bought face masks in bulk from across the globe, when the pandemic had just begun spreading out to the world. More than 2.46 billion masks, protective equipment and other types of PPE kit were inspected by the National Customs in China between January 24 and February 29.[102] As per news reports. Chinese organisations operating in Australia sent bulk medical supplies to China during the height of the crisis. Chinese owned property developer Risland Australia alone reportedly flew tonnes of medical supplies to Wuhan in February, while Greenland Group re-tasked all employees to repurchase face masks, hand sanitisers, thermometers and anti-bacterial wipes. The company bought about three million surgical masks and sent them to China in January and February!

In the current unfolding COVID-19 situation, China sells masks and equipment to the highest bidder in addition to practising medical diplomacy and showcasing its role as a responsible player of the international system. French officials have complained that the masks meant for being sold to France were diverted to the U.S.[103] Jean Rottner, the head of France's Grand Est. region ordered five million masks from China, out of which only two million arrived. Officials complain that the rest has been diverted to the U.S. by China which pays three to four times for the same consignment.

In South Asia, where medical infrastructure in most countries remains poor and shoddy and populaces remain vulnerable to rapid contagion of the virus, similar stories have begun to emanate. In April itself, the government of Nepal cancelled a contract to import testing kits and medical supplies from China. Nepal's Ministry of Health and Population has issued instructions that the COVID-19 Rapid Diagnostic Kit imported from China should not be used after doubts emerged about their reliability.[104] This is going to severely affect testing in the country as the kits imported from China represent about 90 per cent of all the rapid diagnostic testing kits available in Nepal.

In Pakistan, which refused to evacuate its students stuck in Wuhan to show solidarity with China, China has donated 3,00,000 face masks, 10,000 protective suits and USD 4 millions to Islamabad to fight the virus. However, when the consignment from China landed on April 3, it was found that China had sent masks made out of underwear.[105] To make matters worse, the Sindh provincial government had sent the masks to hospitals without verification. In Bangladesh, immediately post Spain's complaint regarding the faulty medical kits, the Chinese Embassy in Dhaka stated that none of the 40,500 test kits sent to Bangladesh was from Shenzhen Bioeasy Biotechnology—the company which was under question by the Spanish government on Thursday for supplying the sub-standard kits. However, Bangladeshi authorities have stated that it will use the Chinese equipment only after thorough examination of the products by its own experts. Dr. Meerjady Sabrina Flora, the director of Bangladesh's Institute of Epidemiology said that if any equipment is found faulty by Bangladesh's medical team, they will be returned.[106]

In India as well, faulty equipment from China emerged, and at the daily government briefing on the COVID-19 situation, Indian Council for Medical Research's Dr. Raman Gangakhedar stated that complaints of faulty equipment have been received and that states have been advised not to use them.[107] India received 170,000 PPE sets from China, out of which at least 90,000 failed quality tests in India.[108] In response, the Chinese Embassy spokesperson in India, Ji Rong said that people are looking at issues with pre-emptive prejudice and that it is unfair to call the equipment faulty.[109]

China is definitely going out of its way to demonstrate its willingness to help those in need in particular, and this includes South Asian countries as well. However, there are more foreign policy calculations behind China's seemingly benign assistance to countries in need. China's rise to the need of the hour- production of medical equipment and masks is driven by concerns regarding its slowing economy, its desire to maintain the leading position in global supply chains and the need to suppress calls for culpability of cover up and spread of the pandemic. China's model of economic development is an export driven one, and China needs the global market to ensure the sustainability of its economic growth rates. Albeit drastically slowed, fact still remains that there is a demand currently for goods- medical goods in particular, to which China is trying its level best to respond and position itself as the central node in the supply of such goods.

In countries like Pakistan, China's narratives about its ability to deal with a pandemic while helping the world would only get amplified. China's soft power would see a tremendous boost. However, given the rising complaints regarding medical equipment, for other countries, the response to China in the world order that emerges post COVID-19 will be very different. Countries across the globe are thinking of recalibrating their relations with China, as is seen in the case of the shutdown of even the last Confucius institute in Sweden in April this year by the government.[110] There is bound to be a new formidable opposition to China's attempts at emerging as the leader in the post COVID-19 world order. For most countries at the moment, including the South Asian ones, the primary concern is that of emerging out of the pandemic with as less economic and medical damages as possible. While China's medical diplomacy will definitely amplify in the next few months to come, it will not be able to garner as many supporters as it would want to through the usage of its soft power.

So far, China has blamed the U.S. for the outbreak of the virus, followed by its claims of the virus first emanating in Italy, followed by its coronavirus narratives aimed against African nationals who are blamed for the spreading of the virus.[111] In addition to this, China has refused calls for independent investigations into the origins of the virus! China has also blocked any research on the origins of the virus! It has cracked down on publication of academic research about the virus' origins, which is the part of an attempt to control the narrative around the pandemic, as revealed by documents published online by Chinese universities.[112] If anything, all of this only works against China's COVID-19 diplomacy and its efforts to project itself as a saviour!

While dealing with the pandemic and searching for means to ensure that growth does not completely get wiped out, countries across the world are also trying to come up with ways and means to hold China responsible. Some independent organisations including lawyers have already petitioned various international forums to seek reparations from China and/or to ensure more accountability from China. In addition to these, what the global community could also consider is a revocation of China's membership of the United Nations Security Council, while putting increased pressure on Beijing to have greater transparency on public health arrangements. Specific Chinese officials' assets could also be frozen and travel prohibitions could be put in place.

While the debate on whether the virus is created purposely by China in a lab rages on, fact remains that China is definitely guilty of the cover up of the initial outbreak. Additionally, biological warfare in the 21st century becomes a part of asymmetric warfare where it is next to impossible to establish culpability. In the current scenario, while evidence maybe disputed, fact remains that a stable global order cannot have another pandemic, in case it can survive this one to begin with. Thus greater responsibility from a player like China is needed. The fact that wet markets continue to exist in China needs greater focus, and till these are not actually shut down, there needs to be more global attention on it.

The world economy has already begun unravelling, with unemployment set to become a problem for countries across the globe. China's economic clout is built on its manufacturing prowess- its export dependent economic growth model. Keeping this in mind, Xi Jinping had said in February itself, much earlier before China succeeded in tackling the pandemic that economic activity must be re-established.[113] Post the end of the pandemic, it will become pertinent for countries to establish supply chains outside China so that such disruptions can be avoided in future.

This remains true for South Asia as well. Indigenous manufacturing needs to be encouraged. Countries should have medical supply chains that are not reliant on China. This is particularly true for India which imports about 70 per cent of its bulk drugs and intermediates from China.[114] India also needs to quickly diversify its import sources to save its industry, consumers and economy from trade breakdown due to dependency on a single partner such as China. As seen in graph 1 on China's South Asia trade, India is China's biggest market in South Asia- clearly implying the extent of India's reliance on China. Indian goods nevertheless face tariff and non-tariff barriers in China. In the post COVID-19 world order, it is imperative that India has supply chains that are not reliant on China. Several questions have emerged on China's relations with South Asian countries in the post COVID world order. In this context, China's relations with Pakistan will not see much of a change, and the two will remain the all-weather friends that they have been so far. However, given the increased suspicion towards China, along with prevailing public perceptions at home, China's South Asia relations, particularly with respect to the Belt and

Road Initiative Projects will undergo a sea change. An example of this is the clash that took place between local Nepalis and Chinese workers amidst the lockdown in March this year. The locals in Nepal's Marsyangdi clashed with the employers of a Chinese company constructing a hydropower plant in Lamjung. The villagers protested the movement of trucks carrying construction materials of Nyadi Hydropower Project. The locals were agitated as the workers had just returned from China![115]

As far as India is concerned, stepping up of aggression by China at the borders is only leading to more antagonism from India, and India in turn is now creating its own form of diplomatic response to this, and example of which is seen in the fact that Members of Parliament of the ruling Party in India- the Bhartiya Janata Party attended the swearing in ceremony of Taiwan's President Tsai Ing-wen in May. As was the case during the Doklam standoff between the Indian and the Chinese armies India will not back down this time as well.

In addition to developments in South Asia, China's projects have been facing problems in Africa as well, as there have been several calls for debt relief from African countries for the BRI projects, China has responded with a tone-deaf attitude, and has even gone to the extent of stating that debt moratorium for under developed countries will not be useful.[116] A high handed approach from China is visible across the globe, and even though the Chinese effort maybe to make hay while the COVID-19 Sun shines, its efforts at attaining the position of a leader through aggression or faulty medical diplomacy will not yield it much.

NOTES

1 Haider Suhasini (2020), "Coronavirus | South Asia remains an outlier in infections", 19 April 2020, https://www.thehindu.com/news/national/coronavirus-south-asia-remains-an-outlier-in-infections/article31378180.ece, accessed online 20 April 2020.

2 Press Trust of India (2020), "COVID-19 to hit South Asia very hard, likely to wipe out gains made in poverty alleviation: World Bank", 12 April 2020, https://www.indiatoday.in/world/story/covid-19-to-hit-south-asia-very-hard-likely-to-wipe-out-gains-made-in-poverty-alleviation-world-bank-1666066-2020-04-12, accessed online 14 April 2020.

3 Ibid.

4 Worldometer (2020), "Countries where COVID-19 has spread", 21 April 2020, https://www.worldometers.info/coronavirus/countries-where-coronavirus-has-spread/, accessed online 21 April 2020.

5 Embassy of India in Beijing of the People's Republic of China, "India-China Trade And Economic Relations", https://www.eoibeijing.gov.in/economic-and-trade-relation.php, accessed online 18 April 2020.

6 Chaudhury Dipanjan Roy (2020), "India, China could explore measures to boost trade hit by Covid-19", 04 April 2020, https://economictimes.indiatimes.com/news/economy/foreign-trade/india-china-could-explore-measures-to-boost-trade-hit-by-covid-19/articleshow/74977563.cms?from=mdr, accessed online 16 April 2020.

7 Press Trust of India (2020), "Coronavirus: Army readying teams for Bangladesh, Bhutan, Sri Lanka, Afghanistan", 21 April 2020, https://economictimes.indiatimes.com/news/defence/coronavirus-army-readying-teams-for-bangladesh-bhutan-sri-lanka-afghanistan/articleshow/75275870.cms?utm_source=contentofinterest&utm_medium=text&utm_campaign=cppst, accessed online 22 April 2020.

8 Worldometers (2020), "Afghanistan", 24 April 2020, https://www.worldometers.info/coronavirus/country/afghanistan/, accessed online 24 April 2020.

9 Cankao News Network (2020), "外媒：阿富汗总统府约 20 名职员感染新冠病毒" (About 20 employees of the Presidential Palace of Afghanistan are infected with the new crown virus), 20 April 2020, https://tech.sina.com.cn/roll/2020-04-20/doc-iircuyvh8788192.shtml, accessed online 22 April 2020.

10 Cankao News Network (2020), "阿富汗释放 1 万名囚犯以遏制新冠病毒传播" (Afghanistan releases 10,000 prisoners to curb spread of new crown virus), 27 March 2020, https://baijiahao.baidu.com/s?id=1662282155758473987&wfr=spider&for=pc, accessed online 21 April 2020.

11 Business Standard (2020), "Covid-19: India gets $5.9 mn US aid; assures Bhutan, Seychelles of help", 17 April 2020, https://www.business-standard.com/article/current-affairs/covid-19-india-gets-5-9-mn-us-aid-assures-bhutan-seychelles-of-help-120041700163_1.html, accessed online 20 April 2020.

12 Quilty Andrew (2020), "With Fake Hand Sanitizer and 12 Ventilators, Afghanistan expects millions of Coronavirus cases", 03 April 2020, https://theintercept.com/2020/04/02/coronavirus-afghanistan/, accessed online 10 April 2020.

13 *Ibid.*

14 Afghan Online Press (2020), "China to Aid Afghans in Coronavirus Fight", 13 March 2020, http://www.aopnews.com/china-afghanistan-relations/china-to-aid-afghans-in-coronavirus-fight/, accessed online 09 June 2020.

15 Xinhua (2020), "China hands over medical supplies to Afghanistan to fight COVID-19", 02 April 2020, http://www.xinhuanet.com/english/2020-04/02/c_138941306_4.htm, accessed online 10 April 2020.

16 The Hindu (2020), "India to use Chabahar port to send assistance to Afghanistan", 13 April 2020, https://www.thehindu.com/news/national/india-to-use-chabahar-port-to-send-assistance-to-afghanistan/article31326064.ece, accessed online 16 April 2020.

17 World Integrated Trade Solution, "Afghanistan exports, imports and trade balance By Country 2018", https://wits.worldbank.org/CountryProfile/en/Country/AFG/Year/LTST/TradeFlow/EXPIMP/Partner/by-country, accessed online 15 April 2020.

18 Voice of America (2020), "Pakistan Closes Border with Afghanistan Over Coronavirus", 16 March 2020, https://www.youtube.com/watch?v=4f90SsMm9Kw, accessed online 10 April 2020.

19 Haider Suhasini and Dinakar Peri (2020), "India temporarily closes 2 consulates in Afghanistan", 08 April 2020, https://www.thehindu.com/news/national/india-temporarily-closes-2-consulates-in-afghanistan/article31291941.ece, accessed online 12 April 2020.

20 Afghanistan Times (2020), "Afghanistan Closes Borders as China's Coronavirus Cases Continue", 05 February 2020, http://www.afghanistantimes.af/afghanistan-closes-borders-as-chinas-coronavirus-continues/, accessed online 10 April 2020.

21 Indo Asian News Service (2020), "Coronavirus outbreak affecting China-Afghan trade", 03 February 2020, https://www.outlookindia.com/newsscroll/coronavirus-outbreak-affecting-chinaafghan-trade/1724645, accessed online 12 April 2020.

22 Daijiworld (2020), "Coronavirus outbreak affecting China-Afghan trade", 03 February 2020, https://www.daijiworld.com/news/newsDisplay.aspx?newsID=670147, accessed online 10 April 2020.

23 Rahim Shoaib A (2020), "What the COVID-19 Outbreak Means for Afghanistan's Troubled

Economy", 11 April 2020, https://thediplomat.com/2020/04/what-the-covid-19-outbreak-means-for-afghanistans-troubled-economy/, accessed online 10 April 2020.

24 *Ibid.*

25 Worldometer (2020), "Bangladesh", 24 April 2020, https://www.worldometers.info/coronavirus/country/bangladesh/, accessed online 24 April 2020.

26 Hossain Iqbal (2020), "Coronavirus in Bangladesh, low testing and quarantine set the scene for a humanitarian disaster", 20 April 2020, https://www.lifegate.com/people/lifestyle/coronavirus-in-bangladesh-health-humanitarian-crisis, accessed online 21 April 2020.

27 Mahmud Faizal (2020), "Hundreds of doctors in Bangladesh infected with coronavirus", 24 April 2020, https://www.aljazeera.com/news/2020/04/hundreds-doctors-bangladesh-infected-coronavirus-200423080515266.html, accessed online 15 April 2020.

28 World Bank (2020), "Physicians (per 1,000 people)", 24 April 2020, https://data.worldbank.org/indicator/sh.med.phys.zs, accessed online 26 April 2020.

29 Saleh Asif (2020), "In Bangladesh, COVID-19 threatens to cause a humanitarian crisis", 06 April 2020, https://www.weforum.org/agenda/2020/04/in-bangladesh-covid-19-could-cause-a-humanitarian-crisis/, accessed online 10 April 2020.

30 Money Control, "Coronavirus impact: Garment exporter in Bangladesh faces $6 bn hit as world retailers cancel orders", 01 April 2020, https://www.moneycontrol.com/news/world/coronavirus-impact-garment-exporter-bangladesh-faces-6-bn-hit-as-world-retailers-cancel-orders-5094181.html, accessed online 10 April 2020.

31 *Ibid.*

32 Konar Debasis (2020), "India-Bangladesh border open amid coronavirus lockdown", 27 March 2020, https://timesofindia.indiatimes.com/city/kolkata/india-bangladesh-border-open-amid-coronavirus-lockdown/articleshow/74853235.cms, accessed online 13 April 2020.

33 Reuters (2020), "Coronavirus impact: Garment exporter in Bangladesh faces $6 bn hit as world retailers cancel orders", 01 April 2020, https://thefinancialexpress.com.bd/economy/bangladesh/tariff-commission-fears-serious-impact-on-trade-with-china-1582602581, accessed online 16 April 2020.

34 Islam Syful (2020), "Tariff commission fears serious impact on trade with China", 25 February 2020, https://thefinancialexpress.com.bd/economy/bangladesh/tariff-commission-fears-serious-impact-on-trade-with-china-1582602581, accessed online 12 April 2020.

35 Xinhua News Agency (2020), "中国向孟加拉国提供紧急抗疫医疗物资援助 (China provides emergency medical aid to Bangladesh", 27 March 2020, https://www.sohu.com/a/383441743_267106l, accessed online 12 April 2020.

36 CGTN (2020), "China ready to send more help to Bangladesh over COVID-19: FM", 08 April 2020, https://news.cgtn.com/news/2020-04-08/China-ready-to-send-more-help-to-Bangladesh-over-COVID-19-FM—Pw8TA3xzFu/index.html, accessed online 12 April 2020.

37 Worldometers (2020), "Bhutan", 24 April 2020, https://www.worldometers.info/coronavirus/country/bhutan/, accessed online 24 April 2020.

38 Dey Sayan and Malati Sunar (2020), "Why Bhutan is an Outlier in the Fight Against Coronavirus, Madras Courier, 03 April 2020, "https://madrascourier.com/opinion/why-bhutan-is-an-outlier-in-the-fight-against-coronavirus/, accessed online 14 April 2020.

39 Rizbal Dhurba (2015), *The Royal Semi-Authoritarian Democracy of Bhutan*, London, Lexington Books, 2015, 65.

40 Interviews with local traders at the Assam-Gelephu border, on 29 April 2017.

41 Varma K.J.M. (2020), "China ready to share its experience to control coronavirus spread with India, provide assistance", 24 March 2020, https://www.livemint.com/news/india/china-ready-to-

share-its-experience-to-control-coronavirus-spread-with-india-provide-assistance-11584965868519.html, accessed online 12 April 2020.

42 Worldometers (2020), "India", 24 April 2020, https://www.worldometers.info/coronavirus/country/india/, accessed online 24 April 2020.

43 Raghunathan Anu (2020), "India Ramps Up Coronavirus Testing, Approves Slew Of Local Test Kit Makers", 20 April 2020, https://www.forbes.com/sites/anuraghunathan/2020/04/16/india-ramps-up-coronavirus-testing-approves-slew-of-local-and-foreign-makers/#6d07406569a5, accessed online 18 April 2020.

44 Biswas Soutik (2020), "肺炎疫情：为什么印度全国封锁后数百万人走路回家 (Coronavirus Pandemic: why millions of people walked home after India 's national blockade)", 31 March 2020, https://www.bbc.com/zhongwen/simp/world-52103978, accessed online 12 April 2020.

45 Narayanan S. (2020), "COVID-19 in India: Time to Reform Labour Laws", 08 May 2020, https://www.isas.nus.edu.sg/wp-content/uploads/2020/05/ISAS-Briefs-No-779.pdf, accessed online 18 May 2020.

46 Press Trust of India (2020), "Trade impact of Coronavirus epidemic for India estimated at 348 million dollars: UN report", 05 March 2020, https://economictimes.indiatimes.com/news/economy/foreign-trade/trade-impact-of-coronavirus-epidemic-for-india-estimated-at-348-million-dollars-un-report/articleshow/74487020.cms?utm_source=contentofinterest&utm_medium=text&utm_campaign=cppst, accessed online 11 April 2020.

47 Bureau of Immigration of the Government of India (2020), "Coronavirus related visa restrictions and conditions for entry into India", 14 February 2020, https://boi.gov.in/content/coronavirus-related-visa-restrictions-and-conditions-entry-india,

48 Global Daily (2020), "印度驻华大使：印度政府即将援助中国一批医疗物资 (Indian Ambassador to China: Indian government is about to assist China with a batch of medical supplies)", 16 February 2020, https://news.sina.cn/global/szzx/2020-02-16/detail-iimxyqvz3334897.d.html?vt=4, accessed online 19 April 2020.

49 Southern Frontier (2020), "又一批中国医疗物资运往印度，印度大使称中国物资"没有问题" (Another batch of Chinese medical supplies was shipped to India, and the Indian ambassador said that the Chinese supplies had "no problem")", 16 April 2020, https://kuaibao.qq.com/s/20200416A0KEXE00?refer=spider, accessed online 02 April 2020.

50 News 18 (2020), "India Will Reject All Faulty PPE Kits Donated by China, Say Govt Sources; 50k of 1.7 Lakh Kits Failed Checks", 16 April 2020, https://www.news18.com/news/india/india-will-reject-all-faulty-ppe-kits-donated-by-china-say-govt-sources-50k-of-1-7-lakh-kits-failed-checks-2580529.html, accessed online 20 April 2020.

51 Srikanth Kondapalli (2020), "Ominous Signals from Beijing", 27 May 2020, https://www.deccanherald.com/opinion/main-article/ominous-signals-from-beijing-842572.html, accessed online 28 May 2020.

52 Worldometers (2020), "Maldives", 26 April 2020, https://www.worldometers.info/coronavirus/country/maldives/, accessed online 26 April 2020.

53 Reuters (2020), "Maldives Confirms First Two Cases of Coronavirus:; two resort locked down", 08 March 2020, https://web.archive.org/web/20200319211647/https://economictimes.indiatimes.com/ news/international/world-news/maldives-confirms-first-two-coronavirus-cases-two-resort-islands-locked-down/articleshow/74535526.cms, accessed online 12 April 2020.

54 Chapple James, "Coronavirus: Four Maldives Resorts Places in Lockdown", 11 March 2020, https://www.ttgmedia.com/news/coronavirus-four-maldives-resorts-placed-in-lockdown-21673, accessed online 05 April 2020.

55 Kwok Caroline (2020), "Maldives builds world's first coronavirus quarantine resort", 12 March

2020, https://www.scmp.com/video/asia/3074862/maldives-builds-worlds-first-coronavirus-quarantine-resort, accessed online 10 April 2020.

56 Gossman Patricia (2020), "Migrant Workers in Maldives at Added Risk from COVID-19", 27 March 2020, https://www.hrw.org/news/2020/03/27/migrant-workers-maldives-added-risk-covid-19, accessed online 12 April 2020.

57 CNBC (2020), "Coronavirus outbreak could have serious consequences for Maldives' local population", 17 March 2020, https://www.cnbc.com/video/2020/03/17/coronavirus-outbreak-could-have-serious-consequences-for-maldives.html, accessed online 13 April 2020.

58 Sudhir Sunjay (2020), "Tackling COVID-19: Experiences from Vietnam and Maldives", 21 April 2020, https://twitter.com/indfoundation/status/1251435445486972928, accessed online 23 April 2020.

59 Worldometers (2020), "Nepal", 26 April 2020, https://www.worldometers.info/coronavirus/country/nepal/, accessed online 26 April 2020.

60 Au Bonnie (2020), "Nepal in full lockdown amid coronavirus pandemic, but finding few Covid-19 cases due to lack of test", 02 April 2020, https://www.scmp.com/video/coronavirus/3078066/nepal-full-lockdown-few-cases-doing-few-covid-19-tests-amid-coronavirus, accessed online 12 April 2020.

61 Kamat Ram Kumar (2020), "Govt told to halt flights to high-risk countries", 02 March 2020, https://thehimalayantimes.com/nepal/government-told-to-halt-flights-to-high-risk-countries/, accessed online 20 April 2020.

62 Prasain Sangam and Prithvi Man Shrestha (2020), "Government bans entry of all passengers, including Nepalis, from midnight March 20", 18 March 2020, https://kathmandupost.com/national/2020/03/18/government-bans-entry-of-all-passengers, accessed online 19 April 2020.

63 Independent Indian scholar based in Nepal, anonymity requested, interview conducted via email on 30 April 2020

64 Prasain Krishana (2020), "Hand sanitisers in short supply due to buying rush sparked by outbreak fears", 04 March 2020, https://kathmandupost.com/money/2020/03/04/hand-sanitisers-in-short-supply-due-to-buying-rush-sparked-by-outbreak-fears, accessed online 09 April 2020.

65 Koirala Bharat (2020), "71 Chinese workers in Pokhara quarantined", 11 March 2020, https://thehimalayantimes.com/nepal/71-chinese-workers-in-pokhara-quarantined/, accessed online 12 April 2020.

66 Xinhua (2019), "Nepal sees rise in number of Chinese tourists in first half", 19 July 2019, http://www.xinhuanet.com/english/2019-07/19/c_138238320.htm, accessed online 02 April 2020.

67 Prasain Sangam (2020), "China's ban on outbound tours certain to affect the Visit Nepal campaign", 27 January 2020, https://kathmandupost.com/money/2020/01/27/china-s-ban-on-outbound-tours-certain-to-affect-the-visit-nepal-campaign, accessed online 19 April 2020.

68 Himalayan News Service (2020), "International flights drop significantly at TIA", 07 March 2020, https://thehimalayantimes.com/business/international-flights-drop-significantly-at-tia/, accessed online 03 April 2020.

69 Shrestha Prithvi Man (2020), "After aviation and tourism, investment and trade fall victim to global Covid-19 outbreak", 15 March 2020, https://kathmandupost.com/money/2020/03/15/after-aviation-and-tourism-investment-and-trade-fall-victim-to-global-covid-19-outbreak, accessed online 15 April 2020.

70 My Republica (2020), "China provides medical aid to Nepal to contain coronavirus", 29 March 2020, https://myrepublica.nagariknetwork.com/news/china-provides-medical-aid-to-nepal-to-contain-coronavirus/, accessed online 12 April 2020.

71 Independent Indian scholar based in Nepal, anonymity requested, email interview, 30 April 2020.

72 Business Today (2020), "What is Pakistan's Smart Lockdown Plan?", 25 April 2020, https://

www.businesstoday.in/latest/trends/coronavirus-impact-what-is-pakistans-smart-lockdown-plan/story/401998.html, accessed online 14 April 2020.

73 Yidianzixun (2020), "巴基斯坦驻华大使反对从武汉撤出巴学生：中国有更好的救治条件 (Pakistani Ambassador to China opposes the evacuation of Pakistani students from Wuhan: China has better conditions for treatment)", 03 February 2020, http://www.yidianzixun.com/article/0OXNViSC?appid=s3rd_didi&s=didi, accessed on April 12, 2020.

74 Chaudhury Dipanjan Roy, "No China link to local coronavirus cases: Pakistan", 31 March 2020, https://economictimes.indiatimes.com/news/international/world-news/no-china-link-to-local-cases-pakistan/articleshow/74904231.cms?utm_source=contentofinterest&utm_medium=text&utm_campaign=cppst, accessed on 25 April 2020.

75 Farmer Ben and Joe Wallen (2020), "India and Pakistan report low cases – but are they underestimating the scale of coronavirus?", 20 April 2020, https://www.telegraph.co.uk/global-health/science-and-disease/india-pakistan-report-low-cases-butare-underestimating-scale/, accessed on 25 April 2020.

76 World Health Organization, "Pakistan" at https://www.who.int/countries/pak/en/, accessed online 20 April 2020.

77 Mangi Faseeh (2020), "Pakistan's Fragile Health System Faces a Viral Catastrophe", 08 April 2020, https://www.bloombergquint.com/businessweek/pakistan-s-fragile-health-system-faces-a-viral-catastrophe, accessed online 12 April 2020.

78 Petersen Hannah Ellis and Shah Meer Baloch (2020), "Pakistan coronavirus camp: 'No facilities, no humanity", 19 March 2020, https://www.theguardian.com/world/2020/mar/19/pakistan-coronavirus-camp-no-facilities-no-humanity, accessed online 12 April 2020.

79 Ebrahim Zofeen T (2020), "China-Pakistan bonhomie in the time of Coronavirus", 30 March 2020, https://www.thethirdpole.net/en/2020/03/30/china-pakistan-bonhomie-in-the-time-of-coronavirus/, accessed online 05 April 2020.

80 Rana Shahbaz (2020), "Pakistan seeks rollover of half of $28b debt", 14 April 2020, https://tribune.com.pk/story/2197495/2-pakistan-seeks-rollover-half-28b-debt/, accessed online 15 April 2020.

81 Desmukh Shreyas Durgadasrao and Arun Sahgal (2020), "Failing COVID-19 Response in Pakistan and Afghanistan", 24 April 2020, https://www.delhipolicygroup.org/publication/policy-briefs/failing-covid-19-response-in-pakistan-and-afghanistan.html#_edn18, accessed online 18 April 2020.

82 International Monetary Fund, " IMF and Policy Responses to COVID-19", https://www.imf.org/en/Topics/imf-and-COVID-19/Policy-Responses-to-COVID-19#I, accessed online 12 April 2020.

83 Press Trust of India (2020), "Coronavirus: Pakistan opens borders with China for medical supplies", 27 March 2020, https://www.businesstoday.in/current/world/coronavirus-pakistan-opens-borders-with-china-for-medical-supplies/story/399418.html, accessed online 19 April 2020.

84 Siddiqui Tahir (2020), "Sindh gets Chinese donation of 500,000 face masks to fight coronavirus", 26 March 2020, https://www.dawn.com/news/1543758/sindh-gets-chinese-donation-of-500000-face-masks-to-fight-coronavirus, accessed online 14 April 2020.

85 Liu Tian and Jiang Chao (2020), "原标题：帮助"巴铁"渡过疫情难关——记解放军抗疫专家组在巴战"疫 (Helping the Pakistani Railways to Get Through the Coronavirus Pandemic: PLA's Anti-epidemic Experts Group in Pakistan)", 06 May 2020, http://m.xinhuanet.com/mil/2020-05/06/c_1210606161.htm, accessed online April 12, 2020.

86 Ebrahim Zofeen T. (2020), "China-Pakistan bonhomie in the time of Coronavirus", 30 March 2020, https://www.thethirdpole.net/en/2020/03/30/china-pakistan-bonhomie-in-the-time-of-coronavirus/ accessed online 12 April 2020.

87 China Daily (2020), "Pakistan donates surgical masks to China", 10 February 2020, https://

www.chinadaily.com.cn/a/202002/10/WS5e410f7fa3101282172765de.html, accessed online 07 April 2020.

88 Haider Mehtab (2020), "CPEC projects may face delay, disruption: report", 25 April 2020, https://www.thenews.com.pk/print/649577-cpec-projects-may-face-delay-disruption-report, accessed online 26 April 2020.

89 Worldometer (2020), "Sri Lanka", 28 April 2020, https://www.worldometers.info/coronavirus/country/sri-lanka/, accessed online 28 April 2020.

90 Srinivasan Meera (2020), "Testing time as Sri Lanka fights virus", 14 April 2020, https://www.thehindu.com/news/international/testing-time-as-sri-lanka-fights-virus/article31341973.ece, accessed online 28 April 2020.

91 Sohu (2020), "斯里兰卡人如何看待中国疫情 (How Does Sri Lanka View the Chinese Epidemic?)", 27 January 2020, https://www.sohu.com/a/369084888_141139, accessed online 27 April 2020.

92 Kuruwita Rathindra (2020), "China to the Rescue in Sri Lanka", 15 April 2020, https://thediplomat.com/2020/04/china-to-the-rescue-in-sri-lanka/, accessed online 18 April 2020.

93 Shazuli Hassan (2020), "Sri Lanka to step up COVID – 19 testing amidst mounting requests", 07 April 2020, https://www.newsfirst.lk/2020/04/07/sri-lanka-to-step-up-covid-19-testing-amidst-mounting-requests/, accessed online 12 April 2020.

94 Kuruwita Rathindra (2020), "China to the Rescue in Sri Lanka", 15 April 2020, https://thediplomat.com/2020/04/china-to-the-rescue-in-sri-lanka/, accessed online 10 April 2020.

95 The Island (2020), "COVID-19 test kits and emergency medical supplies arrive", 12 April 2020, http://www.island.lk/index.php?page_cat=article-details&page=article-details&code_title=221139, accessed online 12 April 2020.

96 The World Bank (2020), "South Asia Must Ramp Up COVID-19 Action to Protect People, Revive Economies", 12 April 2020, https://www.worldbank.org/en/news/press-release/2020/04/12/south-asia-must-act-now-to-lessen-covid-19-health-impacts, accessed online 07 April 2020.

97 Price Water Coopers (2020), "COVID-19 Outbreak: Impact on Sri Lanka and Recommendations", 08 April 2020, https://www.pwc.com/lk/en/assets/COVID-19-Impact-on-Sri-Lanka-PwC.pdf, accessed online 10 April 2020.

98 *Ibid.*

99 Sina Finance (2020), "谢谢你，李文亮医生! (Thank you Dr. Li Wenliang)", 07 February 2020, https://baijiahao.baidu.com/s?id=1657878336127142494&wfr=spider&for=pc, accessed online 17 March 2020.

100 BMJ Publishing Group (2020), "Covid-19: China's president Xi visits Wuhan amid confidence that virus is under control", 11 March 2020, https://www.bmj.com/content/368/bmj.m995, accessed online 12 April 2020.

101 Xinhua News Agency (2020), "国家监委调查组负责人答记者问 (In charge of State Supervision and Administration Commission answers reporters' questions)", 07 February 2020, https://www.thepaper.cn/newsDetail_forward_6588678, accessed online 25 April 2020.

102 Ruiz Karen (2020), "The true scale of China's medical stockpile is revealed: More than TWO BILLION masks were imported into Wuhan in just one month as the coronavirus crisis escalated", 02 April 2020, https://www.dailymail.co.uk/news/article-8178365/China-imported-2billion-masks-peak-coronavirus-crisis.html, accessed online 14 April 2020.

103 Jeffery Lynsey, "German, French Officials Accuse U.S. Of Diverting Supplies", 04 April 2020, https://www.npr.org/2020/04/04/827321294/german-french-officials-accuse-u-s-of-diverting-supplies, accessed online 12 April 2020.

104 Sapkota Ramu (2020), "Nepal to test COVID-19 test kits from China", 01 April 2020, https://

www.nepalitimes.com/latest/nepal-to-test-covid-19-test-kits-from-china/, accessed online 02 April 2020.

105 Asia News International (2020), "COVID-19: China buffoons 'all-weather ally' Pakistan by sending 'underwear' masks", 05 April 2020, https://www.business-standard.com/article/news-ani/covid-19-china-buffoons-all-weather-ally-pakistan-by-sending-underwear-masks-120040500163_1.html, accessed online 12 April 2020.

106 Latif Amir (2020), "Despite concerns, S. Asian countries insist on using Chinese kits", 31 March 2020, https://www.aa.com.tr/en/asia-pacific/despite-concerns-sasian-countries-insist-on-using-chinese-kits/1786131, accessed online 12 April 2020.

107 DTNext (2020), "Faulty equipment, defective results': India to stall use of COVID-19 rapid test kits", 21 April 2020, https://www.dtnext.in/News/National/2020/04/21174315/1226261/Faulty-equipment-defective-results-India-to-stall-.vpf, accessed online 13 April 2020.

108 Outlook (2020), "Over 50,000 Chinese Made PPE Kits Dumped After Failing Quality Test In India", *16* April 2020, https://www.outlookindia.com/website/story/india-news-over-50000-chinese-made-coronavirus-ppe-kits-dumped-after-failing-quality-test-in-india/350853, accessed online 16 April 2020.

109 Basu Nayanima (2020), "China calls it 'unfair and irresponsible' to label as faulty Covid test kits it sent to India", 28 April 2020, https://theprint.in/diplomacy/china-calls-it-unfair-and-irresponsible-to-label-as-faulty-covid-test-kits-it-sent-to-india/410320/, accessed online 29 April 2020.

110 Taiwan News (2020), "Sweden shutters all China-sponsored Confucius Institutes", 23 April 2020, https://www.taiwannews.com.tw/en/news/3921563, accessed online 29 April 2020.

111 Presse Agence-France (2020), "African community targeted in China coronavirus crackdown", 11 April 2020, https://timesofindia.indiatimes.com/world/china/african-community-targeted-in-china-virus-crackdown/articleshow/75092247.cms, accessed online 29 April 2020.

112 Kirchgaessner Stephanie, Emma Graham-Harrison and Lily Kuo (2020), "China clamping down on coronavirus research, deleted pages suggest", 11 April 2020, https://www.theguardian.com/world/2020/apr/11/china-clamping-down-on-coronavirus-research-deleted-pages-suggest, accessed online 12 April 2020.

113 Bloomberg (2020), "China pushes factories to reopen, risking renewed virus spread", 24 February 2020, https://theprint.in/world/china-pushes-factories-to-reopen-risking-renewed-virus-spread/369688/, accessed online 02 April 2020.

114 Bloomberg (2020), "India to boost drug ingredient output to pare China reliance", 14 April 2020, https://m.economictimes.com/industry/healthcare/biotech/pharmaceuticals/india-to-boost-drug-ingredient-output-to-pare-china-reliance/articleshow/75128876.cms, accessed online 14 April 2020.

115 Asia News International (2020), "Go back': Clashes erupt between Nepali locals, Chinese workers amid lockdown", 31 March 2020, https://timesofindia.indiatimes.com/world/south-asia/go-back-clashes-erupt-between-nepali-locals-chinese-workers-amid-lockdown/articleshow/74913551.cms, accessed online 12 April 2020.

116 Yun Sun (2020), "China and Africa's debt: Yes to relief, no to blanket forgiveness", 20 April 2020, https://www.brookings.edu/blog/africa-in-focus/2020/04/20/china-and-africas-debt-yes-to-relief-no-to-blanket-forgiveness/, accessed online 21 April 2020.

15

The COVID-19 Pandemic: China and Southeast Asian Relations

Ambuj Thakur

China in Southeast Asia

As the regional behemoth politically, economically, militarily and demographically, the People's Republic of China's clout in its traditional backyard of Southeast Asia remains unparalleled. Barring the Kachin and the Sagaing regions of Myanmar, the whole of the Southeast Asia lies south of the Tropic of Cancer, and is home to numerous races, cultures and a hot and humid climatic zone. It is more or less geographically divided into two parts – (a) the continental states of Myanmar, Thailand, Laos, Cambodia and Vietnam; and (b) the maritime states of Singapore, Malaysia, Indonesia, the Philippines, and Brunei Dar-us-salam respectively. Collectively grouped into the political entity of the Association of Southeast Asian Nations (ASEAN), covering an area of 4.5 million square kilometres and home to more than half a billion people, the entire region has been touched by Chinese influence in some way or the other throughout history.

The COVID-19 crisis came as a bolt from the blue for the region. It was first detected on a 61-year-old Chinese woman from Wuhan who landed at Bangkok's Suvarnabhumi Airport on January 08, 2020, marking the World's first case outside China.[1] Of the ten ASEAN countries, five of them have directly had their first cases coming from Chinese nationals, including those from Wuhan – Malaysia, the Philippines, Singapore, Thailand and Vietnam. A holistic picture of the pandemic hitting SE Asia can be gleaned from the Tables 1 and 2 given in the subsequent pages. It has also been noted that except for Singapore, Thailand and Malaysia having better healthcare systems and ranked among the top 25 globally, most countries have a long way to go.[2] The highest number of cases so far has been officially reported from Indonesia (54,010), Singapore (43,459) and the Philippines (35,455), whereas the lowest number of cases are from Laos (19), Brunei (141) and Myanmar (299) respectively.[3] What is suggestive here are that the first three are democracies, with institutional mechanisms having a semblance of functionality. However, those with the least reported cases do not necessarily mean that they have robust healthcare systems to face the pandemic. In fact, they have authoritarian political systems in place where governmental supervision or censorship restricts accurate reporting of events and statistics. Incidentally, China has had a closer relationship with authoritarian regimes, where single-party rule without any opposition or military dictatorships. Two exceptions are here. Singapore, despite the People's Action Party (PAP) being in government since independence in 1965, is a capitalist democracy modelled on Western lines and has little affinity with the Chinese Communist Party's vision of a restoration of the Middle Kingdom (*Zhongguo*) centric world order. On the other hand, despite the restoration of a multi-party-political system in Myanmar in 2011, the army (*Tatmadaw*) controls the real levers of state power and the democratic government of Daw Aung San Syu Kyi has to act within the confines set by the former. Therefore, reportage of figures from such countries would be vastly different. But the dark horse here is Vietnam which, though a Communist nation, has the most impressive record in dealing with the pandemic in the entire SE Asian region. A detailed analysis of its COVID-19 response and interactions with China has been presented in a later section of this chapter. Vietnam's policy of *Doi Moi* and mass social discipline has gone a long way in successfully keeping the numbers low so far.

Table 15.1: Showing the number of cases detected and fatalities of all SE Asian countries till June 30, 2020

Country Name	*No. of COVID-19 Cases*	*No. of Deaths*	*First Case detection*
Brunei	141	3	March 09, 2020
Cambodia	141	0	January 27, 2020
Indonesia	54,010	2,754	March 02, 2020
Lao PDR	19	0	March 23, 2020
Malaysia	8,634	121	January 25, 2020
Myanmar	299	6	March 23, 2020
Philippines	35,455	1,244	January 30, 2020
Singapore	43,459	26	January 30, 2020
Thailand	3,169	58	January 08, 2020
Vietnam	355	0	January 23, 2020
SE Asia	**145,682**	**4212**	**January 08, 2020**

Source: WHO.

By early February 2020, most of Southeast Asian countries had been hit by the COVID-19 pandemic, with Myanmar being the last one to register its first case in late March. The state responses were varied and dependent on the nature of their political systems, robustness of their healthcare sectors, economic strength and bilateral relationship with China. A detailed analysis of the Chinese responses to every SE Asian country has been given in the subsequent sections. Broadly, the ten ASEAN members, for the sake of convenience, have been kept under three categories – China's closest allies (Cambodia, Laos and Myanmar); countries, despite differences, reconciling to Chinese leadership in the region (Brunei, Indonesia, Malaysia, the Philippines, and Thailand); and those standing up to China on equal terms but not taking it head on (Vietnam and Singapore).

Table 15.2: Showing the Source of Origin of COVID-19 and Immediate State Responses in SE Asia

Country Name	*Source of Origin*	*Immediate Countermeasures*
Brunei	53 year old Brunei man returning from Kuala Lumpur on March 03.	Treatment starts; contact tracing; 14-day quarantine for those in contact; travel ban on visitors from Italy, Iran and China's Hubei, Zhejiang and Jiangsu provinces; usual safety protocols given by WHO.
Cambodia	38 year old man from Siem Reap coming into contact with Japanese man, who had been in the Philippines and Thailand and detected as positive on returning to Japan	Closing down schools; cancelling Khmer New Year programmes near Angkor Wat complex; shutting down the provincial capital; treatment and usual WHO safety measures; USD 30 million government stimulus; Hun Sen's China visit in February.
Indonesia	64-year-old woman and her 31 year old daughter after contacting a Malaysia-based Japanese national; earlier zero cases from 243 nationals evacuated from Wuhan in early February; many cases subsequently from the cruise liner Diamond Princess docked in Japan	Cancellation of all flights to and from Mainland China; stopping free visa and visa on arrival for Chinese nationals; travel restrictions on people travelling to and from virus hotspots in South Korea, Italy and Iran; thermal and temperature scanners at 135 airport and dock gates in early March; social distancing protocols by mid-March announced by President Widodo; no nationwide lockdown but on a case basis.
Lao PDR	28 year old Laotian man returning from Thailand	National Task Force Committee for COVID-19 Prevention and Control; Two month nationwide lockdown; Government ill-equipped to promote e-learning; border with China closed.
Malaysia	Three Chinese tourists entering from Singapore via Johor; by mid-March every region affected	Movement Control Order promulgated which is similar to a lockdown; prohibition of travel to some regions of China, Iran, Italy, South Korea and Denmark; ramping up testing and treatment facilities; vaccine research led by Institute of Medical Research of Malaysia.

Country Name	Source of Origin	Immediate Countermeasures
Myanmar	36 year-old Myanmarese returning from the USA and a 26 year-old Myanmarese coming from the UK	Government banning mass gatherings, borders closed, Thingyan Festival cancelled; Cinemas closed but bars and restaurants open.
Philippines	38 year old Chinese woman coming from Wuhan	Quarantine measures implemented; 400,000 face masks distributed to pupils in public schools in Manila; drug therapy and vaccine development research; Bayanihan Heal As One Act; partial lockdowns at selective regions.
Singapore	66 year old Chinese man from Wuhan who arrived from Guangzhou with his family on January 20	Contact tracing; intensified border screening, especially for Singaporeans travelling to and from Hubei; cancellation of daily flights to Wuhan by the budget carrier Scoot; adherence to WHO safety measures.
Thailand	61-year-old Chinese woman from Wuhan; world's 1st COVID-19 case outside China	Initially only surveillance and contact tracing; public education on safety guidelines; travel restriction imposed only after March 5 and national emergency declared on March 26 with exponential rise in cases.
Vietnam	66-year-old Chinese man from Wuhan and his 28-year-old son	Immediate lockdown of the Binh Xuyen district of Vinh Phuc province where the first cluster appeared in February; drug therapy and vaccine development; closing border with China, schools and cancellation of all flights to and from Wuhan.

Source: Collated from multiple news and government agencies.

China's relationship with continental SE Asia can be viewed from the vision of both the need for resources and markets on the one hand, and guarding its soft underbelly on the other. It wishes to encompass this region within the ambit of its ambitious Belt and Road Initiative (BRI). Since its inauguration 2013 by Chinese President Xi Jinping, a number of countries have joined the bandwagon for securing easier investments from China. Though many critics have argued that it is a debt trap for poorer countries, yet the BRI maintains its visibility and appeal due to its loans associated with no value-based riders like democratic ideals, freedom of speech etc. propounded by the Western powers. With China still growing its economy despite the pandemic by opening up its factories, the SE Asian countries have a reason to look up to China for its economic prowess and deep pockets. Table 15.3 gives the data on the bilateral trade of each ASEAN nation with China in the year 2018, as compiled by China's National Bureau of Statistics (NBS).

Even if one goes by the figures for 2018 as given in the above table, it becomes evident that China's ~ USD 15 trillion economy enjoyed a decisive advantage in overall trade with all its ASEAN neighbours. While apparently Laos enjoys more favourable trade benefits with respect to China, the trade levels are very low in comparison to the other economies. Myanmar and Cambodia too fall in the zone of low trade with China, but also ending up with big deficits. Bilateral trade with

Table 15.3: China's Trade with ASEAN Countries in 2018

Country Name	*China's Total Imports and Exports in billion USD (2018)*	*China's Total Exports (2018)*	*China's Total Imports (2018)*
Brunei	1.83946	1.59195	0.24751
Cambodia	7.38418	6.00752	1.37666
Indonesia	77.34118	43.19141	34.14978
Lao PDR	3.47215	1.454	2.01815
Malaysia	81.58104	45.37599	36.20505
Myanmar	15.23211	10.54777	4.68434
Philippines	55.64824	35.03664	20.6116
Singapore	82.7644	49.03663	33.72777
Thailand	87.50835	42.87872	44.62964
Vietnam	147.83304	83.87669	63.95635
SE Asia	**560.60414**	**318.99732**	**241.6068**

Source: NBS China; OEC.

Brunei is the lowest in SE Asia, with investments confined to only in infrastructure, agriculture and aquaculture sectors. With Indonesia, the Philippines, Vietnam, Malaysia and Singapore, China enjoys a trade surplus. The only big economy which enjoyed a trade surplus with China in 2018 was Thailand though marginal in terms. The moot point here is that in the near future the world is heading towards a greater recession than 2008. Most of the smaller countries will find it difficult to sustain their economies with projected expenditures rising in the health sector exponentially. Chinese investments are what they will be looking for with Europe in a state of despair and Donald Trump's USA abrogating its responsibilities in the Asia-Pacific Region.

China will definitely try to capture and secure the space emptied by the USA and use its BRI framework as the most potent tool to wield influence. Table 15.4 gives a list of some of the major BRI projects involving China in SE Asia. The notable exceptions are the Philippines, Singapore and Vietnam respectively. While Filipino President Duterte shows his readiness to bend backwards for China on the South China Sea (SCS) related sovereignty issues, he faces opposition from his own bureaucracy and people. So, Chinese claims for the joint development of the Philippines' EEZ in the SCS, under the BRI, will remain stuck in the quagmire for some time to come. Singapore is an economic power on its own and has a range of cooperation ventures with China, even without the BRI. As a city-state also it doesn't stand to gain much from the project. Vietnam, on the other hand, shares a deep mistrust of China, and its domestic policy of self-reliance and self-sufficiency are gelled with its focus on a market-led socialist economy. It wants to retain its historically dominant role in SE Asia, without coming under the Chinese umbrella.

Therefore, Sino-Vietnamese BRI projects look unlikely in the near future. Especially after the economic slump brought in by the COVID-19 pandemic, Vietnam wouldn't like to barter its *Doi Moi* policy for Chinese money.

Table 15.4: Major BRI Projects in SE Asian Countries

Country Name	*Current and Proposed BRI Projects with Chinese Investments*
Brunei	USD 15 billion Pulau Muara Besar Petrochemical Plant and Refinery; Brunei-Guangxi Economic Corridor.
Cambodia	Phnom Penh-Sihanoukville Expressway; new Siem Reap International Airport; Sihanoukville SEZ; 8 bridges and 31 highways amounting to 3,000 kilometres; Lower Sesan Two Hydropower Dam
Indonesia	USD 5.9 billion Jakarta-Bandung High Speed rail; hydropower project at Batang Toru Rainforest; MNC Lido City; Kuala Tanjung Port; Kayan River Hydropower Plant; Lake Toba Tourism District; International Airport at Lembeh.
Lao PDR	Vientiene-Boten Railway; Savannakhet-Lao Bao Railway
Malaysia	Johor Forest City; Melaka Gateway; East Coast Railway; Gemas-Johor Bahru Railway
Myanmar	China-Myanmar Economic Corridor; Dawei Port; Myitsone Dam; Kyaukpyu Deep Sea Tanker Port; Kyaukpyu SEZ; Muse-Mandalay Railway.
Philippines	None
Singapore	None
Thailand	Sino-Thai Railway; Bangkok-Nong Khai Railway; Bangkok-Chiang Mai Railway
Vietnam	None

Source: Collated from various news and government agencies.

For China, the BRI rests on historical foundations besides strategic needs. It's southwest frontier comprising the provinces of Yunnan, Guizhou, Guangxi Zhuang Autonomous Region, Sichuan, and Tibet are not only rich in resources, but also home to a huge ethnic minority population which straddles across international borders. Some of these minority groups are the Tibetans, Dai, Jingpo, Lisu etc. to name a few. Chinese penetration into SE Asia as a whole can also be seen through the securitisation perspective of protecting its own backyard from foreigners, and reflective of their Middle Kingdom psyche of being the hegemon. 'Much of the periphery along national borders of mainland Southeast Asia is inhabited by peoples linguistically and culturally distinct from the populations that dominate the state cores. Alarmingly, they spill promiscuously across national frontiers, generating multiple identities and possible foci of irredentism or secession'.[4] The period from 1839–1949 C.E. has been deeply etched in the memory of the CCP as a *Century of Humiliation* that snatched away China's leadership role and which needs to be corrected, especially in the 21st Century C.E.[5] 'China's most advantageous outlet for its ambitions is in the direction of the relatively weak states of Southeast Asia...likely capital of a Mekong River prosperity sphere, linking all countries of Indochina by road and river traffic, is Kunming in China's Yunnan Province...'.[6] This sums up the moods for China's sensitivities towards the reactions of its southern neighbours to the pandemic.

Countries under China's Direct Security Perimeter

A major case study is Cambodia, which has been one of the few countries maintaining closest connection with China for a long time. Prime Minister Hun Sen has consolidated his hold over Cambodia's political landscape over nearly a quarter of a century, and veered the country towards a closer friendship with China. The COVID-19 crisis has been handled relatively well by the country, if one goes by the official statistics of only 141 cured cases and zero deaths. In a country of 16 million people, such a low incidence of cases raises concerns over the reliability of data on the pandemic. However, proponents of this success story say that extensive contact tracing and more than 16,000 tests since January 2020 helped in containment of the disease. Closing down the borders to foreigners, especially Westerners, as well as educational institutions, cancellation of the Khmer New Year celebrations, banning domestic travel for a week and quarantining 15,000 garment factory workers were some of the drastic measures taken initially.[7] China, Vietnam and Japan have donated medical equipment and supplies, while the USA, Australia, France, Russia and Germany have pledged millions of dollars as aid,[8] including a USD 20 million from the World Bank.[9] Also, the Prime Minister himself set an example of announcing in early April of donating his salary for seven months amounting to USD 17,500 to the National Committee for Combating COVID-19, thereby prompting other officials to follow suit.[10]

It has also been argued that Cambodia's poverty and poor infrastructure has in a way come round to its rescue. Since about 80 percent of the population lives in the rural areas, and owing to poor accessibility and sanitation, people got habituated in wearing masks quite easily not only to save themselves from dust and fumes, but also the COVID-19 disease.[11] The government, moreover, came out with a number of economic stimulus measures for the people. By early April, the Ministry of Economy and Finance came up with task forces to control the supply and prices of strategic goods like rice, salt, vegetable, fish, meat, mask, cleaning alcohol, pharmaceutical and medical equipment, with a view to 'prevent COVID-19 outbreak, stabilise the livelihood of the poor and the vulnerable people and recover and stabilise businesses'.[12] While tourism and industry suffered, the government promoted the growth of the agricultural sector and export of rice and fish were banned in order to cater to domestic needs. Pagodas, restaurants, coffee shops etc. were allowed to function.

But critics argue that Cambodia's economy has been hit severely due to the slump in its tourism industry which contributes about a third of its gross domestic product (GDP) annually. About 1.86 million Chinese tourists visited Cambodia in 2019 amount to 38.7 percent of all foreign tourists,[13] while those visiting the famous Angkor temples amounted to 873,297 respectively.[14] In sharp contrast, Cambodia received only 223,400 foreign tourists in March 2020, a fall of 65 percent in comparison to the same period in 2019.[15] Interestingly Cambodia has banned entry of foreigners from the USA, Germany, Spain, Italy, France and Iran due to the pandemic, but is already formulating its plans to revive the industry by attracting more Chinese tourists under its *China Ready* strategy.[16] Cambodia's garments industry has also suffered badly owing to mass cancellation of orders from the USA and Europe on account of the pandemic and drying up of raw materials from China initially.[17] More than 180 factories have suspended operations jeopardising the livelihoods of nearly 150,000 workers.[18] Moreover, daily wage earners and small businesses, in the informal sector, are having a tough time in repaying their loans to the microfinance institutions.[19]

Prime Minister Hun Sen's visit to China in February 2020 at the peak of the outbreak in the latter signalled the close ties between the countries. He has refused to join the global chorus to hold China responsible for mishandling the pandemic. His promulgation of the *Law on National Administration in the State of Emergency* on 29 April, 2020, has come under much criticism for transferring sweeping powers to the government to curb individual freedoms,[20] including those of the rights to travel freely, that of assembly and privacy. China has remained the biggest source of foreign direct investment in Cambodia since 2013, reaching USD 3.594 billion in 2018 alone,[21] and both the countries have shared a comprehensive strategic partnership of cooperation[22] since 2010. China's support to Cambodia has been reciprocated officially with the latter deciding to remain neutral in the ASEAN-China territorial dispute on the South China Sea recently.[23] Therefore, the COVID-19 crisis is unlikely to bring any major changes in the close Sino-Cambodian bilateral relations in the near future.

A second case study be that of Myanmar, with whom China has shared a love and hate relationship historically, albeit both have been compelled to remain in a close embrace owing to political contingencies in the latter half of the 20th Century C.E. Myanmar following global alerts from the WHO and others, started bracing up for the outbreak of the disease from January 2020 itself, by the end of the month started investigating its first case. Visa on arrival facility was suspended, medical students from Wuhan were evacuated, mass gatherings banned, and mandatory quarantines for foreign travellers were imposed by the middle of March. To bailout the economy, an initial stimulus package of MMK 100 billion (~USD 70 million) was announced by the government, while the first confirmed case came out on March 23.[24] The number of registered cases has been 296 so far, with six deaths and 216 recoveries, and with 71,692 samples tested and 5,878 patients under investigation in a country of nearly 54 million people.[25] Following up on the initial economic stimulus, the government came up with a new COVID-19 Economic Relief Plan (CERP) worth MMK 2.8–4.2 trillion (~USD 2–3 billion) covering monetary policy, tax relief, FDI, trade, financial sector, health, public finances, household sector with an increase in government expenditure.[26] One of the most important features is the plan to reallocate 10 percent of government spending on all ministries to the health sector, thereby signalling a shift in focus away from investing solely on defence so far.[27] However, the flipside is equally true of the Tatmadaw's grip over Myanmar's internal security. Humanitarian groups like the Human Rights Watch (HRW) argue that a year-long exiting internet ban in the conflict-prone north-western Rakhine province has kept the local people unaware of the COVID-19 pandemic and it's a ticking time-bomb.[28]

Having said this, one should recall that in the last three decades the CCP and the Tatmadaw (Myanmar Army) have brought both the countries in a closer embrace defined as the *Paukphaw* or fraternal friendship. This year marks the 70th anniversary of the establishment of diplomatic relations between the People's Republic of China and the Union of Myanmar, and Xi Jinping's visit in mid-January to Naypyidaw to commemorate the event became the first one by a Chinese President in two decades.[29] This relationship was born out of necessity due to their becoming international pariahs following the heavy clampdowns on the pro-democracy movements in both the countries in 1988-89 respectively. It was also born out of China's strategic necessity of opening up its land-locked south-western provinces of Yunnan, Sichuan, Tibet, Guizhou, and the Guangxi Zhuang Autonomous Region to the warm water ports of the Indian Ocean via Myanmar. This thought first found a semblance of official sanction in an article written by Pan Qi, a former top Chinese government official, in the September 02, 1985, issue of the *Beijing Review*.[30] The writer called for the policymakers to explore options to connect China's under-developed but resource-rich periphery with the outside world by developing cross-border trade and transportation networks. He highlighted the importance of Myanmar as a key peg in this strategy of opening up, and also referred to ancient trade routes connecting the region. These routes have been collectively referred to as the Southern Silk Route by the Chinese over time, and many modern-day transportation corridors, including the Stilwell Road of World War II vintage, and the China-Myanmar Economic Corridor (CMEC) respectively.[31]

Xi Jinping's Myanmar visit of January 17-18, 2020, came in the backdrop of the COVID-19 crisis and it was clearly an attempt by China to keep its allies in the neighbourhood within its sphere of influence. He had actually defined Paukphaw in the following words, "Linked by mountains and rivers, the two countries are closely related and mutually dependent with people-to-people bonds, close exchanges, similar encounters and comparable tasks".[32] Seeking a broad consensus on a shared history and commonality of geography and culture, Xi harped on the mutually beneficial win-win cooperation based on the Five Principles of Peaceful Co-existence between the two countries over the past 70 years. A key approach has been to bring the CMEC under the ambit of the Belt and Road Initiative (BRI) since 2013, and Xi impressed upon the Burmese leaders of China's commitment to develop the three pillars of the CMEC namely, New Yangon City, Kyaukphyu Deep-Sea Port and Industrial Zone, and the China-Myanmar Border Economic Cooperation Zone around Ruili-Muse area.[33] Agreements were signed to this effect during the visit, keeping in mind that Myanmar signed a Memorandum of Understanding (MoU) with China to establish the CMEC in 2018 respectively.[34] Interestingly, the Chinese leader kept quiet on the Myitsone Dam issue, a hot potato in Myanmar,[35] focussing mainly in leveraging the advantages of easy access to the Indian Ocean and bypassing the Straits of Malacca. In fact, experts in Myanmar have argued that it remains in China's interests if the CMEC projects could be linked up with the CERP to ensure stability and continuity in a post-COVID-19 future.[36]

The third case is the Laotian People's Democratic Republic or Laos, which also shares a close relationship with China. Diplomatic relations improved after Laotian Prime Minister, Kaysone Phomhivan's state visit to China in 1989 signing four agreements on consular affairs, cultural cooperation, visa exemption and temporary agreement on border affairs respectively.[37] By October 2004, attempts at cross-border cooperation had been furthered with the establishment of a coordination committee on the northern parts of Laos and Yunnan province.[38] Laos is a part of the BRI and by the end of 2016, Chinese financial support for 764 Laotian projects, including 552 wholly funded with the remaining 212 being joint ventures.[39] The showpiece of this cooperation is the 414 kilometre long China-Laos section of the Trans-Asian Railway (TAR) network, with China investing 70 percent of the total bill of USD 5.8 billion.[40] Among all its BRI projects in SE Asia, this is the fastest moving project and also caters to the Laotian governments objective of harnessing it to turn the country 'from a land-locked to a land-linked' one.[41] Chinese interests in the country are protected by the Laotian military despite Northern Laos facing a Hmong insurgency and anti-Chinese sentiments among the local people.[42] Laos falls under the strategy of opening up Southwest China envisaged by Pan Qi in his 1985 article as mentioned earlier.

The first COVID-19 case in Laos was registered on March 24 at Vientiene and it was a 28-year-old returnee from Thailand.[43] Just like other countries of the region, Laos too put in place quarantine measures, lockdowns, as well as closing down border checkpoints and airports, while the people duly cooperated with official directives in maintaining social hygiene.[44] It is estimated by the Asian Development Bank (ADB) that the country's economy would grow only by 3.5 percent in 2020 down from 6.1 percent in 2019[45] respectively. As elsewhere, a big worry remains the status of the education sector with institutions closed down indefinitely due to the crisis. The northern province of Luang Prabang, a UNESCO World Heritage Site, thrives on tourism, and in 2018 alone 655,000 foreigners visited, including a quarter of them being from China, while the total number of Chinese travellers to the country was 800,000 out of 4.1 million tourists.[46] Therefore, people's livelihoods are going to be hit hard, despite the government announcing an economic stimulus package and the World Bank chipping in an amount of USD 18 million to deal exclusively with the pandemic in this country of 7.3 million people mostly inhabiting the rural areas.[47] China sent medical teams, supplies and medicines promptly on a request from the Laotian leadership by March itself.[48] China delivered more than 2000 test kits, while the private Jack Ma Foundation donated 5000 sets of protective clothing with several hundred thousand face masks,[49] something which has recently earned the moniker of 'Face-mask Diplomacy'. With 19 cases detected so far and cured till date, the figures are heartening for this impoverished country as it remains a vital link in China USD 1 trillion BRI project.

These three case studies reflect the broad consensus between their authoritarian political systems with China in maintaining good neighbourly relations. They are China's staunchest allies in the region and the principal means of easing its transportation bottlenecks bypassing the chokepoint of the Malacca Straits. The other countries in the region have had mixed emotions with respect to China, dancing with both the USA, and other regional powers like Japan, South Korea and India as a hedge against her, on the one hand, and also toeing her line in major international issues, including this pandemic in the light of the massive economic investments accruing from such a relationship, on the other. For example, Thailand and the Philippines have traditionally been closer to the USA and both were members of the South East Asian Treaty Organisation (SEATO) before the 1980s. However, today, there is a growing ambivalence towards the West, with the USA under Donald Trump gradually shirking its responsibilities as a global policeman and following a policy of isolationism and transactionism. This has prompted its regional allies to deal with China bilaterally and multilaterally in favourable terms since they can take on its might head on individually. It has given China the upper hand in the region as well as global power relations, and has served it very well during the pandemic.

Countries on China's Outer Periphery

Thailand has for long mastered the art of expertly balancing between major world powers throughout history, with the best examples being able to maintain its independence both during the Anglo-French rivalry over SE Asia in the 19th Century C.E. and the Japanese occupation during World War II. As discussed earlier, the same goes to its relations with China and the USA. The tide tilted gradually towards China when the current Prime Minister of Thailand, Prayuth Chan-ocha captured power through a coup d'état in 2014, and was criticised by the Western powers led by the USA. China's official policy of non-interference in the domestic affairs of other countries, earned it brownie points with the new Thai junta. As a part of the BRI, Thailand has signed a MoU with China in 2014 for the 867-kilometre Sino-Thai Railway project, and both sides jointly inaugurated the construction of the first phase in 2017.[50] The Royal Thai government has a plan to link Bangkok with the four corners of the country in Chiang Mai, Nong Khai, Ra Yong and Padang Besar with Bangkok by 2037 C.E. in a 2,506-kilometre-long high-speed railway network.[51] As a part of the China-Thai Railway corridor, a new agreement for the Bangkok-Nakhon Rathchasima section is scheduled to be signed in October 2020,[52] senior officials from both announced recently.

China was also Thailand's second largest trading partner after the USA in 2018, with bilateral trade amounting to USD 80.14 billion.[53] Both countries had in fact agreed to double their bilateral trade volume to USD 140 billion in 2021 from USD 73.67 billion in 2017 respectively.[54] Interestingly enough, China has delivered medical supplies worth 30 million Baht, including 6000 COVID-19 PCR test kits, 100 infrared thermometers, 10 electrocardiograms etc. to Thailand, a country which has a good healthcare system in the Asia-Pacific region.[55] But within this official show of bonhomie, there are subtle undercurrents of tension between the two countries at the popular level. It became evident with the 'Twitter War' where netizens in China were furious over posts of a Thai internet model, Weeraya Sukaram, with the hashtag #Nnevvy, questioning whether the novel coronavirus originated in China and commenting that Taiwan is not a part of China.[56] This looks funny apparently, but with Chinese netizens insulting the Thai King and the Prime Minister, it shows the belligerent mood of the Middle Kingdom, something that the Thai people would be wary about.

In the case of the Philippines, Chinese presence has been growing ever since incumbent Filipino President Rodrigo Duterte came to power in mid-2016. He has veered the country closer to China, and taking a non-confrontationist approach even in sensitive sovereignty issues like the South China Sea dispute. By mid-2019 he had already made five official visits to China, while not paying a single visit to the USA unlike his predecessors. The Hague Tribunal's ruling in 2016 favouring the Philippines on the South China Sea (SCS) dispute had been rejected by China, and Duterte made no effort to enforce that decision so as to avoid the latter's wrath.[57] He wishes to cooperate with Beijing in a hydrocarbon exploration project that falls within the Philippines' Exclusive Economic Zone (EEZ) in the Reed Bank zone but which the former claims as its own along the infamous 'Nine-dash Line' in the South China Sea. But with growing national unease over Chinese assertiveness in the region, Duterte has his hands tied.

For example, he has rescinded his earlier decision to scrap an existing Mutual Defense Treaty with the USA. This Treaty even if not put into force still acts as deterrence towards Chinese ambitions. Duterte is still pushing for joint exploration of the SCS, but faces problems of harmonising Chinese territorial claims on its EEZ which is treated by the Filipino Constitution as 'an extension of national sovereign territory'.[58] Moreover, China's growing assertiveness in the region amidst the COVID-19 pandemic is making the political class and the people jittery. Duterte has tried to find middle ground, and recently in his talks with Xi Jinping pledged not to allow the Philippines to be a staging ground for anti-China activities, a definite allusion to the USA.[59] At the same time, to keep things under control, the China-backed Asian Infrastructure Investment Bank (AIIB) has approved a USD 750 million loan to the Philippines in dealing with the pandemic.[60] Most importantly, in a telephonic conversation with Duterte lasting 38 minutes on June 11, 2020, Xi promised that 'as a friendly neighbour' the Philippines would be prioritised by China when a COVID-19 vaccine was finally developed by her.[61] Such measures signify that China doesn't want the Philippines to fall back on the US camp again, despite following a carrot and stick policy in relation to its territorial disputes.

The long rage of tropical islands, stretching from the Malacca Straits to the north of the Australian continent, comprising of the modern-day ASEAN member-states of Malaysia, Indonesia, Brunei Dar-us-salam and Singapore, have been home to both Sinic and Indic influences throughout history and have become a melting pot of sorts for cultures and ideas. The Chinese bid for naval supremacy in the region during the Ming dynasty by Admiral Zheng He is well-known. It is also true that after the Chinese state withdrew inwards, the European colonisers took over the entire region for a couple of centuries, only to be briefly replaced by another Asian power, Japan, in the first half of the 20th Century C.E. But with Douglas MacArthur's rallying behind the Chinese Nationalists, Taiwan became what he described in his own words as the USA's 'unsinkable aircraft carrier' in the Pacific, where his target was definitely stemming the tide of Communism in Asia from both China and the Soviet Union. The USA's presence as a security guarantor for

Taiwan, Japan, and the Philippines against China riles the latter. It still feels that to safeguard its own eastern seaboard and to attain its former status of the Middle Kingdom, controlling the SCS region and the sea lanes of communication therein are important. Hence, its exaggerated claims in the region should be read in this light, something which manages to unnerve its SE Asian neighbours too.

Muhyiddin Yassin, the new Malaysian Prime Minister, enjoys a thin majority in Parliament and he is averse to taking any risks in cooling off Sino-Malaysian bilateral relations. He is taking a middle way approach keeping in mind that the USA is in no way to help his people. In fact, Malaysia donated 18 million gloves to China in January 2020 as a part of its COVID-19 diplomacy.[62] On the other hand, the Malaysian branch of the Bank of China in Kuala Lumpur donated a cheque of USD 69,800 to the country's Health Minister, Adham Baba in the second half of April.[63] By the end of March, China had already donated 100,008 COVID-19 Nucleic Acid diagnostic test kits, 100,000 pieces of N95 masks, 500,000 pieces of surgical masks, 50,000 PPE units, and 200 ventilators.[64] Other Chinese agencies like Jack Ma Foundation, Mammoth Foundation, BGI Group, China Enterprises Chamber of Commerce in Malaysia etc. to name a few, have also sent considerable supplies. It should be kept in mind also that Malaysia is home to about 6.6 million ethnic Chinese people comprising 23.4 percent of its population. Though not stated officially, an undercurrent of greater Chinese solidarity may exist among the Mainland Chinese people.

China and Indonesia have also marked the 70th anniversary of the establishment of their diplomatic relations recently, and the bilateral relations have improved considerably since the end of Suharto's rule in 1997 in the latter. China became the second largest investor in 2019, after Singapore, pumping in USD 4.7 billion in 2,130 projects, and accounting for 16.8 percent of the total foreign investments in the country.[65] Chinese tourists accounted for 26.9 percent of all visitors to the popular tourist destination, Bali, in the same period.[66] In 2018, the numbers for foreign and domestic tourists in the country amounted to 15.8 million and 300 million respectively, signifying the scale of the economy's dependence on tourism alone.[67] Chinese investments have come in the sectors like roadways, seaports, railways, mining, technology etc., and policymakers hope that mutually beneficial cooperation with China would allow Indonesia to grow its digital economy to USD100 billion by 2025.[68] With more than 54,000 confirmed cases, 23,000 recoveries and about 2,754 deaths till the end of June 2020, Indonesia has a major uphill task in dealing with the pandemic. By mid-April, China sent 40 tons of medical equipment as assistance. As SE Asia's largest market, and owing to the US and European economies in shambles, China's eyes are firmly set in exploiting its potential for its manufacturing-based export-oriented economy.[69] All projects in the country have been suspended due to the pandemic, including those under the BRI like USD 1.63 billion Morowali Industrial Park, Sulawesi, and USD 5.5 billion Bandung-Jakarta fast train project.[70] However, getting rid of anti-Chinese sentiment may not be easy here, with tempers flaring on China's claims over Indonesia's EEZ in the SCS. It has to be a diplomatic tightrope for both countries. Indonesia, with its fragile health sector, desperately needs Chinese investments and aid to tackle the pandemic.

China and Brunei share a cordial relationship with bilateral trade volumes touching USD 1.8 billion in 2018 and expanding further into aquaculture, agriculture and hydrocarbon sectors under the BRI.[71] China is the main investor in the largest FDI project in Brunei – the USD 15 billion refinery and petrochemical plant, a 70:30 joint venture between China's Zhejiang Hengyi Petrochemical Co. Ltd. and the Brunei government on Pulau Muara Besar.[72] The company has continued running this facility amidst the pandemic since coming into operation in November 2019, and is expected to increase Brunei's GDP by more than USD 1.3 billion and generate 1,600 jobs within a year.[73] According to the national development plan *Wawasan Brunei 2035*, the government has three objectives: to have a well-educated and highly skilled workforce at par with international standards; quality of life counted among the top 10 in the world; and, development of a dynamic and sustainable economy among the top in the world.[74] The last point is important because Brunei's hydrocarbon reserves are going to last at most by another 30 years and diversification is the need of the hour. Brunei attempts to leverage the BRI in realising its 2035 plan. The Brunei-Guangxi Economic Corridor, envisaged in 2014 through a MoU signed between Brunei and the GZAR alongside the 11th China-ASEAN Expo, aims to link ports of the two countries, one of them being the development of the former's Muara port.[75] Moreover, as a part of its COVID-19 reach out, China has also supplied Brunei with 100,000 N95 respirators and 1000 disposable isolation gowns, and the Chinese Embassy in Brunei also donated an amount of USD 42, 158 to the country's COVID-19 Relief Fund.[76]

Vietnam and Singapore: Standing up to China

Last but most importantly, there are two states in SE Asia which have stood up to China in various ways over time and still form a sort of a nucleus in resisting her assertiveness in the region. They are Singapore and Vietnam. Though ethnically Chinese, Singapore has charted its modern history as a city-state since 1965 and followed an avowed blend of Western Capitalism and Asiatic Authoritarianism. Vietnam through its policy of *Doi Moi* since 1986 has attempted to create a socialist market economy following its adoption in the Vietnamese Communist Party's 6th

Party Congress. It came within the backdrop of two momentous changes since unification and US defeat in 1976 – the bloody war with China in 1979, and China's Reform and Opening Up in 1982. The policy allowed for the participation of private sector in small enterprises and creation of a stock exchange for both state and non-state enterprises. Singapore always suffered from an existential fear of getting overrun by the mainland Chinese and therefore have maintained a close military training relationship with Taiwan under the USA's security guarantee provided by the 7th Fleet stationed at Hawaii.[77] She finds a kindred spirit in Taiwan, inhabited by ethnic Chinese but following a western capitalistic democratic model of governance and always living in the fear of taken over by an authoritarian mainland China, most recently witnessed in the gradual repudiation of Hong Kong's Basic Law signed with the UK pledging broad degree of freedom in internal affairs till 2045 C.E. On the other hand, Vietnam has been one of the worst bombed countries on Earth and faced and defeated three mighty superpowers in the 20th Century – France, the USA and China. It has a Communist Party led authoritarian political system too, but shed its past to embrace market-led reforms and countering China's increasing assertiveness in the region. The most unique thing about it is its ability to discard the past and look ahead into the future, something validated by its embracing the USA in 1995 as a part of the normalisation of relations.

The number of COVID-19 cases in Singapore have risen to 43,459 with 26 deaths and 37, 508 recoveries. The corresponding numbers for Vietnam are 355, 0 and 330 respectively. The contrast is very hard to ignore. Vietnam has a population of 95.5 million and a density of 308.1 per square kilometre. Singapore has a population of 5.85 million and a density of 8358 per square kilometre. Vietnam had been well prepared to deal with the pandemic as the Ministry of Health already notified its agencies and hospitals by January 21 to remain prepared. When the first two cases came on January 23, apparently they were Chinese nationals from Wuhan who had arrived on January 13 and travelled throughout Vietnam. Aggressive preventive measures ensured that by February 25 the 16th patient got cured and another 22 days passed before the 17th patient was detected.[78] With the discovery of the elite Bach Mai Hospital as a COVID-19 hotspot, the Prime Minister Phuc declared a limited national lockdown on April 1.

Lacking resources like Taiwan and South Korea in opting for mass testing, Vietnam went for precision-guided lockdowns, aggressive contact tracing and pumping up the production of medical supplies.[79] An exceptional method employed by the state was the intelligent mobilisation of nationalism, where the nCov was framed as a common 'foreign enemy' which the people had to fight united and resolutely, thereby echoing memories of its wartime past in the 20th Century.[80] It has also been successful in marketing its COVID-19 strategy globally through its chairing of the ASEAN Coordinating Council Working Group on Public Health Emergencies (March 31), teleconference with senior ASEAN and US officials (April 1), 25th ASEAN Coordination Council Meeting (April 9) and the Special ASEAN Plus Three Summit (April 14) respectively.[81] Singapore's COVID-19 explosion was mostly a result of its high population density, its globalised connectivity networks and the vast army of poor and marginalised 1 million migrant workers from India, Bangladesh and other countries, whose crowded airless dormitories are perfect breeding grounds for the disease.[82] Cases were galore, when even after the Singapore government announced a lockdown on April 7th no effective measures were taken to ensure physical distancing protocols, temperature screening, distribution of masks and sanitizers etc. by official agencies in the migrant dormitories.[83]

Due to their closely bound economies, China and Singapore have thousands of people working in each other, and therefore, a 'fast lane' arrangement has been put in place from June 8 whereby business travellers will have to undertake a self-paid pre-departure polymerase chain reaction (PCR) test and obtain a document for testing negative for COVID-19.[84] Initially, it has been put in place for travellers between Singapore and Shanghai, Tianjin, Chongqing, Guangdong, Jiangsu and Zhejiang in China.[85] Singapore has been closely associated with China in three official projects namely, China-Singapore Suzhou Industrial Park, Sino-Singapore Tianjin Eco-City, and China-Singapore (Chongqing) Demonstrative Initiative on Strategic Connectivity.[86] More than 50000 Chinese officials came to Singapore since 1990s on study visits and training programmes.[87] It should be noted here that the country is heading for its worst ever recession in two decades with projected GDP growth figures shrinking in the range of 4-7 percent.[88] Singaporean Foreign Minister, Vivian Balakrishnan, in a telephonic conversation with his Chinese counterpart, Wang Yi, on April 28 assured that the latter's migrant workers would be taken care off well.[89] It donated more than 2000 kilograms of medical supplies to China besides contributing USD 1 million in raising funds for the Singapore Red Cross Society.[90] China too supplied Singapore with 500,000 surgical masks and 100,000 KN95 masks.[91]

Due to its successful containment model, Vietnam has been able to offer assistance to its neighbours like Cambodia and Laos. It has given PPE kits, test kits, medical masks worth USD 304,000 to both the countries asserting its traditional leadership over the Indo-China region and SE Asia also.[92] It has also donated 550,000 facemasks to the UK, France, Italy, Germany and Spain, and the USA has purchased 450,000 Vietnamese manufactured DuPont hazmat suits.[93] It has ratcheted up its capacity of producing 7 million fabric masks daily with forty firms involved in the process as also having the capacity to make 5.72 million surgical masks a day.[94] With Chinese manufacturing firms faltering at many instances of maintaining quality controls, Vietnam is stepping in the void and its largest listed firm, the Vingroup, is preparing to make upto 55,000 ventilators monthly.[95] With the country becoming a ray of hope and stability in the region besides Taiwan, many firms are moving parts of their assembly lines from China to its territory.[96] Vietnam has already opened up its tourism sector accounting for 9 percent of its GDP to assure investors and has plans to boosts its small and medium enterprises (SMEs), a sector comprising about 97 percent of total business in the country.[97] Owing to their past animosities, and China's continued belligerence over the SCS, Vietnam has deep insecurities about its northern neighbour. It cancelled all flights to China and sealed the 1,300-kilometre-long international boundary on February 1st itself, much to the latter's annoyance.[98] Interestingly, it has also come to notice, according to a US-based cyber security firm called FireEye, that Vietnamese intelligence agents might have used a group APT32 to hack into Chinese servers to gather more information on the pandemic,[99] though officially Hanoi denies it. The targets include China's Ministry of Emergency Management and Wuhan Municipality websites,[100] and analysts assume that the APT32 has sanction from the Communist Party of Vietnam.

Conclusion

The COVID-19 pandemic has thrown the world into a tizzy leaving the West too weak to check or challenge China's ambition on its periphery, including SE Asia. Regional and local economies are tumbling leaving people increasingly vulnerable to both disease and hunger. States have come up with their respective contingency plans to address the problems. But the sheer magnitude of dealing with an unseen, unknown enemy has made it more difficult to concentrate efforts in defeating it. Some points which this pandemic has brought into focus are, firstly, states were totally unprepared to deal with pandemics despite warning shots being fired a number of times in the past twenty years, like SARS, MERS, Ebola etc. Secondly, though couched in terms of benevolent intentions, governments have tended to appropriate a lot of emergency powers, routed through legislative means, but which have the lesser possibility of being rescinded after the pandemic gets over in future. Thirdly, there is a gradual withdrawal of the Western democracies led by the USA, and this pandemic has shattered their economies more than that of China. Hence, China emerges more powerful in the coming years.

Fourthly, China's recent belligerence on territorial disputes on the SCS, with India and others show that it is not going to back down, where its regime stability is more important than anything else and therefore, would take all necessary steps to maintain that. Fifthly, all SE Asian countries are no match to take on China head on economically, politically and militarily. Even if bandwagoning with India, the USA and Australia are the options, the fact remains that they cannot choose their neighbours and concurrently change international borders, including the disputed ones at will. Sixthly, Chinese leaders know their history and strategic literature well, and they apply their wisdom in dealing with their neighbours accordingly. As argued earlier, with regard to the pandemic, it seems that China is bent on following carrot and stick as well as divide and rule options. It has dealt closely with SE Asia based on their security aspects, clubbing countries, unofficially, into three categories – those within its economic and political grasp like Myanmar, Laos and Cambodia; those it cannot control but nudge favourably in spite of hiccups like Malaysia, Indonesia, Brunei, the Philippines and Thailand; and those like Vietnam and Singapore, with which they have business interests, but have been rivals and having the prospect of disrupting their hegemonistic ambitions by becoming rallying points for extra-regional powers.

Most of these SE Asian countries are members of the BRI and they have a number of big projects coming up with huge Chinese investments. In a way, China holds their economies by the collar and possibilities of debt traps being used as weapons to make them fall inline are always omnipotent. They have no regional security guarantors and China will continue to grow as well as overcome the global backlash over the crisis. Buying into the Chinese line of thinking that they will have to deal with the pandemic together, despite the former being the real culprit, shows to what extent these countries have learnt not only to adjust their behaviour according to China's own but also let its soft power seep into their collective psyche.[101] Chinese propaganda machinery attempts to present China both as the victim of the pandemic and the leading crusader against it, and managed to deploy it to considerable advantage domestically and throughout SE Asia. As of now, with the COVID-19 still at its peak, it will be foolish to predict the future of China's ascendancy in the region by using pre-COVID-19 era concepts and tools. But one thing is clear that for the present, China has mustered the narrative to its advantage and has the upper hand. Cumulatively, it can be said that the Chinese response to the pandemic in SE Asia has been centred firmly on furthering its strategic interest's vis a vis the BRI and cultivating its soft power aggressively. Ratcheting up intractable border problems with its neighbours not only gives the CCP an image makeover as being decisive domestically and externally, but also helps in keeping its neighbours guessing about its next move. This unpredictability coupled with deep pockets bestows China with an aura of invincibility in SE Asia in the face of a weakened Europe and disinterested USA. The COVID-19 pandemic has done more good than bad to China's position in the region. There is only one caveat here. The outcome of the US Presidential election in November 2020 will be an important factor on China's rise. Trump' victory would let it consolidate its position faster in the ensuing years. But a Democratic Presidency under Joe Biden could have semblances of Obama era's US pivot policy in Asia, and that would slow down the Middle Kingdom's march to glory. Some things are better left upon time to unravel!

NOTES

1 Elizabeth Cheung, "Wuhan pneumonia: Thailand confirms first case of virus outside China", *South China Morning Post*, January 13, 2020 at https://www.scmp.com/news/hong-kong/health-environment/article/3045902/wuhan-pneumonia-thailand-confirms-first-case

2 "Coronavirus: how prepared are Asia's healthcare systems?, *Consultancy.asia*, March 23, 2020 at https://www.consultancy.asia/news/3056/coronavirus-how-prepared-are-asias-healthcare-systems. See also, Sukhbir Cheema, "Which Southeast Asian countries have the best healthcare at an affordable rate?", *Mashable SE Asia*, 2018 at https://sea.mashable.com/malaysia/797/which-southeast-asian-countries-have-the-best-healthcare-at-an-affordable-rate#:~:text=Bloomberg%20has%20 just%20 released%20its,the%20biggest%20shocker%20was%20Thailand; Lee J. Miller. and Wei Lu, "These Are the Economies With the Most (and Least) Efficient Healthcare", *Bloomberg*, September 19, 2018 at https://www.bloomberg.com/news/articles/2018-09-19/u-s-near-bottom-of-health-index-hong-kong-and-singapore-at-top.

3 "Novel Coronavirus Map", *Channel News Asia* at https://infographics.channelnewsasia.com/covid-19/map.html

4 James C. Scott, *The Art of Not Being Governed: An Anarchist History of Upland Southeast Asia* (New Haven and London: Yale University Press, 2009), p. 9.

5 Ambuj Thakur, *Sub-regional Initiatives of China in South and Southeast Asia, 1999–2012*, Unpublished Ph.D Thesis (New Delhi: Jawaharlal Nehru University, 2014), p. 207.

6 Robert D. Kaplan, *The Revenge of Geography: What the map tells us about coming conflicts and the battle against fate* (New York: Random House, 2012), p. 207.

7 Kimkong Heng, "What lies behind Cambodia's surprise coronavirus success?, *Nikkei Asian Review*, June 02, 2020 at https://asia.nikkei.com/Opinion/What-lies-behind-Cambodia-s-surprise-coronavirus-success.

8 Ibid.

9 Kimkong Heng, "Cambodia COVID-19 success and economic challenges", *East Asia Forum*, June 12, 2020 at https://www.eastasiaforum.org/2020/06/12/cambodias-covid-19-success-and-economic-challenges/

10 Kimkong Heng, "What lies behind Cambodia's surprise coronavirus success?, *Nikkei Asian Review*, June 02, 2020 at https://asia.nikkei.com/Opinion/What-lies-behind-Cambodia-s-surprise-coronavirus-success

11 Ibid.

12 "Cambodia: Government and institution measures in response to Covid19", *KPMG*, May 27, 2020 at https://home.kpmg/xx/en/home/insights/2020/04/cambodia-government-and-institution-measures-in-response-to-covid.html

13 "Chinese tourists to Cambodia, big opportunity for small Businesses", *GMA*, December 10, 2019 at https://www.chinesetouristagency.com/2020-3millions-chinese-tourists-will-travel-to-cambodia-big-opportuny-for-small-businesses/#:~:text=%202020%20%3A%20Chinese%20tourists

%20to%20 Cambodia%2C%20big,attract%20Chinese%20Tourists%E2%80%A6%20 contact %20us..%20%20More%20; Wu Qin, "Chinese tourists to Cambodia up 38.7 pct in H1 of 2019", *Xinhua*, August 07, 2019 at http://www.xinhuanet.com/english/2019-08/07/c_138290915.htm

14 Xinhua, "Cambodia's famed Angkor welcomed 873,297 Chinese tourists last year", *Borneo Bulletin*, January 13, 2020 at https://borneobulletin.com.bn/2020/01/cambodias-famed-angkor-welcomed-873297-chinese-tourists-last-year/

15 Nguon Sovan and Mao Pengfei, "Spotlight: Cambodia expects Chinese tourists to drive its tourism growth after COVID-19 outbreak", *Xinhua*, May 16, 2020 at http://www.xinhuanet.com/english/2020-05/16/c_139062205.htm

16 Ibid.

17 David Hutt, "Cambodia poised to be big Covid-19 loser", *Asia Times*, May 12, 2020 at https://asiatimes.com/2020/05/cambodia-poised-to-be-big-covid-19-loser/

18 Ibid.

19 Phorn Bopha and Khan Sokummono, "For Many Cambodians, Debt Repayment Bigger Threat Than COVID-19", *Voice of America*, May 22, 2020 at https://www.voanews.com/south-central-asia/many-cambodians-debt-repayment-bigger-threat-covid-19

20 Sun Narin, "National Assembly Passes 'State of Emergency' Law; Travel Ban Conditions Tweaked", *Voice of America*, April 10, 2020 at https://www.voacambodia.com/a/national-assembly-passes-state-of-emergency-law-travel-ban-conditions-tweaked-/5367066.html; "The Draft Law in the State of Emergency", *AMCHAM Cambodia*, at https://amchamcambodia.net/covid-19-update-state-of-emergency-draft-law/

21 Hin Pisei, "China still No1 source of FDI", *The Phnom Penh Post*, September 23, 2020 at https://phnompenhpost.com/business/china-still-no1-source-fdi?__cf_chl_jschl_ tk__= 4be05e2f30f27388b6f9f04d3fb1dda268b53b6b-1593428991-0-AQYNwbixW8CXmYgzU3KNWCFTuLi1TeUMZBGiZ2ULXuGtYkrve50C4lEDwWibwhgCx86f_ktogSWNwwXpU2t_Iz8qHSSBlaQ9kyHxGjYj9B_3lnnfet NsSs Wa5lu2DUKxscs RM17U2VZ x8jysqHvA _Vij5g6_wN j9KwijtJlmzbGGRm_uLnC1GNIp-0TgolUq3314ofZPcTBYI2yLslwWcv4uKwelfIl7Ezx9zgAD1sGFWJhxVa9n28RngUcZ—uwO0ukqxdTM-ccezXpXvvQMZK7H4JMuna NQ8HDDx Ueu3fs2 EGTVynMzA5kQzg0cORzMw

22 People's Daily Online, "China, Cambodia agree to build comprehensive strategic partnership", *People's Daily*, December 13, 2010 at http://en.people.cn/90001/90776/90883/7229822.html.

23 Ry Sochan, "Cambodia to remain neutral on ASEAN-China territorial dispute", *The Phnom Penh Post*, June 25, 2020 at https://www.phnompenhpost.com/national-politics/cambodia-remain-neutral-asean-china-territorial-dispute

24 Nan Lwin, "Time: Myanmar's Government Responses to the COVID-19 Pandemic", *The Irrawaddy*, May 26, 2020 at https://www.irrawaddy.com/specials/myanmar-covid-19/timeline-myanmars-government-responses-to-the-covid-19-pandemic.html.

25 Aseanplus News, "Covid-19: Cases in Myanmar increasing – total now 296 confirmed infections cases", *The Star*, June 28, 2020 at https://www.thestar.com.my/aseanplus/aseanplus-news/2020/06/28/covid-19-cases-in-myanmar-increasing—total-now-296-confirmed-infections-cases.

26 Nan Lwin, "Myanmar Prepares COVID-19 Relief Package Worth up to Several Billion Dollars", *The Irrawaddy*, April 28, 2020 at https://www.irrawaddy.com/specials/myanmar-covid-19/myanmar-prepares-covid-19-relief-package-worth-several-billion-dollars.html; Government of the Union of Myanmar, "Overcoming as One: COVID-19 Economic Relief Plan" *EUROCHAM, Myanmar*, April 27, 2020 at https://eurocham-myanmar.org/uploads/7a892-cerp—final-report-(1)5713756333092471786.pdf.

27 Ibid.

28 Jason Slotkin, "Parts Of Myanmar Unaware Of COVID-19 Due To Internet Ban, Rights Advocates Say", *NPR.org*, June 24, 2020, at https://www.npr.org/sections/coronavirus-live-updates/2020/06/24/882893419/parts-of-myanmar-unaware-of-covid-19-due-to-internet-ban-advocates-say.

29 "China-Myanmar's 'Paukphaw' friendship in 70 years", *CGTN*, January 15, 2020 at https://news.cgtn.com/news/2020-01-15/China-Myanmar-s-Paukphaw-friendship-in-70-years-NdOswxpJdu/index.html

30 Pan Qi, "Opening the Southwest: An Expert Opinion", *Beijing Review*, 35, 22-23.

31 Ambuj Thakur, "The BCIM Forum: tracing the historical basis" in G. Das and C. J. Thomas (eds.), *BCIM Economic Cooperation: Interplay of Geo-economics and Geo-politics* (London: Routledge, South Asia Edition, 2019), pp. 98–121.

32 "China-Myanmar's 'Paukphaw' friendship in 70 years", *CGTN*, January 15, 2020 at https://news.cgtn.com/news/2020-01-15/China-Myanmar-s-Paukphaw-friendship-in-70-years-NdOswxpJdu/index.html.

33 Nan Lwin, "China pushes BRI projects as Myanmar rolls out COVID-19 Economic Relief Plan", *The Irrawaddy*, May 07, 2020 at https://www.irrawaddy.com/news/burma/china-pushes-bri-projects-myanmar-rolls-covid-19-economic-relief-plan.html.

34 Ibid.

35 Kyaw Zwa Moe, "Beyond the Cliche' of 'Paukphaw', China and Myanmar need each other", *The Irrawaddy*, January 17, 2020 at https://www.irrawaddy.com/opinion/commentary/beyond-the-cliche-of-pauk-phaw-china-and-myanmar-need-each-other.html.

36 Nan Lwin, "China pushes BRI projects as Myanmar rolls out COVID-19 Economic Relief Plan", *The Irrawaddy*, May 07, 2020 at https://www.irrawaddy.com/news/burma/china-pushes-bri-projects-myanmar-rolls-covid-19-economic-relief-plan.html.

37 Linda de Hoyos, "Beijing reaps profit from 'China White'", *EIR, 1990*, 17(10), 8-9 at https://larouchepub.com/eiw/public/1990/eirv17n10-19900302/eirv17n10-19900302_008-beijing_reaps_profit_from_china.pdf; "(KPL) Laos-China cooperation continues to grow (part1)", *Embassy of the PRC in Lao PDR*, April 23, 2013 at http://la.china-embassy.org/eng/news/t1034300.htm.

38 "(KPL) Laos-China cooperation continues to grow (part2)", *Embassy of the PRC in Lao PDR*, April 24, 2013 at http://la.china-embassy.org/eng/news/t1034827.htm.

39 Yang Zi, "Securing China's Belt and Road Initiative", *United States Institute of Peace*, 436, p.3.

40 Ibid.

41 Selina Ho, "Can the China-Laos Railway keep on track?", *East Asia Forum*, July 12, 2019 at https://www.eastasiaforum.org/2019/07/12/can-the-china-laos-railway-keep-on-track/.

42 Yang Zi, "Securing China's Belt and Road Initiative", *United States Institute of Peace*, 436, p. 4.

43 "Ministry of Health and WHO respond to first case of Covid-19 in Laos", *WHO*, March 24, 2020 at https://www.who.int/laos/news/detail/24-03-2020-ministry-of-health-and-who-respond-to-first-case-of-covid-19-in-laos#:~:text=The%20Ministry%20of%20Health%20%28MoH% 29%20of%20 Lao%20People%E2%80%99s,23%20March%20and%20is%20currently%20in%20stable%20 condition.

44 Ekto Vongphakdy, "Impact of the Covid-19 pandemic in Laos", *Institute of Strategic and International Studies Malaysia* May 26, 2020 at https://www.isis.org.my/2020/05/26/impact-of-the-covid-19-pandemic-in-laos/; Jasmina Yap, "Laos Suspends Visas At Checkpoints Bordering China" *The Laotian Times* February 02, 2020 at https://laotiantimes.com/2020/02/02/laos-suspends-visas-at-checkpoints-bordering-china/.

45 Ibid.

46 Nathan Thomson, "Claims of a Coronavirus-Free Laos are Probably Fiction" *Foreign Policy* March 20, 2020 at https://foreignpolicy.com/2020/03/20/laos-coronavirus-free-claims-probably-fiction/; Yang Han, "Laos sets outs its stall to attract growing influx of visitors from China" *China Daily* October 14, 2019 at http://www.chinadaily.com.cn/global/2019-10/14/content_37515248.htm.

47 "Covid-19: The Lao PDR Government Announces New Economic Policy Measures" *VDB Loi* April 03, 2020 at http://www.vdb-loi.com/laos_publication/covid-19-the-lao-pdr-government-announces-new-economic-policy-measures/; "Lao PDR: Emergency Financing for COVID-19 Response Project" *The World Bank* April 07, 2020 at https://www.worldbank.org/en/news/press-release/2020/04/08/lao-pdr-emergency-financing-for-covid-19-response-project.

48 "President Xi Jinping Exchanges Messages with Bounnhang Vorachit on China-Laos Cooperation Against COVID-19" *Ministry of Foreign Affairs, PRC* June 15, 2020 at https://www.fmprc.gov.cn/mfa_eng/zxxx_662805/t1789190.shtml.

49 Bertil Lintner, "China comes to the COVID-19 rescue in Laos" *Asia Times* April 10, 2020 at https://asiatimes.com/2020/04/china-comes-to-the-covid-19-rescue-in-laos/.

50 "CHINA-Thailand railway project: The route and key events" *CGTN* August 13, 2019 at https://news.cgtn.com/news/2019-08-01/China-Thailand-Railway-INqEbn7Suc/index.html; "China, Thailand to enhance cooperation" *State Council, PRC* April 26, 2019 at http://english.www.gov.cn/premier/news/2019/04/26/content_281476630266138.htm.

51 "China–Thailand Railway Cooperation" *Belt & Road News* April 13, 2019 at https://www.beltandroad.news/2019/04/13/china-thailand-railway-cooperation/.

52 "China–Thailand Railway Agreement likely to be signed in October: Thai Transport Minister" *Xinhuanet* May 25, 2020 at http://www.xinhuanet.com/english/2020-05/25/c_139087013.htm.

53 "Statistics on China-Thailand Trade in January-December 2018" *Ministry of Commerce, PRC* March 19, 2019 at http://english.mofcom.gov.cn/article/statistic/lanmubb/ASEAN/201903/20190302844902.shtml#:~:text=March%2019%2C%202019%20%2D%2014%3A,%243.82%20 billion%2C%20up%200.2%25.

54 Phusadee Arunmas, "Thai-China trade pact signed" *Bangkok Post* November 08, 2018 at https://www.bangkokpost.com/business/1572030/thai-china-trade-pact-signed.

55 Wassana Nanuam, "China gives more gear to fight Covid" *Bangkok Post* May 13, 2020 at https://www.bangkokpost.com/thailand/general/1917024/china-gives-more-gear-to-fight-covid.

56 "China-Thailand coronavirus social media war escalates" *Al Jazeera* April 14, 2020 at https://www.aljazeera.com/news/2020/04/china-thailand-coronavirus-social-media-war-escalates-200414121313775.html.

57 Yen Nee Lee, "Philippine President Duterte says he'll stand up to China – he might not deliver" *CNBC* August 27, 2019 at https://www.cnbc.com/2019/08/28/philippines-duterte-in-china-meets-xi-jinping-to-talk-south-china-sea.html.

58 Richard Javad Heydarian, "Philippines challenging China in South China Sea" *Asia Times* June 27, 2020 at https://asiatimes.com/2020/06/philippines-challenging-china-in-south-china-sea/.

59 Kinling Lo and Kunal Purohit, "China and Philippines pledge mutual support after Rodrigo Duterte's U-turn on scrapping US alliance" *South China Morning Post* June 12, 2020 at https://www.scmp.com/news/china/diplomacy/article/3088885/china-and-philippines-pledge-mutual-support-after-rodrigo.

60 "China-backed AIIB approves $750 million loan for Philippines' COVID-19 response", *Reuters*, May 29, 2020 at https://in.reuters.com/article/us-health-coronavirus-aiib-philippines/china-backed-aiib-approves-750-million-loan-for-philippines-covid-19-response-idINKBN2350B8.

61 Associated Press, "China promises Philippines will get vaccine against COVID-19", *Financial Express*, June 12, 2020 at https://www.financialexpress.com/lifestyle/health/china-promises-philippines-will-get-vaccine-against-covid-19/1989553/.

62 Shannon Teoh, "China & Malaysia Coronavirus Diplomacy", *Belt & Road News*, April 30, 2020 at https://www.beltandroad.news/2020/04/30/china-malaysia-coronavirus-diplomacy/.

63 Xinhua, "Bank of China donates funds to Malaysia to fight COVID-19", *People's Daily Online*, May 01, 2020 at http://en.people.cn/n3/2020/0501/c90000-9686386.html.

64 Veena Babulal, "China delivers medical equipment to Malaysia to aid Covid-19 fight", *New Straits Times*, March 28, 2020 at https://www.nst.com.my/news/nation/2020/03/579028/china-delivers-medical-equipment-malaysia-aid-covid-19-fight.

65 Randy Mulyanto, "After 70 years of ties, China and Indonesia have a fruitful, complicated relationship", *South China Morning Post*, April 12, 2020 at https://www.scmp.com/week-asia/politics/article/3079446/after-70-years-ties-china-and-indonesia-have-fruitful.

66 Ibid.

67 James Guild, "In Indoneia, Will COVID-19 Trigger Another Asian Financial Crisis?", *The Diplomat*, May 21, 2020 at https://thediplomat.com/2020/05/in-indonesia-will-covid-19-trigger-another-asian-financial-crisis/.

68 Randy Mulyanto, "After 70 years of ties, China and Indonesia have a fruitful, complicated relationship", *South China Morning Post*, April 12, 2020 at https://www.scmp.com/week-asia/politics/article/3079446/after-70-years-ties-china-and-indonesia-have-fruitful.

69 Muhammad Zulfikar Rakhmat and Dimas Rizki Permadi, "Two reasons why China needs to expand its help to Indonesia to deal with COVID-19", *The Conversation*, April 17, 2020 at https://theconversation.com/two-reasons-why-china-needs-to-expand-its-help-to-indonesia-to-deal-with-covid-19-136245.

70 Ibid.

71 "Two-way trade between China, Brunei up 80% in 2018", *The Scoop*, June 17, 2020 at https://thescoop.co/2019/06/17/two-way-trade-between-china-brunei-up-80-in-2018/.

72 Ibid.

73 People's Daily Online, "Chinese companies in Brunei help boost local economy amid epidemic", *People's Daily*, April 07, 2020 at http://en.people.cn/n3/2020/0407/c90000-9676846.html.

74 Stephen Druce and Abdul Hai Julay, "The Road to Brunei's Economic Diversification: Contemporary Brunei-China Relations", January 2019 at https://www.researchgate.net/publication/337222630_The_Road_to_Brunei%27s_Economic_Diversification_Contemporary_Brunei-China_Relations, p.141.

75 Ibid., p. 143.

76 Xinhua, "Brunei receives medical material donations from China", *Global Times*, April 24, 2020 at https://www.globaltimes.cn/content/1186640.shtml.

77 Robert D. Kaplan, *The Revenge of Geography: What the map tells us about coming conflicts and the battle against fate* (New York: Random House, 2012), p. 209.

78 Minh Vu, and Bich T.Tran, "The Secret to Vietnam's COVID-19 Response Success", *The Diplomat*, April 18, 2020 at https://thediplomat.com/2020/04/the-secret-to-vietnams-covid-19-response-success/.

79 Ibid.

80 Ibid.

81 Ibid.

82 Shashank Bengali, "From 'gold standard' to a coronavirus 'explosion': Singapore battles new outbreak", *Los Angeles Times*, April 14, 2020 at https://www.latimes.com/world-nation/story/2020-04-14/coronavirus-surges-migrant-workers-in-singapore; See also, Tan Tarn How, "Surreal life in Singapore, from Covid-19 to 'circuit breaker' and migrant worker's plight", *South China Morning Post*, April

26, 2020 at https://www.scmp.com/week-asia/opinion/article/3081538/surreal-life-singapore-covid-19-circuit-breaker-and-migrant.

83 Ibid.

84 Zhaki Abdullah, "Business and official travellers on Singapore-China 'fast lane' arrangement must get COVID-19 swab tests", *Channel News Asia*, June 03, 2020 at https://www.channelnewsasia.com/news/singapore/singapore-china-fast-lane-covid-19-swab-tests-business-travel-12798518.

85 Ibid.

86 "People's Republic of China: Overview", *Ministry of Foreign Affairs, Singapore*, at https://www.mfa.gov.sg/SINGAPORES-FOREIGN-POLICY/Countries-and-Regions/Northeast-Asia/Peoples-Republic-of-China.

87 Ibid.

88 Press Trust of India, "COVID-19: Singapore heads towards worst-ever recession in nearly two decades", *The Hindu*, May 26, 2020 at https://www.thehindu.com/news/international/covid-19-singapore-heads-towards-worst-ever-recession-in-nearly-two-decades/article31677797.ece.

89 Clement Yong, "Coronavirus: China donates 600,000 masks to Singapore", *The Straits Times*, May 05, 2020 at https://www.straitstimes.com/singapore/coronavirus-china-donates-600000-masks-to-singapore.

90 Ibid.

91 Ibid.

92 Prashanth Parameswaran, "What's in Vietnam's New Coronavirus assistance to Cambodia and Laos?, *The Diplomat*, April 06, 2020, at https://thediplomat.com/2020/04/whats-in-vietnams-new-coronavirus-assistance-to-cambodia-and-laos/.

93 James Pearson, "Vietnam challenges China's monopoly on virus diplomacy", *Reuters*, April 10, 2020 at https://in.reuters.com/article/health-coronavirus-vietnam-diplomacy/vietnam-challenges-chinas-monopoly-on-virus-diplomacy-idINKCN21S0E4.

94 Ibid.

95 Ibid.

96 Dezan Shira & Associates, "Covid-19 Contingencies: Assistance with Relocating China Assembly to Vietnam", *China Briefing*, February 18, 2020 at https://www.china-briefing.com/news/covid-19-contingencies-assistance-with-relocating-china-assembly-vietnam/.

97 Pankaj Jha, "Opportunities for Vietnam's economy in post-COVID-19 phase", *Modern Diplomacy*, June 23, 2020 at https://moderndiplomacy.eu/2020/06/23/opportunities-for-vietnams-economy-in-post-covid-19-phase/.

98 Bac Pham and Bennett Murray, "Behind Vietnam's COVID-19 Response, Deep Distrust of China", *The Diplomat*, May 14, 2020 at https://thediplomat.com/2020/05/behind-vietnams-covid-19-response-deep-distrust-of-china/.

99 Ibid.

100 "Covid-19, Vietnamese hackers attack China to harvest information", *Asianews.it*, April 28, 2020 at http://www.asianews.it/news-en/Covid-19,-Vietnamese-hackers-attack-China-to-harvest-information-49934.html.

101 Sophie Boisseau du Rocher, "What COVID-19 Reveals About China-Southeast Asia Relations", *The Diplomat*, April 08, 2020 at https://thediplomat.com/2020/04/what-covid-19-reveals-about-china-southeast-asia-relations/.

16

COVID-19 and Sino-Australian Relations: Testing Stability

Mrittika Guha Sarkar

Introduction

The COVID-19 has struck the global health, economic structure, and the international order in an unprecedented manner. The exponential spread of the novel coronavirus, in entirety, has been questioning the legitimacy and capabilities of international institutions and global governance regimes. The pandemic has been pushing the globalized world order into uncertainty; the consequences on human health might seem temporary, but the economic and political upheavals unleashed by the virus could last for years. In the backdrop of this, the effects of the COVID-19 pandemic on Sino-Australian relations would be grave. The crisis, if anything, is bolstering the fault lines of an already fluid bilateral relationship between both the countries.[1]

In this regard, the chapter would be focussing on the China-Australia bilateral ties amidst the COVID-19, which have relegated substantially. While doing so, the chapter would try to understand the various nuances of the ties which have been affected by the pandemic. The chapter would also put in perspective the current Sino-Australian rift through various factors unravelling since the past few years, only to comprehend the current situation more extensively.

Impact of COVID-19 in Australia

The Australian government's official position since the primary stages of COVID-19 spread in the territory has been to start 'early-stage modelling'[2], which has helped the Federal government to take early measures to contain the virus. In retrospect, while China witnessed its first case of COVID-19 as early as in December 2019 in Wuhan, Hubei province, Australia reported its first case only on January 25, 2020, in Melbourne. The government had started taking early precautions- taking note of the Chinese situation of COVID-19, and listing the novel Coronavirus pandemic potential under the Biosecurity Act of 2015 which enabled it to take border measures in Australia.[3] Additional border measures were in place by the very next day, while the government levelled up the travel advice for visiting Wuhan to level four: "do not travel" by January 24, 2020.

Post the first reported case in Australia, as a part of the *Australian Health Sector Emergency Response Plan for Novel Coronavirus (COVID-19)*; the government has been conducting weekly reports on the spread of the virus while taking initial actions to minimize the diffusion across Australia. Such has been pertaining towards refusal of direct flights from Hubei Province, China; health checks on people arriving at Australia's international borders from countries posing a high virus spread risk; and isolating people with symptoms or in close contact with the infected.[4] In terms of preparing the health systems to handle increased numbers of patients, the Australian government has developed strategies to increase the number of health care staffs who have substantial experience in working with Intensive Care Units (ICU) and establish clinics designated to specialize in dealing with the COVID-19. Further, to learn more about the virus and how it behaves in the Australian community, the government, besides adding the novel virus into the national disease tracking database, has been analyzing the various trends of the virus; and assessing the details of infected patients- such as his/her travel history, the severity of the disease, transmission to people with close contact with the infected and more.[5] The government moreover, has developed health guidelines to the public and provided information to experts in accordance with the WHO recommendations; and provided fact sheets to general practitioners, EDs, pathology providers and healthcare managers. Lastly, regular media updates regarding the spread of the virus and the developing hotspots have been provided to the public, and guidelines regarding necessary hygiene behaviour- such as wearing masks, gloves, sanitizers and more- to contain the virus have also been shared. [6] In the purview of the current developments, the Australian government has delivered an economic support package worth $17.6 billion to encourage investment and sustain employment; and a further $2.4 billion health package to protect its population. It further has provided $669 million to expand Medicare-subsidized telehealth services to enable its citizens to access quality healthcare from home; and deliver support to Australians experiencing domestic, family and sexual violence due to the fallout of the virus.

In the backdrop of the current policies in place, the official data of COVID-19 cases in Australia had suggested towards a plateauing trend and decreasing number of new cases since the beginning of April (See Table 16.1). However, cases seem to be rising since the end of June. Australia has currently reported 10. 3 per cent of its COVID-19 cases as a result of community transmission, 27.9 per cent of the cases are contacts of confirmed cases, and 61.4 per cent have been acquired overseas.[7]

Figure 16.1: COVID-19 Trend in Australia

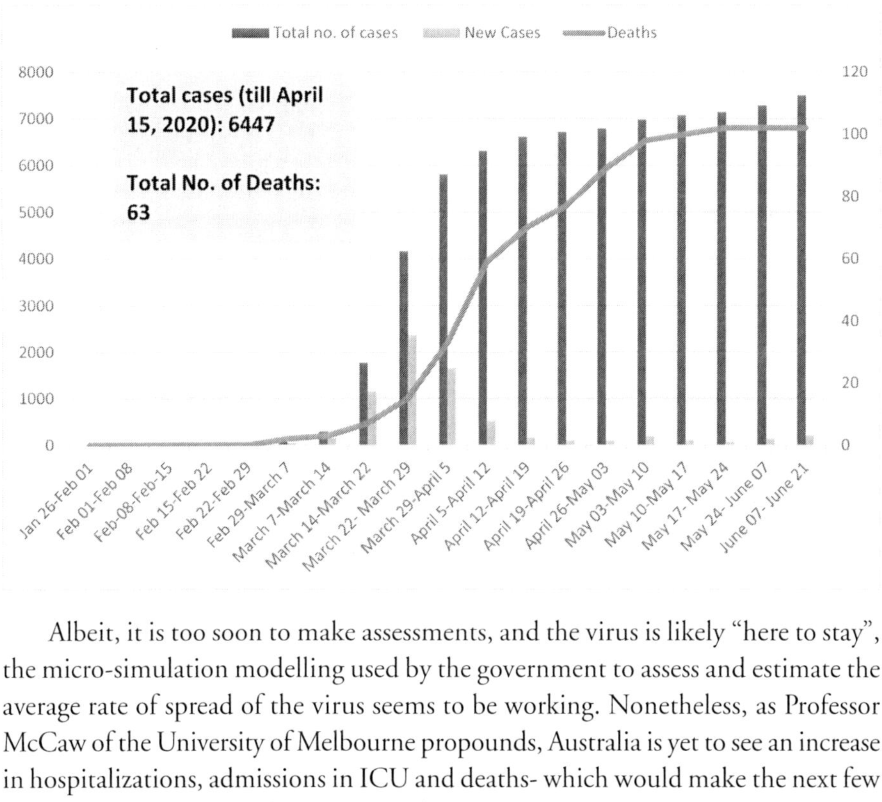

Albeit, it is too soon to make assessments, and the virus is likely "here to stay", the micro-simulation modelling used by the government to assess and estimate the average rate of spread of the virus seems to be working. Nonetheless, as Professor McCaw of the University of Melbourne propounds, Australia is yet to see an increase in hospitalizations, admissions in ICU and deaths- which would make the next few weeks "absolutely critical" for the country.[8] These scenarios, according to epidemiologist James Trauer, could result in either bad health outcomes or "extensive long-term lockdowns" in Australia.[9] This has materialized in the Metropolitan Melbourne as it witnessed the highest daily increase of the virus since the pandemic began on July 03, 2020. As a result, the Melbourne has been led into a six-week lockdown from July 06, 2020, with stage 3 restrictions- people would only be allowed to leave their houses for work, education, exercise, for necessary goods or services or medical or compassionate reasons until August 19, 2020.[10]

However, as COVID-19 is resonating the preparedness, decisiveness and determination of the Australian government to respond to the pandemic, it is also revealing pitfalls in the policies which revolve around unclear and mixed information from the government, blame-shifting between state governments and political point-scoring.[11] Such has sullied the confidence of a substantial part of the population towards the information circulated by the media and government; while leading one-third of the population to believe that there has been an overreaction towards the threat of COVID-19.[12] Invariably, a growing amount of lack of trust amongst people towards the government in Australia is leaving a part of the population confused and unaware about the policies regarding the COVID-19.

Consecutively, rising numbers of Novel Coronavirus cases in the country have also alarmed doctors working on the frontline, raising an immediate need for renewed lockdowns to avert a disaster. Such comes at the backdrop of the government levelling up its stimulus packages while lifting restrictions and allowing education facilities and large workplaces remain open and functional.[13] Further, a demand for greater severity in social distancing and lockdown is deemed necessary to avoid severe health crisis. At the same time, further efforts are required to prepare the health system for a surge in COVID-19 in critical stages.

Tracing the Sino-Australian Partnership Amidst the COVID-19 crisis

Australia's foreign policy, more often than not, has been guided by its dilemma of striking the correct balance between its defence partner the US and its economic partner China. With this dilemma at the backdrop, Australia has often debated how to best sustain Canberra's strategic autonomy.[14] For long, this conundrum was gently muted under the benefits of mutually advantageous economic relations between Australia and China, particularly as the 'China miracle'[15] allowed Beijing to situate itself at the centre of regional supply chain networks, and its trade and investment expansion became the driving forces of its rapid economic development and industrialization. However, even as the economic relations between both the nations developed, China gradually started translating its economic might into strategic and political influence in Australia. In retrospect, the very first instance of Beijing's political influence on Canberra was indicated when the Chinese diplomat Chen Yonglin defected to Australia in 2005 which signalled towards CCP's interference in Australia through 'a network of 1000 Chinese Government informants in Australia'[16] to 'infiltrate the country in a systematic way'.[17] Arguably, China had already started utilizing its friendship with Australia to obtain political mileage. Nonetheless, this argument started becoming glaringly evident with Xi Jinping coming to power. After years of Beijing's 'peaceful rise'[18], Australia seemed to be facing an increasingly assertive, proactive and nationalistic China.

Consequently, even as trade between China and Australia grew every year, the fundamental differences of national interests increasingly started floating at the surface level. By the end of 2017, this took to the front seat as the federal government, and largely the public started discussing the widespread interference of China in the Australia's domestic politics. Moreover, China's intrusions in Australia's cyber realm, the latter's arguably growing dependence on Beijing in terms of trade, tourism and education were gradually being deliberated. In this context, many policies were undertaken by Australia to protect its interests, sovereignty and autonomy had been viewed by China to be unfair and discriminatory. To this, China, though not overtly, had responded assertively while viewing Australia's policies to be influenced by the US. If anything, power-politics and difference of opinions and approaches had pushed the Sino-Australian bilateral ties towards greater complications. This is particularly reiterated as irrespective of Australia and China sharing a 'Comprehensive Strategic Partnership' having elements of enhanced two-way trade, corporate connections, and people-to-people ties; the political differences between both the countries had become starker. With the onset of COVID-19 pandemic, the Sino-Australian bilateral ties have been driven towards a greater test for stability. The pandemic has, in fact, amplified and accelerated several trends in the bilateral relations which were already underway before the disease emerged in Wuhan late last year.

Australia's Demand for an Independent Inquiry: The Beginning of a New Low

Arguably, the Sino-Australian relations started witnessing greater tensions amidst the pandemic since Australia announced its decision to lead the call for an independent investigation into China's role as the origin of COVID-19.[19] In this regard, on April 20, just a day after Australia's Minister of Foreign Affairs Marise Payne called for an independent review of the spread of the virus[20], Canberra received strong responses from China, particularly as the Foreign Ministry spokesperson Geng Shuang dismissed her comments as baseless and influenced by 'a certain country'.[21] Post this event, the strategic community in China expressed its discontent through numerous articles on *Global Times*, *CGTN*, *China Daily* and more, accusing Australia of not following an independent foreign policy. In fact, Australia was described as a "gum stuck on the bottom of China's shoe", by the Global Times editor Hu Xijin.[22] Chinese Embassy officials too, expressed their discontent while reiterating their perspective of Canberra acting in accordance with instructions from Washington and cooperating with the US in its 'propaganda war against China'.[23] However, a sign of a probable economic conflict between both the partner countries arose during Ambassador Cheng Jingye's interview with the Australian Financial Review political correspondent Andrew Tillet.[24] Notably, the interview reflected a peculiar evolution in China's approach towards Australia which was shaping to be more confrontation-oriented rather than focussing on cooperation. This was significantly reiterated with Ambassador Cheng's reply to one of Tillet's questions which stated:

> 'Chinese public is frustrated, dismayed and disappointed with what you are doing now. In the long term, for example, I think if the mood is going from bad to worse, people would think why we should go to such a country while it's not so friendly to China. The tourists may have second thoughts. Maybe the parents of the students would also think whether this place, which they find is not so friendly, even hostile, is the best place to send their kids to. So it's up to the public, the people to decide. And also, maybe the ordinary people will think why they should drink Australian wine or eat Australian beef.'[25]

The statement by ambassador Cheng, if anything, was resonating a coercive approach by China towards Australia; which, if not explicitly alluding in Ambassador Cheng's statement, was subtly suggestive of the 'wolf-warrior diplomacy'[26] under the Xi government.

However, further to China's dismay, a group of more than 100 countries had come to back the Australian government to establish the enquiry at the World Health Assembly (WHA). This development, most importantly, had reflected on Australia's leadership efforts at the WHA. Essentially, Australia had utilized its three-year term on the WHO executive board to push for an investigation for the source of the pandemic.[27] For Australia, it was reasonable to demand an "impartial, independent and comprehensive evaluation" of a pandemic which had ensued immense health and economic crisis. This investigation was also important for Australia as two of the Chinese scientists who worked for the Wuhan Institute of Virology, Shi Zhengli and Peng Zhou, studied bats at Australia's national science agency – the Commonwealth Scientific and Industrial Research Organization (CSIRO) facility as a part of a jointly funded research by Australian and Chinese governments. Dr Zhengli currently is the director of the Centre for Emerging Infectious Diseases at the Chinese Academy Sciences' Wuhan Institute of Virology.[28] At the same time, Dr Zhou remains the head of the Bat Virus infection and Immunity Project at the Wuhan Institute of Virology.[29] Notably, the Wuhan Institute of Virology has been at the centre of controversies since allegations were made by the US Secretary of States Mike Pompeo for its 'accidental' origin of the virus.[30] However, even as the WHA adopted the Corona inquiry resolution, the Chinese embassy in Australia dismissed the latter's role and stated that the draft resolution at the WHA on independent investigation into the pandemic was "totally different from Australia's proposal of an independent international review".[31] Clearly, Australia had been witnessing provocative responses from China which, if nothing else, was a prognosis of the bilateral relations taking a grim turn.

Effects on the Agriculture Sector

Within a few weeks of Ambassador Cheng's coercive remarks on Australia's independent enquiry move, China banned beef exports from four Australian abattoirs[32] and announced an 80 per cent tariff on barley, only to reiterate the implicitly assertive and blunt responses by the ambassador.[33] Most importantly, even as the Chinese official statements explained their policy changes as a requirement due to the violations by Australian beef companies in inspection and quarantine requirements; and as antidumping remedy measures against Australia's $1.5 billion barley exports to China; it is China's discontent over Australia's political noises which moved Beijing to undertake a policy approach which would serve Canberra as a warning.[34] Arguably, this pressure tactic by China has a possibility to also target other export products by Australia, including seafood, dairy goods, Australian wine, oatmeal, fruits and more if Canberra is not willing to change its policies which are going against Beijing's interests.[35]

As a matter of fact, this approach by Beijing is not new. China has used such economically coercive approaches towards Australia earlier on several occasions. The first instance took place on account of the former Prime Minister Malcolm Turnbull's initiation of foreign interference laws which implicitly targeted China. As a result, arguably, six Australian wine companies faced delays at Chinese customs in 2018.[36] Similar incidents took place with several Chinese ports restricting or delaying Australian coal imports in early 2019. Even though the official Chinese response mentioned the need for environmental checks for the imported coal, a larger consensus was built over China's discomfort towards Australian policies questioning Beijing's aggressive posture in the South China Sea;[37] and Canberra blocking Chinese telecommunication giants such as Huawei and ZTE from rolling out in the country's 5G network due to security concerns. Further, factors involved were the barring of the Chinese billionaire and major political donor Huang Xiangmo from Australia on account of a pro-Beijing lobby group;[38] and Australia's accusations towards a 'state actor' responsible for cyber-attacks on political parties targeting China.[39]

However, China's current aggressive behaviour is distinguishable from before. Particularly as its aggressiveness displayed earlier was less overt. Even as China had criticized or complained about Australia's policy behaviours, those remained tacit and of a low magnitude. Instead, China's current diplomatic and political behaviour through economic pressures amidst the COVID-19 has been reaching a higher degree. Certainly, China's foreign policy has witnessed significant changes amidst the pandemic where the current approach resonates greater assertiveness to sustain China's global image of a 'strong power' and domestic image of competent and firm leadership.

This foreign policy behaviour by China has pushed Australia towards a greater economic challenge, particularly at the backdrop of Canberra entering into recession for the first time in 29 years.[40] Beijing's assertive approach has further put the Australian government to test as it was due to the former's miraculous performance during the Global Financial Crisis (GFC) and its strong demand which served as one of the factors assuaging Canberra's dwindling export sector, underpinning the resilience of the Australian economy.[41] However, the current scenario categorized by tense bilateral relations between Australia and China puts the increasing trade and economic relations between both the countries through an enormous ordeal.

Notably, China's current economic move to increase tariffs and boycott certain Australian exports also remain significant as the particular sectors form a serious chunk of Australia's prosperity (See Figure 16.2).

Figure 16.2: Australia's Exports with China (By Category)

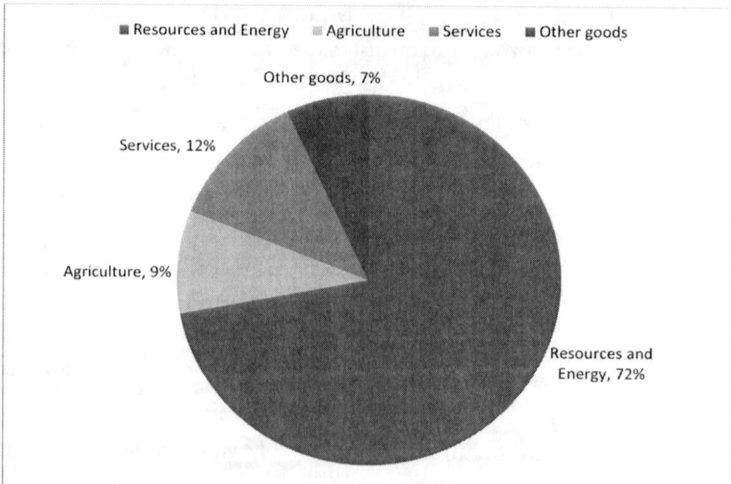

Source: Australian Bureau of Statistics (ABS) at https://www.abs.gov.au/; Australian Bureau of Agricultural and Resource Economics and Sciences (ABARES) at https://www.agriculture.gov.au/abares; and Reserve Bank of Australia (RBA) at https://www.rba.gov.au/.

Inferring from Figure 16.2, even as the agriculture sector doesn't occupy the major portion of Australia's exports to China, it still remains as one of the most internationally competitive sectors of the Australian economy, comprising of 9 per cent of its exports to China out of which approximately AU$ 1 billion[42] is held by beef and AU $ 1.3 billion is comprised of barley exports.[43] Importantly, two-thirds of Australia's agriculture produce is exported- which accounts for 49 per cent of the total barley, and 28 per cent of the total beef produce exported to China; only to increase the economic stakes for Australia further.[44] To put in perspective, China has targeted two of Australia's most economically powerful sectors of agriculture through bans and tariffs, only to result in greater economic problems for the particular sector of the country which is already going through depression due to the pandemic. From a larger perspective, China's assertive move has a possibility to hurt the Sino-Australian bilateral trade in general, which has been growing at a comfortable level since the past few years. (Figure 16.3)

Figure 16.3: China's Trade with Australia (2009-2019)

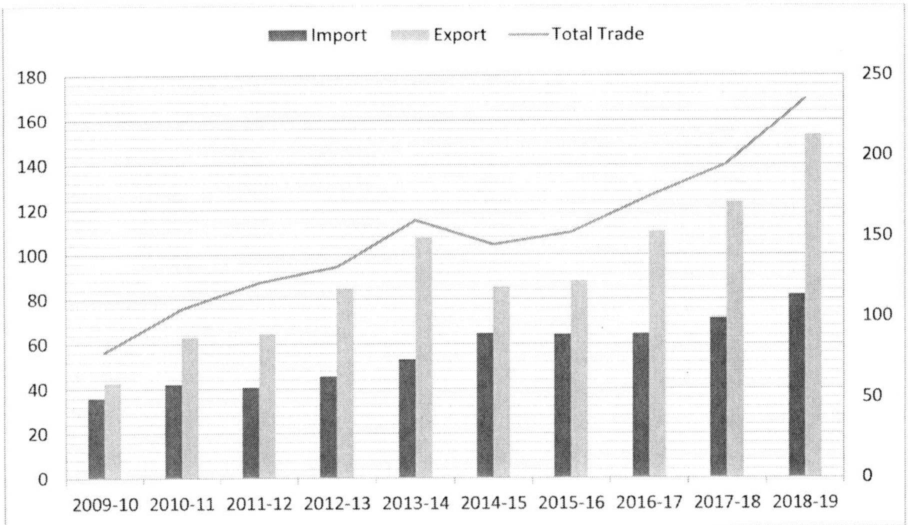

Source: Australian Trade and Investment Commission at https://www.austrade.gov.au/

It is important to note that China has been Australia's largest trading partner and accounts for 32.6 percent of its exports. Its mines have provided iron ore, coal and gas to stimulate China's industrialization and growth. However, products like barley and beef are not as exclusive to Australia and thus, are prone to greater political vulnerability. In fact, China's resolute decision to restrict beef and barley from Australia can pave the way for Beijing to enhance imports of the two products from the US instead, helping China to meet the obligations stated under the Phase One trade deal,[45] particularly to mollify the rising pressures from Washington.[46]

Moreover, considering China's strategic community suggesting towards greater economic aggression by China if Australia continues with its current policies towards Beijing, such a scenario could further be detrimental to Canberra's economic sector as the trade surplus between both the countries has traditionally been in favour Australia.[47]

Effects on the Service Sector

Another important element of Ambassador Cheng's statement was the gesture towards a possible change in the Chinese approach for Australia's service sector, particularly education and tourism. Significantly, it was the move by China's Education Bureau to warn Chinese students about applying or continuing their studies in Australia on account of the 'racist incidents' during the COVID-19 pandemic, which reiterated an assertive sentiment through the wolf warrior diplomacy of the Xi Jinping administration.[48] The statement by the education minister reminding 'overseas students to conduct a good risk assessment and be cautious about choosing to go to Australia or return to Australia to study' showcased a shift in the Sino-Australian relations through China's suggestively confrontational approach and Beijing's overt critiques through official and diplomatic mediums.[49] A similar approach was witnessed as the Chinese Ministry of Culture and Tourism issued a travel alert to its citizens on June 6 propounding risks of travelling to Australia due to significant increase in racist attacks on 'Chinese and Asian people'.[50] Arguably, the Chinese alerts have not been completely unwarranted. Fran Martin, Associate Professor in Cultural Studies at Melbourne University during an interview titled 'Expectations and Experiences of Chinese University Students in Australia' with the Australia-China Relations Institute (ACRI) on May 03, 2018, raised significant issues of racism experienced by Chinese students in Australia, apart from social barriers of language proficiency, exclusion from certain work opportunities and more.[51] Certainly, with the COVID-19 originating out of China (arguably), the number of racist attacks on Chinese, as well as Asian people have risen even as Australian authorities, and university officials deny[52] such accusations.[53] However, even as the warnings highlight China's increasing displeasure towards racist acts in Australia, it also emphasizes on the bigger picture of worsening ties. No doubt, Beijing has every right to issue a warning to its citizens over discrimination; however, the timing of the statement suggests political motivations.[54]

It must be noted that Beijing issued a similar safety warning to all Chinese students in Australia in 2018 after the then Australian Minister for International Development and the Pacific Concetta Fierravanti-Wells accused Chinese infrastructure aid to the Pacific islands as 'White Elephant' projects.[55] The accusations had underlying concerns about debt sustainability regarding Chinese projects in many less developed countries in the Pacific.[56] It can be argued that China's economically coercive moves are typically initiated towards actors whose policies go against China's interests to keep them in check. In the purview of the current times, China's assertive moves can be assumed to be evolving into a strategic orientation, seeking for political gains. This argument can be best be substantiated with the articles by the Chinese scholarly community inferring Australia's denials towards accusations for racist attacks as a response to its 'nervousness' due to a possible reduction in Chinese tourism and educational sources.[57] The Chinese assertiveness, if anything, suggest towards a trend within China's coercive policies which acknowledges Australia's underlying economic vulnerability to China and focusses on specific sectors where China has the upper hand.

Undeniably, China has been the biggest source of international students and visitors to Australia; and in the past few years, the numbers have just been increasing. In the last decade, Australia has witnessed a massive growth in the number of tourists and students, which has substantially contributed to Australia's economy. The amount spent by the Chinese has increased from AU$ 3 billion in 2009 to AU$ 12.4 billion in terms of tourism, and AU$ 4.4 billion to AU$ 12 billion in terms of education (See Figure 16.4). Moreover, Chinese nationals make up for roughly 38 per cent of Australia's international students and 15percent of its tourists.[58]

Figure 16.4: China's Contribution to Australia's Service Sectors ($Aud Billion)

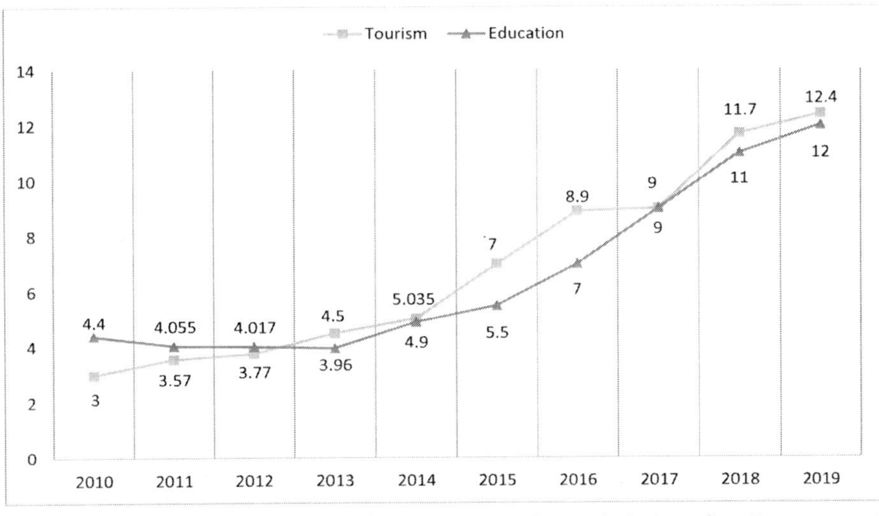

Source: Australian Tourism Industry (https://www.australia.com/en); Australian Department of Education, Skills and Employment (https://www.education.gov.au/)

Interestingly, however, China has rarely issued statements or generated policies which would be catering to its iron ore imports from Australia. China remains heavily reliant on Australia for iron ore which contributes to its steel industry.[59] Steel, on the other hand, remains the backbone of China's infrastructure development, and thus China's national goals of urbanization and modernization. In this context, Australia does hold leverage in this area by being one of the largest producers of iron ore in the world.[60] At the same time, Canberra also holds leverage due to its geographical proximity to China which considerably eases shipping and transportation costs. Thus, it can be argued that China would continue its assertive posture towards Australia, but through a measured approach which would ensure the sustainability of its economy. However, this factor should not deter the acknowledgement of a changed Australia policy where the Xi administration is increasingly viewing Australia more as an adversary power, rather than a comprehensive strategic partner amidst Canberra's leading call for an independent inquiry.

It is thus, important to understand the nuances of this changed policy which throws light on the underlying tensions in the Sino-Australian relations which have been developing since the past few years. These tensions as the undercurrents highlight the fundamental contradictions of the bilateral ties which best pose as factors to understand the current Sino-Australian tensions amidst COVID-19.

Understanding the Underlying Fault lines in the Sino-Australian Ties

Tensions between China and Australia are not new, and viewing the current strains in the bilateral ties in isolation would be abrupt. Instead, tensions between both the countries were building up at least since 2015; until which, security concerns regarding China's intrusive behaviour were muffled underneath Beijing's powerful business lobby and the profitable relation Canberra had shared with Beijing.

The Factor of the Port of Darwin

It was not until 2015 when the Northern Territories government in Australia signed an agreement to hand over the port of Darwin to the Landbridge Industry for a lease of 99 years, that the security concerns regarding China started figuring overtly.[61] A reason for the same was the Landbridge Industry being a subsidiary of China's Shandor Landbridge group with whom the Australian government signed a deal worth AU$ 506 million. Importantly, the owner of the company Ye Cheng had close links with the CCP as well as the PLA, which held significance in view of the US using the same port for the deployment of its many marines each year. The concerns only kept increasing from there, particularly as during an interview in Beijing in 2016, Mr Ye expressed how the port of Darwin would fit in the company's strategy to expand its shipping and energy interests.[62] He also propounded how the port served China's foreign policy goal of the BRI, particularly as the Commonwealth of Australia had not become a part of the infrastructural initiative yet. To put in perspective, the NT government had allowed the lease of one of Australia's most important strategic assets to China, only allowing Beijing to intrude in Canberra strategically. Post this, the rules were changed to prevent something similar from happening again; however, several incidents on the same pattern kept cropping up such as the S. Kidman Property case, the Ausgrid case[63] and more.

Expanding Footprints into Australian Party Politics

For a long time, the Australian government had desired to segregate its core national security concerns from its economic interests. However, it is China's reported role in fostering political corruption in the country which initiated a wave of revelations, forcing Australia to reassess its bilateral relations with China. China's covert political involvement in Australia, most importantly, played a significant role in highlighting the fundamental differences in the ideological, political and security perspectives of both the countries, according it as a major juncture in the Sino-Australian bilateral relationship.[64]

It mainly started with the revelations of Huang Xiangmo in Australia's political and media circles in 2016, which highlighted financial links between the Chinese business and Australian political world. Huang Xiangmo was a property developer from China who moved to Australia and quickly gained political clout and momentum. Importantly, he was a major donor to both Labor and Liberal parties on the one hand, and Australian universities on the other.[65] He had, in fact, donated AU$ 1.8 million to the University of Technology Sydney in 2014 to set up the Australian-China Relations Institute (ACRI).[66] Huang was also the director of the United Front Work Department (UFWD)-linked Australian Council for the Promotion of Peaceful Reunification of China (ACPPRC).[67] Although the ACPPRC was claimed to be an independent organization, its linkages to the UFWD which remains the core of the CCP with being led by the members of the Politburo Standing Committee, unravelled concerns of Chinese involvement in Australian party-state affairs.

However, Huang first came under political scrutiny when during a press conference organized by the ACPPRC for the young Labor Party Senator from New Whales, Sam Dastyari who, in the presence of Huang, expressed the necessity to treat the South China Sea (SCS) as 'China's Affair'.[68] He further explicated the importance for Australia to 'respect China's decision' regarding the SCS and 'as a friend of China', not get involved in the disputed region.[69] This surprisingly was contradictory to the positions taken by the Labor Party Shadow Minister Stephen Conroy who condemned China's assertive expansion in the SCS and stated the Labor government's decision to authorize the Defence Force to conduct freedom of navigation activities in the SCS region if it deemed 'necessary and safe'. [70] Moreover, Dastyari's statements were contrary to Australia's official view at large, which has, more often than not, opposed China's militarization in the SCS. [71] The image of Dastyari supporting China's national interests which conflicted with Australia's viewpoint, along with news reports of another Chinese donor with CCP links paying a travel bill for Dastyari, created a political outcry and forced the young Senator to apologize and step down from the party position.[72] The Dastyari affair led many media investigations to unravel the linkages between CCP and Australian politicians. Reportedly, Huang Xiangmo had given AU$ 100,000 in cash to the Secretary-General of the NSW Labour Party and AU$ 2 million to major political parties through his companies.[73] Further, Huang Xiangmo had threatened to cancel a promised AU$ 400,000 to the Labor Party if it did not soften its positions on the SCS issue in response to Conroy's firm position seeking freedom of navigation in the SCS.[74] It was supposedly, in relation to this threat, that Dastyari's remarks suggested support for China's adventurism in the disputed region. Largely, businesses linked to China had given more than $5.5 million between 2013 and 2015,[75] even as the Australian Security Intelligence Organisation (ASIO) had warned several top party officials regarding the underlying national security concerns of the contributions.[76]

Significantly, these political scandals shed light on the various ways the CCP, and its linked donors have sought to exert pressure on Australia to influence the country from within. Notably, these links have not just been in Australian politics, but also academic and research institutions, within the Chinese community in Australia and other individuals. Reports of overseas Chinese students being encouraged to spread patriotic and pro-CCP sentiments in the campus, while inhibiting dissent serve as a ploy. In this context, there had been several incidents where the academic staff in Australian universities were made to apologize for comments which were 'deemed offensive' to ethnic Chinese students. A reference for the same were instances where a professor at the University of Newcastle had to apologize for his reference to Taiwan as an independent country; a professor at the University of Sydney was slammed for showing Arunachal Pradesh, Ladakh and Aksai Chin as part of India; and similar incidents took place in Australian National University and Monash University.[77]

The deluge of allegations and revelations on Chinese influence activities sparked an intensive national debate in Australia which led the then Prime Minister Malcolm Turnbull to announce the introduction of draft legislation to counter foreign interference and espionage on December 7, 2017.[78] Subsequently, the growing concern in the government regarding the increasing instances of foreign interference in universities led Australia to set up a task force in August 2019, which would ensure universities to remain free of foreign influences. The minister of education, Dan Tehan, stated that the task force would:

> '...deter and detect deception, undue influence, unauthorized disclosure or disruption to our research, intellectual property and research community, while protecting academic freedom.'[79]

The task force was further supported by four working groups working to protect the cybersecurity, research and intellectual property, foreign collaboration and culture and communication both in the university sector as well as across the government.

Arguably, these steps saw two sides of the debate where either the business and academic communities were supporting the legislation acknowledging the growing Chinese interferences in Australian affairs, or they were opposing the decision as an exaggeration of Chinese influence in the country which could possibly lead to a rift in the bilateral relations.[80] Irrespective, the political and public mood, in general, seemed to change post this incident, with greater support for firm policies against foreign interferences. However, notwithstanding the reports and allegations, Australia witnessed strong responses from China. The Chinese scholarly and strategic community, in particular, condemned Australia's new law for targeting the Chinese business community and students for political donations which were registered and transparent, and accusations which were baseless.[81] For China, Australia's political moves had pushed the bilateral ties towards greater volatility, while having a possibility to affect the academic, business and cultural exchanges between both the countries. As discussed earlier, Australia's law faced economic retaliation from China as the six of its wine companies faced delays at Chinese customs.

For China, the law came as a surprise as Australia was one of the first countries which reformed its national security laws and policies to limit foreign political interference. This enabled China to perceive Australia beyond the influences of the US. More importantly, Australia was an attractive destination for donations and expansion of Chinese influences as the country had immense strategic value for being one of US' closest allies. Chinese influences in Australia, allowing it to soften Canberra's approach on important disputes such as the SCS would have provided Beijing with political gains and support towards its core strategic interests. This would have only allowed Beijing to pursue its ambitions in SCS more broadly, further strengthening the Chinese leadership legitimacy.

Further, for China, Australia remained a trade partner who was economically dependent on Beijing for its growth. China's support for Australia's business community and academic circles enabled it to strengthen the Comprehensive relationship both the countries shared. However, at the same time, China's growing financial support to Australian businesses, political parties, university campuses and research institutes accounted for Canberra's financial dependence on Beijing. To put in perspective, Australia's democratic structure not prohibiting campaign donations from foreigners, its large community of ethnic Chinese Australian citizens, and its increasingly profitable trade and business relations with China only enhanced Canberra's China dilemma. This dilemma, significantly, has only been growing as Australia meddles between China as an economic partner and a security concern.

5G and the establishment of China's Security Threats

In August 2018, Australia became the first country and the first member of the Five Eyes Intelligence Sharing alliance (comprising of the US, Australia, UK, Canada, and New Zealand) to bar the Chinese telecommunication giant Huawei from providing 5G technology in Australia.[82] It issued security guidance to prevent its telecommunication carriers from buying 5G equipment and services from both Huawei and ZTE. This was reiterated through a joint statement by the then acting Home Affairs Minister Scott Morrison and Communications Minister Mitch Fifield:

> 'The Government will continue to engage and support Australians, including the telecommunications industry, to manage national security risks.'[83]

While not overtly targeting the Chinese telecommunication companies, Australia's ban emphasized on companies which are "likely subject to extrajudicial directions" clearly directing towards China's National Intelligence Law introduced in 2017.[84] The law obligates the Chinese companies to "support, assist and cooperate with the state intelligence-gathering work", reiterating the possibility of national security information to be passing through the CCP as a legal mandate.[85] In fact, the Huawei's founder Ren Zhengfei being a member of the CCP makes an even more established case for Australia to enact such a law.[86]

Australia also placed equal importance on the possibility of espionage through unauthorized access or sabotage by limiting Chinese participation in the periphery network.[87] In this context, the act aimed to protect the 'confidentiality of communications carried on, and of information contained on, telecommunications networks or facilities'. At the same time, it highlighted national security considerations, including the long-term risk to 'the security of critical infrastructure' from sabotage.[88]

Not surprisingly, China retaliated firmly to this move by Australia. An official response from Ambassador Cheng to the media suggested China's view of the ban to be politically motivated amidst a global campaign led by the US. He went on to say:

> 'It is discrimination against a Chinese company. At the same time, it doesn't serve the best interests of Australian companies and consumers… it has become a sore point, or thorny issue, in bilateral relations as it damages mutual trust between the two sides.'[89]

China also stated its response to Australia at the World Trade Organization in April 2019 about its 'discriminative' policies which appears to go against the global trade rules.[90] The Chinese media took a step ahead and suggested towards a counteraction from China as accusations towards Huawei remain inconclusive. Articles in *Global Times* stating 'Australia is bound to pay the price for its unwise decisions' only re-established a potential aggressive response from China, which was on the way.[91] This presumption materialized when Beijing delayed Australian coal imports through the northern ports on the claims of quality checks. However, it could be argued that China was targeting Australia's coal imports to China, which account for 3.7 per cent of Australia's GDP, in response to the Canberra's recent 5G policy.[92]

Viewing this development from the Chinese perspective, the 5G technology and Huawei held immense significance to China's foreign policy and restrictions for the same only added to China's discontent. For China, technological capability is something Beijing has been harnessing since decades; however, by retaining distinctive characteristics of authoritarianism and party control. Under Xi, China has sought to develop the 5G technology to mark its presence as the technological leader in the global order, and Huawei has been central to the construction of the particular technology. However also, under the Xi administration, the government has enhanced its control over private companies through heavy regulations, which has blurred the lines between public and private businesses. These regulations have only strengthened post the 2017 National Intelligence Law; while the CCP's domestic practice of control is casting a shadow on its companies, leading the global community to perceive them as a national security threat increasingly.

Nonetheless, the unfavourable policies towards Chinese technology and companies by countries like Australia are leading Beijing to view Canberra through confrontational lenses. Apart from Australia's conduct towards China's 5G technology, the former's condemnation of China's treatment of Uighur people; and Australia's critique of China's new National Security Bill in Hong Kong has also received sharp criticisms by Beijing. In fact, Australia had joined a group of 23 countries including the UK, the US, Germany, Japan and Canada in 2019 to condemn China's treatment of Uighur and other minorities in the Xinjiang region.[93] The group pushed for urgent implementation of recommendations by independent UN experts on the situation in China. Subsequently, Australia expressed its deep and growing concerns over China's imposition of the new National Security bill in Hong Kong, which would have clear implications for the human rights in Hong Kong.[94] Australia even considered options for providing citizenship to people from Hong Kong.[95] In the purview of the current times, Australia's policies, if anything, are threatening China's strategic core strategic goals and national security interests. From the Chinese perspective, the policies are also tarnishing China's role in the global community, at the same time, interfering in China's internal affairs with Hong Kong and Xinjiang as a pretext.

Amidst the COVID-19, the above factors have only heightened the fault lines present in the bilateral relations. The worsening relations are also affecting the people's perspectives towards the other country. In this context, the people-to-people ties, which were a foundational element in the Sino-Australian bilateral relations, are being affected with mutual trust being at an all-time low.[96]

Diminishing Public Opinion

While both Australia and China grapple with the COVID-19, a trend is increasingly emerging within the public, which point towards growing criticism against the other nation. Such surrounds downgrading bilateral relations amidst the pandemic due to unfavourable policies undertaken by both the countries towards each other.

In terms of Australia, it is China's efforts to intrude and influence the Australian polity and community in general; and its confrontational response coupled with economic coercion towards Australia's policies which are leading the Australian public to perceive China negatively. Moreover, it also the latter's not so-early response towards the containment of the virus, penalizing the whistle-blowers such as Dr Li Wenliang, and covering up for its late reactions to intimate the WHO, and largely the international community for the virus spreading inside its territory which is enabling the people to view China as an irresponsible power. If anything, the Australian government, as well as its people, have been questioning the lack of transparency, accountability and responsibility in China's global governance model; which is likely to influence the Sino-Australian bilateral relations to a great extent.

The above rhetoric could best be reflected by an online article published in *The Daily Telegraph* which stated the point-by-point rebuttal of the Chinese consul-general's criticism over the paper's coverage of the pandemic by general Australian audiences.[97] The responses came at the backdrop of the Chinese consul-general stating:

> 'Recently, certain Australian media outlets have been pushing the argument that China should be held "responsible" for the spread of the COVID-19 pandemic, even claiming to demand compensation from China. These claims lack scientific and factual evidence, are full of arrogance and prejudice, and are simply unconvincing.'[98]

The reactions by the Australian government humorously expressed the growing feeling of scepticism and discontent among the general population of Australia against China. The very fact that the article was one of the most-read pieces in recent times comes as a reference to the above argument.

A larger emphasis on the growing displeasure over China and its actions were reiterated through the Lowy Institute Poll of 2020.[99] According to the polls, the trust factor in China as a major power went down from 56 per cent in 2010 to 23 per cent in 2020. (See Figure 16.5) China's coercive responses to Australia's policies, coupled with China banning Australian beef and putting high tariffs on barley have presumably played a major factor. As a result, feelings towards China amidst the COVID-19 has substantially turned negative; according to the polls, feelings for China have fallen from 54 per cent in 2010 to 39 per cent in 2020, taking the range of 0 to 100 to represent feelings starting from 'very cool to 'very warm'. (See Figure 16.6)

Figure 16.5: Trust in China as a Global Power

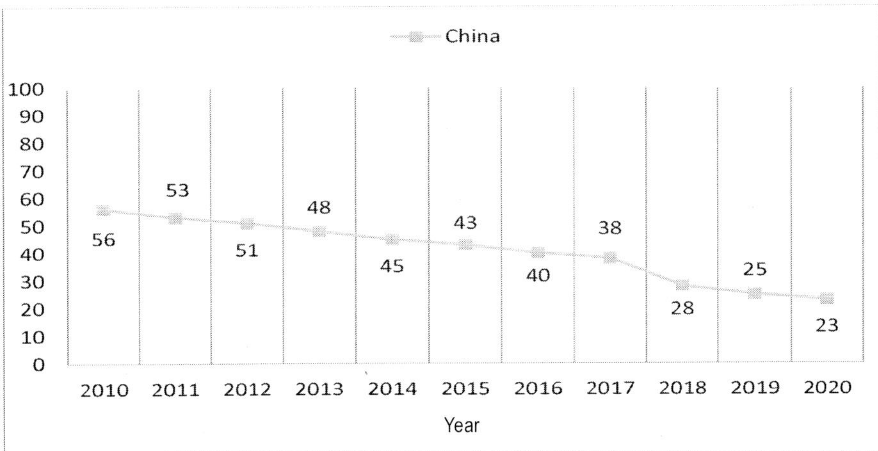

Source: Lowy Polls Institute 2020

Figure 16.6: Feelings Towards China

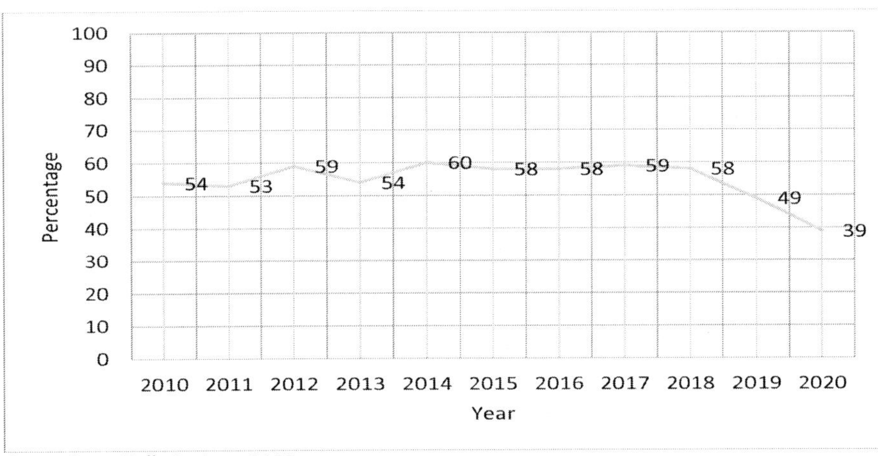

Source: Lowy Polls Institute 2020

Further, the polls have also represented views by the Australian public in regards to their confidence in China's governance system in handling the COVID-19 pandemic, where 68 per cent of the people have shown 'less favourable' views. (See Figure 16.7) Indeed, reports of China's late response to the Novel Coronavirus spread, and the penalization of early whistle-blowers have held significance in that respect.

Figure 16.7: Confidence in China's System of Government in Handling the COVID-19

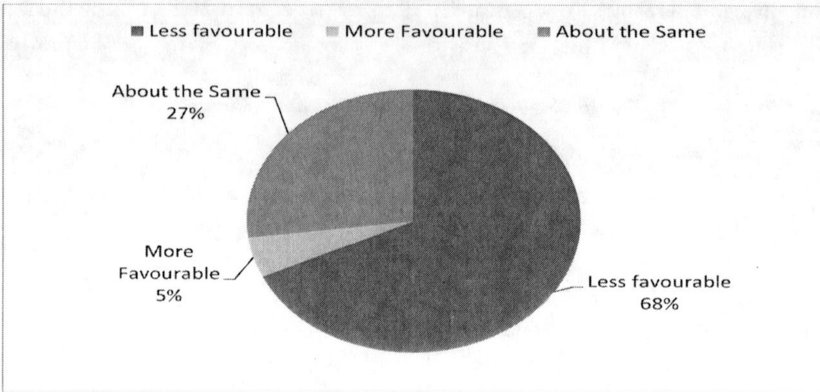

Source: Lowy Polls Institute 2020

However importantly, the polls also represented the people voicing Australia's China dilemma, with the percentage of people considering China' more as an economic power' falling to 55 percent in 2020 from 77 per cent in 2015; and the percentage of people considering China' more as a security threat' rising from 15 per cent in 2015 to 41 per cent in 2020. (See Figure 16.8) Even as the percentage of people considering China more as a security threat remains less than the category of people considering China more as an economic power, the rise in the former category indicates towards a gradual shift in the sentiments of people towards China.

Figure 16.8: China: An Economic Power or a Security Threat

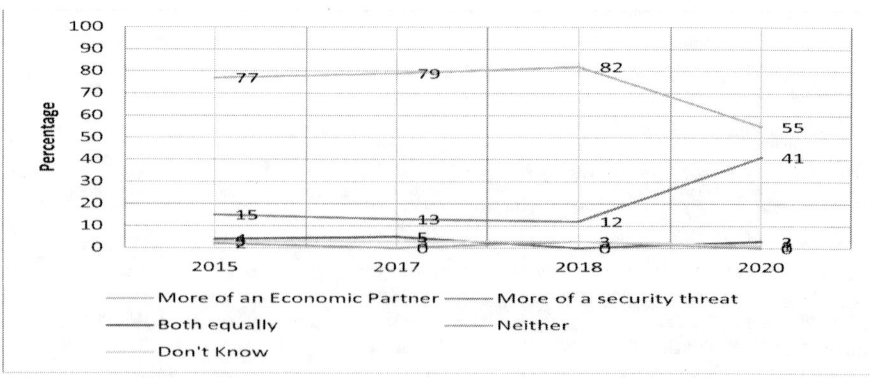

Source: Lowy Polls Institute 2020

Predictably, similar sentiments were visible within China towards Australia in a survey conducted by the public opinion department of the Global Times and the Australian Studies Centre at Beijing Foreign University.[100] According to the findings, a large number of respondents didn't view Australia favourably. A reason can be the mounting reports of racist attacks on the Chinese population in Australia. In fact, China had been worried about an increasing anti-China sentiment brewing in Australia since a while. The public opinion regarding China had been becoming less favourable post the reports of China's political interference in Australia. The Chinese media had thus, warned Australia regarding the diminishing mutual trust between both the countries which could affect the bilateral ties. However visibly, the mutual trust has been diminishing even after efforts were undertaken by both the governments to resolve tensions.[101]

It must be noted, that diminishing mutual trust can be an element of apprehension between two countries even as it might not play a dominant factor. Mutual trust and favourability towards the other country plays a significant role in laying the foundation of the bilateral ties. A non-favourable approach towards a country can influence multiple elements of bilateral relations. Putting in the perspective of the Sino-Australian ties, diminishing mutual trust and favourability could affect various sectors in both countries such as trade, education, tourism and more, which remain interdependent. As discussed above, Australia remains dependent on China for tourism, education, as well as trade for many commodities. China too remains dependent on Australia for imports such as iron ore, coal, food and more. China and Australia share an economically mutual profitable relation, and the current scenario between both the countries, if continued, can significantly affect the above elements.

Conclusion

The COVID-19 has brought substantial changes to the Sino-Australian bilateral ties where the current tensions have only been emblematic to the foundational fault lines between both the countries. For Australia, it is not a rising and a more powerful China which has become the problem, but it is Beijing's more authoritarian, nationalistic and ideological foreign policy approach under the current leadership which has evolved as a contradiction in relation to Canberra's values of sustaining a liberal democratic order harbouring freedom and transparency. It is also China's overtly confrontational approach towards Australia, which has re-emphasized the latter's China dilemma; is China more of an economic partner or a security threat? This dilemma has evolved to be further convoluted as China threatens Australia with economic coercion in response to the latter's call for an independent inquiry.

For China, on the other hand, it is Australia's recent policies and particularly its political moves during the pandemic, which has threatened its core strategic interests, as well as questioned its global governance system. This has invariably led China to view Australia as an adversary rather than a comprehensive strategic partner. More so, as the global criticisms amidst the COVID-19 pandemic have already tainted China's image as a responsible power, only to further hinder the Chinese dream of National Rejuvenation.[102] In this context, China is already reeling from immense domestic pressure to ensure economic growth and sustainability amidst a global economic crisis.[103] Importantly, the sustainability of economic growth holds huge stakes for the stability of the CCP, as well as leadership. The greater challenge for Xi in the current scenario surrounds its ability to endure China's economic growth to sustain its dominant position in the global order. This, however, is being threatened with the global call for diversification, to which Australia contributes substantially.

Certainly, the COVID-19 would change many trends in the global order, as it already has; but not the fundamental fault lines between Australia and China. More so, as China's governance system and geo-political goals would only turn more authoritarian and ambitious post the COVID-19 era.[104] Thus, China would further tighten its control over the technology arena and try to suppress any forms of internal dissent or external critiques more firmly. This might only complicate Australia's choices towards China even more. In the post-COVID-19 period, Australia might not bring significant changes in its policies of foreign interference and 5G network. It might continue to follow a domestic and foreign policy which would cater to its interests and protect its national security. In this context, the major point of contention between both the countries would continue to exist in the post-COVID-19 period too, only to hold further significant implications for the Sino-Australian bilateral ties.

However, on the face of an increasingly assertive by China, Australia would want to diversify away from Beijing. Australia's efforts to diversify away from China have been going on since a while; its desire to strengthen relations with the US, Japan and India through the Quadrilateral Initiative;[105] its involvement in the US-led infrastructural initiative such as the Blue Dot Network;[106] and Canberra's efforts to strengthen ties with the Pacific Island community through the 'Pacific Step-Up' program[107] can be established as a ploy. Domestically, Australia has called for 'market diversification' to reduce its economic dependence on China on the account of latter's aggressive policies posing as a threat.[108] It has sought to branch out and encourage its Australian producers to sell their products to other buyers, as well as businesses to spread their risk across numerous markets.[109] However, this has witnessed its share of debates and deliberations with many economists warning Australia of a low possibility of finding an alternative which would share similar demand levels.[110] At the least, these initiatives might not result in forming an alternative for the relations Australia shares with China.

In this context, Australian states and businesses should not stop looking towards opportunities with China. At the same time, they should also not overlook the risks of dealing with a more aggressive and nationalistic China. It must be noted that the Sino-Australian bilateral ties do hold a possibility to deteriorate further if substantial measures are not taken; however, these conflicts would be unlikely to completely breakdown the bilateral ties.[111] Thus, a clearer understanding of the risks involved and the factors which shape the federal government's policies towards Beijing can be an effective response from Canberra.[112] If this scenario can be achieved, a workable relationship with China would be in Australia's interests to protect its economic pursuits and at the same time, not compromise on its sovereignty. Australia also might want to demand greater fairness and reciprocity in relations with Australia.[113] Reciprocity and fairness have been iron principles in the foreign policy practice which Australia swears by. In this regard, a reciprocal and fair relationship between both the countries in terms of each other's security perceptions and ambitions can be helpful. Reciprocity could also be an important element in terms of investment access to China's companies and enterprises.[114] China has been responsible for providing limited access to other countries in Chinese companies, especially state-owned enterprises. Australia might want to access its responses accordingly and seek to establish a mutually fair and profitable relationship with China. Even though such an outlook towards China might not allow for a trouble-free bilateral relationship, a cooperative element in the bilateral ties would serve Australia's national interests better than a permanent shift to complete hostility.

NOTES

1 China and Australia have completed 48 years of their diplomatic relations, but their engagement goes way back to 1949 when PRC was formed. In fact, Chinese presence and influence in Australia began back in history from the colonial times. Since then, the bilateral relations have witnessed the impacts of the changes and continuities in both Australian and Chinese foreign policy which have birthed many high points as well as trigger points. This has been aptly reflected in many scholarships such as James Reilly and Jingdong Yuan (eds), *Australia and China at 40*, (Sydney: UNSW Press, 2012); Wang Yi, *Australia-China Relations Post 1949: Sixty Years of Trade and Politics*, (New York: Routledge, 2012); Robert Macklin, *Dragon and Kangaroo: Australia and China's Shared History from the Goldfields to the Present Day*, (Sydney: Hachette Australia, 2017); Lachlan Strahan, *Australia's China: Changing Perceptions from the 1930s to the 1990s*, (New York: Cambridge University Press, 1996). However, there is lack of enough scholarship which would trace the implications of the deepening strategic and economic engagement between Australia and China. Clive Hamilton, *Silent*

Invasion: China's Influence in Australia, (London: Hardie Grant Books, 2018) has been one of the few scholarly works which has reflected on the investigative reporting which revealed the Chinese influence in Australian politics and institutions; and the connections between Chinese Australians and Chinese intelligence agencies. Importantly, this book sparked controversy in Australia as the government assessed its policies towards China to protect its sovereignty and democracy.

2 The 'early stage modelling' amidst the COVID-19 has been a method to allow the government authorities to gain an understanding of the likely effectiveness of treatment alternatives under different circumstances. In terms of Australia, the utilization of the early stage modelling has enabled the Morrison government to take early measures to fight against the disease. See Sophie Scott, "Coronavirus data modelling has Australia in good position, but COVID-19 'here to stay'." *ABC News*, April 07, 2020, at https://www.abc.net.au/news/2020-04-07/coronavirus-government-COVID19-modelling-experts-on-response/12128950

3 "Update on Novel Coronavirus: Joint media release with Professor Brendan Murphy, Chief Medical Officer, about Novel Coronavirus", *Department of Health, Government of Australia*, January 31, 2020, at https://www.health.gov.au/ministers/the-hon-greg-hunt-mp/media/update-on-novel-coronavirus

4 "Australian Health Sector Emergency Response Plan for Novel Coronavirus (COVID-19)", *Department of Health, Government of Australia*, March 2020, https://www.health.gov.au/sites/default/files/documents/2020/03/australian-health-sector-emergency-response-plan-for-novel-coronavirus-COVID-19-short-form-the-australian-health-sector-emergency-response-plan-for-novel-coronavirus-short-form.pdf

5 Ibid.

6 Ibid.

7 Paige Cockburn, "How community transmission is very different to locally acquired coronavirus", *ABC News*, June 27, 2020, at https://www.abc.net.au/news/health/2020-06-28/what-exactly-is-community-transmission-and-how-is-it-curbed/12397296

8 Sophie Scott no. 2

9 Ibid.

10 "Coronavirus Australia: Melbourne in six-week lockdown after Victoria records 191 new cases", *The Guardian*, July 07, 2020, at https://www.theguardian.com/australia-news/2020/jul/07/coronavirus-victoria-update-191-new-COVID-19-cases-as-community-transmission-soars

11 Matthew Sussex, "Public messaging, trust and Covid-19: some pointers for policymakers", *Asia & The Pacific Policy Society*, March 25, 2020, https://www.policyforum.net/public-messages-COVID-19/

12 Katherine Murphy, "guardian Essential Poll: one-third ay there has been an overreaction to coronavirus", *The Guardian*, March 23, 2020, https://www.theguardian.com/australia-news/2020/mar/24/guardian-essential-poll-one-third-say-there-has-been-an-overreaction-to-coronavirus

13 Melissa Davey, "Thousands of Australian doctors call on government to ramp up coronavirus response", *The Guardian*, March 17, 2020, https://www.theguardian.com/world/2020/mar/17/thousands-of-australian-doctors-call-on-government-to-ramp-up-coronavirus-response; Mike Head, "Australian Doctors Condemn Government Response to Covid-19 'disaster,'" *World Socialist Website*, March 19, 2020 https://www.wsws.org/en/articles/2020/03/19/doct-m19.html

14 David Brophy, "Australia's China Debate in 2018", *Power*, Jane Golley, Linda Jaivin, Paul J. Farrelly and Sharon Strange (eds), (Australian National University Press: 2018), pp. 155-158

15 Ibid.

16 "Chinese defector wins permanent residency", *The Sydney Morning Herald*, July 09, 2005, at https://www.smh.com.au/national/chinese-defector-wins-permanent-residency-20050709-gdlnno.html

17 Peter Hartcher, "Insidious: Former ASIO boss warns on Chinese interference in Australia", *The Sydney Morning Herald*, November 22, 2019, https://www.smh.com.au/politics/federal/insidious-former-asio-boss-warns-on-chinese-interference-in-australia-20191121-p53cv2.html

18 Since the Third Plenary Session of the Eleventh Central Committee of the Chinese Communist Party in 1978, China under the leadership of Deng Xiaoping delved into a new strategic path concentrating on economic development. This approach to development emphasized on a more prosperous life for its people driven by capital, technology, and resources acquired through peaceful means instead of invasion, expansion or colonization. In other words, China established a new strategic path to development which suit its national conditions while deterring to move away from its movements of the past. This approach first debuted in the global arena in 2003 at the Boao Forum where Zheng Bijian delivered a speech titled "The new road of China's peaceful rise and the future of Asia". In this speech, Zheng highlighted China's desire to rise but not by seeking hegemony. This approach would also ensure that China avoids confrontation with major powers. See Zheng Bijian, "China's Peaceful Rise to Great-Power Status", *Foreign Affairs*, 84(5), September-October 2005, pp. 18-24; Yi Xiaoxiong, "Chinese Foreign Policy in Transition: Understanding China's 'Peaceful Development", *Journal of East Asian Affairs*, 19(1), Spring/Summer, 2005, pp. 74-112. However, debates soon started ensuing with people assessing its implications of the approach of 'peaceful rise' in regard to China's relations with other countries. At the same time, people were questioning the possibility of the motto not allowing China to behave aggressively if the need arose. Nevertheless, since 2012, China's assertive actions in the South China Sea (SCS) through militarization of the islands, in East China Sea (ECS), Taiwan Straits, and with the recent India-China border conflicts, it can be argued that China's foreign policy approach has shifted from a peaceful rise to a more aggressive and assertive rise. Please see, Christopher Primiano, "The end of China's term limits and its 'Peaceful Rise'?" *The Asia Dialogue*, April 26, 2018, at https://theasiadialogue.com/2018/04/26/the-end-of-chinas-term-limits-potential-implications-for-its-peaceful-rise/; Bonnie S. Glaser and Evan S. Medeiros, "The Changing Ecology of Foreign Policy-Making in China: The Ascension and Demise of the Theory of 'Peaceful Rise", *The China Quarterly*, June 2007(190), pp. 291-310.

19 Ton Fowdy, "Australia at a crossroads in its relationship with China", *China Daily*, April 30, 2020, at https://www.chinadaily.com.cn/a/202004/30/WS5eaa7a39a310a8b241152fa8.html; Paul Karp, "China bristles at Australia's call for investigation into Coronavirus origin", *The Guardian*, April 29, 2020, at https://www.theguardian.com/world/2020/apr/29/australia-defends-plan-to-investigate-china-over-COVID-19-outbreak-as-row-deepens

20 Brett Worthington, "Marise Payne calls for global inquiry into China's handling of the Coronavirus outbreak", ABC News, April 19, 2020, at https://www.abc.net.au/news/2020-04-19/payne-calls-for-inquiry-china-handling-of-coronavirus-COVID-19/12162968; "Coronavirus: Australia can lead the way for a global response", *Minister for Foreign Affairs, Minister for Women*, April 22, 2020, at https://www.foreignminister.gov.au/minister/marise-payne/news/coronavirus-australia-can-lead-way-global-response

21 "Foreign Ministry Spokesperson Geng Shuang's Regular Press Conference on April 20, 2020", *Ministry of Foreign Affairs of the People's Republic of China*, April 20, 2020, at https://www.fmprc.gov.cn/mfa_eng/xwfw_665399/s2510_665401/t1771576.shtml

22 Lily Kuo, "Australia called 'gum stuck to China's shoe' by state media in coronavirus investigation stoush", *The Guardian*, April 28, 2020, at https://www.theguardian.com/world/2020/apr/28/australia-called-gum-stuck-to-chinas-shoe-by-state-media-in-coronavirus-investigation-stoush

23 "Chinese Embassy's Spokesperson Responding to a Question by Global Times on Mr. Dutton's

Remarks", *Embassy of the People's Republic of China in the Commonwealth of Australia*, April 21, 2020, at http://au.china-embassy.org/eng/sghdxwfb_1/t1771892.htm

24 "Transcript of Chinese Ambassador Cheng Jingye's interview with Australian Financial Review political correspondant Andrew Tillet", *Embassy of the People's Republic of China in the Commonwealth of Australia*, April 27, 2020, at http://au.china-embassy.org/eng/gdtp_16/t1773741.htm

25 Ibid.

26 The recent 'Wolf Warrior diplomacy' has been a new foreign policy approach of the Xi Jinping administration which reflects a shift from an implicit, and a low-key profile to an assertive, proactive, and high-profile diplomatic response tone from China. Owing its name to the two Chinese blockbusters, *Wolf Warrior* and *Wolf Warrior II* reflecting China's special operation forces, the Wolf Warrior diplomacy has been China's diplomatic style towards countries such as the US and Australia to defend Beijing's national interests in a confrontational way. Please read, Zhu Zhiqun, "Interpreting China's 'Wolf-Warrior Diplomacy", *The Diplomat*, May 15, 2020, at https://thediplomat.com/2020/05/interpreting-chinas-wolf-warrior-diplomacy/

27 Daniel Hurst, "Australia making its presence felt at WHO while backing calls for major reform", *The Guardian,* May 16, 2020, at https://www.theguardian.com/world/2020/may/16/australia-making-its-presence-felt-at-who-while-backing-calls-for-major-reform

28 Brittany Chain, "How Australia partly funded two Chinese scientists from the Wuhan lab linked to the COVID-19 outbreak to study bat viruses at a CSIRO lab", *Daily Mail Online*, April 28, 2020, at https://www.dailymail.co.uk/news/article-8261201/Australia-funded-Chinese-scientists-research-bats.html

29 Angelica Snowden, "Coronavirus: Trade Minister Simon Birmingham denies knowledge of investigations into Wuhan scientists who worked in Australia", *The Australian*, April 28, 2020, at https://www.theaustralian.com.au/world/coronavirus-wuhan-scientists-worked-in-australia/news-story/e18ba52f59a9d32479bf12c5dfa5733b

30 Julian Borger, "Mike Pompeo: 'enormous evidence' coronavirus came from Chinese lab", *The Guardian*, May 03, 2020, at https://www.theguardian.com/world/2020/may/03/mike-pompeo-donald-trump-coronavirus-chinese-laboratory; "The Wuhan Lab Theory", Wall Street Journal, May 06, 2020, at https://www.wsj.com/articles/the-wuhan-lab-theory-11588806940

31 Chen Qingqing and Liu Xin, "Australia gets 'slap to the face' as global community welcomes China-sponsored resolution on COVID-19", *Global Times*, May 19, 2020, at https://www.globaltimes.cn/content/1188817.shtml

32 "China suspends beef imports from four Australian firms", *Xinhua*, May 12, 2020, at http://www.xinhuanet.com/english/2020-05/12/c_139051057.htm

33 Chu Daye and Wang Bozun, "China imposes punitive duties on Aussie barley, more products could be probed", *Global Times*, May 19, 2020, at https://www.globaltimes.cn/content/1188857.shtml

34 Ibid.

35 Ibid.

36 "Australian wine shipments held up at Chinese ports amid political tensions: report", *The Sydney Morning Herald*, June 15, 2018, at https://www.smh.com.au/business/the-economy/australian-wine-shipments-held-up-at-chinese-ports-amid-political-tensions-report-20180615-p4zloj.html

37 Gareth Hutchens, "Australia concerned over China's 'aggressive tactics' in South China Sea", *The Guardian*, October 03, 2018, at https://www.theguardian.com/world/2018/oct/03/australia-concerned-over-chinas-aggressive-tactics-in-south-china-sea

38 Christopher Knaus, "Australia is a 'giant baby', banned billionaire Huang Xiangmo says", *The Guardian*, February 12, 2019, at https://www.theguardian.com/australia-news/2019/feb/12/australia-is-a-giant-baby-banned-billionaire-huang-xiangmo-says

39 Michelle Grattan, "State actor makes cyber-attack on Australian political parties", *The Conversation*, February 18, 2019, at https://theconversation.com/state-actor-makes-cyber-attack-on-australian-political-parties-111993

40 Katherine Murphy, "Australia enters first recession in 29 years after blow from bushfires and Coronavirus", *The Guardian*, June 03, 2020, at https://www.theguardian.com/business/2020/jun/03/australia-enters-first-recession-in-29-years-after-blow-from-bushfires-and-coronavirus

41 Tony McDonald and Steve Morling, "The Australian economy and the global downturn Part 1: Reasons for resilience", *Economic Roundup Issue 2, 2011, Treasury, Government of Australia*, April 02, 2020, at https://treasury.gov.au/publication/economic-roundup-issue-2-2011/economic-roundup-issue-2-2011/the-australian-economy-and-the-global-downturn-part-1-reasons-for-resilience

42 Michael Smith, "Australian beef exports threatened as Chinese buyers look to US", *Financial Review*, June 21, 2020, at https://www.afr.com/world/asia/australian-beef-exports-threatened-as-chinese-buyers-look-to-us-20200619-p554bn; Ashley Townshend, "China's Pandemic-Fueled Standoff with Australia", *War on the Rocks*, May 20, 2020, at https://warontherocks.com/2020/05/chinas-pandemic-fueled-standoff-with-australia/

43 "China to levy 80.5percent in tariffs on Australian barley", *CGTN*, May 18, 2020, at https://news.cgtn.com/news/2020-05-18/China-to-levy-80-5-in-tariffs-on-Australian-barley-QBiL2GzQ5O/index.html

44 Tan Su-Lin, "China's restrictions on Australian beef, barley seen as retaliation for support of coronavirus investigation", *South China Morning Post*, May 12, 2020, at https://www.scmp.com/economy/global-economy/article/3084062/chinas-restrictions-australian-beef-barley-seen-retaliation

45 The Phase One Deal between the US and China was signed on January 15, 2020 after approximately two years of trade war, marking a potential truce between both the countries. This deal obligated the cancellation of new tariffs on China and reduction of the existing ones on behalf of the US if Beijing commits to increase purchases from the US and adopts global trade norms. However, the schisms between both the countries have continued even after the deal, and instead have enhanced amidst the COVID-19 pandemic. Please read, "What's Inside the US-China Phase One Deal?", *Center for Strategic & International Studies(CSIS)*, January 15, 2020, at https://www.csis.org/analysis/whats-inside-us-china-phase-one-deal

46 Michael Smith, "China steps up warnings, buys US barley, Russian beef", *Financial Review*, May 15, 2020, at htatps://www.afr.com/world/asia/china-steps-up-warnings-buys-us-barley-russian-beef-20200515-p54tag

47 "Chinese demand drives record Australian trade surplus in March", *Xinhua*, May 07, 2020, at http://www.xinhuanet.com/english/2020-05/07/c_139037978.htm; David Uren, "Australia's booming trade with China will shape strategic policy", *The Strategist*, September 03, 2019, at https://www.aspistrategist.org.au/australias-booming-trade-with-china-will-shape-strategic-policy/

48 "MOE issues first warning statement in 2020 for students preparing to study abroad", *Ministry of Education, The People's Republic of China*, June 10, 2020, at http://en.moe.gov.cn/news/press_releases/202006/t20200619_467021.html

49 Ibid.

50 "China's warning against travel to Australia based on adequate facts: FM", *People's Daily*, June 09, 2020, at http://en.people.cn/n3/2020/0609/c90000-9698861.html

51 "Expectations and Experiences of Chinese University Students in Australia- With Fran Martin", *Australia-China Relations Institute*, May 03, 2018, at https://www.australiachinarelations.org/content/expectations-and-experiences-chinese-university-students-australia-fran-martin-0; Andrew Markus,

"Racism and international students in Australia", *Monash University*, at http://books.publishing.monash.edu/apps/bookworm/view/A+Home+Away+from+Homepercent3F+International+Students+in+Australian+and+South+African+Higher+Education/175/OEBPS/c06.htm

52 Weizhen Tan, "Australian official urges international students to consider studying in the country as China claims racism", *CNBC*, June 12, 2020, at https://www.cnbc.com/2020/06/12/australia-tensions-with-china-amid-racism-warning-to-students.html

53 Zhang Han, Liu Caiyu and Xu Keyue, "Evidence of Aussie racism mounts", *Global Times*, June 10, 2020, at https://www.globaltimes.cn/content/1191204.shtml; Zhang Han, "China's travel warning a result of Australian animosity, rocky bilateral ties", *Global Times*, June 07, 2020, at https://www.globaltimes.cn/content/1190827.shtml

54 Adam Carey, Fergus Hunter and Matt Bungard, "Chinese students see political motive in Beijing's call to stay away", *The Sydney Morning Herald*, June 11, 2020, at https://www.smh.com.au/national/chinese-students-see-political-motive-in-beijing-s-call-to-stay-away-20200611-p551rk.html; Bang Xiao and Samuel Yang, "Chinese international students defend Australia as a 'safe' educational destinational", *ABC News*, June 10, 2020, at https://www.abc.net.au/news/2020-06-10/chinese-international-students-defend-australia/12340820

55 Agence France-Presse, "China funding white elephant infrastructure projects in the Pacific, says Australian minister", *South China Morning Post*, January 10, 2018, at https://www.scmp.com/news/china/diplomacy-defence/article/2127626/china-funding-white-elephant-infrastructure-projects

56 Ibid.

57 "Tourism loss may be just tip of iceberg in China-Australia row", *Global Times*, June 07, 2020, at https://www.globaltimes.cn/content/1190849.shtml

58 Cheng Mingming, "We depend on Chinese travellers, so how will coronavirus travel bans impact our economy?", *SBS News*, February 12, 2020, at https://www.sbs.com.au/news/we-depend-on-chinese-travellers-so-how-will-coronavirus-travel-bans-impact-our-economy

59 Rory Medcalf, "*Contest for the Indo-Pacific: Why China Won't Map the Future*", (Carlton, Victoria: La Trobe University Press, 2020), p. 212

60 Chan Lai-Han, "Can Australia Flatten the Curve of its Economic Dependency on China?" T*he Diplomat*, May 22, 2020, at https://thediplomat.com/2020/05/can-australia-flatten-the-curve-of-its-economic-dependence-on-china/

61 "Lease of the Port of Darwin to the Landbridge Group", *Parliament of Australia*, at https://www.aph.gov.au/Parliamentary_Business/Committees/Senate/Economics/Foreign_Investment_Review/Interimpercent20Report/c02

62 Christopher Walsh, "How and why did the Northern Territory lease the Darwin Port to China, and at what risk?", *ABC News*, March 12, 2019, at https://www.abc.net.au/news/2019-03-12/why-did-northern-territory-sell-darwin-port-to-china-what-risk/10755720; Michael Forsythe, "Australia Defends Port's Lease to Chinese Company with Military Ties", *The New York Times*, November 13, 2015, at https://www.nytimes.com/2015/11/14/world/australia/darwin-port-australia-chinese-military.html

63 Post the Darwin deal which led to a change of rule demanding the jurisdiction of the Foreign Investment Review Board to extend the sale of strategic assets to state governments, the first incident of sale of a land holding in Australia to a foreign company came when the then Treasurer Scott Morrison blocked the sale of S. Kidman holdings to a Chinese consortium led by Hunan Dakang Pasture Farming and Shanghai CRED Real Estate Co. The sheer size of the holdings (100,000 sq. km) had demanded for a scrutiny of the deal, which finally then was acquired by the Australian billionaire Gina Reinhart with minority Chinese investments. Please see, Jamie Smyth, "Australia to

block vast land scale to China-led consortium", *Financial Times*, April 29, 2016, at https://www.ft.com/content/d4a5c5fa-0dc5-11e6-9cd4-2be898308be3. Similarly, during a sale of a New South Wales (NSW) electricity distribution company in Ausgrid to the Chinese State Grid for AU$ 1 billion, the treasury under Scott Morrison had to intervene and veto it. Viewing from the national security point of view, Ausgrid used to operate secure fibre cables to the NSW police headquarters. The deal thus, was finally vetoed on the account of being "contrary to national Security", while a new Critical Infrastructure Centre was set up to assess such investments in future. Please see, Peter Hartcher, "Revealed: Why the sale of Ausgrid to Chinese buyers was vetoed", *The Sydney Morning Herald*, May 28, 2018, at https://www.smh.com.au/opinion/revealed-why-the-sale-of-ausgrid-to-chinese-buyers-was-vetoed-20180528-p4zhxh.html

64 For more arguments, please read, Clive Hamilton, *Silent Invasion: China's Influence in Australia*, (London: Hardie Grant, 2018), pp. 137-258

65 Tan Su-Lin, "Banned billionaire Huang Xiangmo to Liberal and Labor: I want my money back", *Financial Review*, February 08, 2019, at https://www.afr.com/politics/banned-billionaire-huang-xiangmo-to-liberal-and-labor-i-want-my-money-back-20190208-h1b0e0

66 Matthew Knott and Heath Aston, "Don't become 'propaganda vehicles' for China: universities warned over donations", *The Sydney Morning Herald*, September 08, 2016, at https://www.smh.com.au/politics/federal/dont-become-propaganda-vehicles-for-china-universities-warned-over-donations-20160908-grc1as.html

67 Grant Wyeth, "Why did Australia Push Out a Chinese Communist Party-Linked Billionaire?", *The Diplomat*, February 09, 2019, at https://thediplomat.com/2019/02/why-did-australia-push-out-a-chinese-communist-party-linked-billionaire/

68 "Sam Dastyari defended China's policy in South China Sea in defiance of Labor policy, secret recording reveals", *ABC News*, November 29, 2017, at https://www.abc.net.au/news/2017-11-29/sam-dastyari-secret-south-china-sea-recordings/9198044?nw=0

69 Ibid.

70 Louise Yaxley, "Election 2016: Federal Labor would green-light South China Sea military exercise: Conroy", *ABC News*, June 16, 2016, at https://www.abc.net.au/news/2016-06-16/labor-would-approve-south-china-sea-military-exercise/7518330?nw=0

71 "South China Sea: Australia raises alarm over possible Chinese military build-up on contested Spartley Islands", *ABC News*, June 1, 2015, at https://www.abc.net.au/news/2015-06-01/australia-takes-tough-stance-against-chinas-island-moves/6510540?nw=0

72 Katherine Murphy, "Sam Dastyari told to resign from Senate positions after China revelation", *The Guardian*, November 29, 2017, at https://www.theguardian.com/australia-news/2017/nov/30/sam-dastyari-told-to-resign-from-senate-positions-after-china-revelation

73 Jamelle Wells and Nick Dole, "Chinese billionaire Huang Xiangmo gave $100,000 to NSW Labor official, ICAC hears", *ABC News*, August 26, 2019, at https://www.abc.net.au/news/2019-08-26/icac-hears-huang-xiangmo-gave-100k-to-nsw-labor-official/11447622; Dan Conifer and Stephanie Borys, "Australia denies citizenship to Chinese political donor Huang Xiangmo and strips his permanent residency", *ABC News*, February 06, 2019, at https://www.abc.net.au/news/2019-02-06/australia-denies-citizenship-chinese-businessman-huang-xiangmo/10784512

74 Kelsey Munro, "China cabinet: Huang Xiangmo's visa strife, and outlook downbeats", *The Interpreter*, February 07, 2019, at https://www.lowyinstitute.org/the-interpreter/huang-xiangmo-visa-strife-and-outlook-downbeats

75 Chris Uhlmann, "Australian businesses with close ties with China donated $5.5 to political parties, investigation shows", *ABC News*, August 22, 2016, at https://www.abc.net.au/news/2016-08-21/

australian-groups-strong-ties-china-political-donations/7768012; Nick McKenzie and Chris Uhlmann, "A man of many dimensions: the big Chinese donor now in Canberra's sights", *The Sydney Morning Herald*, February 06, 2019, at https://www.smh.com.au/politics/federal/a-man-of-many-dimensions-the-big-chinese-donor-now-in-canberra-s-sights-20190206-p50vzt.html

76 Chris Uhlmann, "Domestic spy chief sounded alarm about donor links with China last year", *ABC News*, September 01, 2016, at https://www.abc.net.au/news/2016-09-01/asio-chief-sounded-alarm-about-donor-links-with-china-last-year/7804856

77 Navdeep Suri, "Australia-China relations: The Great Unravelling", *ORF Issue Brief*, No. 366, June 02, 2020, at https://www.orfonline.org/research/australia-china-relations-the-great-unravelling-67204/#_edn38; Josh Horwitz, "Australian professors and universities are being shamed into apologizing for offending Chinese students", *Quartz*, August 29, 2017, at https://qz.com/1064435/australian-professors-and-universities-are-being-shamed-into-apologizing-for-offending-chinese-students/

78 "National Security Legislation Amendment (Espionage and Foreign Interference) Bill 2017", *Parliament of Australia*, June 28, 2018, at https://www.aph.gov.au/Parliamentary_Business/Bills_Legislation/bd/bd1718a/18bd134#:~:text=Thepercent20Billpercent20waspercent20introducedpercent20into,Australia'spercent20politicalpercent20andpercent20electoralpercent20systems.

79 The University Foreign Interference Taskforce- Guidelines to counter foreign interference in the Australian University sector", *Department of Education, Skills and Employment*, Australian Government, August 28, 2019, at https://www.education.gov.au/ufit; "Framework for the development of principles-based guidelines to counter foreign interference in the Australian university sector", *Government of Australia*, at https://docs.education.gov.au/system/files/doc/other/uni_sector_cfi_framework_final_unclassified.pdf

80 Amy Searight, "Countering China's Influence Operations: Lessons from Australia", *Center for Strategic and International Studies (CSIS)*, May 08, 2020, at https://www.csis.org/analysis/countering-chinas-influence-operations-lessons-australia

81 Han Feng, "Can China-Australia ties override strains?", *Global Times*, July 02, 2018, at http://www.globaltimes.cn/content/1109169.shtml

82 Michael Slezak and Ariel Bogle, "Huawei banned from 5G infrastructure rollout in Australia", *ABC News*, August 23, 2018, at https://www.abc.net.au/news/2018-08-23/huawei-banned-from-providing-5g-mobile-technology-australia/10155438

83 "Joint Media Release: Government Provides 5G Security Guidance to Australian carriers", *Government of Australia*, August 23, 2018, at https://www.minister.communications.gov.au/minister/mitch-fifield/news/government-provides-5g-security-guidance-australian-carriers

84 Tim Biggs and Jennifer Duke, "China's Huawei, ZTE banned from 5G network", *The Sydney Morning Herald*, August 23, 2018, at mitch-fifield/news/government-provides-5g-security-guidance-australian-carriers

85 "National Intelligence Law of the People's Republic of China_中国人大网", *The National People's Congress of the People's Republic of China*, June 27, 2017, at https://cs.brown.edu/courses/csci1800/sources/2017_PRC_NationalIntelligenceLaw.pdf

86 Jagannath P. Panda, "India must stay alert to Beijing's techno-national gambit", *Sunday Guardian*, may 23, 2020, at https://www.sundayguardianlive.com/news/india-must-stay-alert-beijings-techno-national-gambit

87 "Australia, Huawei and 5G ", *IISS Strategic Comments*, 25(28), October 2019, at https://www.iiss.org/-/publication/0063b52b-5ae5-4705-81bd-a8e8e305fb48/australia-huawei-and-5g.pdf

88 Ibid.

89 Fergus Hunter, "Huawei ban a 'thorny issue' hurting China-Australia relations, says ambassador", *The Sydney Morning Herald*, February 17, 2020, at https://www.smh.com.au/politics/federal/huawei-ban-a-thorny-issue-hurting-china-australia-relations-says-ambassador-20200217-p541ic.html

90 "China warns Australia at WTO about 5G restrictions", *Reuters*, April 12, 2019, at https://www.reuters.com/article/us-huawei-australia-china-wto/china-warns-australia-at-wto-about-5g-restriction-idUSKCN1RO20H

91 Li Qingqing, "Australia to pay for 5G restrictions on Huawei", *Global Times*, April 15, 2019, at https://www.globaltimes.cn/content/1146018.shtml

92 Kalinga Seneviratne, "China's squeeze on Australian coal nothing to do with Huawei's 5G ban. Really?", *South China Morning Post*, March 05, 2019, at https://www.scmp.com/week-asia/geopolitics/article/2188701/chinas-squeeze-australian-coal-nothing-do-huaweis-5g-ban; Jason Scott and Dan Murtaugh, "China Restricts Australian Coal Imports in Likely Retaliation to Huawei 5G Ban", *Fortune*, February 21, 2019, at https://fortune.com/2019/02/21/china-australia-coal-imports/

93 Paul Karp, "Australia 'deeply concerned' about China's treatment of Uighur people", *The Guardian*, July 15, 2019, at https://www.theguardian.com/world/2019/jul/15/australia-deeply-concerned-about-chinas-treatment-of-uighur-people; Rob Harris, "Australia among 23 nations to condemn China on human rights at the UN", *The Sydney Morning Herald*, October 30, 2019, at https://www.smh.com.au/politics/federal/australia-among-23-nations-to-condemn-china-on-human-rights-at-the-un-20191030-p535wx.html

94 Max Walden, "Australia joins UK, Japan in expressing concern over China's treatment of Uyghurs, Hong Kong", *ABC News*, July 01, 2020, at https://www.abc.net.au/news/2020-07-01/australia-statement-condemn-china-over-hong-kong-uyghur-abuses/12409268

95 Matt Coughlan and Daniel McCulloch, "China warns Australia over Hong Kong visas", *Canberra Times*, July 03, 2020, at https://www.canberratimes.com.au/story/6817420/china-warns-australia-over-hong-kong-visas/?cs=14231#gsc.tab=0

96 "Mutual trust between Australia and China at all-time low", *Global Times*, June 25, 2020, at https://www.globaltimes.cn/content/1192669.shtml

97 Tim Blair, "Via Local Commie Underlings, Beijing Officially Disapproves", *Daily Telegraph*, April 04, 2020, at https://www.dailytelegraph.com.au/blogs/tim-blair/via-local-commie-underlings-beijing-officially-disapproves/news-story/491b415795fbbdc526d33d5b569134a4

98 "Statement from the Spokesperson of the Chinese Consulate General in Sydney", *Consulate General of the People's Republic of China in Sydney*, April 15, 2020, at http://sydney.chineseconsulate.org/eng/xwdt/t1769912.htm

99 Natasha Kassam, "Lowy Institute Poll 2020", *Lowy Institute*, June 24, 2020, at https://poll.lowyinstitute.org/report/

100 *Global Times*, no. 96

101 V Wood, "Time for a whole-of-government China strategy to build trust with China", *Ministry of Defence, Government of Australia*, 2016, at https://www.defence.gov.au/ADC/Publications/IndoPac/Wood_IPSP_Building_trust_with_China.pdf; "Chinese premier calls for China-Australia ties to normal back", *Xinhua*, November 04, 2019, at http://www.xinhuanet.com/english/2019-11/04/c_138525878.htm

102 Jagannath P. Panda, "Five Reasons Why Xi's 'Peking Model' Will Struggle Post-Covid-19", *PacNet*, April 07, 2020, at https://pacforum.org/wp-content/uploads/2020/04/20200407_PacNet_19-1.pdf

103 Bao Huaying, "China's Daunting Post-COVID Challenges", *The Diplomat*, May 08, 2020, at https://thediplomat.com/2020/05/chinas-daunting-post-COVID-challenges/; Ananth Krishnan, "Analysis: For China's Xi, the coronavirus challenge comes laden with economic costs and political risks", *The*

Hindu, February 05, 2020, at https://www.thehindu.com/news/international/analysis-for-chinas-xi-biggest-challenge-yet-comes-laden-with-risks/article30742980.ece

104 M. Taylor Fravel, "Has Covid-19 Changed How China's Leaders Approach National Security?" *A ChinaFile Conversation*, June 03, 2020, at https://www.chinafile.com/conversation/has-COVID-19-changed-how-chinas-leaders-approach-national-security

105 Jason Scott, "Australia's Leader backs Revived Quad as Counter to China", *Bloomsberg*, October 03, 2019, at https://www.bloomberg.com/news/articles/2019-10-03/australia-s-leader-backs-revived-quad-as-counter-to-china

106 Stephen Kuper, "Australia joins Blue Dot Network in attempt to counter Beijing's Belt and Road", *Defence Connect*, November 13, 2019, at https://www.defenceconnect.com.au/key-enablers/5137-australia-joins-blue-dot-network-in-attempt-to-counter-beijing-s-belt-and-road

107 The Pacific Step-up was introduced as one of the prime foreign policy priorities and fundamental importance to Australia in the Pacific Island Forum Leader' Meeting in September 2016. The initiative was undertaken with the goal of bolstering economic, political and cultural development in the pacific island community and enhance Australia's regional and global stature. This initiative further emphasised on in Australia's Foreign Policy White Paper of 2017 Defence White Paper of 2016, as an effort for Canberra to further engage in the region. Please see, "Stepping-up Australia's engagement with our Pacific family", *Department of Foreign Affairs and Trade*, Government of Australia, September 2019, at https://www.dfat.gov.au/sites/default/files/stepping-up-australias-engagement-with-our-pacific-family.pdf.

108 Paul Karp, "Australian trade minister says 'risk' of trade with China may drive businesses to other markets", *The Guardian*, May 17, 2020, at https://www.theguardian.com/australia-news/2020/may/17/australian-trade-minister-says-risk-of-trade-with-china-may-drive-businesses-to-other-markets

109 Ibid.

110 Euan Black, "Peak Stupidity: alls to diversify Australian exports criticised", *The New Daily*, May 17, 2020, at https://thenewdaily.com.au/finance/finance-news/2020/05/17/china-barley-exports-diversification/; "Coronavirus: Cutting reliance on China to hit jobs", *The Australian*, June 03, 2020, at https://www.theaustralian.com.au/nation/politics/coronavirus-cutting-reliance-on-china-to-hit-jobs/news-story/487fae74afc4cebd9333ffacbf18aed3

111 "Tensions run high, but all-out China-Aussie confrontation low", *Global Times*, July 08, 2020, at https://www.globaltimes.cn/content/1193933.shtml

112 Shiro Armstrong, "Don't decouple, better manage risks of China trade", *Financial Review*, March 15, 2020, at https://www.afr.com/policy/economy/don-t-decouple-better-manage-the-risks-of-china-trade-20200315-p54a6f

113 Rory Medcalf, "China's economic leverage: perception and reality", *Policy Options Paper,* No. 2, March 2017, National Security College, Australian National University, at https://nsc.crawford.anu.edu.au/sites/default/files/publication/nsc_crawford_anu_edu_au/2017-05/policy_papers.pdf; Rory Medcalf, "*Contest for the Indo-Pacific: Why China Won't Map the Future*", (Carlton, Victoria: La Trobe University Press, 2020), pp. 212-213

114 Ibid.

17

COVID-19 and Latin America

Shaheli Das

The COVID-19 pandemic is one of the worst crisis in human history. Its severity can be deciphered from its expansion across the globe as well as the death toll caused by it. Beijing, besides being the origin of the virus, is also the worst affected nation so far. Not to mention the country has also utilised this crisis in its favour to make deeper inroads into the so-called United States' (US) "backyard" and strengthen its ground there. In this context, this chapter explores the following topics and questions: the various schools of thought prevalent in China with regard to its foreign policy and the perspective which best define China's outreach to Latin America. The questions addressed in this chapter are as follows, what is at stake for China in Latin America?, what is the impact of COVID-19 on Latin America?, what kind of aid and assistance China has offered to the Latin American countries (LACs), and finally are the LACs blaming China for the spread of the virus and its containment strategies?

China's Foreign Policy: The Various Schools of Thought

The People's Republic of China (PRC) has re-emerged at the global stage from being a relatively poor nation to the second largest economy of the world today. Over time the country's foreign policy aspirations have multiplied and the government has widened the purview of its activities, both regionally as well as internationally. At present, the PRC is amidst the process of regulating its foreign policy preferences and charting a new path in international affairs, renouncing its traditional policy of relative restraint (Merics) and engaging into what may be referred to as proactive diplomacy. It is as part of such a new foreign policy stance that the country has made deep inroads into Latin America in the twenty first century.

David Shambaugh in his book *China Goes Global: The Partial Power* has discussed in detail about the various schools of thought within China that have offered their analysis on what the PRC's identity as well as position as a major power should be. They include the Nativists, the Realists, Major Powers, Asia First, Global South, Selective Multilateralists and the Globalists. In this section a detailed discussion on the perspectives of these schools of thought has been made.

The **Nativists** comprise of the populists, Marxists and the nationalists. They are sceptical of the external world, and perceive global multilateral engagement as "traps" (set by the West) to enmesh and mire the PRC in expensive commitments abroad. They are boisterous opponents of the West; with certain analysts in this group possessing a formidable traditional Marxist inclination. In domestic policy arguments, the followers of this group act as twins of the "New Left" and uphold that the "reform and opening" strategy of the last three decades has cost the country its socialist veracity, impaired the country's culture with undesirable foreign influences, and has imperilled the country's sovereignty and independence in international affairs.

The **Realists** are firm nationalists, but of a less fanatical and more pragmatic variety. They could also be identified as rigid "China Firsters", who do not ascribe much importance to the concerns of the other nations or constituencies in international matters. This is a predominant school in Chinese IR discourse at present.

The PRC's realists view the nation-state as the core unit of study. They endorse the value of state sovereignty above everything else, dismissing discussions that transnational problems infiltrate across borders. They view the global environment as uncertain and anarchic. They are largely pessimistic of the PRC's external surroundings, especially of the US. They perceive an intrinsic competitive – even antagonistic – force at work in Sino-US relations.

The realists may be divided into "hard" and "soft" realists, and the offensive" and "defensive" realists. The hard-power realists contend for bolstering the comprehensive national power (综合国力), but more specifically the military and the economic components. On the other hand, the soft power realists underscore the diplomacy along with cultural (soft) power. The offensive realists put forth that the PRC must utilise its freshly developed military capability, diplomatic influence and most importantly the country's economic strength.

The **Major Powers School** contends that the PRC must focus its diplomacy on administering its ties with the major powers and blocs of the world, namely the

US, Russia and possibly the European Union, while not paying much consideration to the emerging economies or to multilateralism. The principal catchphrases of this group are *daguo shi shouyao* (major powers are of chief importance).

These analysts argue and emphasize that if the PRC's relations with other major powers is hinged then it would be detrimental to a number of interests of the PRC and would consequently impede Beijing's other regional ties. A chief reason for the major power inclination is called for by the PRC's modernization drive: the Western nations are a chief source of advanced technology together with capital and investment.

The **Asia First school** of thought calls for greater focus of China's diplomacy on its immediate periphery as well as the Asian neighbourhood. They contend that if the country's neighbourhood is unstable, then it would be a chief barrier to China's growth as well as national security. Since China is strategically positioned in Asia, bordering as many as fourteen nations by land and several others by sea, therefore the analysts of this school claim that it is difficult to undervalue the significance of the Asian neighbourhood for the PRC.

An important subgroup of this school of thought are the proponents who support "multilateral regionalism" as well as East Asian community building, as discrete from a more state-based approach. This school of thought does not underscore the PRC's relations within Asia at the cost of exclusion of the country's ties with other nations and regions; instead they appeal for Asia to be given weightage relative to the major powers or the PRC's ties with the developing nations. However, the Asia Firsters do consider in offering Asia relatively greater weightage over Beijing's ties with the developing world or the major powers.

Another school of thought are the **Selective Multilateralists** who consider that the PRC must bolster its international engagements over time, but only on those matters in which the country's national security interests are precisely involved. They view contributions to global governance as a *tactic*, rather than a *philosophy*. Interestingly, the Selective Multilateralists are not inclined towards multilateralism per se. Rather than working in institutions, they are in favour of engaging closely within small adhoc group of countries. The Sextet on Iran (USA, China, Russia, UK, France, Germany) and the Six Party Talks on North Korea (USA, China, Japan, North Korea, Russia, South Korea) are key illustrations to this end.

The **Globalists** are of the opinion that the PRC should bear a larger accountability to focus on a broad spectrum of issues of global governance, that is proportionate with its size, influence and power. Globalization is the starting point of their analysis. The proponents believe that in the age of globalization, the idea of sovereignty has its confines as several "non-traditional" challenges frequently traverse borders and such issues must be managed multilaterally. Thus, non-traditional security issues such as smuggling, human security, counter-terrorism, piracy, economic security, are the prime areas of analytical focus of this school.

This school of thought promotes the PRC's increased engagement in various regional diplomatic groupings across the world and the country's increased activism in the UNSC. Finally, the Globalists also display a fondness for soft power. They contend that the PRC has much to offer to global norms from its traditional philosophy as well as culture.

The **Global South** school of thought contends that given China's historical encounter with colonialism and imperialism, as well as the fact that China is a developing nation, the country's key global identity and liability rests with the developing world. Advocates of this school are of the opinion that the PRC must continue to view itself as a developing nation in the years ahead, and the country would continue to be liable to cooperate with the emerging powers for the purpose of common development, despite the fact that it has already attained the global power status. According to this school of thought, it is necessary for Beijing to identify itself as a developing nation so as to secure diplomatic support from the developing world. Such a strategy is important to ward off the West on matters such as human rights, climate change, Tibet and Taiwan to name a few.

Proponents of this group call for a fundamental reconstitution of the international system in order to reallocate economic resources, institutional influence, as well as power from the North to the South. They discern the present global institutional system to be unfair and prejudiced in favour of the developed nations. From this perspective, the PRC is a disgruntled and a revisionist power, and not a gratified and status quo one. Thus, not unexpectedly advocates of this school are firm sponsors of the BRICS group, and robust advocates of the G-20, with an objective to promote global multipolarity and bolster South-South solidarity.[1]

Having discussed the various perspectives on China's foreign policy, the country's engagement with Latin America can be analysed from the perspective of the Global South school of thought. Indeed as has been the historical experience and the national narrative of China suffering a "Century of Humiliation" at the hands of Great Powers in the nineteenth and the twentieth centuries, the leadership of the country continues to view the PRC as a developing nation even today. Despite the fact that the country is the second largest economy of the world today, the leadership maintains that the PRC has a long way to go before it attains the 'developed' nation status. Given the shared stance on matters of global importance as well as having played its developing nations card, the PRC has over time developed close ties with the LACs. Thus, it is this school of thought which is most suitable to analyse

Chinese foreign policy towards the region of Latin America. A lot is at stake for China in the region, owing to which the country is taking bigger strides to make deep inroads here. This has been discussed in detail in the next section.

What is at Stake for China?

Quite unlike the past, in the recent years China's presence in US 'backyard' has profoundly increased. The country's foreign policy strategy has undergone a visible shift from Deng Xiaoping's dictum "lie low, bide your time" to one of power projection and active engagement under President Xi Jinping. Although the region of Latin America is not strategically as important to China as South Asia or East Asia, bonhomie between the two sides has considerably increased in the recent years.

China's interest in Latin America can be broadly divided into two categories: maximalist objectives and the minimalist objectives. The maximalist goal refers to China's desire to attain a great power status. There are two aspects to this goal: economic and political. Interestingly, Latin America is valuable to fulfil this objective from both the angles. Economically, in order to sustain its domestic economic boom and as a resource-intensive nation, China seeks to attain raw materials from the LACs and diversify the source of such imports. The region is also viewed by the Chinese as a stable market for the export of its manufactured goods. Consequently, Chinese investors have ventured into the region to obtain stakes in the natural resource firms, offer loans to petroleum and mining investors, and preparing long term procurement contracts for mineral and oil in Latin America.

Politically, in order to attain its twin centenary goals of instituting a moderately prosperous society by 2020 as well as developing a moderately socialist nation by the middle of the 21st century, China adheres to an independent foreign policy. Consequently, China seeks to construct a new type of international relations. At the core of this strategy is the idea of development of constructive ties with the other developing nations across the world. Quite alike the nations of Latin America, China identifies itself as a developing nation and attempts to restore solidarity with the LACs based on a common historical experience and the idea of shared demands and desires. Also, given the ongoing Sino-US power transition, China seeks to construct a multipolar world that would comprise of restructuring the global order, reformation of international financial institutions and bodies of global governance such as the IMF, World Bank and the UN. To this end, the Belt and Road Initiative (BRI), construction of multilateral development banks such as the Asian Infrastructure Investment Bank (AIIB) and New Development Bank (NDB) may be recognized as chief contributions to global governance reform. As founding member of these key projects and institutions, China seeks to surge its influence in shaping the norms of global governance and consequently accomplish its objective of becoming a principal player in the international arena. Latin America comprises of 33 nations, off which China maintains diplomatic ties with as many as 24 countries – a number that is big enough for Beijing to identify this region with great importance in its foreign policy agenda. Therefore, China seeks active engagement and participation of the LACs in its landmark projects and initiatives.

The minimalist objective refers to displacing the Republic of China (ROC), popularly known as Taiwan, in Latin America through the announcement of the One-China policy as the basis of its diplomatic relations with the countries in the region. Essentially, China has used economic diplomacy to lure the LACs towards it through arrangements such as foreign direct investment (FDI), loans and funding large scale infrastructure projects in the region. Given the fact that China has emerged as the largest creditor of the LACs that have instituted diplomatic relations with the country, the remaining nations in the region have started viewing their engagement with China as a beneficial prospect. A case in point is the recent trend of Latin American countries namely Panama (2017), Dominican Republic (2018), and El Salvador (2018) switching diplomatic ties with the PRC. Table 17.1 comprises a list of LACs that instituted diplomatic relations with the PRC post-2000.

Table 17.1: List of Latin American countries that instituted Diplomatic Relations with the PRC post 2000

Sl. No.	*Country*	*Year of Establishment of Diplomatic Relations*
1	The Commonwealth of Dominica	23 March 2004
2	The Republic of Costa Rica	1 June 2007
3	The Republic of Panama	13 June 2017
4	Dominican Republic	1 May 2018
5	Republic of El Salvador	21 August 2018

Given the fact that Latin America is of key importance to China owing to the above mentioned reasons, it is interesting to understand the manner in which Latin America has been affected by the coronavirus pandemic, which is said to have its origin in the PRC.

Impact of COVID-19 on Latin America

While the coronavirus has affected almost every nation of the world including the PRC, the US and other wealthier countries of Europe, its ripple effect has touched the borders of Latin America as well. As of 1st April, 2020 Latin America comprises of a total number of 14,000 or more of confirmed cases of COVID-19, off a global total of approximately 850,000.[2] Lockdowns have been announced and imposed by several Latin American governments such Argentina, Colombia, Bolivia, Ecuador, Chile, Guatemala, El Salvador, Uruguay, Peru, while several others have undertaken voluntary isolation. Table 17.2 demonstrates a comparison of the gradual rise of COVID-19 cases in China and the LACs in the month of January-May 2020. The data in the tables below are derived from the World Health Organization.

Table 17.2: Comparison of the Gradual Rise of COVID-19 cases in China and the Latin American Countries (January-May 2020)

Name of Country	*Cases on 31 January, 2020*	*Cases in 29 February, 2020*	*Cases in 31 March, 2020*	*Cases on 30 April, 2020*	*Cases on 23 May, 2020*
People's Republic of China	**9,720**	**79,389**	**82,545**	**84,373**	**84,522**
The Republic of Cuba	0	0	170	1,467	1,916
The Republic of Chile	0	0	2,449	14,885	61,857
The Republic of Peru	0	0	852	31,190	108,769
The United States of Mexico	0	2	993	16,752	59,567
The Argentine Republic	0	0	820	4,201	9,931
The Cooperative Republic of Guyana	0	0	8	75	127
Jamaica	0	0	36	381	534
The Republic of Trinidad and Tobago	0	0	82	116	116
The Bolivar Republic of Venezuela	0	0	129	329	882
The Federative Republic of Brazil	0	1	4,256	71,886	310,087
The Republic of Suriname	0	0	8	10	11
Barbados	0	0	33	80	90
The Republic of Ecuador	0	1	1,962	24,675	35,828
The Republic of Colombia	0	0	702	5,949	18,330
Antigua and Barbuda	0	0	7	24	25
The Multinational States of Bolivia	0	0	97	1,053	5,187
Grenada	0	0	9	19	22
The Oriental Republic of Uruguay	0	0	309	625	749
The Commonwealth of Bahamas	0	0	14	80	97
The Commonwealth of Dominica	0	0	11	16	16
The Republic of Costa Rica	0	0	314	705	903
The Republic of Panama	0	0	989	6,200	10,116
Dominican Republic	0	0	901	6,652	13,989
Republic of El Salvador	0	0	30	377	1,725

Source: World Health Organization.[3]

The tables reflect that while COVID-19 cases were on the rise since January in China, the cases of the virus in Latin America were mostly on the rise since the month of March, reaching a peak in May for both China and the LACs. It can also be derived that while the LACs were not as badly affected as China, yet the nations most affected in the region were Chile, Peru, Mexico, Brazil and Ecuador.

Impact on Health Sector

The pandemic has thrown the biggest challenge to the health sector in the region of Latin America. The region which has witnessed decades of underinvestment in the health sector, is now left nowhere near equipped to deal with a pandemic. The per capita average yearly healthcare spending of Latin America is $949 – a number less than one-fourth of the average expenditure across the Organization for Economic Cooperation and Development.[4] Till date, the region comprises of limited coverage as well as access to healthcare, especially for the rural and the poorest section of the population in Latin America. The healthcare system of the region has already been stretched way beyond the requirements of a "normal" year; heading into a crisis. Alike in other places of the world, respirator capacity and hospital beds have not been able to meet the requirement of this pandemic. Infact, in countries like Haiti, Venezuela and Honduras, the ratio of beds to patients is not even equivalent to one bed per 1000 patients. On the other hand, in countries like Mexico, Colombia and Peru the ratio is less than two beds. In Venezuela, its existent humanitarian crisis together deficiency of healthcare facilities has been deteriorating to an extent that President Maduro's government has offered to work with opposition President Juan Guaido to combat the COVID-19 pandemic.

Impact on Economy

Apart from health risks, COVID-19 has had an economic impact on the region as well. With the influx of the virus in the region, shock waves have reached out on all domains. Since February 26th when Brazil testified the first confirmed case of COVID-19, the nation's currency lost as much as 20 percent of its value.[5] However, contrary to the forecast of the economists for the major European countries whereby it was envisaged that the economies of these nations would suffer a negative growth, the region of Latin America might have been somewhat less impacted.

The Economic Commission for Latin America and the Caribbean (ECLAC) has projected a 1.8 percent contraction in the gross domestic product (GDP) of the region. This could in turn bring about a hike in the region's unemployment rate by 10 percent and propel a tragic increase in the count of people living in poverty. In other words, of a total population of 620 million inhabitants in Latin

America, the number of people residing in poverty is likely to rise from 35 million to approximately 220 million. To add to it, the number of people living under extreme poverty could witness a rise from 67.4 million to 90 million.[6] Further, the ECLAC has suggested that Latin America's export to the PRC could observe a decline of 10.7 percent in value.

Owing to the fact that China is the number one trading partner of several countries in the region as well as a destination for the export of goods, quite clearly the region is to a great extent economically reliant on China. Thus, falling rate of exchanges with the PRC has made countries like Brazil, Peru and Chile principally vulnerable. Alberto Ramos, head of Latin American research at Goldman Sachs has stated, "The key source of downside risk [the financial risk associated with losses] to Latin America is a deterioration of the terms of trade triggered by deep long-lasting impact of a China slowdown on commodity prices".[7]

Undoubtedly, there would be an immense impact on global supply chains, especially in Latin America, owing to the fact that the PRC is the second largest trading partner of the region as a whole. For instance, due to the PRC's rising demand for blueberries, grapes and avocados, Peru and Chile have emerged as vital markets in the recent times. However, as Sebastian Osman of Araya & Cia have rightly mentioned, "There are two principal problems; the transportation of the product and the delays, on taking it from the exporter to the final customer, and the low prices of those products in the market."[8]

Thus, the Latin American economies stand vulnerable at the moment. The Chilean President Sebastian Piñera has predicted that the COVID-19 outbreak would have a sizeable economic impact on the country owing to the falling prices of copper across the globe and the fact that half of the country's copper export is sent to Beijing. The Chilean Commission on Copper has said that copper exports would not only witness a decline in value but also quantity this year. Consignments to the PRC have already been rescheduled.

Peru has also witnessed a sharp fall in its exports to the PRC, which is its principal foreign market. According to Asociación de Exportadores (ADEX), the leading business association of Peruvian foreign trade, in January alone, the country's exports declined by 16 percent compared to 2019, principally affecting two fundamental goods: fishmeal and minerals. To add to it, Peru's manufacturing sector is likely to be affected by the shortage of inputs from Beijing. In this context Erik Fischer, ADEX president has said, "There is going to be a drop in Chinese demand and that the pharmaceuticals and textiles industries here that rely on Chinese raw materials and that are not receiving them in normal conditions will have less productivity and less sales".

Brazilian officials have stated that the country's exports have already begun to suffer the setback, falling 6.2 percent in comparison to the previous year. There has been a decline of commodities exports over 20 percent, primarily as a result of economic crisis in the PRC, which is the biggest trading partner of this South American nation. However, industry lobby experts have estimated that soybean exports would witness a sale of 73 million tonnes this year and that its export would not suffer a setback due to the crisis. The picture in the stock market stands quite on the contrary to the economic crisis suffered by the Brazilian companies as a consequence of the pandemic. BRF, a chief food company of Brazil, has lost 56.5 percent of its market value in the present year.

Other countries that have been affected are Argentina, Uruguay and Ecuador to name a few. Given the fact that Argentina is already on the threshold of a new sovereign default, declining export of goods and lower prices signify a big blow for the country. Abeceb, a business consultancy has mentioned in its report that, "The main direct effect of coronavirus is manifested on the export of commodities, such as soybeans and, above all, meats", "China is Argentina's second market so fewer purchases from there would have a big effect on our economy". In January, beef exports declined 32.8 percent in comparison to the last quarter of 2019. According to Argentine beef trade chamber CICCRA, the PRC accounts for 75 percent of the country's beef exports and consequently fewer consignments there could fundamentally explain the decline.

Similar has been the case of Uruguay where exports declined 18.7 percent in the month of February as against the same month last year. According to government data, this has been the case primarily due to declining sale of dairy products, beef, cellulose and wood to China.[9]

The Rise of Cybercrime

Latin America has a high number of internet users but is ill-equipped to negate cybercrime. As governments in the region impose stringent quarantine measures to combat the pandemic, corporations, individuals as well as critical infrastructure remain vulnerable and at risk to attacks. Online scams, phishing email schemes and ransomware attacks have breeded and propagated in Latin America amidst the COVID-19 pandemic, unmasking the perils that hackers pose to governments, people and banks.

In second half of March, a ransomware application named COVIDLock, proliferated across the South American nation of Costa Rica, targeting companies as well as individuals. The application banked on the people's anxiety of the pandemic alleging to prevent contamination by offering interactive maps of the spread of the virus.

The app instead hijacked the devices of the victims and claimed a ransom in the cryptocurrency bitcoin.

Similarly criminals in the South American nations of Guatemala, Puerto Rico and Mexico have manipulated apprehensions of financial and health crisis to wreak phishing scams intended at compiling sensitive information which permitted them to perpetrate identity and insurance frauds. The emails draw the attention of people with assurances of government stimulus money, coronavirus tests as well as vaccines.

In this context, Charity Wright, an analyst at the IntSights Cyber Intelligence firm has stated that nations in the region with big economies such as Brazil, Colombia, Mexico as well as Argentina are the likely targets of these hackers. He said,

> "They have the money, a huge population and are adopting new technology quickly, but at the same time these countries are very much behind the rest of the world in implementing cyber defense mechanisms, regulation and compliance policies across the board."[10]

Fall in Air Traffic

The region has witnessed a 91 percent drop in air traffic in April 2020 compared to last year owing to the outbreak of the pandemic. Two of Latin America's largest airlines have been fully grounded and nearly all other flights have been cancelled.[11] The latest data of the International Air Transport Association demonstrates that the region will experience one of the steepest fall in traffic, second to that of Europe. Most airlines of Latin America have ceased to operate as nations in the region close their borders so as to combat the proliferation of the pandemic.[12] This has led to a huge loss of revenue generated from the aviation sector.

Thus, by and large the LACs have been hard-hit by the COVID-19 pandemic. Owing to the fact that a lot is at stake for China in the region, it is of relevance to understand whether Beijing has indeed offered any substantial aid and humanitarian assistance to the region of not. The following section seeks to explore this issue in detail.

China's Aid to Latin America

Undoubtedly, COVID-19 has generated critical economic, political as well as social impacts across multiple countries of the world. While there has been a serious yearning amidst the global community to boost cooperation against the pandemic, China has shown much readiness to coordinate efforts with various nations across the world to contain the pandemic.[13]

The country has extended help and assistance to the affected nations in four areas. First, intergovernmental assistance. In all, the PRC has announced provision of aid to as many as 82 nations, the African Union (AU) and the World Health Organization (WHO). Such assistance comprises of masks, testing reagents as well as protective masks. Second, medical technological cooperation. Beijing has shared its experience of the COVID-19 treatment with the other nations of the world, held video conferences with healthcare specialists from various international organizations and countries, as well as sent medical teams to these affected nations. Third, sub-national assistance. Local governments in the PRC have offered provisions to cities in Italy, Republic of Korea and Japan. Fourth, non-governmental assistance. Civil organizations and enterprises in China have also bestowed donations to the countries affected by the pandemic.[14]

The PRC has offered timely help to Latin America. Governments from the Southern Cone to Central America have obtained a varied range of donations, spanning from testing kits to ventilators. Thus, a new face of Chinese soft power and diplomacy has evolved, which is gaining recognition as "facemask diplomacy".

Experts from China have held a video conference with their counterparts in Latin America, to confront the pandemic. In the video-conference, Chinese experts discussed in detail regarding the characteristic of the virus as well as shared Chinese know-how of disease control, community-based quarantine and clinical treatment. Experts from the PRC also responded to questions raised by their South American counterparts. It replicated the doctrine of holding public health and safety as a principal priority that has enabled the PRC to undertake effective measures to curtail the proliferation of the virus, and which continues to be relevant and applicable in the region of Latin America at this crucial juncture.

From Mexico to Argentina, Brazil to Peru, various Latin American countries have acknowledged offers of support from Beijing as the count of COVID-19 cases have soared across the region, amidst mounting fears about the lack of preparedness of their healthcare systems. In this context, Chinese Ambassador Zou Xiaoli has discussed the manner in which the Asian giant has displayed readiness to aid Argentina combat the pandemic by donating gloves, masks, protective suits and thermometers. The Chinese embassy has announced its donations by publishing pictures on Twitter of big trucks carrying a mobile hospital, which was instituted inside a military base near the Argentine capital. Such assistance has come at a critical juncture for the country, when Argentina is wrestling with acute financial crisis and bargaining $110 billion in foreign debt with creditors, which comprises of the International Monetary Fund (IMF) as well. A spokesman of Argentina's foreign ministry has said, "This is part of the link we have with China, which is a solid relationship of mutual respect and ties that go beyond strong trade."[15]

China has left no effort to swiftly brace the LACs to combat the health emergency, by adhering to practical as well as competent measures to allay the impact of the virus in the region. Venezuela was one of the first nation in the region to obtain Beijing's medical supplies, as a shipment transporting 4,015 COVID-19 testing kits, together with chemical reagents, gloves, air purifiers and masks, arrived on March 19. Given the massive Chinese assistance, shortly after the IMF declined President Nicolas Maduro's appeal for a loan worth $15 billion to bolster the country's collapsing health system, the Venezuelan Vice-President Delcy Rodriguez stated, "We want to thank President Xi Jinping, his government and his people from the bottom of our Bolivarian heart." She also proclaimed that the COVID-19 response team of the government was holding online meetings with specialists from the PRC. Another shipment arrived in Venezuela from Beijing in the last week of March which comprised of '500,000 rapid testing kits, 70,000 infrared thermometers and a delegation of medical specialists'.[16]

Argentina too has received aid from the PRC to combat the pandemic in the form of health and equipment supplies, medical supplies together with technical advice from specialists in the PRC through video conference. The Alberto Fernández government has obtained over 50,000 test kits, 200,000 face masks, 10,000 disposable protection suits, 2000 protection goggles, 20,000 disposable gloves, 550 digital thermometers, and 10 respirators, with more to come.[17]

In Chile, the PRC has agreed to send 1000 ventilators. However, the case is quite opposite with regard to Uruguay. This Latin American nation first offered donations to Beijing and later received donations from the PRC in kind.

Not only the Chinese government, but also Jack Ma, one of the wealthiest citizen of the PRC and the founder of Chinese multinational company Alibaba, which specialises in e-commerce, IT and retail has also come forward to the rescue of Latin America. Ma announced a donation of medical provisions to 24 nations of the region on Twitter. The donation comprised of 400,000 testing kits, 2 million masks and 104 ventilators as well as tendered to cover transportation costs. Amongst the countries that benefitted are Mexico, Ecuador, Argentina, Peru and Brazil.[18]

Latin America's largest nation Brazil too looked up to Beijing for assistance. The states in Brazil most affected by the pandemic are Sao Paulo, Rio de Janeiro and Ceara. While certain Brazilian officials such as President Jair Bolsonaro's lawmaker son and Brazilian education minister condemned the PRC for its management of the crisis, governors and some mayors of a number of Brazilian states opted to bypass President Jair Bolsonaro and seek assistance from the Chinese government. Meanwhile the country's then Health Minister Luiz Henrique Mandetta stated that Brazil was confronting a "serious problem" securing sufficient mechanical ventilators and also spoke to the Chinese ambassador to ensure the fulfilment of these orders. Mandetta was later removed from the post owing to a series of differences with President Bolsonaro with regard to government endeavour to lift the lockdown and reactivate the country's economy.[19] With regard to assistance, the Beijing-based New Development Bank administered by the BRICS nations, has demonstrated readiness to release a loan worth US$ 1 billion to Brazil so as to bolster the country's social and health infrastructure.

Mexico has instituted a network of thermographic cameras manufactured by China, to screen for fevers, a chief symptom of the infection. The Artificial Intelligence (AI)-enabled cameras that utilise infrared sensors to determine body temperature from a distance, have been set up outside financial and business centres in Mexico's capital as well as in other big cities like Guadalajara and Monterrey.[20]

Thus the shared efforts between the PRC and countries in Latin America to resist COVID-19 is critical for the region, as it has a feeble health system, which by now has been stretched thin in managing the growing cases. Infact, the above-mentioned instances underscore that the proposal to develop a China-Latin America community with a shared future bears greater relevance at present than ever before, as human beings are confronting a common enemy that identifies no race or borders.[21]

The Taiwan Factor

Taiwan, an island nation located 150 miles away from the coast of mainland China, has appeared as a model for successful pandemic response with the nation suffering merely six deaths from the novel coronavirus so far. Infact the ROC's COVID-19 response has led to the international community, inclusive of the US, championing the case of granting observer status to the island-nation at the World Health Organization (WHO). Such a verdict would by all means enrage the PRC that deems the island-nation as a legal component of its territory.

Given the country's quick response in combating the virus, transparency in informing the public about the situation, competence in mapping out the contact history of the confirmed COVID-19 patients, as well as guidance to the people for the usage of face masks in public places have won applaud for the healthcare specialists in containing the virus. Stephen Tan, president of a private think tank Cross-Strait Policy Association has said,

> "The relatively low infections and deaths in Taiwan have impressed many countries – especially after the pandemic spread in the US and Europe, and many of them have felt that it would be unfair not to allow Taiwan to join the WHO, given its medical strength and ability to check the pandemic".[22]

With regard to Latin America, China has utilised the Belt and Road Initiative to lure nations in the US "backyard" and strengthen its foothold there. However, the outbreak of the pandemic has offered an opportunity to the ROC to drive back Beijing and reinforce the present alliances in the region in what may perhaps be the island-nation's conclusive stand.

Since President Tsai assumed power in 2016, as many as seven diplomatic partners of Taiwan have switched sides to China, which comprises of three nations from the region – the Dominican Republic, Panama and El Salvador. However, President Tsai has tendered the remaining allies of the ROC in the region a high rank in her foreign policy agenda. She makes frequent sojourns to countries like St. Lucia, Haiti, St. Nevis as well as Kitts, while also making an opportune stopover at the US. To add to it, the nation's International Cooperation and Development Fund (ICDF) continues to offer funds to its allies in the region to bolster their energy, agriculture and technology sectors.

With regard to Taipei's assistance to the LACs during the pandemic, it may be said that the ROC has displayed much readiness to offer assistance to its allies in Latin America and the Caribbean as it has done across the world. The country has taken this situation as an opportunity to project itself as an effective global power in the region vis-à-vis China. Doctors and health experts at six hospitals in the island-nation have engaged in video conferences with their counterparts in the Latin America and the Caribbean, imparting information on their experience of combating the novel coronavirus and the measures they have undertaken in their hospitals to contain the spread of the virus. The video conferences were organized within the framework of bilateral medical cooperation agreements that the ROC had signed with its allies in the South American continent.[23] The country has donated 40,000 face masks, forehead thermometers, and six thermal imaging body detection instruments to Saint Lucia. Thermal imaging devices and 40,000 face masks were also donated to St. Vincent and Grenadines. Guatemala received as many as 180,000 masks, expensive ultrasound and X-ray machinery from Taiwan.[24]

Thus, at a time when the world is pointing fingers towards the PRC for being the place of origin of the novel coronavirus, Taiwan has put in place its health diplomacy to reach out to nations in the farthest extent of the world, create a space for itself and make its voice heard. But does it mean that the LACs are outrightly blaming China for the outbreak and management of the pandemic and considering developing ties with the ROC? This question has been explored in detail in the following section.

Are Latin Americans Blaming China?

The coronavirus pandemic has derived a range of responses towards China from across the world. The U.S.-China ties have touched an all-time low, since the aftermath of the Tiananman massacre in June 1989. While both nations have experienced massive loss of human life together with a sharp financial slowdown, political officials in both nations have worked on safeguarding their respective domestic standing by holding the other's government responsible. The U.S. President Donald Trump has gone as far as referring to the coronavirus as the "Chinese virus". On the other hand, state media and senior Chinese officials have propelled a theory that the virus was created by the U.S. and planted in the PRC last fall.[25]

Another school of thought identifies the COVID-19 crisis as the "opportunity of the century" for China to strengthen its position as a world power. Even in the past, the Asian giant has embraced opportunities to enhance its place in the world. A case in point is its role during the 2008 financial crisis and its assistance to the European debt market. In this regard, Keyu Jin, associate professor of economics at London School of Economics has said,

> "I think this is the opportunity of the century for China to build trust in the world, which it has found so difficult to come by as a rising nation, and to rebuild its international image – China doesn't (want to) waste an opportunity like this."[26]

Thus, there are two distinct schools of thought in the world at present regarding China's role in the spread of the coronavirus pandemic. Latin America, home to 620 million people, stands divided on this issue. Tensions have been simmering between China and certain countries in the region as they strive to contain the pandemic. Presidents of Mexico and Brazil, which together comprise of more than half the region's population as well as economy have strikingly dismissed appeals to restrict public life and shut down business.

Several officials from the Brazilian government have raised fingers at China. Infact, relations between the two nations became even more strained when Brazil's Education Minister Abraham Weintraub associated the pandemic to Beijing's "plan for world domination" and the Brazilian President's son and federal lawmaker Eduardo Bolsonaro referred to COVID-19 coronavirus as the "Chinese virus" in a tweet. While Eduardo condemned Beijing's "dictatorship" for the manner in which it dealt with the pandemic in March, Weintraub suggested that the PRC was behind the global health catastrophe. He impersonated a Chinese accent and raised the questions, "Geopolitically, who will come out stronger from this global crisis?", "Who in Brazil is allied with this infallible plan for world domination?", on Twitter.

The Chinese embassy in Brazil denounced the tweet as "absurd and despicable" and referred to it as "highly racist".[27] Amidst this diplomatic spat, the Brazilian President Jair Bolsonaro on his part has explicitly denied the necessity to implement social distancing, which has put him in contention with mayors and governors in Brazil. To add to it, he has referred to lockdowns as a "crime" and identified governors as "job killers".[28]

Apart from allegations being leveraged against China, the outbreak of the pandemic has led to questions being raised by many in the region of South America. Officials from several Latin American nations have questioned their ties with the PRC vis-a-vis the ROC. For instance, Dragos Dolanescu, a legislator who represents Social Christian Republican Party in Costa Rica has said,

> "I find it unfortunate that Ambassador Tang Heng, the highest diplomatic representative of the People's Republic of China in Costa Rica, considers it appropriate to seek the Ministry of Foreign Affairs to put an end to my protests and comments on incontrovertible events such as the first outbreak of COVID-19 originated in the city of Wuhan, so that Costa Rica does not speak of Taiwan (a nation with which we had a close relationship until 2007 and that we share respect for democracy)".

Further he mentioned,

> "To deny the existence of Taiwan, a country with a democratic tradition like ours and with an important cultural presence in Costa Rica, is to blind itself to the reality of the world, since Taiwan is recognised by several countries in the world. Using diplomatic channels to prevent a deputy from exercising his constitutional right to political control (article 121 of our Political Constitution) is, to use the same terms as Ambassador Tang, "touch the red line" on the exogenous influence of internal affairs of the operation of the Republic of Costa Rica."[29]

Deliberating in favour of Taiwan, Pelegrin Castillo, leader and opinion maker at the ProNacion think tank in the Dominican Republic has stated,

> "Experience shows that open societies are more adept than closed societies at dealing with these crises than those which appeal to autocratic and totalitarian strategies. Taiwan and Israel are two such nations which have shown the way."[30]

While Beijing has been subject to criticism by many in the region, the country has been lauded by several others in Latin America. Chinese aid and assistance to several countries in the region has won the country much applaud from the local people of the region. When China was worst hit by the pandemic in February, the Venezuelan government expressed solidarity with China. The Ministry of Foreign Affairs of the Bolivarian Republic of Venezuela issued a statement,

> "The whole world is amazed at the energetic determination with which the Chinese Government has been complying with the health protocols recommended by international health organizations to control the spread of the virus, leaving for human history multiple testimonies of its titanic effort to protect its people, breaking all existing records in response speed, from the development of health infrastructures to the efforts to disseminate relevant information to the universal scientific community to favor research and early development of specific vaccines."[31]

China has offered steady assistance to Peru to fight against the pandemic in a timely manner. Based on President Xi's vision of a community with a shared future for mankind, Beijing has shared its experience in epidemic control and prevention without reservation, as well as expedited export channels for the transit of anti-epidemic supplies to support Peru, and other Latin American nations, in their containment efforts.[32] Lauding the Chinese endeavour, the Peruvian President Martin Vizcarra appreciated Beijing's organizational ability as well as the "useful experience" that the nation has imparted to the pandemic affected nations. He also hailed the close diplomatic ties between the two nations and expressed gratitude to China for the assistance and support the country extended to Peru to combat the pandemic.[33]

Antonio Ortega, secretary general of Broad Front Party of Costa Rica, too has expressed his appreciation for Beijing's generous help to this Latin American nation in their struggle against the pandemic. He stated that such generosity validated the friendship and solidarity that the people of the two nations shared.[34]

On April 1st, Marcelo Ebrard, foreign minister of Mexico, tweeted "Gracias China!!!" together with a photograph of a plane that transported 100,000 masks, five ventilators and 50,000 test kits donated by the PRC. Few days later on April 13th, Felipe Solá, foreign minister of Argentina, expressed his gratitude for China upon the receipt of a large shipment of vital necessities to combat the pandemic namely masks, protective suits and gloves. The delivery cartons were embellished with Argentine as well as Chinese flags and a quote about brotherhood in Spanish from an Argentine poem "El Gaucho Martin Fierro" written by Jose Hernandez.[35]

Thus, China has received a mixed bag of responses from the LACs in terms of the assistance it has offered to support their containment measures. While officials of some countries in the region have questioned Chinese management of the pandemic as well as their ties with the PRC vis-à-vis the ROC, many others have appreciated the Chinese humanitarian assistance to their respective countries.

Conclusion

It is not the first time in history that Beijing has offered a lending hand to Latin America. In 2008, following the Great Depression, Beijing which funded a global stimulus representing seven percent of the PRC's GDP, sustained the economies of Latin America by importing products such as timber, oil and metallic minerals in huge amount. At present, the PRC is the second largest trading partner of the LACs, and the country has surpassed the US to rank as the top trading partners of several major economies of the region namely Brazil, Peru, Chile as well as Uruguay. The country's adherence to medical diplomacy amidst the coronavirus pandemic maybe deemed as a natural off-shoot of this budding relationship. It may also be viewed as a victory for a region that has over a prolonged period invested too little in healthcare infrastructure.

As nations in this hemisphere are confronted with the challenge of a rising public health crisis, the virtual silence of the US is thunderous. To add to it, US' inward looking strategy at present to address the pandemic crisis situation within its borders, has left unstable and increasingly desperate countries in its own hemisphere jostling to attain humanitarian as well as medical assistance from elsewhere. Such state of affairs has offered China with the opportunity to make deeper inroads into the US "backyard".

The other aspect is that of the one-China policy. While the region of Latin America is of key importance to China both economically as well as strategically, the PRC has founded its ties with every country in the region on the basis of its one-China principle. Even at a time, when China has offered massive humanitarian and medical assistance to countries affected by the pandemic across the globe, it continues to abide by this principle. Whereas Beijing has offered aid and assistance to numerous countries in the region, Paraguay has not received any aid to combat the pandemic, from China. The reason being, unlike countries like Chile, Venezuela, Argentina and the like, Paraguay does not enjoy formal diplomatic relations with China. This sends out a strong message to all those nations in the region which have not yet formally recognised the one-China principle, and instituted diplomatic ties with the PRC. Such a strategy would compel them to contemplate on considering the PRC as a more reliable diplomatic partner vis-à-vis the ROC.

The third aspect is that of foreign policy decision making in China. Decision makers in the country are likely to be influenced by the nationalist as well as selective multilateralist school of thought. While China continues to be sceptical of Western "traps", it seeks to bolster its international engagements. A case in point is the Chinese antagonism with the US with regard to the outbreak of the pandemic and the country's approach to offer humanitarian assistance to countries across the world to strengthen its position in the international arena.

Thus, despite the fact that China has by far been the worst affected nation of the world by the COVID-19 crisis, the country has very ingeniously utilised this crisis as an opportunity in its favour. By offering humanitarian assistance and aid to countries across the world, as is in the case of Latin America, China has lived up to its image of being a responsible stakeholder and a pre-dominant global force. To add to it, through its tactful strategies of offering aid to only those nations with which it shares formal diplomatic relations, China has very skilfully reinforced its adherence to the one-China principle on the global map. The crisis has acted in the country's favour in terms of strengthening its grounds in Latin America as also in the rest of the world. Therefore, once again China has utilised its economic power to attain its strategic objectives in the region.

NOTES

1 Shambaugh David, *China Goes Global: The Partial Power*, USA, OUP USA, 2013.

2 Collyns Dan (2020), "How will the Coronavirus affect Latin America's economic growth and the fight against poverty?", 02 April 2020, https://newsus.cgtn.com/news/2020-04-01/Latin-American-countries-close-borders-for-COVID-19-Pkc4P9sQFO/index.html, accessed online 3 April 2020.

3 World Health Organization (2020), "WHO Coronavirus Disease (COVID-19) Dashboard", 13 June 2020, https://covid19.who.int/, accessed online 13 May 2020.

4 Mead Walter Russell (2020), "The Coronavirus Threat South of the Border", 6 April 2020, https://www.hudson.org/research/15902-the-coronavirus-threat-south-of-the-border, accessed online 13 May 2020.

5 Ceurvels Matteo (2020), "COVID-19's Impact on Businesses and Consumers in Latin America", https://www.emarketer.com/content/COVID-19-s-impact-on-businesses-and-consumers-in-latin-america, accessed on 13 May 2020.

6 Collyns Dan (2020), "How will the Coronavirus affect Latin America's economic growth and the fight against poverty?", 2 April 2020, https://newsus.cgtn.com/news/2020-04-01/Latin-American-countries-close-borders-for-COVID-19-Pkc4P9sQFO/index.html, accessed online 3 April 2020.

7 Ceullar Alejandra, Fermin Koop, Manuela Andreoni, Andres Bermudez Lievano (2020), "Coronavirus takes toll on Latin American economies", 30 March 2020, https://dialogochino.net/en/trade-investment/34547-coronavirus-takes-toll-on-latin-american-economies/, accessed online 3 April 2020.

8 CGTN (2020), "Coronavirus is having a ripple effect in Latin America", 19 February 2020, https://newsus.cgtn.com/news/2020-02-19/Coronavirus-is-having-a-ripple-effect-in-Latin-America-OaRiA94qJ2/index.html, accessed online 3 April 2020.

9 Ceullar Alejandra, Fermin Koop, Manuela Andreoni, Andres Bermudez Lievano (2020), "Coronavirus takes toll on Latin American economies", 30 March 2020, https://dialogochino.net/en/trade-investment/34547-coronavirus-takes-toll-on-latin-american-economies/, accessed online 3 April 2020.

10 Austin Anastasia (2020), "Latin America Under Threat of Cybercrime Amid Coronavirus", 8 April 2020, https://www.insightcrime.org/news/analysis/threat-cyber-crime-coronavirus/, accessed online 3 April 2020.

11 Rochabrun Marcelo (2020), "Air Traffic in Latin America Falls 91% Due to the Coronavirus Outbreak", 16 April 2020, https://www.reuters.com/article/us-health-coronavirus-latam-airlines/air-traffic-in-latin-america-falls-91-due-to-the-coronavirus-outbreak-idUSKBN21Y2VS, accessed online 3 April 2020.

12 CAPA (2020), "COVID-19 : Time is Running Out for Distressed Latin Airlines", https://centreforaviation.com/analysis/reports/COVID-19-time-is-running-out-for-distressed-latin-airlines-519212, accessed on 3 April 2020,

13 Ministry of Foreign Affairs of the People's Republic of China (2020), "President Xi Jinping to Attend G20 Extraordinary Virtual Leaders' Summit on COVID-19", 26 March 2020, https://www.fmprc.gov.cn/mfa_eng/wjbxw/t1761663.shtml, accessed online 3 April 2020.

14 Ministry of Foreign Affairs of the People's Republic of China (2020), "Foreign Ministry Spokesperson Geng Shuang's Regular Press Conference on March 20, 2020", 21 March 2020, https://www.fmprc.gov.cn/mfa_eng/xwfw_665399/s2510_665401/t1758992.shtml, accessed online 3 April 2020.

15 Garrison Cassandra (2020), "With U.S. Hit by Virus, China Courts Latin America with Medical Diplomacy", 26 March 2020, https://www.reuters.com/article/us-health-coronavirus-latam-china-featur/with-u-s-hit-by-virus-china-courts-latin-america-with-medical-diplomacy-idUSKBN21D346, accessed online 3 April 2020.

16 Koop Fermin, Manuela Andreoni, Andres Bermudez Lievano, Alejandra Cuellar (2020), "Latin America seeks Chinese medical aid to fight coronavirus", 6 April 2020, https://dialogochino.net/en/trade-investment/latin-america-chinese-medical-aid-to-fight-coronavirus/, accessed online 3 April 2020.

17 Ibid.

18 Ibid

19 XinhuaNet (2020), "Brazil's COVID-19 death toll nears 2,000 as over 30,000 test positive", 17 April 2020, http://www.xinhuanet.com/english/2020-04/17/c_138983328.htm, accessed online 3 April 2020.

20 XinhuaNet (2020), "LatAm doubles down on efforts to contain COVID-19, with help from China", 28 March 2020, http://www.xinhuanet.com/english/2020-03/28/c_138926274.htm, accessed online 3 April 2020.

21 XinhuaNet (2020), "Timely help amid COVID-19 outbreak highlights China-LatAm community with shared future", 27 March 2020, http://www.xinhuanet.com/english/2020-03/27/c_138921706.htm, accessed online 3 April 2020.

22 Chung Lawrence (2020), "Taiwan Offers Masks and Medical Aid to Foreign Countries, Angering Beijing", 5 April 2020, http://www.europe-solidaire.org/spip.php?article52832, accessed online 3 April 2020.

23 Trieste John Van (2020), "Taiwan Helping Latin American Allies Fight COVID-19", 1 April 2020, https://en.rti.org.tw/news/view/id/2002997, accessed online 3 April 2020.

24 Ward Jared (2020), " Taiwan's Medical Diplomacy in the Caribbean : A Final Stand Against Beijing", 11 May 2020, https://thediplomat.com/2020/05/taiwans-medical-diplomacy-in-the-caribbean-a-final-stand-against-beijing/, accessed online 3 April 2020.

25 Bremmer Ian (2020), "China and America's Blame Game Over COVID-19 Hurts Everyone", 26 March 2020, https://time.com/5810493/coronavirus-china-united-states-governments/, accessed online 3 April 2020.

26 Taylor Chloe (2020), "'Opportunity of the century': How the coronavirus crisis could establish China as a global leader", 31 March 2020, https://www.cnbc.com/2020/03/31/how-the-coronavirus-crisis-could-establish-china-as-a-global-leader.html, accessed online 3 April 2020.

27 New Straits Times (2020), "Brazil minister says COVID-19 part of China's 'plan for world domination'", 07 April 2020, https://www.nst.com.my/world/world/2020/04/582029/brazil-minister-says-COVID-19-part-chinas-plan-world-domination, accessed on 3 April 2020.

28 VIA News (2020), "Divided Latin America Scrambles to Survive Coronavirus Onslaught", 9 April 2020, https://via.news/south-america/divided-latin-america-scrambles-to-survive-coronavirus-onslaught/, accessed online 3 April 2020.

29 Vargas Dinia (2020), "Dragos Dolanescu Responds to China That Ethical Democracy Does Allow It to Speak", https://www.crhoy.com/nacionales/dragos-dolanescu-le-responde-a-china-que-democracia-tica-si-le-permite-hablar/, accessed online 3 April 2020.

30 Boronat, Orlando Gutierrez (2020), "Coronavirus Failures Lead Latin America To Question Growing Ties To China", 21 March 2020, https://www.caribbeannewsglobal.com/coronavirus-failures-lead-latin-america-to-question-growing-ties-to-china/, accessed online 3 April 2020.

31 Ministry of Foreign Affairs of the Bolivarian Republic of Venezuela (2020), "Communique", 3 February 2020, http://mppre.gob.ve/en/comunicado/venezuela-expresses-solidarity-china-coronavirus/, accessed online 3 April 2020.

32 Xinhua (2020), "China pledges continuous support for Peru in COVID-19 fight: Xi", 1 May 2020, http://www.xinhuanet.com/english/2020-05/01/c_139022067.htm, accessed online 3 April 2020.

33 CGTN (2020), "Xi Jinping: China Willing to Enhance Global Cooperation To Curb COVID-19 Spread", 30 April 2020, https://news.cgtn.com/news/2020-04-30/President-Xi-holds-phone-calls-with-Czech-Peruvian-presidents-Q7nzsh2XaE/index.html, accessed online 3 April 2020.

34 Xinhua (2020), "Foreign Party Leaders Praise China for Practicing Concept of Community With Shared Future in Anti-Epidemic Cooperation", 28 March 2020, http://www.xinhuanet.com/english/2020-03/28/c_138926483.htm, accessed online 3 April 2020.

35 Angelo Paul and Rebecca Bill Chavez (2020), "'Gracias China!'", 21 April 2020, https://www.nytimes.com/2020/04/21/opinion/china-latin-america-covid.html, accessed on 3 April 2020.

18

China-Africa Relations Amidst COVID-19

Abhishek Kumar Darbey

China needs Africa for various reasons such as for political support at the international forum, to have reliable economic partners, for uninterrupted oil supplies, for Chinese investments under Belt & Road Initiative, and for its military expansion. China's President Xi Jinping declared "China Dream" cannot be achieved without the African resources, land, people and market. China Dream is about achieving the Two Centenaries: the material goal of China becoming a "moderately well-off society" by 2021, the 100th anniversary of the Chinese Communist Party, and the modernisation goal of China becoming a fully developed nation by 2049, the 100th anniversary of the founding of the People's Republic of China. In this context, COVID-19 outbreak in Africa has tested China's commitments to the continent. The outbreak of the disease in the continent is certainly an economic concern for all major foreign investors including China. According to the China Investment Global Tracker (2019), China's investment and contracts in sub-Saharan Africa is estimated to be US$ 299 billion from 2005-2018. In addition, in 2018, Xi Jinping vowed to invest a further US$ 60 billion into Africa. China may face serious challenges and losses if the pandemic severely affects the social and economic lives in Africa. The pandemic will certainly impact the ongoing Chinese projects in Africa and further escalation of the disease will result in heavy losses and delay of the projects. China will have to help Africa within its capacity in containing the coronavirus to avoid the losses of its stakes and interests in the continent. China will face the challenges to meet the high expectations of 54 African governments during the pandemic.

Africa and COVID-19

As per June 18, 2020, the total numbers of confirmed cases in Africa was 268,662 and among them 145,520 are still active cases with 7,221 deaths, and the reports of the coronavirus confirmed cases are from 54 countries in Africa. On February 14, 2020, the 1st confirmed case of COVID-19 was diagnosed in Egypt, Africa, and the 1st confirmed case of COVID-19 in the sub-Saharan Africa was diagnosed in Nigeria. In the months of February, March and April in 2020, the growth rate of the Coronavirus cases were less for instance, according to the figures published by John Hopkins University, by April 30, 2020, the number of confirmed cases in Nigeria, South Africa, Ghana, Kenya were 1,728 cases/51 deaths, 5,647 cases/103 deaths, 2,074 cases/17 deaths, 396 cases/17 deaths respectively.[1] As per May 2020, the most affected African countries of COVID-19 pandemic are South Africa, Egypt, Nigeria, Algeria, Ghana, Morocco and Cameroon, but in the case of Morocco the COVID-19 patients' recovery rate is fast with only 628 active cases. At present, the African countries with COVID-19 active cases of more than 1000 are Egypt, South Africa, Nigeria, Ghana, Sudan, Democratic Republic of Congo, Cameroon, Algeria, Gabon, Djibouti, Kenya, Somalia, Ethiopia, Central Africa Republic, Equatorial Guinea and Guinea-Bissau. African countries with the higher numbers of deaths are Egypt (1,198), South Africa (952) and Algeria (698).

So far, the COVID-19 pandemic in Africa is relatively at better position than many parts of the world, but given the very poor health care and medical infrastructure in the continent many experts have raised their concerns about the possible escalation of the pandemic in the region, and it's devastating impacts on social and economic lives of the Africa people. On April 8, 2020, Matshidiso Moeti, Director of the WHO Sub-Saharan Africa Regional Office said, "The new Coronavirus pandemic may not only cause tens of thousands of deaths, but will also cause economic and social damage. The spread of the virus to areas outside major cities means the fight against epidemic has entered a new stage."[2]

Matshidiso suggested, "To enhance community participation, provincial and district government must have sufficient resources to fight the local epidemic." He added that the WHO in Africa is working in key areas, detection, isolation, close contact tracing, infection prevention and control, and patient management. Ahmed Al-Mandhar, Director of the WHO Eastern Mediterranean Region said, "Africa still has the opportunity to reduce cases and slow down transmission. All countries must quickly expand the scale of operations, implement comprehensive response, and use proven and effective public health and social distancing measures, while effectively containing the spread of the virus."[3] It is suggested that the Sub-Saharan

Africa's economy will be contracted by 1.6 percent in 2020. Abebe Aemro Selassie, Director of the African Department at the International Monetary Fund (IMF) said, "The region is facing a sharp decline in global growth, financial austerity, a sharp drop in the price of major exports, and severe damage to the economic activities. Therefore, we now expect the Sub-Saharan Region economic growth rate this year will be contracted by 1.6 percent."[4]

Abebe Aemro Selassie made few suggestions for the Sub-Saharan Africa as follows:

First, make every effort to increase public health expenditure to control the epidemic. Second, substantial and timely support is essential, including cash transfers or physical support for vulnerable families, including informal workers, and targeted temporary support for the hardest hit areas. The ability of countries in sub-Saharan Africa to respond appropriately will depend to a large extent on their access to preferential funding from the international community. Third, monetary and financial policies can also play an important role in maintaining companies and employment. To support these domestic measures, the coordinated efforts of all development partners will be key. The IMF will provide approximately $11 billion in funding to the 32 sub-Saharan countries that have requested assistance in recent weeks and has already provided funds to Burkina Faso, Chad, Gabon, Ghana, Madagascar, Niger, Rwanda, Senegal and Togo.[5]

On the basic health infrastructure of Africa, few studies suggest the situation in the continent is much more fragile. Denis Chopera, Africa Health Research Institute underlines that Africa is already plagued by HIV–AIDS and tuberculosis, and diabetes is in the process of spreading in Africa, and therefore, these existing diseases may seriously threaten the health of people infected with new coronavirus. Sub-Saharan Africa inhibits about 27.5 million approximately 70 percent of people living with HIV worldwide and also, around 25 percent of tuberculosis patients in the globe. According to the WHO, in 2018, 93 percent of an estimated 228 million cases of malaria worldwide are in Africa. Although, it should be a reasonable assumption that patients infected with HIV and/or tuberculosis are at greater risk of being infected with the Coronavirus and also the case fatality rate is higher among these group of people. However, so far, the rate of spread of the Coronavirus is slower in the areas seriously plagued with HIV and tuberculosis.[6]

On April 2, 2020, Wang Xiaochun, senior consultant at the African Center for Disease Control and Prevention (CDC) pointed out, "In the beginning, most African countries reported COVID-19 confirmed cases were imported, but recently more and more countries in Africa are at a stage of community-transmitted, and there is a trend of potential coronavirus pandemic in the region." He added, "As of 9:30

a.m. on April 2, 2020, Eastern Africa time, the number of confirmed cases in Africa reached 6,213, with 221 deaths, and the case fatality rate reached 3.56 percent." He highlights that among the 54 member countries in Africa, the five countries namely South Africa, Egypt, Algeria, Morocco, and Tunisia are the most affected, accounting for 64 percent of the total reported cases across Africa. Except South Africa, the other four countries are located in northern Africa.[7] He further said, "Comparing the situation in Africa with that of Europe in the first 50 days after the first confirmed case report, we can see the total number of confirmed case increased significantly 30 days after the first report in Europe but in the case of Africa the growth rate of cases is much slower." He believes that measures taken by the African countries to prevent and control coronavirus were effective. Of the 54 member countries in Africa, 32 countries have completely closed their borders, 9 countries have closed international airports, and 5 countries have restricted travel to and from specific countries.[8]

He said, two temporary organisations have been established within the Africa CDC. One is the African Working Group on Coronavirus Response to carry out surveillance, nosocomial infection prevention and control, clinical management, laboratory diagnosis, risk communication, and supply chain and medical supplies procurement; the other is the Africa CDC emergency management system, which connects 54 AU member states and conduct regular communication every week.

Africa CDC have developed detailed plans for working in three areas: Preventing the spread of Coronavirus; preventing deaths caused by Coronavirus; and preventing social unrest and harm caused by the Coronavirus. By early April 2020, 43 countries in Africa were facilitated to carry out testing and diagnosis of the Coronavirus.

Tedros Adhanom, WHO Director-General on Africa Day May 25 2020 at the WHO media briefings on COVID-19 said, Africa is least-affected region globally in terms of number of COVID-19 confirmed cases and deaths, and so far, the continent has just 1.5 percent of the world's reported cases of COVID-19, and less than 0.1 percent of the total deaths. He said, Africa CDC and WHO are working together to provide COVID-19 detection training for the African laboratory technicians and to build up the national capacity across the region.[9] He reports that at present, 48 African countries have a community engagement plan in place, and 51 countries have lab-testing capacity for COVID-19. The WHO has shipped millions of personal protective equipment (PPE) and lab testing kits to 52 African countries. He also raised his concerns on the gaps and vulnerabilities in the continent that only 19 percent of countries in the region have an infection prevention and control programme, and standards for water, sanitation and hygiene in health facilities.[10]

Higherlife Foundation co-founder Strive Masiyiwa along with philanthropists

Sir Richard Branson and Jeff Skoll have come together to expedite the availability of critical medical equipment, including ventilators and breathing support devices in Africa.[11] In late May 2020, Masiyiwa was appointed as an AU Special Envoy to mobilise the private sector response to COVID-19 pandemic in Africa. Their initial plan is to start the production of 1,000 bridge ventilators, which will be offered to the healthcare facilities at a lower price than standard ventilators. Strive Masiyiwa said: "We have found a major South African company called Invicta Holdings that can mass produce these bridge ventilators and oxygen helmets. Any country that wants them can buy them at cost from that company. This is a not-for-profit venture for us as philanthropists."[12] Therefore, Africa is largely dependent on international communities and organisations to effectively fight against COVID-19.

China's Health Care Development and Medical Assistance to Africa

Since the 1960s, health care development and medical assistance have been one of the main successful areas of cooperation between China and Africa. From the early 1960s to 2005, China have sent medical teams to 47 African countries and more than 15,000 Chinese doctors travelled to Africa and have treated more than 170 million patients. For the United Nations-backed Global Fund to Fight AIDS, Tuberculosis and Malaria, in 2007, China approved $1.1 billion, of which 66 percent was dedicated to Africa.[13] In June 2006, Chinese officials handed over a 150 bed modern hospital with a capacity to handle 400 patients to the government of the Democratic Republic of Congo (DRC).[14]

In the White Paper on China's Africa Policy 2006, then Chinese Foreign Minister Li Zhaoxing brought out renewed Chinese engagement with African health systems. This new Policy pledges to support African national efforts to enhance government capacity in areas of health, and major declarations made were, the Chinese financial assistance to African governments will be increased to support for national health system; enhancing the exchange of medical personnel and information between China and African nations; establishing resident medical teams in the region; building and improving health care facilities; and training domestic medical personnel.[15] It also included the investments on infectious diseases such as, HIV and malaria, and promises to increase exchanges focused on Chinese traditional medicine and emergency medical responses. The policy is based on parallel frameworks to China's Eight Principles of Foreign Aid formulated in 1964 and also with the political string of 'One China Policy' attached to it. China's foreign aid in the African health sector increased drastically after the implementation of it's Africa health diplomacy and the grant increased from US$ 1.54 billion in the period 2004-2008 to US$ 3.8 billion in 2009-2013. Larger percentage of the grant was invested in building health infrastructure, equipment and medicine supplies, and in sending Chinese medical teams to Africa.[16]

China's new roles and opportunities in Africa at the peak of the COVID-19 pandemic

On February 14, 2020, Egypt health ministry announced the first case in the country at the Cairo International Airport involving a Chinese national. This is also the first confirmed cases of COVID-19 in Africa. The patient was placed in quarantined isolation in hospital and the Egyptian authorities had notified the World Health Organisation (WHO).[17] The joint statement from Egypt's health and population ministries said the patient was not from Egypt and also did not revealed the nationality of the person as well as about his recent travel history.[18] On February 17, 2020, Algeria registered the first confirmed case of COVID-19 and the Ministry of Health, Population and Hospital Reform of Algeria reported to the WHO also indicated the patient's nationality as Italian.[19]

China pretends to have found new roles and responsibilities in Africa at the peak of the pandemic but in fact, it has certainly seems to be looking for new opportunities to replace other major donors or players in the continent and to further deepen the China-Africa relations at all levels, including people to people relations. With the escalation of the COVID-19 pandemic, most African nations including the AU have been expecting to get medical supplies from China, and China responded to their concerns on time with major initiatives to donate medical and other necessary supplies to Africa at various platforms. Other immediate cause for the Chinese government rapid response to the African countries was the ongoing efforts led by the United States and the West to blame China for the possible unleash of the Coronavirus and also for concealing the actual data and the nature of the outbreak in Wuhan. China uses multiple channels to provide the necessary medical supplies and equipment to Africa.

Government Level Initiatives

Soon after, the emergence of COVID-19 cases in Africa, the Chinese government top leaders as well as the other leaders/ officials responsible for the Chinese diplomacy to African countries ramped up their efforts to communicate with the African leaders/officials through various diplomatic channels. President Xi Jinping had telephonic conversations with few Heads of African countries and Foreign Minister Wang Yi calls on phone to most of the African countries' Foreign Ministers. On May 18, 2020, Xi Jinping's speech at the World Health Assembly (WHA), in particular highlights the fragile health situations Africa and draws the attention of the world for greater support to the continent. On April 28, 2020, Wang Yi attended the extraordinary meetings of BRICS Foreign Ministers, where he highlighted about China's measures to support Africa in COVID-19 response and also, urged the WHO for greater support for the continent. On March 20, 2020, Wang Yi at the telephone conversation with Moroccan Minister of Foreign Affairs and International Cooperation Nasser Bourita said, China will donate essential medical supplies, share response experience and send medical expert teams to help countries affected by the disease.[20] On April 13, 2020, Wang Yi at phone conversation with Chairperson of the AU Commission Moussa Faki Mahamat said, China and Africa are comprehensive strategic and cooperative partners and therefore, must fight the pandemic together through closer coordination and cooperation. He underlines that China is sending much needed medical supplies to the AU and African countries through various channels. He said that China will provide more medical supplies and send medical expert teams to Africa. Faki underlines that Africa will not forget the support and assistance from China for Africa's national independence and liberation, fight against apartheid and economic and social development, and also expressed deep appreciation for China's emergency assistance to Africa's COVID-19 response. He ensured that Africa will always stand firmly with China.[21]

During the outbreak in China, there were cases of racial violence against the Africans in Guangdong, and therefore, in order to address the issue Assistant Foreign Minister Chen Xiaodong on 13 April 2020 conducted a group meeting with ambassadors and representatives from 20 African countries.[22] He stated that Africans will be treated in a fair, just and friendly manner and Foreign Ministry will stay in close contact with Guangdong to earnestly address the legitimate concerns of the African side.[23] On 18 April 2020, Xi Jinping congratulates Zimbabwean President Emmerson Mnangagwa on the 40th anniversary of the establishment of China-Zimbabwe diplomatic relations.[24] He pointed out that China and Zimbabwe have reached the important consensus on establishing and developing the comprehensive strategic cooperative partnership. He stated that the Chinese side stands ready to boost cooperation with the Zimbabwean side to overcome the ongoing challenges of the COVID-19 epidemic. Emmerson Mnangagwa responded by saying, Zimbabwe followed the One China policy and actively participates in the Belt and Road Initiative, and will continue to resolutely push for deeper development of the comprehensive strategic cooperative partnership between the two countries.[25] On April 17, 2020, Wang Yi spoke with Senegalese Foreign Minister Amadouba said, as FOCAC co-chairs, China will work with Senegal to follow through on the outcomes of the FOCAC Beijing Summit, with particular attention to China-Africa joint response to COVID-19.[26]

Amadou Ba conveyed appreciation for China's assistance to Senegal's epidemic response, and expressed hope and belief that China will continue to extend strong supports to Africa in its fight against COVID-19 pandemic.[27] On May 11, 2020, Wang Yi spoke by phone with Ethiopian Foreign Minister Gedu Andargachew and the Angolan Foreign Minister Tête António, and he said China will stand firm with Africa in the fight against COVID-19. He also pointed out that the attempts by some to blame China for their own ineffective response are set to be rejected and opposed by the international community, including African countries.[28] He expressed confidence that Angola and Ethiopia will guard against attempts to use virus as an excuse to discredit China or sow discord between China and Africa. He expected Africa to join China in giving staunch support to the WHO. Gedu reaffirmed Ethiopia's commitment to the One China Policy and its readiness to stand with China on the international stage.

On March 31, 2020, Premier Li Keqiang spoke with Algerian Prime Minister Abdelaziz Djerrad expressed the hope that Algeria will protect and provide the essential need of Chinese citizens there.[29] Djerrad expressed the hope for China's continued support in terms of containment supplies, equipment and medical treatment, and cherished the bilateral comprehensive strategic partnership.[30] On April 11, 2020, Wang Yi had telephone conversation with Mauritanian Foreign Minister Ismael Ould Chiekh Ahmed and underlined that two China aided projects in Mauritania, namely the renovation of China-Mauritania Friendship Hospital and the infectious and tropical diseases treatment center of Nouakchott National Hospital were delivered ahead of schedule. China will continue to support Mauritania and encourage Chinese companies and social groups to donate supplies.[31] On April 16 2020, Li Keqiang took a call from Sudanese Transitional Prime Minister Abdalla Hamdok, and Li said China will stand firmly with Sudan and provide support and help as best as they can. Li added that the Chinese people will work with people in Africa and the wider world in solidarity and partnership in this trying time to safeguard global public health security.[32]

On April 3, 2020, Xi Jinping in telephone conversation with Namibian President Hage Geingob said, China will step up assistance to Namibia and other African countries and will continue to share its experience in COVID-19 prevention and control with African countries and enhance health cooperation. He emphasised that the friendship between China and Namibia and the other African countries will be deepened in the fight against the outbreak. Hage Geingob thanked Chinese government for taking care of 500 Namibian students in China during the pandemic and for its aid and supports to African countries, and calls China the "best friend" of Namibia and Africa.[33] On May 15, 2020, Xi Jinping in telephone conversation with South African President Cyril Ramaphosa made the remarks that the international community to step up support for Africa's fight against the COVID-19 pandemic and actively participate in the initiative endorsed by the Group of 20 (G20) to suspend debt services payments for the world's poorest countries.[34] He assures the South African President all forms of medical support within China's capacity, and boost coordination on multilateral platforms such as BRICS, the G20 and the United Nations, so as to push for greater development of China-South Africa comprehensive strategic partnership and jointly safeguard the fundamental interests of the two and also other developing countries. Xi Jinping summarises China's medical support to African Union and African countries, and other actions taken to help Africa in their COVID-19 responses. He suggested for combating the disease in solidarity and jointly overcome the crisis, and also the two sides support the United Nations and the World Health Organisation (WHO) in playing their active roles in coordinating global anti-epidemic cooperation. Ramaphosa convinced and assured Xi Jinping that South Africa supports China's core interests and will work closely with China to safeguard the two countries' common interests.

According to China's National Health Commission, by April 7, 2020, more than 1,000 Chinese medical personnel working in Africa and the agency has directed them to help local health organisations stem the spread of the coronavirus. For instance, since March 2020, Chinese medical expert Jiang Yuandong in Zimbabwe trained more than 140 health workers and introduced China's experience in containing the outbreak. Kitojo Wetengere, a consultant professor of economic diplomacy and former lecturer with the Tanzania-Mozambique Center for Foreign Relations in Dar es Salaam said, "By sending medical experts and medical supplies to other countries to contain the COVID-19 pandemic, China has proved to be a friend in need."[35] On March 18, 2020, China at the video conference with 24 African countries and the African Union (AU) Center for Disease Control and Prevention expressed its commitment of sharing experience and supporting Africa in the fight against the epidemic.[36] According to Africa CDC, by March 18, 2020, the total number of coronavirus confirmed cases in 33 out of the 55 AU members were slightly above the 500. Dai Bing, Director-General of the Department of African Affairs of China's Foreign Ministry was chairing the video conference said, China will share its best experience with African countries as part of the Chinese commitment to supporting and assisting Africa in their response to the pandemic. After the videoconference, Ahmed E. Ogwell Ouma, Deputy Director of Africa CDC stated, Chinese government has placed its experience on the table for African countries to be able to see and use in the fight against the epidemic. He said convincingly that "The experience that China has undergone is very important for us, because our is just starting, while in China it is ending. That experience is very important." He revealed that Africa CDC is working very closely with China CDC to ensure that Africa CDC is better prepared to support countries in the region, and also to ensure that African countries are learning from China's experience. Few representatives from the African countries raised their concerns for the shortage of medical equipment in their countries, for instance, Isaac Phiri, Deputy Director for epidemiology and disease control in the Ministry of Health said, "We require personal protective equipment. That is one of the most important equipment that we need. We also need laboratory equipment, rapid test kits and the new medication that China is using." Kenya's Cabinet Secretary for Health Mutahi Kagwe said, "This is an extremely important step in terms of knowledge sharing and it gave us a tremendous amount of knowledge which we believe will also go a long way to assisting our people."[37]

On April 6, 2020, China's medical supplies for 18 countries in Central and West Africa arrived at Accra Airport in Ghana.[38] By April 6, 2020, Ghana had more than 9,000 COVID-19 confirmed cases with 400 deaths. Besides Ghana, the other beneficiary African countries are Nigeria, Senegal, Gabon, Sierra Leone, Guinea-Bissau, Guinea, Cote d'Ivoire, Gambia, Liberia, Mali, Burkina Faso, Republic of Congo, Equatorial Guinea, Togo, Benin, Cape Verde, and Sao Tome and Principe. This batch of crucial Chinese medical supplies include Personal Protective Equipment (PPEs), N95 face masks, medical protective suits, goggles, gloves, temporal artery thermometers, and ventilators. Wang Shiting, Chinese Ambassador to Ghana said, "This effort shows China's firm commitment to the China-Africa relations and further strengthen the strong historical bonds between China and Africa. Shirley Ayorkor Botchwey, Ghana's Minister for Foreign Affairs and Regional Integration, said the donation came at a crucial time when many of the beneficiary countries needed them most to curb the spread of the pandemic.[39] On April 23, 2020, another batch of China's medical supplies for 12 African countries arrives in Addis Ababa, Ethiopia.[40] Officials and Representatives from African Union (AU) and the Africa CDC attended the delivery ceremony held at the Ethiopian Airlines Cargo Terminal in Addis Ababa. Tan Jian, Chinese Ambassador to Ethiopia, present at the ceremony said, "A friend in need, is a friend indeed. The China-Africa cooperation in fighting COVID-19 is a telling testament to our friendship." This batch of the Chinese medical supplies include facial masks, disposable protective clothing, forehead thermometers, medical protective goggles, gloves and shoe covers for medical use. Beneficiary African countries of the Chinese donations are Angola, Cameroon, Central African Republic (CAR), Chad, Djibouti, Lesotho, Madagascar, Namibia, Niger, Rwanda, Somalia as well as Tanzania's Zanzibar. It is said that is the second batch of China's medical supplies to Ethiopia. According to Africa CDC, by April

23, 2020, the number of COVID-19 confirmed cases in Africa reached to 25,937 with 1,242 deaths. Dawit Yirga, Director General of Asia and Oceania Affairs at the Ethiopian Ministry of Foreign Affairs said, "Africa and China are all weather friends and the Sino-Africa strategic partnership has shown vitality and strength in this time of unprecedented challenges."[41]

Military Level Initiatives

On May 8, 2020, medical experts from China's People's Liberation Army (PLA) and their South African counterparts held a video conference to share experience of combating COVID-19.[42] During the video conference, valuable experiences on subjects such as Treatment of COVID-19 patients, Analysis of Important Cases, Management and Control of COVID-19 in Hospitals, and COVID-19 Testing Technology and Methods, etc. were shared by seven Chinese military medical experts and officers from the Medical services Directorate of the Logistics Support Department of the Central Military Commission. They also discussed about the vaccine development, asymptomatic patients examination, anti- COVID-19 medication, the usage and sensitivity of the testing kits, disinfecting materials, etc. with experts from South African National Defence Force (SANDF).[43] From June 2-5, 2020, PLA sent medical supplies to 20 countries including the five African countries such as Ethiopia, Mozambique, Tunisia, Angola, Egypt etc.[44]

Since 2008, PLA began participating in UN led escort operations in the Gulf of Aden and East Africa to safeguard their commercial ships against the piracy. With the growing Chinese investments and strong presence of Chinese citizens and companies in Africa, the Chinese military presence is also increasing in the continent such as PLA soldiers participating in UN led peacekeeping operations, disaster relief operations and in various naval escort missions. On September 28, 2015, Xi Jinping delivered a speech at the 70th Session of the United Nations General Assembly. Xi announced that China has decided to establish a 10-year, US$ 1 billion China-UN peace and development fund to support the UN's work and promote the multilateral cooperation cause. China will join the new UN peacekeeping capability readiness system, take the lead to set up a permanent peacekeeping police squad and build an 8,000 strong standby peacekeeping force. He also said that China will provide US$ 100 million of free military assistance to the African Union in the next five years to support the establishment of the African Standby Force and the African Capacity for Immediate Response to Crisis.[45] On August 1, 2017, PLA officially open it's first overseas Support Base in Djibouti, which is operated by PLA Navy. On September 22, 2017, PLA conducted the first live fire exercises at the base. In May 2018, China began constructing a large-scale pier of over 330 meters in length at the base. The presence of the Chinese base has created geopolitical tensions in the area with the other traditional players such as the US, Japan and France. Incidents of military confrontations are reported between China and the traditional players for instance, in 2018, the US Department of Defense issued a NOTAM reporting instances of laser attacks against pilots flying near the base.[46] Many experts now anticipate more Chinese bases in the years to come. Recent developments show the base includes personnel from various branches such as marines and Special Forces. In May 2020, it has also built a 660-metre-long pier, where large and heavier PLA ships will soon be able to moor. It is said that the base also has underground cyber and electronic warfare facilities.[47] PLA Navy troop training in Djibouti aim to enhance combat capability and prepare for counter-terrorism operations and possible evacuations of overseas Chinese nationals.

On July 15, 2019, the first China-Africa and Security Forum kicked off in Beijing, and it was attended by 100 senior representatives from the defense departments of 50 African countries and the African Union, including 15 defense ministers and chiefs of general staff, to discuss new approaches of China-Africa security cooperation in the new era.[48] Major General Song Yanchao, Deputy Director of the Office for International Military Cooperation of China's Ministry of National Defense said, "In face of new situations, the common languages, aspirations and interests of China and Africa in peace and security field have been increasing. Closer cooperation between the two sides is embracing new precious historical opportunities." Hamed Bakayoko, Defense Minister of Cote d'Ivoire said he hopes the forum will help strengthen China-Africa cooperation in peace and security, so that the two sides will jointly safeguard in Africa and the world.[49] On July 17, 2019, State Councillor and Minister of National Defense Wei Fenghe said at the Forum, China and Africa should make new progress in peace and security cooperation and contribute to the development of China-Africa comprehensive strategic and cooperative partnership.[50] Arms sale to Africa is a key issue on the agenda because in recent years, China is a major arms supplier to Africa. According to Cobus van Staden of the South African Institute of International Affairs, China is the second largest arms supplier to the continent. According to Stockholm International Peace Research Institute, from 2013 to 2017, China's arms exports to Africa surged 55 percent from the previous five-year period of 2008 to 2012.[51] Over the same period, China's share of total African arms imports rose 8.6 percent to 17 percent. According to United Nation Register of Conventional Arms (UNROCA), China exported 24 battle tanks to Tanzania and 30 to Chad in 2013. Since 2007, China exports Armoured combat vehicles to African countries, for instance, in 2009, Ghana and Namibia imported 76 and 21 respectively, and Kenya imported 32 in 2007. Other buyers in the continent are Rwanda, Burundi, Mozambique, Chad and Gabon.[52] JF-17 single-engine jet was developed jointly by the Pakistan Aeronautical Complex and the Chengdu Aircraft Corporation of China. In March 2020, Air Marshal Sadiq Abubakar, Chief of Air Staff of the Nigerian Air Force (NAF) announced that the NAF will receive its three JF-17 Thunder multi-role fighters in November 2020. In March 2019, Pakistan Economic Coordination Committee (ECC) approved the sale of three JF-17s to Nigeria at the price of US$184 million.[53] In March 2020, Morocco receives delivery of a number of WS 2D Multiple Rocket Launchers from China. Launched in 2004, the WS-2 is manufactured by China National Precision Machinery Corporation (CPMIEC).[54] On April 8, 2020, the Nigerian Army (NA) bought 17 military vehicles consisting of VT-4 main battle tank (MBT), ST-1 wheeled tank destroyer and two types of self-propelled howitzers from the China North Industries Corporation (NORINCO). Lieutenant General Lamidi Adeosun, NA Chief of Policy and Plans (CPPLANS) said that Nigeria and the NORINCO signed a package contract in 2019.[55]

So, PLA has two long terms goals in Africa, one is to provide security for its investments, infrastructures, companies and nearly 1 million Chinese nationals living in the continent. Prior to 2017, the presence of PLA troops in the continent were in the form of UN Peacekeepers but today, about 10,000 marine corps and special forces with combat readiness and capability are deployed in Africa. Second, bilateral military engagements will provide greater scope for China's arms sale to the African country. China's arms market in Africa is growing rapidly, which will certainly boost its defense industry.

Jack Ma Foundation Initiatives

Jack Ma has long term business goals in Africa and he finds the crisis of COVID-19 in Africa as an opportunity to expand the Alibaba Group in the continent. On January 10, 2020, Jack Ma said, "Today's Africa is the China of 20 years ago!" and by relying on the digital revolution, it is possible to turn Africa into a global hub. Jack Ma visited Kenya and Rwanda in 2017 as Special Advisor to the United Nations Conference on Trade and Development, and he found that most young Africans are primarily looking for stable, salaried employment in sectors such as banking, energy or mining rather than to be an entrepreneur. He also figures out that Africa is ripe for radical transformation. He said, digital revolution has the potential to bring tremendous prosperity to the continent, provided it has the entrepreneurs and businesses capable of carrying it out. On the inadequacy of African infrastructure, he said, in this new world, heavy infrastructure is of little use.[56] He believed that Africa can do even better than China, and the lack of infrastructure is an asset there. Africa has the advantage of its 1.3 billion inhabitants, 40% of whom are under 16 years old. Six of the ten fastest growing economies in the world are in Africa, and the number of smartphones per capita is growing rapidly. After his first trip to Africa in 2017, Jack Ma created the Africa Netpreneur Prize Initiative (ANPI) aims to support the next generation of African entrepreneurs. In its inaugural year 2019, nearly 10,000 entrepreneurs from 50 African countries applied for ANPI. The Jack Ma Foundation has committed to running the competition for 10 years. In 2019, the prize money of US$ 1 million was distributed among the top 10 entrepreneurs in Africa.[57]

The top three finalists were:

- Temie Giwa-Tubosun, founder and CEO, LifeBank (Nigeria) – First Place, winning $250,000
- Dr. Omar Sakr, founder and CEO, Nawah-Scientific (Egypt) – Second Place, winning $150,000
- Christelle Kwizera, founder, Water Access Rwanda (Rwanda) – Third Place, winning $100,000

Jack Ma explores new channels and platforms to interact with the African governments at the peak of the pandemic. Jack Ma and Alibaba Foundations' medical supplies donations to all 54 African countries will have far reaching impacts on his business expansions in the continent.

On March 29, 2020, a press release issued by Jack Ma Foundation and Alibaba Foundation and the Prime Minister of Ethiopia, Abiy Ahmed, committed to provide medical supplies and medical equipment to each of the 54 countries in Africa.[58] Medical supplies such as 20,000 test kits, 100,000 face masks, 1,000 sets of protective clothing, and 1,100 sets of protective shields will be donated directly to the governments in each of the 54 African countries. Respective governments are responsible for arranging collection and distribution of the equipment. On March 22, 2020, the first flight of 100 MT of medical supplies arrived in Addis Ababa on Ethiopian Airlines. Ethiopian Airlines is responsible for providing cargo facilities of the donated medical supplies to the rest of the African countries. The Ethiopian Federal Ministry of Health and the African Union CDC are providing technical guidelines and diplomatic linkages with the African countries.

On April 8, 2020, second batches of COVID-19 donations from Jack Ma Foundation and Alibaba Foundation arrive in Africa. This medical supplies was distributed to all the 54 African countries.[59] On April 6, 2020, the Jack Ma Foundation and Alibaba Foundation said in a statement "Batches of medical supplies for Africa are en route with 500 ventilators, 200,000 suits and face shields, 2,000 thermometers, a million swabs and extraction kits, and 500,000 gloves." It also said, they are connecting African medical professionals with doctors from China and around the world to collaborate online and exchanges experiences in the treatment and prevention of the COVID-19.[60] On April 14, 2020, among the first United Nations "Solidarity Flight" donations, a large quantity of personal protective equipment donated by the Jack Ma Foundation and Alibaba Foundation to all countries in Africa.[61]

Table: 18.1: 1st Batch of Jack Ma Medical Supplies Donations to Africa

Date	*No. of Countries*	*Jack Ma Donations to the African countries*
March 23, 2020	2	Sudan, Ethiopia
March 24, 2020	13	Djibouti, Somalia, Tanzania, South Sudan, Uganda, Rwanda, Burundi, Kenya, Nigeria (Lagos), Zimbabwe, Zambia, South Africa, Togo
March 25, 2020	8	Comoros, DRC, Gabon, Ghana, Madagascar, Malawi, Mauritius, Seychelles
March 26, 2020	8	Mozambique, Cameroon, Angola, Equatorial Guinea, Eswatini, Lesotho, Botswana, Namibia
March 27, 2020	10	Sierra Leone, Algeria, Chad, Liberia, Guinea Bissau, Guinea, Tunisia, Cote D'Ivoire, Cape Verde, Mali
March 28, 2020	8	Burkina Faso, Mauritania, Gambia, Senegal, Republic of Congo, Sao Tome, Niger, Benin
March 29, 2020	1	Central Africa Republic

Sources: WFP WHO.

On April 27, 2020, the Africa CDC received the third round of medical equipment and supplies donated by the Jack Ma and Alibaba foundations at the Addis Ababa airport. The medical supplies includes 406 million masks, 500,000 swabs and test kits, 300 ventilators, 200,000 sets of protective clothing, 200,000 face shields, 2,000 temperature guns, 100 body temperature scanners, and 500,000 pairs of gloves. On the donations, AU Commission Chairperson Moussa Faki Mahamat said, "These vital supplies will enhance the Africa CDC's strategic stockpile to assist member states in the COVID-19 fight." Ahmed Ogwell, Deputy Director of Africa CDC said that "this is a partnership that works. The Africa CDC values friends of Africa." On April 28, 2020, the Jack Ma Foundation along with Africa CDC organised a special webinar entitled "Global MediXChange for Combating COVID-19 (GMCC): The Experience of China".

Loans Moratorium for the indebted African nations

According to Deborah Drautigam (2019), from 2000-2017, the Chinese government, banks and contractors signed US$ 146 billion in loan commitments to African countries and their SOEs. Angola is the top recipient of Chinese loan, with US$ 43 billion over 17 years. Angola, Zambia, Sudan and the Republic of Congo (Brazzaville) are among those seeking debt relief, arguing they need to reallocate funds to health care and equipping hospitals to fight the coronavirus.[62] Oil producers such as Angola, Nigeria, the Republic of Congo, Equatorial Guinea and South Sudan are hit hard due to plunge in oil prices. Tourism dependent countries such as Seychelles and Mauritius face recessions, while Zambia, Botswana, the Democratic Republic of Congo, South Africa and Zimbabwe suffers due to drop in demand for commodities they produce.

In early June 2020, Linda Calabrese – research fellow and development economist at the Overseas Development Institute in London explains the impact of COVID-19 on African countries' debt vis-à-vis China. Linda says, the African countries will face health as well as economic challenge: Many African countries are burdened by their debt, which they are paying back what they borrowed and therefore, have very little room to divert these resources towards more pressing health and economic needs. China is the largest bilateral creditor to Africa and it is estimated that the Chinese government banks and SOEs are estimated to hold 17 percent to 24 percent of Africa's external debt.[63] Linda said that Zambia and Djibouti owe most of their debt to China. Many African countries have also borrowed from other bilateral, multilaterals or the private sector and therefore, countries such as Ethiopia, Nigeria, and Kenya spend more money to pay back private creditors than the Chinese government and policy banks. The Chinese government support debt service relief for the poorest countries by contributing to the IMF's Catastrophe Containment and Relief Trust. Moreover, as part of the G-20, China took part to the eight-month debt moratorium (payment suspension) agreed for poor countries. Generally, China do not use the multilateral initiatives for providing debt-relief, and the Chinese Ministry of Foreign Affairs said that they are "keeping in contact" with poor countries bilaterally on debt issue, but so far, no initiative have been taken by China. Based on China's past total debt portfolio, Linda speculates that relief of Chinese debt will be limited, and that further suspensions of payment or some form of restructuring are more likely outcomes. In last few decades, China's lending to low-income countries has increased dramatically and the renewed interest that the US and the UK have shown towards Africa in the last few years is partly due to their fear that China will replace them in their traditional sphere of influence.[64] On April 7, 2020, Chinese foreign ministry on the debt relief for Africa said, "The origin of Africa's debt problem is complex, and the debt profile of each country varies. We are aware that some countries and international organisations have called for debt relief programmes for African countries, and we are willing to study the possibility of it jointly with the international community."[65] In early April 2020, Ghanaian Foreign Minister and Economist Ken Ofori-Atta said to the Washington based Center for Global Development, "my feeling is that China has to come on stronger, and I think our Africa debt to China is over US$ 145 billion, about US$ 8 billion in payments required this year." In May 2020, Yun Sun, a fellow with the Africa Growth Initiative at the Brookings Institution in Washington, said Beijing was unlikely to take a unilateral approach to debt forgiveness. Sun added, "rather than outright relief, postponement of loan payments, debt restructuring, and debt/equity swap are more likely in China's playbook." On June 17, 2020, Xi Jinping at the extraordinary China-Africa Summit said, China will exempt some African countries from repaying zero-interest rate loans due at the end of 2020.[66] He also said, under the framework of the China-Africa cooperation forum, China will further extend loan payment forbearance for some countries including African countries.

Conclusion

Undoubtedly, China has long term goals in Africa and therefore, it has immediate urgency to take care of Africa. For instance, China's medical supplies and other forms of assistance to the continent were ramped up soon after US President Donald J Trump called Coronavirus as the 'Chinese virus'. China lab origin theory about the Coronavirus forced the Chinese leadership at all levels to increase their communications with all diplomatic partners in order to discredit the theory. During these telephone conversations between the Chinese and the counterpart leaders, China's assurance of medical supplies and assistance to the other side was compulsions as well as an opportunity. At the peak the pandemic, China commits for free aid and assistance to Africa countries is its compulsion because Chinese government generally avoids donations or free aid. Most of the beneficiary countries of Chinese donated medical supplies in Africa expressed their immediate support for China against the forces propagating China lab origin theory. China's proactive attitude to help countries across the globe with crucial medical supplies helped to overcome the blames and narrative of unleash of virus from the Wuhan lab. The opportunity to depict as a responsible major power was smartly used by the Chinese government. China used multiple channels to help African countries in their COVID-19 response such as, government to government, people to people, military to military, Chinese companies' initiative etc. China enjoys reliable bilateral relations with most of the African countries but there is serious anti-China feeling among the Africans and local companies. There are regular cases of racial violence against the Chinese citizens as well as entrepreneurs in the continent. In early June 2020, three Chinese factory bosses were murdered and burnt in Zambia, where there are 80,000 Chinese national lives. The killings of Chinese citizens in Zambia also occurred in 2006 and 2010. African resentment is due to China's growing presence in the continent. Most of the Chinese embassies in Africa were proactive since March 2020 to facilitate the Chinese citizens in distributing medical supplies and food in several countries in Africa. For instance, in early May, Chinese communities distributed packed meat and fish to Africans living in Hong Ning Chinese Aged Home in Johannesburg. In April 2020, during the lockdown a local farm run by the Chinese distributed vegetable to the African living in that area in South Africa. On May 27, 2020, local Chinese communities donated 100,000 face masks to the Health Bureau of Johannesburg Municipal. Similarly, apart from Jack Ma other companies such as Huawei, TikTok provided medical supplies to African countries. These donations of medical supplies by Chinese communities and companies will help in developing people to people relations between Chinese and African. Africans are in dire need of these crucial medical supplies and therefore, they cannot reject or boycott these Chinese donations. Larger goals of the Chinese government depend on expansion of Chinese companies and stronger presence of the Chinese communities in the Continent. Very few countries such as South Africa maintain military to military exchanges with China. So, the channel of PLA and SANDF was also used to train the South African military personnel as front-line worker in the pandemic. Based on the saying 'Friend in need is a friend indeed', Chinese is actively working to develop closer ties with Africa at all levels.

In the post-COVID-19 world order, China-Africa relations might gain further momentum as we saw, none of the government in Africa credited the China lab origin theory. Most of the African governments reiterated their position of all-weather friends of China. Africa finds a special priority in China's foreign policy and most African government understand its significance. China is also one among the other traditional players in Africa, who has political and economic interests, but there is a higher degree of reliability in China-Africa bilateral relations. At present, both sides also enjoy greater coordination and cooperation, and quick response for each other's call. China has not stopped it's BRI projects in Africa, which might have affected due to the pandemic but once the virus is contained, the projects will gain it's momentum. Both sides government is looking forward to overcome the disease and resume the projects with the same momentum as it was. Therefore, it doesn't seem that the bilateral relations will be affected due to the pandemic.

NOTES

1 Coronavirus Africa news summary: cases and deaths" DIARIO AS April 30, 2020 at https://en.as.com/en/2020/04/30/other_sports/1588268567_267942.html

2 "10,000 Cases And 500 Deaths In Africa. Health Officials Say It's Just The Beginning" *National Public Radio*, April 8, 2020 at https://www.npr.org/sections/coronavirus-live-updates/2020/04/08/830209940/10-000-cases-and-500-deaths-in-africa-health-officials-say-its-just-the-beginnin

3 2019 冠状病毒病疫情：非洲病例破万 [Coronavirus disease outbreak in 2019: African cases break ten thousand] April 8, 2020 at https://news.un.org/zh/story/2020/04/1054502

4 Ibid.

5 2019 冠状病毒病大流行——对非洲发展的空前威胁 [Coronavirus pandemic-an unprecedented threat to Africa's development] April 10, 2020 at https://news.un.org/zh/story/2020/04/1055102

6 非洲能否承受 2019 年冠状病毒疫情? [Can Africa withstand the 2019 coronavirus epidemic?] March 24, 2020 at https://www.project-syndicate.org/commentary/africa-covid19-advantages-disadvantages-by-denis-chopera-2020-03-2020-03/chinese

7 确诊病例超 7000、蔓延至 50 多国，非洲情况不容乐观 [The number of diagnosed cases exceeds 7000 and spread to more than 50 countries. The situation in Africa is not optimistic] April 5, 2020 at https://zh.al-ain.com/article/africa-corona-virus-pandemic

8 Ibid.

9 "WHO Director-General's opening remarks at the media briefing on COVID-19," *WHO*, 25 May, 2020 at https://www.who.int/dg/speeches/detail/who-director-general-s-opening-remarks-at-the-media-briefing-on-Covid-19—25-may-2020

10 Ibid.

11 "Covid-19: Philanthropists to manufacture medical equipment in Africa," *VERDICT*, May 28, 2020 at https://www.medicaldevice-network.com/news/philanthropists-medical-equipment-africa/

12 Ibid.

13 "COVID-19 Pandemic in Africa" at https://en.wikipedia.org/wiki/Africa%E2%80%93China_relations

14 "China hands over hospital to DR Congo," *Xinhua*, June 2, 2006 at https://reliefweb.int/report/democratic-republic-congo/china-hands-over-hospital-dr-congo

15 "Chinese Global Health Diplomacy in Africa: Opportunities and Challenges," *National Center for Biotechnology Information*, October 1, 2019 at https://www.ncbi.nlm.nih.gov/pmc/articles/PMC6447313/#:~:text=Chinese%20health%20diplomacy%20also%20helped,the% 20legitimate %20 government %20of%20 China.&text= While%20Wes tern%20donors%20 often %20provided,%2C%20equipment%2C%20and%20logistical%20support.

16 Ibid.

17 COVID-19 pandemic in Egypt at https://en.wikipedia.org/wiki/COVID-19_pandemic_in _Egypt

18 "Africa confirms first case of coronavirus," *Duowei*, February 15, 2020 at https://www.dw.com/en/africa-confirms-first-case-of-coronavirus/a-52384446

19 "A second COVID-19 case is confirmed in Africa," *Afro WHO,* 25 February 2020 at https://www.afro.who.int/news/second-covid-19-case-confirmed-africa

20 "State Councillor and Foreign Minister Wang Yi Had Phone Calls with Foreign Ministers of Hungary, Greece and Morocco," *Ministry of Foreign Affairs*, March 20, 2020 at https://www.fmprc.gov.cn/mfa_eng/zxxx_662805/t1759148.shtml

21 "Wang Yi: Rock-solid China-Africa Friendship Will Not Be Affected by Isolated Incidents" *Ministry of Foreign Affairs*, April 13, 2020 at https://www.fmprc.gov.cn/mfa_eng/wjb_663304/zzjg_663340/fzs_663828/xwlb_663830/t1769661.shtml

22 "MFA: Assistant Minister Chen Xiaodong Meets with African Diplomatic Envoys to China" *Ministry of Foreign Affairs*, April 13, 2020 at https://www.fmprc.gov.cn/mfa_eng/wjb_663304/zzjg_663340/fzs_663828/xwlb_663830/t1769665.shtml

23 Ibid.

24 "Xi Jinping and Zimbabwean President Emmerson Mnangagwa Exchange Congratulatory Messages on the 40th Anniversary of the Establishment of China-Zimbabwe Diplomatic Relations," *Ministry of Foreign Affairs*, April 18, 2020 at https://www.fmprc.gov.cn/mfa_eng/wjb_663304/zzjg_663340/fzs_663828/xwlb_663830/t1771806.shtml

25 Ibid.

26 "Wang Yi Speaks with Senegalese Foreign Minister Amadou Ba on the Phone," *Ministry of Foreign Affairs*, April 18, 2020 at https://www.fmprc.gov.cn/mfa_eng/wjb_663304/zzjg_663340/fzs_663828/xwlb_663830/t1771190.shtml

27 Ibid.

28 "Wang Yi Spoke by Phone with Ethiopian Foreign Minister Gedu Andargachew," *Ministry of Foreign Affairs*, May 12, 2020 at https://www.fmprc.gov.cn/mfa_eng/wjb_663304/zzjg_663340/fzs_663828/xwlb_663830/t1778391.shtml

29 "Premier Li Keqiang Talks by Phone with Algerian Prime Minister Abdelaziz Djerrad," *Ministry of Foreign Affairs*, March 31, 2020 at https://www.fmprc.gov.cn/mfa_eng/wjb_663304/zzjg_663340/xybfs_663590/xwlb_663592/t1764847.shtml

30 Ibid.

31 "Wang Yi Speaks by Phone with Mauritanian Foreign Minister Ismael Ould Cheikh Ahmed" *Ministry of Foreign Affairs*, April 11, 2020 at https://www.fmprc.gov.cn/mfa_eng/wjb_663304/zzjg_663340/xybfs_663590/xwlb_663592/t1768577.shtml

32 "Premier Li Keqiang Speaks by Phone with Sudanese Transitional Prime Minister Abdalla Hamdok," *Ministry of Foreign Affairs*, April 16, 2020 at https://www.fmprc.gov.cn/mfa_eng/wjb_663304/zzjg_663340/xybfs_663590/xwlb_663592/t1770813.shtml

33 "Xi Jinping: China to continue COVID-19 support for Namibia, Laos," *CGTN*, April 5, 2020 at https://news.cgtn.com/news/2020-04-03/Xi-Jinping-holds-phone-talks-with-Namibia-s-President-Hage-Geingob-PogrH779iE/index.html

34 "Xi calls for more international support for Africa's COVID-19 fight," *Xinhua*, May 16, 2020 at http://www.xinhuanet.com/english/2020-05/16/c_139060522.htm

35 "Xinhua Headlines: From factories in east China to hospitals across Africa, Chinese help boosts confidence in COVID-19 fight," *Xinhua*, April 7, 2020 at http://www.xinhuanet.com/english/2020-04/07/c_138954932.htm

36 "Africans hail China's efforts in curbing COVID-19, keen to learn its experience," *Xinhua*, March 19, 2020 at http://www.xinhuanet.com/english/2020-03/19/c_138892667_2.htm

37 Ibid.

38 "China sends medical supplies to 18 African countries," *CGTN*, April 7, 2020 at https://newsaf.cgtn.com/news/2020-04-07/China-delivers-37-6-tons-of-medical-supplies-to-Ghana-PtMR3Oy3iE/index.html

39 Ibid.

40 "Africa welcomes latest Chinese donation of medical supplies to fight COVID-19," *Xinhua,* April 24, 2020 at http://www.xinhuanet.com/english/2020-04/24/c_139005359.htm

41 Ibid.

42 "Chinese military medical experts share experience of combating COVID-19 with S. African counterparts," *Xinhua*, May 9, 2020 at http://www.xinhuanet.com/english/2020-05/09/c_139043823.htm

43 Ibid.

44 "PLA sends anti-virus supplies to militaries of 20 countries," *Xinhua*, June 5, 2020 at http://www.xinhuanet.com/english/2020-06/05/c_139117131.htm

45 中国国家主席习近平联大一般性辩论发言：以史为鉴才能避免重蹈覆辙 [Chinese President Xi Jinping's speech at the UN General Assembly: Use history as a mirror to avoid repeating the mistakes] United Nations September 28, 2015 at https://news.un.org/zh/story/2015/09/243472

46 "Chinese People's Liberation Army Support Base in Djibouti" Wikipedia at https://en.wikipedia.org/wiki/Chinese_People%27s_Liberation_Army_Support_Base_in_ Djibouti #:~:text= The %20Chinese%20People's%20Liberation%20Army,cost%20of%20US% 24590%20million

47 "China's Djibouti naval base increasing its power," *East Asia Forum*, May 16, 2020 at https://www.eastasiaforum.org/2020/05/16/chinas-djibouti-naval-base-increasing-its-power/

48 "Feature: Overview of 1st China-Africa Peace and Security Forum," *China Military Online*, July 17, 2019 at http://eng.mod.gov.cn/news/2019-07/17/content_4846012.htm

49 "1st China-Africa peace, security forum opens in Beijing," *Xinhua*, July 15, 2019 at http://www.xinhuanet.com/english/2019-07/15/c_138228749.htm

50 "State councillor meets representatives from China-Africa peace, security forum," *Xinhua*, July 18, 2019 at http://english.www.gov.cn/statecouncil/weifenghe/201907/18/content_WS5d2fe17cc6d00d362f66872c.html

51 "Everything you need to know about the weapons China sells to Africa," *South China Morning Post*, 8 July, 2018 at https://www.scmp.com/news/china/diplomacy-defence/article/2154189/everything-you-need-know-about-weapons-china-sells

52 Ibid.

53 "Nigeria will take Delivery of Jf-17 Fighters in November 2020," *Quwa Defence News & Analysis*, March 1, 2020 at https://quwa.org/2020/03/01/nigeria-will-take-delivery-of-jf-17-fighters-in-november-2020/#:~:text=The%20Nigerian%20Air%20Force's% 20(NAF, role%20 fighters%20 in%20November%202020.

54 "Morocco apparently operating Chinese multiple rocket launchers," *defenseWeb*, March 13, 2018 at https://www.defenceweb.co.za/land/land-land/morocco-apparently-operating-chinese-multiple-rocket-launchers/

55 "China-made VT-4 MBT delivered to Nigeria," *China Military Online*, April 4, 2020 at http://eng.chinamil.com.cn/view/2020-04/10/content_9789120.htm

56 Jack Ma: "Today's Africa is the China of 20 years ago!," *Africa Report*, January 10, 2020 https://www.theafricareport.com/22056/jack-ma-todays-africa-is-the-china-of-20-years-ago/#:~:text=The%20barriers%20that%20slow%20down,Africa%20into%20a%20global%20hub.

57 "$1 Million Awarded to African Entrepreneurs in Grand Finale of the Jack Ma Foundation Africa Netpreneur Prize Initiative," *Businesswire*, November 17 2020 at https://www.business wire.com/news/home/20191117005049/en/1-Million-Awarded-African-Entrepreneurs-Grand-Finale

58 "PM Abiy, Jack Ma Foundation and Alibaba Foundation Initiative to Reverse COVID-19 from Africa," *Reliefweb*, March 29 2020 at https://reliefweb.int/sites/reliefweb.int/files/resources/Update%20%236%20Reverse%20COVID-19%20%2829%20March% 202020%29.pdf

59 "Jack Ma Foundation, Alibaba Foundation make second round of COVID-19 donations to Africa," *Xinhua*, April 8, 2020 http://www.xinhuanet.com/english/2020-04/08/c_138958284. htm

60 Ibid.

61 "Factsheet: Jack Ma Foundation and Alibaba Foundation's Global Donations and Efforts to Combat COVID-19," *Alizila*, April 15, 2020 at https://www.alizila.com/factsheet-jack-ma-foundation-alibaba-foundations-coronavirus-donations-and-efforts/

62 "Africa has a question for Beijing: will you forgive us our debt?," *South China Morning Post*, May 7, 2020 at https://www.scmp.com/news/china/diplomacy/article/3082832/africa-has-question-beijing-will-you-forgive-us-our-debt

63 "COVID-19: The Impact on China-Africa Debt Insights from Linda Calabrese," *The Diplomat,* June 02, 2020 at https://thediplomat.com/2020/06/Covid-19-the-impact-on-china-africa-debt/

64 Ibid.

65 "China in the driver's seat amid calls for Africa debt relief," *The Economic Times,* April 13, 20 at https://economictimes.indiatimes.com/news/international/business/china-in-the-drivers-seat-amid-calls-for-africa-debt-relief/articleshow/75118832.cms?from=mdr

66 "China will exempt some African countries from repaying certain loans," *Reuter,* June 17, 2020 at https://www.reuters.com/article/health-coronavirus-china-africa/china-will-exempt-some-african-countries-from-repaying-certain-loans-idUSL4N2DU37W

ANNEXURE

Charts

Effect of COVID-19 on Environment

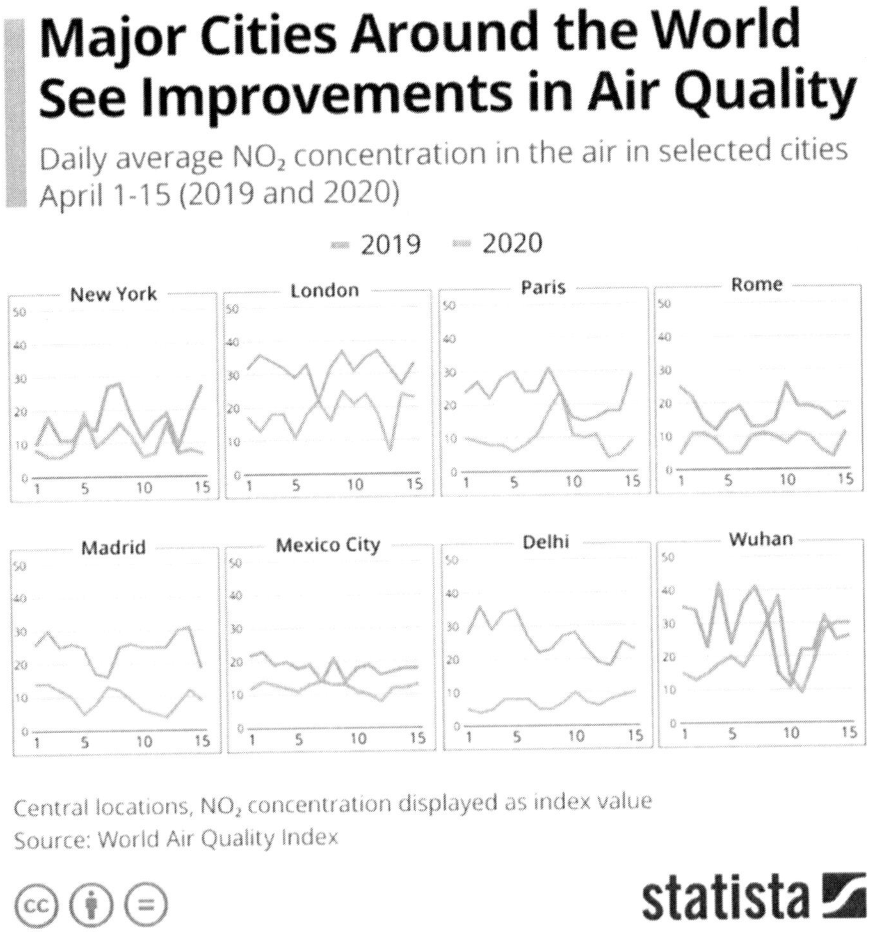

Source: https://www.weforum.org/agenda/2020/05/coronaviris-covid-19-air-quality-cities-lockdown/

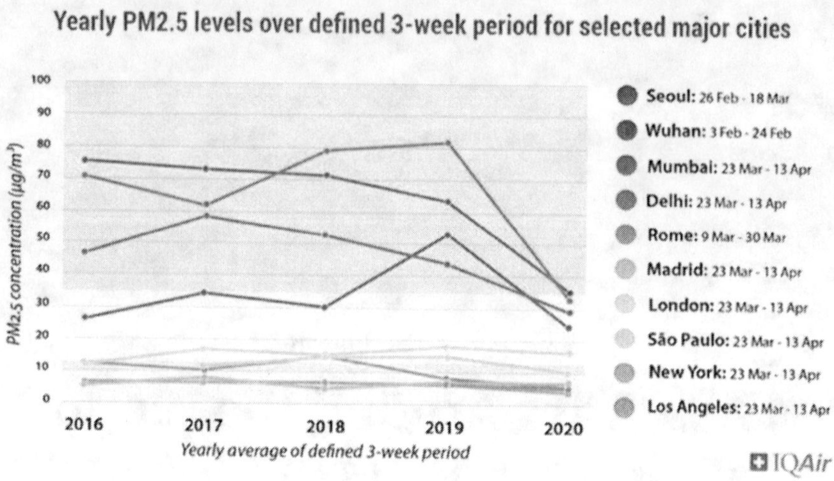

Source: https://www.eco-business.com/news/how-the-coronavirus-pandemic-is-changing-people-and-our-planet/

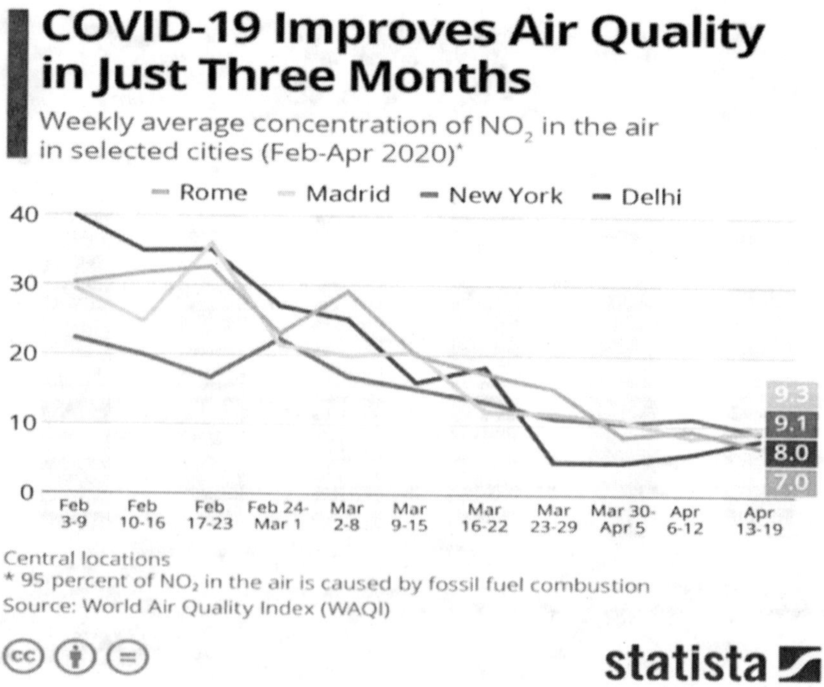

Source: https://www.statista.com/chart/21495/no2-in-the-air-selected-cities/

Energy prices Down Due to Covid-19

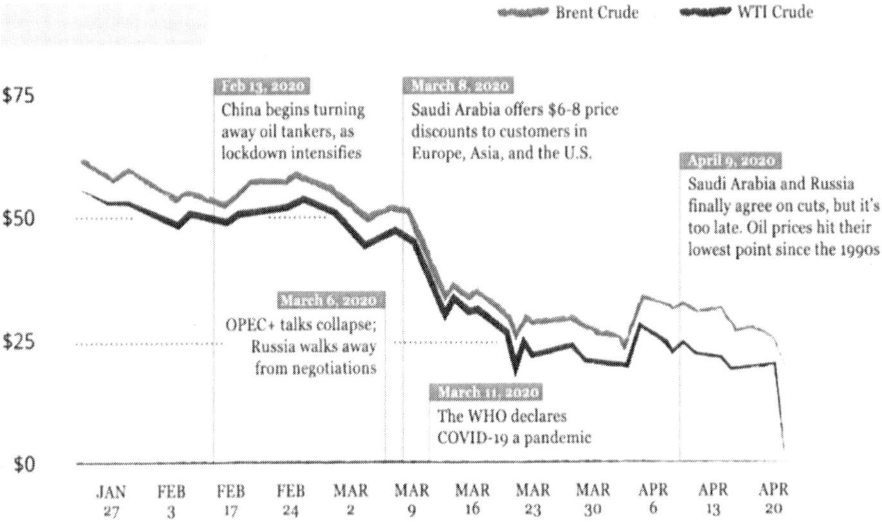

Source: https://www.visualcapitalist.com/subzero-oil-price-crash-covid-19/

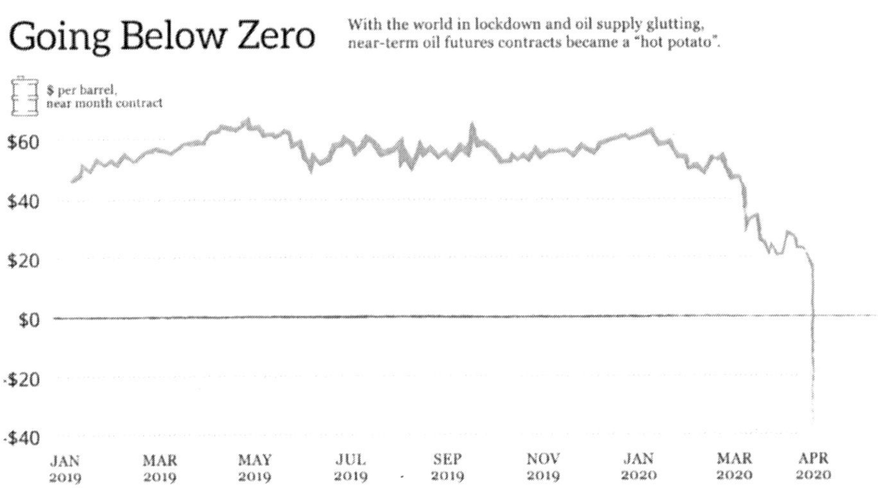

Source: https://www.visualcapitalist.com/subzero-oil-price-crash-covid-19/

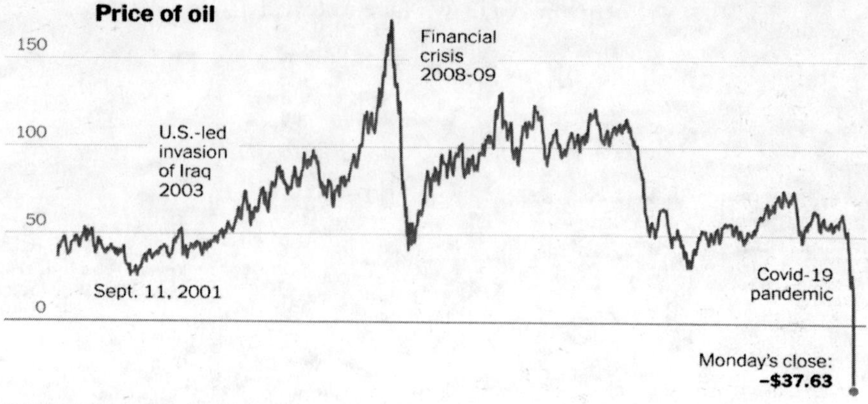

Source: https://www.google.com/search?sxsrf=ALeKk00wqZGw8MRlV4gNt9p4eU7yVbsMCg :1595346185596&source=univ&tbm=isch&q=effect+of+COVID-19+on+energy+prices+-+chart&sa=X&ved= 2ah UKEwjinb7V197qAhWNA3IKHSTWCaQQsAR6 BAg KEAE & biw=1517&bih =730#imgrc=g1Rw_RpUSdahKM

Impact of Covid-19 on Healthcare

Epidemics and Pandemics since Middle ages

Starting year	Event	Geographic extent	Estimated direct morbidity or mortality	Estimated economic, social, or political impact
1347	Bubonic plague (Black Death)	Eurasia	30–50% mortality of the European population	Likely hastened end of the feudal system in Europe
Early 1500s	Introduction of smallpox	Americas	More than 50% mortality in some communities	Destroyed native societies, facilitating the hegemony of European countries
1881	Fifth cholera pandemic	Global	More than 1.5 million deaths (9.7 per 10,000 persons)	Sparked attacks on Russian tsarist government and medical officials
1918	Spanish flu influenza pandemic	Global	20 million–100 million deaths (111–555 deaths per 10,000 persons)	GDP loss of 3% in Australia, 15% in Canada, 17% in the United Kingdom, 11% in the
1957	Asian flu influenza pandemic	Global	0.7 million–1.5 million deaths (2.4–5.1 deaths per 10,000 persons)	GDP loss of 3% in Canada, Japan, the United Kingdom, and the United States
1968	Hong Kong flu influenza pandemic	Global	1 million deaths (2.8 deaths per 10,000 persons)	$23 billion–$26 billion direct and indirect costs in the United States
1981	HIV/AIDS pandemic	Global	More than 70 million infections, 36.7 million deaths	2–4% annual loss of GDP growth in Africa
2003	SARS pandemic	4 continents, 37 countries	8,098 possible cases, 744 deaths	GDP loss of $4 billion in Hong Kong SAR, China; $3 billion–$6 billion in Canada; and $5 billion in Singapore
2009	Swine flu influenza pandemic	Global	151,700–575,500 deaths (0.2–0.8 per 10,000 persons)	GDP loss of $1 billion in the Republic of Korea
2012	MERS epidemic	22 countries	1,879 symptomatic cases, 659 deaths	$2 billion loss in the Republic of Korea, triggering $14 billion in government stimulus spending
2013	West Africa Ebola virus epidemic	10 countries	28,646 cases, 11,323 deaths	$2 billion loss in Guinea, Liberia, and Sierra Leone
2015	Zika virus pandemic	76 countries	2,656 reported cases of microcephaly or CNS malformation	$7 billion - $18 billion loss in Latin America and the Caribbean

Adapted from: Patel, V., D. Chisholm., T. Dua, R. Laxminarayan, and M. E. Medina-Mora, editors. 2015. Mental, Neurological, and Substance Use Disorders. Disease Control Priorities, third edition, volume 4. Washington, DC: World Bank

Source: https://www.expresspharma.in/guest-blogs/long-term-impact-of-covid-19-pandemic-on-healthcare-scenario-in-india/

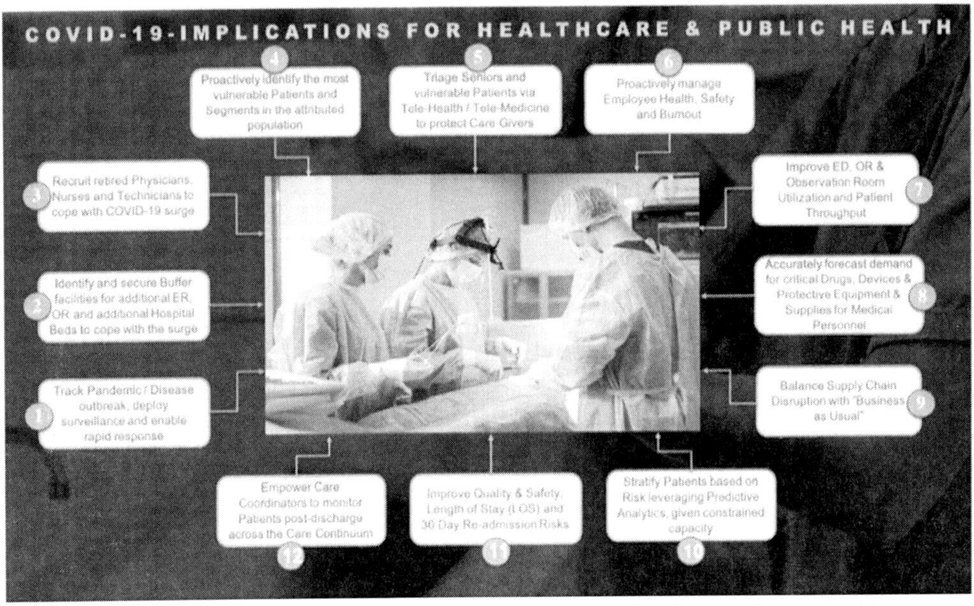

Source: https://www.alteryx.com/input/covid-19-and-its-impact-on-healthcare-and-public-health

Stocks Decline Amidst COVID-19

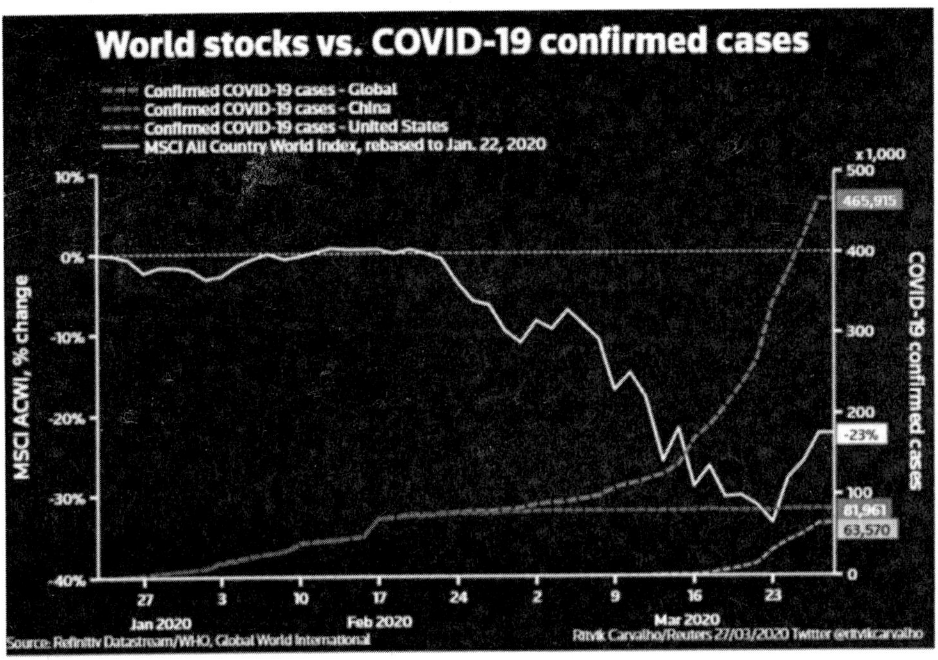

Source: https://www.weforum.org/agenda/2020/03/take-five-quarter-life-crisis/

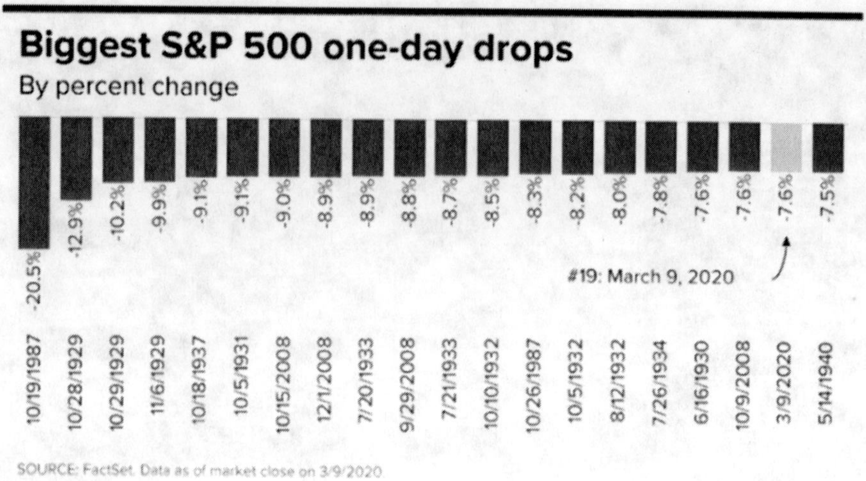

Source: https://www.cnbc.com/2020/03/08/dow-futures-drop-700-points-as-all-out-oil-price-war-adds-to-coronavirus-stress.html

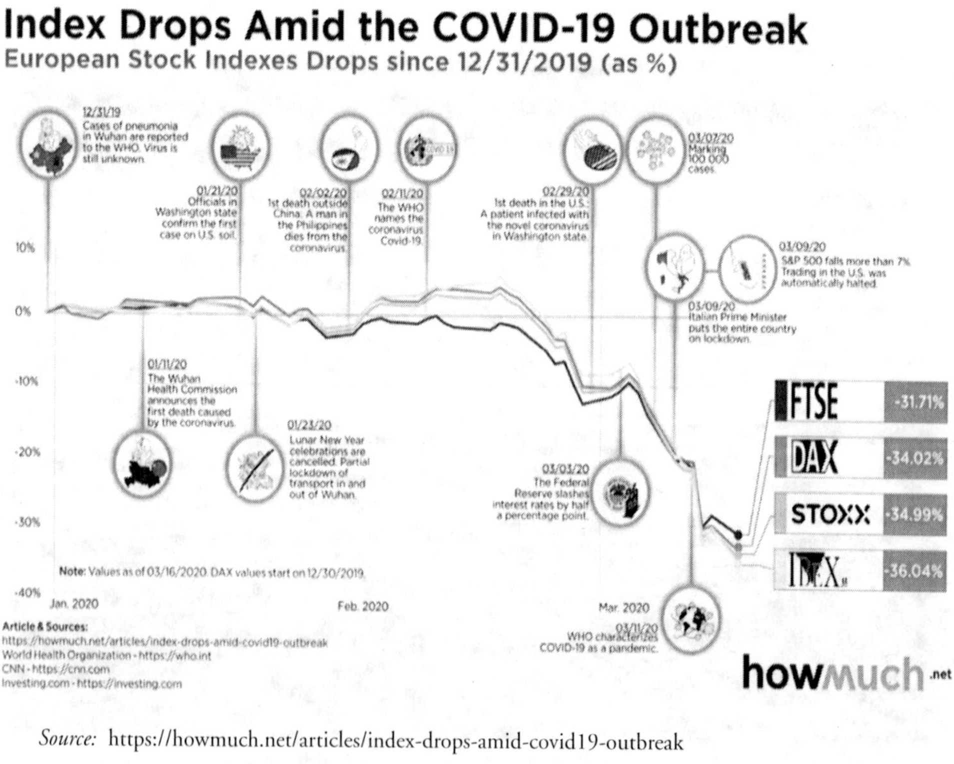

Source: https://howmuch.net/articles/index-drops-amid-covid19-outbreak

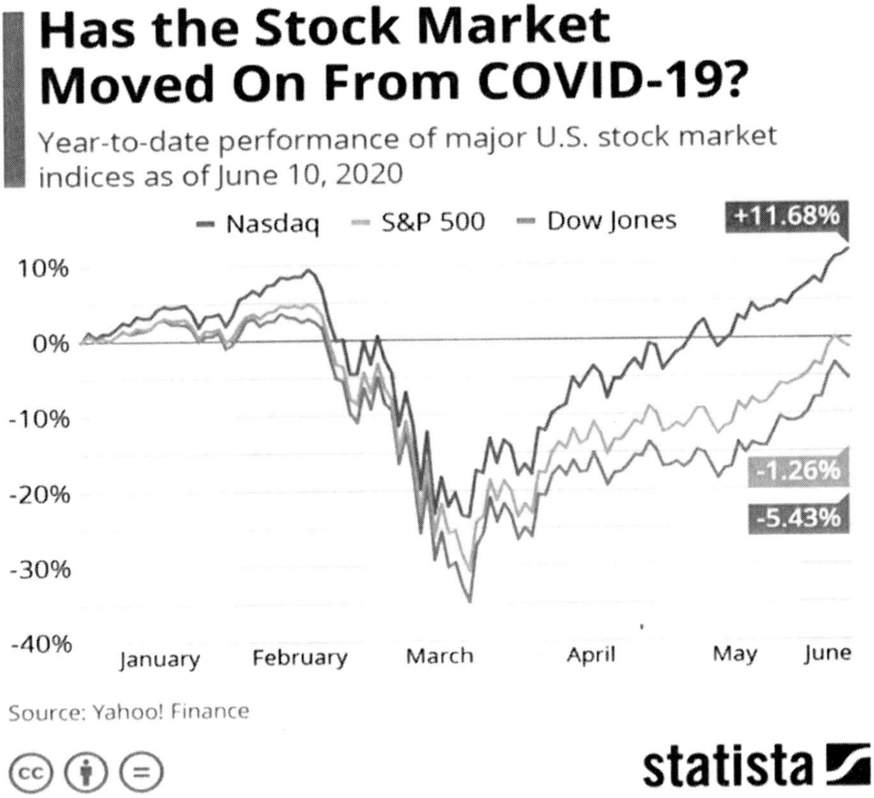

Source: https://www.statista.com/chart/20939/year-to-date-performance-of-major-us-stock-market-indices/

Aviation Industry Down Due to Covid-19

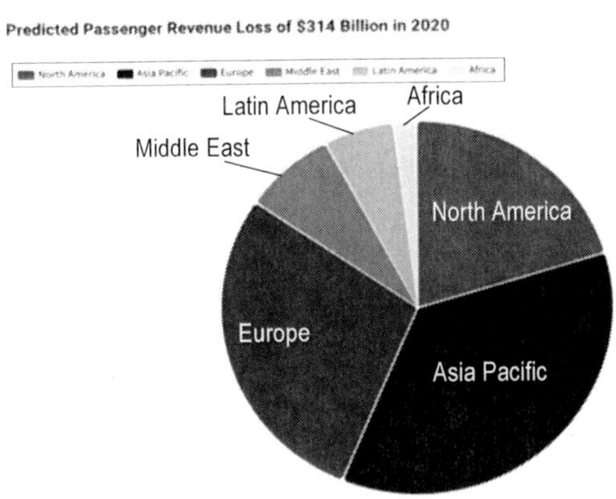

Source: https://www.smartertravel.com/how-hard-covid-hit-air-travel/

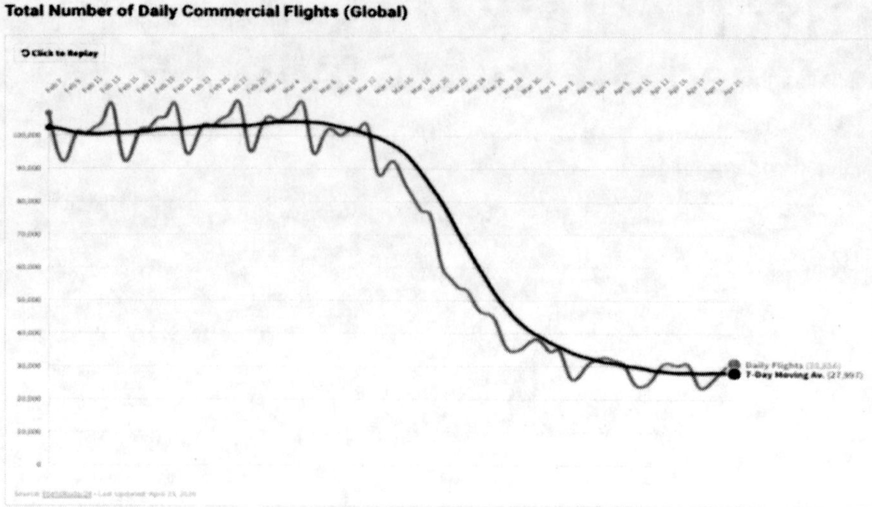

Source: https://www.smartertravel.com/how-hard-covid-hit-air-travel/

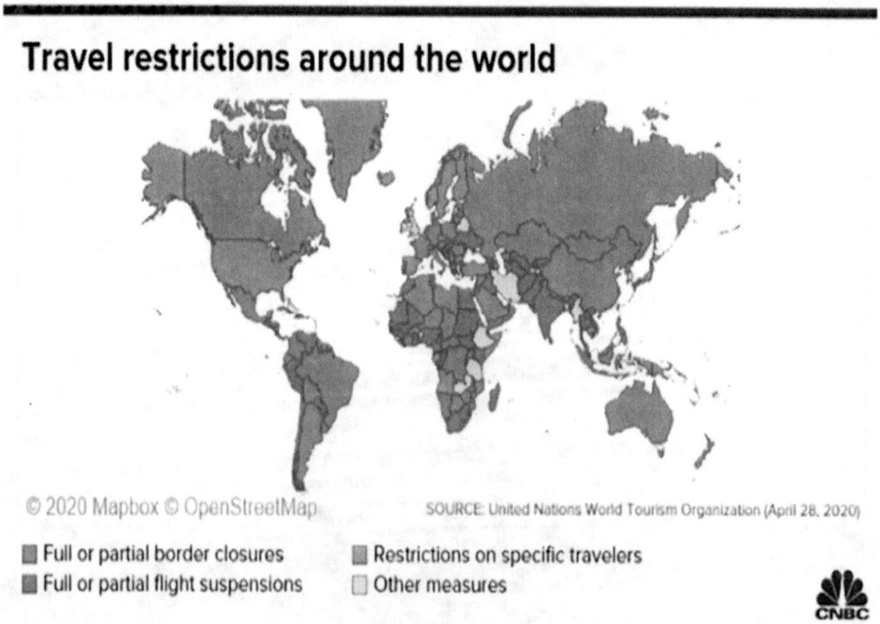

Source: https://www.cnbc.com/2020/05/06/coronavirus-pandemics-impact-on-travel-tourism-in-5-charts.html

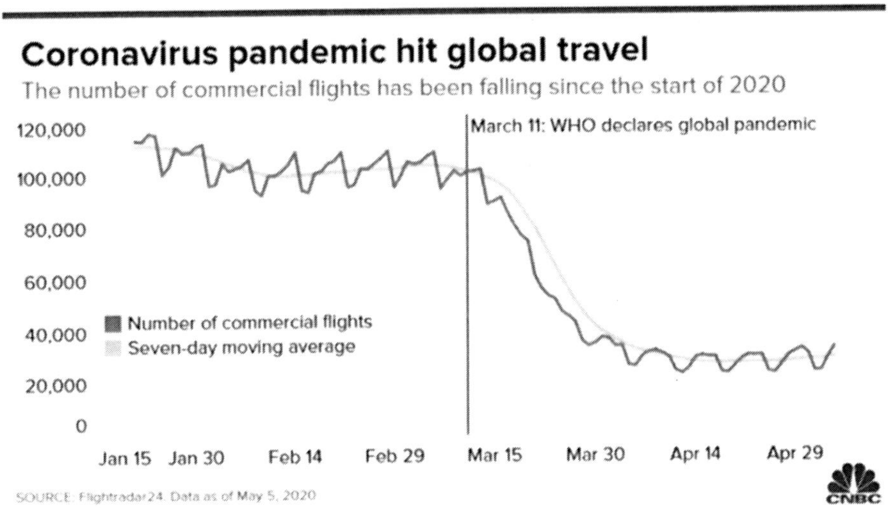

Source: https://www.cnbc.com/2020/05/06/coronavirus-pandemics-impact-on-travel-tourism-in-5-charts.html

Spread of Covid-19 Cases Across the World

Sr No	*Country*	*31 January, 2020*	*29 February, 2020*	*31 March, 2020*	*30 April, 2020*	*31 May, 2020*	*30 June 2020*	*15 July, 2020*
1.	China	9,720	79,389	82,545	84,373	84,570	85,227	85,677
2.	USA	7	62	140,640	1,003,974	1,734,040	2,537,636	3,344,783
3.	Australia	9	25	4,557	6,746	7,185	7,767	10,251
4.	India	1	3	1,251	33,050	182,143	566,840	936,181
5.	Pakistan	0	4	1,865	16,117	69,496	209,337	255,769
6.	Afghanistan	0	1	166	2,171	15,094	31,238	34,940
7.	Bangladesh	0	0	49	7,667	47,153	141,801	190,057
8.	Sri Lanka	1	1	122	649	1,630	2,042	2,665
9.	Maldives	0	0	17	396	1,672	2,337	2,801
10.	Russian Federation	2	2	1,837	106,498	405,843	647,849	746,369
11.	Austria	0	10	9,618	15,364	16,638	17,666	19,060
12.	Denmark	0	3	2,577	9,008	11,633	12,751	13,061
13.	Hungary	0	0	447	2,775	3,867	4,145	4,263
14.	Malta	0	0	156	463	616	670	674
15.	Slovenia	0	0	763	1,418	1,473	1,585	1,859
16.	Belgium	0	1	15,301	49,741	58,592	61,427	62,781
17.	Estonia	0	1	715	1,666	1,865	1,987	2,015
18.	Ireland	0	0	2,910	20,253	24,929	25,462	25,670
19.	Netherlands	0	6	11,750	38,802	46,257	50,223	51,091
20.	Spain	0	32	85,195	216,476	238,415	248,452	256,619
21.	Bulgaria	0	0	359	1,447	2,513	4,831	7,645
22.	Finland	1	2	1,313	4,906	6,826	7,209	7,293
23.	Italy	2	1,128	101,739	203,591	232,664	240,436	243,344
24.	Poland	0	0	2,055	12,640	23,571	34,154	38,457
25.	Sweden	1	13	4,028	20,302	37,113	67,667	76,001
26.	Croatia	0	7	790	2,062	2,246	2,725	3,827
27.	France	6	100	43,977	127,066	148,436	156,930	162,390
28.	Latvia	0	0	376	849	1,065	1,117	1,178
29.	Portugal	0	0	6,408	24,505	32,203	41,912	47,051
30.	Cyrus	0	0	231	843	943	996	1,022
31.	Germany	7	57	61,913	159,119	181,482	194,259	199,726
32.	Lithuania	2	2	1,837	106,498	405,843	647,849	746,369
33.	Romania	0	3	1,952	11,978	19,133	26,582	33,585
34.	Czechia	0	0	3,002	7,579	9,230	11,805	13,341
35.	Greece	0	3	1,212	2,576	2,915	3,390	3,883
36.	Luxembourg	0	0	1,988	3,769	4,016	4,256	5,056
37.	Slovakia	0	0	336	1,391	1,521	1,665	1,908
38.	Myanmar	0	0	14	150	224	299	337
39.	Thailand	19	42	1,651	2,954	3,081	3,171	3,232
40.	Laos	0	0	9	19	19	19	19
41.	Cambodia	1	1	107	122	125	141	165
42.	Vietnam	5	16	203	270	328	355	373
43.	Singapore	16	102	879	15,641	34,366	43,661	46,630

Sr No	Country	31 January, 2020	29 February, 2020	31 March, 2020	30 April, 2020	31 May, 2020	30 June 2020	15 July, 2020
44.	Malaysia	8	24	2,626	5,945	7,762	8,637	8,729
45.	Indonesia	0	0	1,528	10,118	26,473	55,092	78,572
46.	Philippines	1	3	1,546	8,212	18,086	36,438	57,545
47.	Brunei Darussalam	0	0	127	138	141	141	141
48.	Cuba	0	0	170	1,467	2,025	2,340	2,432
49.	Chile	0	0	2,449	14,885	94,858	275,999	319,493
50.	Peru	0	0	852	31,190	148,285	279,419	330,123
51.	Mexico	0	2	993	16,752	84,627	216,852	304,435
52.	Argentina	0	0	820	4201	14,702	59,993	103,265
53.	Guyana	0	0	8	75	150	230	300
54.	Jamaica	0	0	36	381	575	696	759
55.	Trinidad and Tobago	0	0	82	116	116	126	133
56.	Venezuela	0	0	129	329	1,370	5,297	9,707
57.	Brazil	0	1	4,256	71,886	465,166	1,344,143	1,884,967
58.	Suriname	0	0	8	10	12	492	780
59.	Barbados	0	0	33	80	92	97	103
60.	Ecuador	0	1	1,962	24,675	38,571	55,665	69,570
61.	Colombia	0	0	702	5,949	26,688	91,769	154,277
62.	Antigua and Barbuda	0	0	7	24	25	65	74
63.	Bolivia	0	0	97	1,053	8,731	31,524	49,250
64.	Grenada	0	0	9	19	23	23	23
65.	Uruguay	0	0	309	625	816	929	989
66.	Bahamas	0	0	14	80	101	104	113
67.	Dominica	0	0	11	16	16	18	18
68.	Costa Rica	0	0	314	705	1,022	3,130	8,036
69.	Panama	0	0	989	6,200	12,531	31,686	47,173
70.	Dominican Republic	0	0	901	6,652	16,908	31,816	46,305
71.	El Salvador	0	0	30	377	2,395	6,173	10,303
72.	Egypt	0	1	656	5,537	23,449	66,754	83,930
73.	South Africa	0	0	46	128	758	2,138	5,343
74.	Nigeria	0	1	111	1532	9855	25133	33616
75.	Ghana	0	0	152	1671	7768	17351	24,988
76.	Sudan	0	0	7	375	4800	9258	10417
77.	Congo	0	0	98	500	2965	6938	8134
78.	Cameroon	0	0	139	1,806	5659	12592	15173
79.	Algeria	0	1	511	3848	9267	13,571	20216
80.	Gabon	0	0	7	276	2613	5394	5942
81.	Djibouti	0	0	31	1089	3194	4659	4979
82.	Kenya	0	0	51	384	1888	6190	10,971
83.	Somalia	0	0	3	601	1916	2904	3076
84.	Ethiopia	0	0	23	130	1063	5846	8181
85.	Central African Republic	0	0	6	50	874	3613	4321
86.	Equatorial Guinea	0	0	14	315	1,043	1,043	1,043
87.	South Africa	0	0	1,326	5,350	30,967	144,264	298,292
88.	Guinea-Bissau	0	0	8	77	1256	1654	1902

Timeline of COVID-19

2019

Nov 9:	Wuhan Institute of Virology publish a study revealing they created a new virus in the lab from SARS-CoV.
Dec 6:	Five days after a man linked to Wuhan's seafood market presented pneumonia-like symptoms, his wife contracts it, suggesting human to human transmission.
Dec 8:	The first case of novel coronavirus was reported.
Dec 12:	The first patient affected by the novel coronavirus was hospitalised.
Dec 24-Feb 3:	In another study of 70 genomes of virus strains from China and other places a group of scholars – Li Xingguang and others suggested that COVID-19 did not originate from pangolins but was due to human-to-human transmission.
Dec 26-30:	Evidence of new virus emerges from Wuhan patient data.
Dec 27:	China's health authorities told a novel disease, then affecting some 180 patients, was caused by a new coronavirus. Vision Medicals, which constructed the genome structure of the new virus, found that it has similarities with the SARS, and shared the data with Wuhan officials and Chinese Academy of Medical Sciences, but it fell on deaf ears.
Dec 30:	The National Health Commission (NHC) observes the outbreak of a viral pneumonia in the city of Wuhan and sends out a national working group as well as a team of experts to advice and assist its containment and treatment. According to the Wuhan Municipal Health Commission, the first case was traced and confirmed on December 8, 2019.
Dec 31:	The Wuhan Municipal Health Commission testifies that the 27 cases of pneumonia in Wuhan were diagnosed as viral pneumonia, and all cases were identified to be linked to a local seafood market. The commission stated that patients noted symptoms of difficulty in breathing and fever. While authorities examined the hygiene condition of the market, every patient received quarantined medication. The World Health Organization China Country Office was notified.

Chinese internet authorities begin censoring terms from social media such as Wuhan Unknown Pneumonia.

Taiwan alerted the WHO about the possible human-to-human transmission of a SARS-like virus in Wuhan through an email to International Health Regulations (IHR).

Sensing the threat, Taiwan began to screen flights arriving from Wuhan.

2020

Jan 1: Authorities in Wuhan shut down the local Huanan Seafood Wholesale market.

The Chinese administration directs testing to end and samples to be demolished.

The government of the PRC publicly criticizes eight doctors on account of "rumour mongering" on national television.

Jan 2: The Chinese Center for Disease Control and Prevention (China CDC) and the Chinese Academy of Medical Sciences (CAMS) obtained the first set of samples of patients from the province of Hubei and initiated pathogen identification.

The NHC proposed a series of directives on early discovery, early diagnosis as well as early quarantine for the containment of the viral pneumonia.

Shi Zhengli the well-known scientist at the Wuhan Institute of Virology, reconstructed the entire genome structure of the new virus.

Jan 3: Dr. Li Wenliang denounced by local police in Wuhan for disseminating supposedly false statements regarding the outbreak online.

The Wuhan Municipal Health Commission revised information on its website regarding the state of the viral pneumonia, reporting the occurrence of as many as 44 cases of viral pneumonia.

China's top health authority issues a gag order.

Jan 4: The WHO, in its first public remark, tweeted, "China has reported to WHO a cluster of pneumonia cases – with no deaths – in Wuhan, Hubei Province".

Jan 5: Wuhan Municipal Health Commission stops releasing daily updates on new cases. Continues until January 18.

Laboratory test findings dismissed respiratory pathogens, namely influenza, adenovirus, avian influenza, the Middle East Respiratory Syndrome and Severe Acute Respiratory Syndrome, as the cause.

59 cases of COVID-19 were confirmed.

Feb 7: Visitors from Mainland China, Hong Kong and Macau were barred to enter Taiwan if they had a prior history of visit to these places within a span of 14 days.

Jan 8: An expert evaluation squad from the NHC identified the pathogen as a new coronavirus, which was the cause of the epidemic.

World's first case of COVID-19 outside China detected in a 61-year-old Chinese woman from Wuhan who landed at Bangkok's Suvarnabhumi Airport.

Jan 9: *Caixin* published two stories citing CCTV and the World Health Organisation (WHO) which for the first time mentioned about the possibility of the new infections being caused due to "an emerging type of coronavirus".

Jan 10: PRC official Wang Guangfa says outbreak "under control" and mostly a "mild condition".

Jan 11: In an official bulletin, the Wuhan Health Commission stated that no new cases have been detected since January 3, no human to-human transmission had taken place and that they diagnosed 41 cases of "unexplained viral pneumonia" patients mainly from the procurement section of the Huanan Seafood market.

Chinese state media broadcasted the first death due to the novel coronavirus of a 61 year old man who had gone to the live animal market in Wuhan city.

Jan 11-12: China's National Health Commission informed the WHO that the outbreak was associated with the Seafood Market at Wuhan, while it shared the genetic sequence of the virus with the WHO.

Jan 11-Feb 27: Hu Zixin and others from Shanghai and Houston based on the modified stacked auto-encoder (MAE) model and utilising artificial intelligence methods for real-time forecasting data argued that the COVID-19 epidemic would be over by April 2020.

Janu12: The Wuhan Municipal Health Commission for the first time, altered the name "viral pneumonia of unknown cause" to "pneumonia caused by the novel coronavirus", in a briefing.

Dr. Li Wenliang was hospitalized with syndrome of the novel coronavirus.

Professor Zhang Yongzhen's lab in Shanghai is closed by authorities for "rectification", one day after it shares genomic sequence data with the world for the first time.

Jan 13: Incubation period of 2019-nCoV was identified as fourteen days.

Ministry of Public Health, Thailand announced the first imported case of the novel coronavirus (2019-nCoV) from Wuhan city in China.

Jan 14: PRC National Health Commission chief Ma Xiaowei privately warns colleagues the virus is likely to develop into a major public health event.

Jan 15: Ministry of Health, Labour and Welfare, Japan (MHLW) announced an imported case of lab-confirmed 2019-nCoV from Wuhan city in China.

Jan 16: US announced passenger screening for those arriving in the country from Wuhan.

Jan 18: The Wuhan Health Commission declares four fresh cases of the virus, but plays down the danger of human-to-human transmission, permitting 40,000 families to congregate for a potluck dinner on the occasion of Lunar New Year.

Jan 19: Pulmonologist Zhong Nanshan revealed human-to-human spread.

Baibuting neighbourhood in Wuhan city celebrates Lunar New Year banquet.

Jan 20: National IHR Focal Point (NFP) for Republic of Korea announced the first case of 2019-nCoV in the Republic of Korea.

The PRC affirmed people-to-people transmission of the virus as well as cases of infection of the medical workers.

The NHC declared that it would adhere to containment measures exercised for Category A transmittable diseases. Pneumonia resulting from the 2019-nCoV was categorised as a Category B transmittable disease as well as quarantinable disease at the border.

Annual Spring Festival travel flow commenced in Hubei Province.

Jan 20-21: Experts from the China as well as the Western Pacific regional offices of the WHO carried out a brief field sojourn to Wuhan.

The CDC issued the travel advisory to Taiwanese citizens asking them to take necessary measures while travelling to Wuhan by raising the travel notice level for Wuhan to Level 2.

Jan 21: U.S Centres for Disease Control and Prevention (U.S. CDC) declared the first case of novel coronavirus in the U.S, in a patient who travelled back from Wuhan on January 15, 2020.

The local authorities gave permission to a gala to usher in the Year of the Golden Rat, which reveals them downplaying the outbreak.

The National Health Commission noted the detection of cases outside of Wuhan, including faraway places like Beijing,Shanghai, Hainan, Yunnan, Jilin and Guangdong provinces as well as in Thailand, Japan and South Korea.

The first positive case of COVID-19 was detected in Taiwan.

Xi's written instructions on 20th January to openly report the coronavirus related cases and prioritise the health and safety of people was reported prominently by the People's Daily.

Jan 22: The State Council Information Office hosted a press conference on the deterrence and containment of the epidemic, with Li Bin, Vice Minister of NHC, addressing the media.

Jan 23: Wuhan brought under quarantine.

The National Health Commission bulletin for the first time gave an elaborate clinical diagnosis of 17 patients who passed away succumbing to the virus.

First two cases of COVID-19 detected in Vietnam of Chinese nationals from Wuhan who had arrived on January 13 and travelled throughout Vietnam.

PLA's Su-30 and Y-8 aircraft flew to the Western Pacific through the Bashi Channel south of Taiwan.

Jan 24: Officials in Beijing prevent the Wuhan Institute of Virology from sharing sample isolates with the University of Texas.

President Trump praised Chinese efforts to tackle the disease in a tweet.

The Australian government levelled up the travel advice for visiting Wuhan to level four: "do not travel".

Jan 25: President Xi chaired a party meeting on the deterrence and containment of the novel coronavirus epidemic. In the meeting, fresh strategies for the medication of the patients were discussed.

Taiwan raised the warning level to 3 for the entire province of Hubei and 2 for the rest of Mainland China.

Australia reported its first case of COVID-19.

Jan 26: A week long Spring Festival break, supposed to end on January 30, was further extended till February 2, in order to contain the epidemic.

Jan 28: President Xi Jinping and WHO Director General Tedros Adhanom Ghebreyesus met in Beijing.

Taiwan raised the warning level to 3 for Mainland China.

Jan 29: Four Pakistani students tested positive for COVID-19 in China.

A Caixin report questioned the inevitable: "Was there a cover-up?" The content of the subhead made it amply evident, that there indeed was a cover up.

Jan 30: WHO announced "public-health emergency of international concern".

Two Chinese tested positive in Rome.

Russia was one of the first countries to close its border with China.

January 30, 2020 saw the first case in India in Kerala's Thrissur District.

Jan 31: The Trump government restricted travel from the PRC.

The number of infections in China are nearly five times the figures quoted by the Chinese side at 58,000 as against the official count of 12,000.

Feb 1: Member of CAS heads squad to assist Wuhan.

Vietnam cancelled all flights to China and sealed the 1,300-kilometre long international boundary.

Feb 2: The first case of novel coronavirus death reported outside the PRC in Philippines.

Philippines enforced a travel ban on tourists coming in from China, Macao and Hong Kong, as well as a fourteen day period of quarantine for residents of Philippine.

The US had banned entry to travellers from China and those with recent travel history to the country.

The official Chinese media highlighted that the CPC members were a "vanguard" against COVID-19.

Feb 3: WHO publishes the global community's Strategic Preparedness and Response Plan to assist in safeguarding states with fragile health systems.

China commences a clinical trial of Gilead Sciences' antiviral medicine remdesivir, formerly examined on patients with Ebola, and now against the novel coronavirus, soon after Huoshenshan hospital in Wuhan began operation. The hospital was constructed over a brief period of ten days and is devoted to treating novel coronavirus cases.

The Shanghai Stock Exchange plunges 8 percent, with its fallout reflected in global domains as well.

Russian Prime Minister Mikhail Mishustin said that foreigners testing positive would be sent back.

Feb 4: Hong Kong reported its first case of death of a patient due to novel coronavirus. The patient was a 39 year old man who had a travel history from Wuhan city of China.

Belgium announced its first case of novel coronavirus.

The CPC's Propaganda Department announced sending 300 journalists to ensure that the rhetoric regarding the control and prevention of COVID-19 remains under its control.

Feb 5: Diamond Princess cruise ship, docked in Yokohama, Japan quarantined thousands.

Diagnostic principles of 2019-nCoV expanded.

The Bill & Melinda Gates Foundation declared funding worth $100 million to back up the response as well as preparedness efforts vis-à-vis the 2019-nCoV epidemic.

Russia was the first country to send a delegation of five epidemic prevention experts team to help China in fighting the epidemic and for technical exchanges on epidemic prevention.

Feb 6: Japan declares its contribution worth $10 million to the WHO's novel coronavirus outbreak response fund to assist nations with fragile health systems as these countries get ready for the possible spread of the virus.

China's internet watchdog tightens controls on social media platforms.

The US' Centre for Disease Control and Prevention issued its first travel advisory for China, related to the spread of respiratory illness in Wuhan.

Feb 7: The Asian Development Bank approves of a fund worth $2 million to aid the response capacity endeavour against the novel coronavirus epidemic in the Asia Pacific region.

WHO announced that 28 nations in the African continent now possessed the competence to diagnose the virus – up from originally two.

The U.S vows a fund worth $100 million to the novel coronavirus response.

Dr. Li Wenliang, China's whistleblower doctor who tried to raise the alarm against the virus, died.

Feb 8: Criticising the height of misinformation at a press conference, WHO Director General Tedros Adhanom Ghebreyesus stated, "we're not just battling the virus; we're also battling the trolls and conspiracy theorists that push misinformation and undermine the outbreak response". Further, he said that WHO was making an endeavour to engage with social networking platforms such as Facebook, Twitter, Google, Baidu, TikTok, Tencent, Weibo and Pinterest to advance precise briefing about 2019-nCoV.

Five British nationals test positive for the 2019-nCoV at a ski camp in eastern France.

The State Council emphasised on the safety of workers and public health, although in the next two days partial onsite production activities in medical equipment manufacturing, energy, grain, transportation and logistics were encouraged.

The only working thermal scanner at Tribhuvan International Airport stopped working.

Feb 9: 3,187 medical workers sent to Hubei province of China.

Citizen-journalist and local businessman Fang Bin disappears.

The protection rate in Wuhan is lower till this date mostly due to the mixing of the susceptible to the infectious cases and that the infectious cases spreading to rest of China is far higher.

Russia sent 23 tonnes of medical assistance to China.

Feb 10: A team of experts for the WHO-led 2019-nCoV global mission depart for China.

The U.K.'s health department announced the novel coronavirus as an "imminent threat" to public health, permitting the administration to compulsorily quarantine individuals.

168 labs across the world now possess the competence to diagnose the 2019-nCoV.

19 provinces in China associate with 16 cities in Hubei province for help and support.

After his first public inspection of COVID-19, Xi called for a "people's war against novel coronavirus".

Feb 11: The WHO suggested an official name for the novel coronavirus: COVID-19, a short form of coronavirus disease 2019.

WHO Director General refers to the epidemic as a "very grave threat for the rest of the world".

Travel restriction was extended to foreigners even transiting through Mainland China, Hong Kong and Macau, and it was mandatory for anyone who visited China to self-quarantine for two weeks.

All Chinese newspapers led by Xinhua, CPC mouthpiece People's Daily and official broadcaster CCTV showed Xi wearing mask and inspecting a hospital in Beijing.

Feb 11-12: WHO organised the Research And Innovation Forum on the outbreak of the novel coronavirus. The forum was attended by over 400 experts as well as funders from across the world, and it comprised of presentations by George Gao, Director General of China CDC as well as Wu Zunyou, the chief epidemiologist of China CDC.

Feb 12: At the Politburo Standing Committee meeting Xi stated that "positive changes" occurred in tackling the COVID-19 cases due to "hard-won progress made by all sides".

Feb 13: The third case of death due to COVID-19 outside mainland China reported from Japan. The previous cases of death took place in Philippines and Hong Kong.

WHO stated that as many as 17 countries in the African continent now possessed the capability to examine for COVID-19. This was a clarification from the announcement made in February 7th, when WHO had claimed that 28 nations in the continent possessed the capacity for the same.

Feb 14: Wuhan requests the patients who have recovered from COVID-19 to donate plasma.

The first confirmed case of COVID-19 in the sub-Saharan Africa was diagnosed in Nigeria.

Egypt announced its first case of the novel coronavirus.

Feb 15: France confirms first death due to COVID-19.

Feb 16-24: The WHO-China Joint mission that comprises of Germany, Canada, Japan, Republic of Korea, Nigeria, Singapore, the US (CDC, NIH), Russia stayed at Beijing and also visited two other cities in China. They interacted with scientists, health officials as well as medical workers in various health facilities.

Feb 16: Taiwan confirms the country's first death due to COVID-19, indicating the fifth death owing to the virus outside mainland China.

Feb 17: Algeria registered the first confirmed case of COVID-19 and the Ministry of Health, Population and Hospital Reform of Algeria reported to the WHO that the patient's nationality as Italian.

Feb 18: A total of 92 COVID-19 cases documented in 12 nations across the world apart from the PRC in which people-to-people transmission of the novel coronavirus had occurred.

Liu Zhiming, director of the Wuchang Hospital in the city of Wuhan, passed away due to COVID-19.

Feb 19: Iran confirmed first case of COVID-19.

Feb 20: In two days, Iran confirmed five cases of COVID-19, of which two patients died. These were the first cases of death in the Middle East due to the novel coronavirus.

Peng Yinhua, a young respiratory doctor in the city of Wuhan, passed away due to COVID-19.

The first case of COVID-19 was reported in Lodi in north-western Italy.

Feb 21: More than 500 cases of novel coronavirus could be located in four prisons in the PRC.

Israel and Lebanon confirmed first cases of COVID-19 in their countries respectively.

Feb 23: Instances of COVID-19 in Italy witnessed an incessant rise in what could be identified as the biggest outbreak in a country away from Asia.

South Korean President Moon Jae-in declared the highest-level of alert in the country after the number of COVID-19 cases cross 340 in South Korea.

Feb 24: The PRC prohibited trade and intake of animals. It also delayed the annual parliamentary meeting.

European Commission declared a fresh aid package worth €232 million for global readiness as well as response to COVID-19.

With regard to the report of Russian authorities checking passport of Chinese citizens in public places and other measures, the Chinese embassy stated that Russian authorities should be moderate and non-discriminative against Chinese as only Chinese citizens were inspected.

The first case of COVID-19 in Afghanistan.

Feb 25: Algeria, Croatia, Switzerland and Austria confirm their first cases of COVID-19.

Feb 26: Brazil reports the country's first case of COVID-19, indicating the first such case in South America.

Georgia, Greece, Norway, Macedonia, Romania, Norway and Pakistan confirm their first cases of novel coronavirus.

The Asian Development sanctioned another $2million in order to aid countries in the Asia-Pacific to bolster their resilience and brace them to combat the COVID-19 well.

Feb 27: Denmark, San Marino, Estonia and the Netherlands confirm their first cases of COVID-19.

Feb 28: WHO raises the international risk of the proliferation of the virus from "high" to "very high".

New Zealand, Nigeria, Mexico, Belarus, Ireland, Azerbaijan, Lithuania as well as Iceland confirm their first cases of the virus.

Feb 29: China-WHO joint investigation report on novel coronavirus published.

Ecuador, Monaco, Qatar as well as Luxemburg confirm the first cases of the novel coronavirus.

WHO revised its directions with regard to travel restrictions.

March 1: The United Nations sanctions $15 million from the body's Central Emergency Response Fund to UNICEF and WHO to bolster weaker nations in spheres comprising of ministering the proliferation of the virus, investigating cases as well as managing laboratories.

Armenia, Czech Republic as well as Iceland confirm their first cases of the COVID-19.

Dominican Republic confirmed the first case of the virus. This marks the first confirmed case of COVID-19 in the Caribbean.

A US national in Bhutan tested positive for COVID-19.

March 7: Two confirmed cases were reported in Maldives.

March 8: More than 100 nations across the world report cases of the novel coronavirus.

Three people tested positive for the COVID-19 in Bangladesh. Two of these three people returned from Italy.

March 10: 71 Chinese workers who were employed in the construction of the Pokhara Airport, who had returned from China after undergoing a 14-day long quarantine were put into quarantine for another 14 days.

The Chinese President Xi Jinping took a celebratory "victory lap" by visiting the epicentre of virus in Wuhan, the capital of Hubei province, indicating that the worst of the outbreak was over, and that China has successfully contained the virus as compared to the major Western nations.

March 11: WHO classified COVID-19 as a pandemic.

The first positive case was reported in Sri Lanka. The infected 52-year-old tour guide had come in contact with Italian tourists.

March 12: China's first team arrived in Rome with essential medical supplies and equipment and later helped the hard-hit Spain with the same resources.

March 13: COVID-19 Solidarity Response Fund introduced to obtain donations corporations, private individuals as well as institutions.

Chinese foreign ministry spokesman Zhao Lijian provided semi-official support to the theory that the origin of the COVID-19 may not be Wuhan, but the United States.

March 16: US President Donald Trump in a tweet referred to the novel coronavirus as the "Chinese virus".

Pakistan closed its borders with Afghanistan in its bid to control the spread of the Coronavirus.

March 18: China at the video conference with 24 African countries and the African Union (AU) Center for Disease Control and Prevention expressed its commitment of sharing experience and supporting Africa in the fight against the epidemic.

March 19: Venezuela was one of the first nation in the region to obtain Beijing's medical supplies, as a shipment transporting 4,015 COVID-19 testing kits, together with chemical reagents, gloves, air purifiers and masks, arrived on this date.

President Putin appreciated measures taken by China to counter the spread of infection.

March 20: Wang Yi in a telephone conversation with Nasser Bourita, Moroccan Minister of Foreign Affairs and International Cooperation, said China will donate essential medical supplies, share response experience and send medical expert teams to help countries affected by the disease.

Sri Lanka imposed a nation-wide curfew.

March 22: The first flight of 100 MT of medical supplies arrived in Addis Ababa on Ethiopian Airlines.

March 23: First confirmed case in Myanmar.

March 24: SAARC had reported just 1536 cases in total, and 22 deaths due to the virus.

Indian Prime Minister Narendra Modi announced a three-week long lockdown.

March 25: The G-7 foreign ministerial meeting failed to come out with a statement, divided as it were by the name of the virus again.

March 27: Pakistan opened its borders with China for a day to accept Chinese medical supplies to fight the growing coronavirus outbreak.

March 29: A press release issued by Jack Ma Foundation and Alibaba Foundation and the Prime Minister of Ethiopia, Abiy Ahmed, committed to provide medical supplies and medical equipment to each of the 54 countries in Africa.

March 30: Taiwan announced that on the basis of reciprocity, while it will receive alcohol required for manufacturing hand sanitisers from Australia, it will export non-woven fabric for mask production to the country.

April 1: A report carried by Bloomberg quoted unnamed sources as alleging that the US intelligence community had concluded that China had concealed the extent of the spread of the disease.

Latin America comprised of a total number of 14,000 or more of confirmed cases of COVID-19, off a global total of approximately 850,000.

Marcelo Ebrard, foreign minister of Mexico, tweeted "Gracias China!!!" together with a photograph of a plane that transported 100,000 masks, five ventilators and 50,000 test kits donated by the PRC.

April 2: Ursula von der Leyen, EU Commissioner tweeted thanking Taiwan for the donation of 5.6 million masks.

China sent 25.5 tons of medical supplies to Russia.

China handed over the first batch of China-aided medical supplies to Afghanistan.

April 6: China's medical supplies for 18 countries in Central and West Africa arrived at Accra Airport in Ghana.

Ghana had more than 9,000 confirmed cases COVID-19 with 400 deaths.

April 7: Japanese Prime Minister Shinzo Abe declared a "state of emergency" in accordance with article 32 of the Act on Special Measures, with effect in seven prefectures of Tokyo, Kanagawa, Saitama, Chiba, Osaka, Hyogo and Fukuoka.

The Japanese government adopted its biggest-ever emergency economic package of $990 billion (108 trillion yen).

April 8: Second batch of COVID-19 donations from Jack Ma Foundation and Alibaba Foundation arrive in Africa.

April 11: A 10-member medical team was sent by China to Russia to assist the country on the prevention, control, diagnosis and treatment of COVID-19.

A 10-member medical team was sent by China to Russia to assist the country on the prevention, control, diagnosis and treatment of COVID-19.

April 13: Felipe Solá, foreign minister of Argentina, expressed his gratitude for China upon the receipt of a large shipment of vital necessities to combat the pandemic namely masks, protective suits and gloves.

India sent a ship through Iran's Chabahar port carrying a major consignment of wheat and hydroxychloroquine, which is being used in the fight against the coronavirus pandemic.

April 14: Among the first United Nations "Solidarity Flight" donations, a large quantity of personal protective equipment was donated by the Jack Ma Foundation and Alibaba Foundation to all countries in Africa.

April 16: Russian Prime Minister issued an order to use the Chinese drug Hydroxychloroquine which is still not registered in Russia.
India received its much-delayed order of 650,000 tests from China

April 17: Wuhan belatedly raises its official fatalities by 1290.

Apr 17-May 6: Japanese Prime Minister Shinzo Abe declared a nationwide state of emergency

April 19: Cai Wei and his partner who had participated in "Terminus 2049", a Github project which preserved censored news stories, videos and articles from individuals shared on social media apps like WeChat since January 2018 on the coronavirus outbreak, were arrested by the Beijing police and were accused of "picking quarrels and provoking trouble", a commonly used charge against dissidents in China.

April 22: Costa Atlantica, an Italian cruise ship docked for repairs in Nagasaki carrying 623 crew members (with no passengers) reported 34 COVID-19 cases- making it second such incident after Diamond Princess.

April 23: Another batch of China's medical supplies for 12 African countries arrives in Addis Ababa, Ethiopia.
The number of confirmed cases COVID-19 in Africa reached 25,937 with 1,242 deaths.
At least 251 doctors tested positive for coronavirus in Bangladesh according to the Bangladesh Doctors Foundation (BDF).
Twenty-five years old Li Zehua, who went missing in Wuhan after he posted a video on YouTube on 20 February showing porters being hired for transporting corpses of people who likely died of coronavirus, was released only after weeks of what appears to be a forced quarantine.
Michael Pompeo's press statement characterized Beijing's actions in the South China Sea as part of "long-term threats to...shared security" and called attention to China's exploitation of the COVID-19 crisis.

April 24: Afghanistan reported 1279 cases of coronavirus infections with 42 deaths.

April 25: Pakistani Prime Minister Imran Khan announced a 'smart lockdown', under which areas where outbreaks have taken place will be closed, while certain economic activities continue to take place.

April 27: The Africa CDC received the third round of medical equipment and supplies donated by the Jack Ma and Alibaba foundations at the Addis Ababa airport.

April 28: The Jack Ma Foundation along with Africa CDC organised a special webinar titled "Global MediXChange for Combating COVID-19 (GMCC): The Experience of China".
A request by the Department of Foreign Affairs and Trade, Australia on instituting an independent international investigation of the origin of the pandemic was turned down by the Chinese Ambassador to Australia Cheng Jingye on grounds of it being a 'political manoeuvre' and requested the Australian government to put aside ideological bias and stop political games.

April 29: Cambodian Prime Minister Hun Sen promulgates the *Law on National Administration in the State of Emergency* and is criticised for transferring sweeping powers to the government to curb individual freedoms, including those of the rights to travel freely, that of assembly and privacy.

April 30: The number of confirmed cases in Nigeria, South Africa, Ghana, Kenya were 1,728 cases/51 deaths, 5,647 cases/103 deaths, 2,074 cases/17 deaths, 396 cases/ 17 deaths respectively.

The US Office of the Director of National Intelligence issued a press statement concurring with the scientific opinion that the COVID-19 virus was not manmade although it did not rule out accidental leak from the laboratory in Wuhan.

New China TV – the official YouTube channel of Chinese state news agency Xinhua- released a short satirical video titled "Once upon a virus..." mocking US allegations against China on the handling of the coronavirus outbreak.

May 1: While the number of Chinese confirmed cases remained constant at around 84,000, the number of COVID-19 cases in the US had risen exponentially to over 1 million with over 50,000 deaths – the largest of any country in the world.

May 3: Fran Martin, Associate Professor in Cultural Studies at Melbourne University during an interview titled 'Expectations and Experiences of Chinese University Students in Australia' with the Australia-China Relations Institute (ACRI) raised significant issues of racism experienced by Chinese students in Australia, apart from social barriers of language proficiency, exclusion from certain work opportunities and more.

May 5: Indian and Chinese troops engaged in non-lethal face offs and skirmished along the India-China border.

May 8: Medical experts from China's People's Liberation Army (PLA) and their South African counterparts held a video conference to their share experience of combating COVID-19.

May 11: Wang Yi had a telephonic conversation with spoke by phone with Gedu Andargachew, Ethiopian Foreign Minister and Téte António, the Angolan Foreign Minister, whereby he emphasized that China will stand firm with Africa in the fight against COVID-19.

May 14: In the meeting of the Politburo of the CPC, the role of Xi Jinping was strongly commended. President Xi in turn stressed on the need to manage the serious and complex situation overseas and the still daunting task of preventing domestic resurgence of CCOVID-19 cases.

May 18: Xi Jinping's speech at the World Health Assembly (WHA), in particular highlights the fragile health situations Africa and draws the attention of the world for greater support to the continent.

May 22: Premier Li Keqiang in his address to the 13th NPC declared a "decisive victory" against coronavirus in Hubei, and praised the contribution of media personnel, among others.

May 25: Tedros Adhanom, WHO Director-General at the WHO media briefings on COVID-19 said, Africa is least-affected region globally in terms of number of COVID-19 confirmed cases and deaths, and so far, the continent has just 1.5 percent of the world's reported cases of COVID-19, and less than 0.1 percent of the total deaths.

June 2-5: PLA sent medical supplies to 20 countries including the five African countries such as Ethiopia, Mozambique, Tunisia, Angola, Egypt.

June 5: The Inter-Parliamentary Alliance on China (IPAC) was launched to foster deeper collaboration between like-minded legislators to work towards reforms on how democratic countries should approach China.

June 7: China issued a white paper on COVID-19 and sought to project a picture of being swift, timely, open and transparent, centralised and efficient, well-coordinated.

June 11: In a telephonic conversation with Philippines President Rodrigo Roa Duterte, Xi promised that 'as a friendly neighbour' the Philippines would be prioritised by China when a COVID-19 vaccine was finally developed by the country.

June 17: Xi Jinping at the extraordinary China-Africa Summit said, China will exempt some African countries from repaying zero-interest rate loans due at the end of 2020.

July 6: Melbourne has been led into a six-week lockdown with stage 3 restrictions-people would only be allowed to leave their houses for work, education, exercise, for necessary goods or services or medical or compassionate reasons until August 19, 2020.

Sources:

1. Sharri Markson, "Coronavirus NSW: Dossier lays out case against China bat virus program", 02 May 2020, https://www.dailytelegraph.com.au/coronavirus/bombshell-dossier-lays-out-case-against-chinese-bat-virus-program/news-story/55add857058731c9c71c0e96ad17da60
2. Xinhua, "China Publishes Timeline on COVID-19 Information Sharing, Int'l Cooperation", 06 April 2020, http://www.xinhuanet.com/english/2020-04/06/c_138951662.htm
3. John Hopkins University and Medicine, "Hubei Timeline", 02 May 2020, https://coronavirus.jhu.edu/data/hubei-timeline
4. Committee on Coordination of Statistical Activities, " How COVID-19 is Changing the World", 19 May 2020, https://www.uneca.org/sites/default/files/PublicationFiles/ccsa_covid19_final.pdf
5. Congressional Research Service, "COVID-19 and China: A Chronology of Events (December 2019-January 2020)", 13 May 2020, https://crsreports.congress.gov/product/pdf/R/R46354.
6. Ravelo, Jenny Lei and Sara Jerving, "COVID-19-A Timeline of the Coronavirus Outbreak", 4 June 2020, https://www.devex.com/news/covid-19-a-timeline-of-the-coronavirus-outbreak-96396
7. WHO, "WHO Timeline-COVID-19", 27 April 2020, https://www.who.int/news-room/detail/27-04-2020-who-timeline--covid-19.

Index